Medical Imaging: Diagnostic Techniques

Medical Imaging: Diagnostic Techniques

Edited by Mckinsey Harper

hayle medical

New York

Hayle Medical,
750 Third Avenue, 9th Floor,
New York, NY 10017, USA

Visit us on the World Wide Web at:
www.haylemedical.com

ISBN: 978-1-63241-504-2

The publisher's policy is to use permanent paper from mills that operate a sustainable forestry policy. Furthermore, the publisher ensures that the text paper and cover boards used have met acceptable environmental accreditation standards.

Printed in China.

Cataloging-in-Publication Data

Medical imaging : diagnostic techniques / edited by Mckinsey Harper.
p. cm.
Includes bibliographical references and index.
ISBN 978-1-63241-504-2
1. Diagnostic imaging. 2. Imaging systems in medicine. 3. Diagnostic imaging--Equipment and supplies.
4. Diagnostic imaging--Digital techniques. I. Harper, Mckinsey.

RC78.7.D53 M43 2018
616.075 4--dc23

Table of Contents

Preface

Cardiac magnetic resonance imaging (CMR) is a technique used in the imaging, diagnosis and assessment of the diseases related to the cardiovascular system. CMR technique is minimally invasive and is seen as a safe way to carry out cardiovascular assessment. Modern scanners are able to capture high-resolution images in extremely short durations, leading to comprehensive snapshots of the heart and the cardiovascular system. The acquiring of 3D data sets as a results of the CMR technique has led to the effective diagnosis of coronary artery disease. The aim of this book is to present researches that have transformed this discipline and aided its advancement. It is an essential guide for both academicians and those who wish to pursue this discipline further.

This book has been the outcome of endless efforts put in by authors and researchers on various issues and topics within the field. The book is a comprehensive collection of significant researches that are addressed in a variety of chapters. It will surely enhance the knowledge of the field among readers across the globe.

It gives us an immense pleasure to thank our researchers and authors for their efforts to submit their piece of writing before the deadlines. Finally in the end, I would like to thank my family and colleagues who have been a great source of inspiration and support.

Editor

Clinical Criteria Replenish High-Sensitive Troponin and Inflammatory Markers in the Stratification of Patients with Suspected Acute Coronary Syndrome

Barbara Elisabeth Stähli[1], Keiko Yonekawa[1,2], Lukas Andreas Altwegg[1], Christophe Wyss[1], Danielle Hof[3], Philipp Fischbacher[4], Andreas Brauchlin[1], Georg Schulthess[4], Pierre-Alexandre Krayenbühl[2], Arnold von Eckardstein[3], Martin Hersberger[5], Michel Neidhart[6], Steffen Gay[6], Igor Novopashenny[7], Regine Wolters[7], Michelle Frank[1], Manfred Bernd Wischnewsky[7], Thomas Felix Lüscher[1], Willibald Maier[1]*

1 Department of Cardiology, Cardiovascular Center, University Hospital Zurich, Zurich, Switzerland, **2** Division of Internal Medicine, University Hospital Zurich, Zurich, Switzerland, **3** Institute of Clinical Chemistry, University Hospital Zurich, Zurich, Switzerland, **4** Department of Internal Medicine, Hospital Männedorf, Männedorf, Switzerland, **5** Institute of Clinical Chemistry and Biochemistry, Childrens Hospital Zurich, Zurich, Switzerland, **6** Center for Experimental Rheumatology, Department of Rheumatology, University Hospital Zurich, Zurich, Switzerland, **7** FB Mathematics and Computer Science, University of Bremen, Bremen, Germany

Abstract

Objectives: In patients with suspected acute coronary syndrome (ACS), rapid triage is essential. The aim of this study was to establish a tool for risk prediction of 30-day cardiac events (CE) on admission. 30-day cardiac events (CE) were defined as early coronary revascularization, subsequent myocardial infarction, or cardiovascular death within 30 days.

Methods and Results: This single-centre, prospective cohort study included 377 consecutive patients presenting to the emergency department with suspected ACS and for whom troponin T measurements were requested on clinical grounds. Fifteen biomarkers were analyzed in the admission sample, and clinical parameters were assessed by the TIMI risk score for unstable angina/Non-ST myocardial infarction and the GRACE risk score. Sixty-nine (18%) patients presented with and 308 (82%) without ST-elevations, respectively. Coronary angiography was performed in 165 (44%) patients with subsequent percutaneous coronary intervention – accounting for the majority of CE – in 123 (33%) patients, respectively. Eleven out of 15 biomarkers were elevated in patients with CE compared to those without. High-sensitive troponin T (hs-cTnT) was the best univariate biomarker to predict CE in Non-ST-elevation patients (AUC 0.80), but did not yield incremental information above clinical TIMI risk score (AUC 0.80 vs 0.82, $p = 0.69$). Equivalence testing of AUCs of risk models and non-inferiority testing demonstrated that the clinical TIMI risk score alone was non-inferior to its combination with hs-cTnT in predicting CE.

Conclusions: In patients presenting without ST-elevations, identification of those prone to CE is best based on clinical assessment based on TIMI risk score criteria and hs-cTnT.

Editor: Tanja Zeller, Medical University Hamburg, University Heart Center, Germany

Funding: This study has partially been supported by grants of the Swiss National Research Foundation (http://www.snf.ch/E/Pages/default.aspx; no. 3200B0-112661, Special Programme University Medicine: Grant Nr 33CM30-1241112/1 and 3100-068118.02/1) and Roche Diagnostics GmbH. The funders had no role in study design, data collection and analysis, decision to publish, or preparation of the manuscript.

Competing Interests: The authors have read the journal's policy and have the following conflicts. Dr. Maier and Dr. Altwegg report receiving consulting fees from Roche Diagnostics GmbH. No other potential conflict of interest was reported.

* E-mail: karmaiew@usz.uzh.ch

Introduction

Acute coronary syndromes (ACS) are a major cause of death worldwide [1]. In emergency rooms, patients with chest pain and symptoms suggestive of ACS account for a large part of medical admissions [2]. However, a wide spectrum of clinical presentations may be associated with cardiac ischemia. Hence, in these patients, rapid identification, risk stratification, and appropriate selection for early percutaneous coronary revascularization (PCI) or coronary artery bypass grafting (CABG) are crucial for prognosis [3–7].

Recently, testing for high-sensitive cardiac troponin (hs-cTnT) has been shown to be even more sensitive compared to conventional assays [8,9]. However, designed to improve the detection of minimal myocardial injury and to minimize the number of unidentified ACS patients, high-sensitive assays show decreased specificity. Indeed, various cardiac and non-cardiac conditions including tachyarrhythmias, hypertensive episodes, congestive heart failure, pulmonary embolism, sepsis, and high-intensity training have been associated with a rise in hs-cTnT [10–12]. Thus, despite the ability of clearly ruling-out the likelihood of ACS in patients with chest pain, the increased number of individuals testing positive for troponin has hampered decision making in daily clinical practice. Particularly, the decision when to perform coronary angiography in individuals without obvious ST-segment elevations (Non-ST-elevation patients) remains challenging and calls for complementary rule-in parameters to identify those at particular risk of impending cardiac events (CE). Accordingly, for the purpose of this study, CE comprise not only the conventional endpoints of subsequent myocardial infarction and cardiovascular death, but, by operational definition, also the need for coronary revascularization established by means of coronary angiography.

Besides sensitive indicators of myocardial injury such as heart-type fatty acid-binding protein (H-FABP) [13,14], markers of coronary plaque activation and/or instability appear most promising in such context. Several groups, including our own, have recently suggested myeloid-related protein 8/14 (MRP 8/14), a marker of phagocyte activation – highly expressed in coronary thrombi – as a candidate marker for the early detection of atherothrombosis and ACS [15–17]. Early indicators of coronary plaque instability also include pregnancy-associated plasma protein A (PAPP-A), a metalloproteinase exhibiting pro-atherosclerotic effects, and myeloperoxidase (MPO), an oxidative leukocyte enzyme, which has been shown to predict CE even in patients who are negative for troponin T [18,19]. Yet, the complexity of the molecular pathways in the chain of events leading to ACS, as well as the heterogeneity in clinical presentation, imply that a single-marker strategy is most likely inferior to a multi-marker approach. Indeed, multi-marker testing adds useful prognostic information to that of individual markers, both for the prediction of early and long-term outcomes in patients with suspected ACS [20–22]. However, the potential of different novel cardiac biomarkers in comparison to and combined with clinical assessment in predicting CE in individuals presenting with symptoms suggestive of ACS has not been fully elucidated.

Thus, we investigated within a prospective single-center study, initially designed to assess the diagnostic role of MRP 8/14 in patients presenting with suspected ACS – *My*eloid *R*elated Protein 8/14 *i*n the Evaluation of *A*cute Chest Pain in the Emergency *D*epartment (MyRiAD study) – the predictive value of 15 biomarkers, stand-alone or in combination with established clinical parameters, for CE within 30 days.

Methods

Study design and patient enrollment

This single-centre, prospective observational study included patients presenting to the emergency room from July 2007 to April 2008 with symptoms suggestive of ACS and for whom conventional troponin (c-cTnT) measurements were requested on clinical grounds. Exclusion criteria were the onset of symptoms > 24 hours, clinical signs of infection, and refusal or inability of the patient to give informed consent. Of 538 patients screened, 377 patients were included in the final analysis.

Assuming an event rate of 30% and an area under the curve (AUC) of 0.8 for MRP 8/14 to predict CE (according to the initial MyRiAD study hypothesis), a minimal number of 326 patients was calculated in order to obtain a power of 80% and an alpha-level of 0.05. The study was carried out according to the principles of the Declaration of Helsinki and approved by the institutional ethics committee of the University Hospital Zurich. Written informed consent was obtained from all patients.

Patient management

All patients underwent the regular emergency room assessments including detailed clinical history taking, physical examination, 12-lead electrocardiogram (ECG), and the pertinent blood analysis routine (see below). Subsequent clinical management, in particular as to additional examinations (i.e. coronary angiography) and therapies, was based on current practice and left at the discretion of the treating physicians. Routine markers including c-cTnT, myoglobin, creatine kinase (CK), creatine kinase-myocardial band (CK-MB), N-terminal pro-brain natriuretic peptide (NT-proBNP), and D-dimers were available to the treating physicians. There were no study-specific interventions. Details on screening, enrollment, and patient management are summarized in the study flow chart (figure 1).

Biomarker analysis

Blood samples were harvested in serum, heparin plasma, and citrate plasma tubes and immediately processed by the Institute of Clinical Chemistry. Subsequently, routine markers for the assessment of myocardial infarction were directly assessed, and the remaining samples deep-frozen and stored (-70°C) for later analysis of specific biomarkers.

Routine markers included c-cTnT, myoglobin, CK, CK-MB, and NT-proBNP, which were analyzed from heparin plasma (maximal inter-assay variation 3.7%, 2.5%, 1.8%, 2.8%, and 4.4%, respectively; limit of detection of 10 ng/L, 21 µg/L, 7 U/L, 3.0 U/L, and 5.0 ηg/L with a functional assay sensitivity of 10%). D-dimers were determined from citrate plasma on a Roche Modular Analytics System using commercial assays from Roche Diagnostics (Rotkreuz, Switzerland).

Study specific blood analyses were limited to the sample collected on admission and included MRP 8/14, H-FABP, high-sensitive C-reactive protein (hs-CRP), interleukin-6 (IL-6), MPO, PAPP-A, insulin-like growth factor 1 (IGF-1), and fibrinogen. Interleukin-6 and hs-CRP were determined from heparin plasma, and IGF-1 from serum on an Immulite 2000 chemiluminescence analyser using commercial assays from Siemens Healthcare Diagnostics GmbH (Deerfield, USA; maximal inter-assay variation of 2.7%, 3.1%, and 4.5%, respectively; limit of detection of 1.5 ηg/L, 0.3 mg/L, and 3.0 µg/L with a functional assay sensitivity of 10%). Pregnancy-associated plasma protein A was measured immunochemically by Time Resolved Amplified Cryptate Emission (TRACE) from serum on a Kryptor analyzer from Brahms AG (Hennigsdorf, Germany; maximal inter-assay variation of 4.7%; limit of detection of 0.004 U/L with a functional assay sensitivity of 10%). Fibrinogen was determined on a CA7000 analyzer from Siemens Healthcare Diagnostics GmbH using commercial assays (maximal inter-assay variation of 4.8%). Myeloid-related protein 8/14 was determined from serum using assays from Buehlmann Laboratories (Schoenenbuch, Switzerland; limit of detection of 0.4 µg/mL; cut-off value of 4.7 µg/mL). Heart-type fatty acid-binding protein was measured from serum using assays from Hycult biotechnology (Uden, The Netherlands; limit of detection of 0.1 ηg/mL, cut-off value of 5 ηg/mL). Samples were tested in double determination, if the two values differed by more than 10%, the sample was repeated, unless absorbance was <0.1 or both concentration values were clearly within the normal range. Concentrations of hs-cTnT were analyzed from serum with the Elecsys assay from Roche Diagnostics (Mannheim, Germany; limit of detection 5 pg/mL, cut-off value of 13 pg/mL). Myeloperoxidase was measured from heparin plasma using assays from Immundiagnostik (Bensheim, Germany; limit of detection of 1.6 ng/mL).

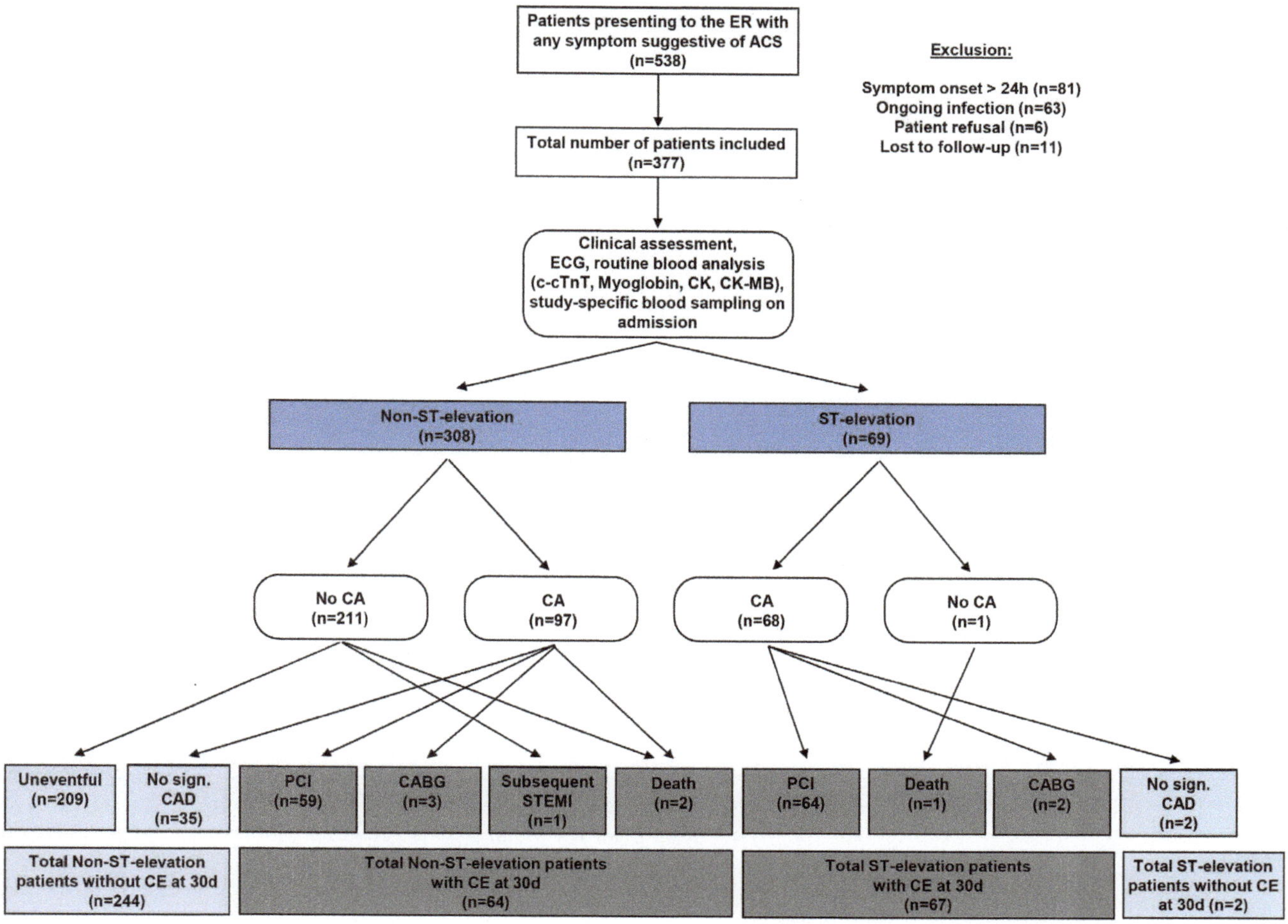

Figure 1. Study flow chart of the prospective, observational MyRiAD study. Abbreviations: ER, emergency room; CA, coronary angiography; CAD, coronary artery disease; CE, cardiac events (composite of early coronary revascularization by percutaneous coronary intervention [PCI] or coronary artery bypass grafting [CABG], subsequent myocardial infarction or cardiovascular death); c-cTnT, conventional cardiac troponin T; CK, creatine kinase; CK-MB, creatine kinase-myocardial band.

Patient assessment and outcome measures

Assessment of patients with suspected ACS was primarily based on ECG, notably the presence of new or presumed new ST-elevation ≥0.2 mV in ≥2 contiguous leads, as an indicator of likely acute total coronary artery occlusion necessitating immediate invasive reperfusion strategies (ST-elevation patients). In Non-ST-elevation patients, pretest probability of ACS was assessed by the TIMI risk score for unstable angina/Non-ST myocardial infarction, which allows stratification into those at low, intermediate, and high risk of adverse CE. The original TIMI risk score includes 7 predictor variables: 1) age ≥65 years, 2) ≥ 3 risk factors for coronary artery disease, 3) documented significant coronary artery disease on previous coronary angiography (i.e. coronary artery stenosis ≥ 50%), 4) persistent ST depression of ≥ 0.05 mV, 5) ≥ 2 episodes of angina in the last 24 hours, 6) aspirin use within the last 7 days prior to admission, and 7) elevated cardiac biomarkers, with each adding 1 point (score 0-7 points) [23]. If aspirin was administered by the emergency physician or afterwards, it was not included in the clinical TIMI risk score calculation. For the particular purpose of this study, namely to assess the incremental predictive value of singular specific cardiac biomarkers over established clinical risk parameters, the original calculation of the TIMI risk score was modified by including all predictor variables except the one 'elevated cardiac biomarkers'; hence, the TIMI risk score utilized in the present study is named the "clinical TIMI risk score".

To allow comparison between different risk scoring systems in ACS, in all patients, the Global Registry of Acute Coronary Events (GRACE) score was calculated. This score includes age, heart rate, systolic blood pressure, creatinine, Killip Class, cardiac arrest at admission, ST-segment deviation, and elevated cardiac enzymes [24]. According to the "clinical TIMI risk score", the original calculation of the GRACE risk score was modified by including all predictor variables except the one 'elevated cardiac enzymes'; hence, the GRACE risk score utilized in the present study is named the "clinical GRACE risk score".

In analogy to the endpoints in the TIMI risk score validation study, the main outcome measure was CE, for the purpose of this study specifically and operationally defined as a composite of early coronary revascularization by PCI or CABG, cardiovascular mortality, and subsequent myocardial infarction requiring revascularization within 30 days [23,25].

Data collection and statistical analysis

All data and imaging records including coronary angiographies and interventions were reviewed and entered into a dedicated, individually designed, and web-based database. Before the final analysis, data were monitored and cross-validated according to clinical trial center standard operating procedures.

Continuous variables are presented as medians and interquartile range as they were not normally distributed as assessed by the Shapiro-Wilk W test. Categorical variables are given as frequencies and percentages. Continuous variables were tested for differences with the Wilcoxon signed-rank test or the Mann-Whitney U test as appropriate. The independence of two categorical variables was tested by the Pearson's Chi-square test. Receiver-operator-characteristic (ROC) curves were constructed to assess AUCs, sensitivity, and specificity of cardiac biomarkers in predicting CE at 30 days.

For multivariate analysis we used decision tree technique allowing multi-level splits based upon adjusted significance testing (Bonferroni testing). The goal was to create a model that predicted the value of the target variable "CE within 30 days" based on several input variables (clinical parameters and biomarkers). Each interior node corresponds to one of the input variables, each leaf represents a value of the target variable given the values of the input variables represented by the path from the root to the leaf.

Binary logistic regression with and without bootstrapping as well as standard generalized linear models for the logistic regression models were used to test predictors of the outcome variable and to establish two risk prediction models (model I: clinical TIMI risk score, and gender; model II: clinical TIMI risk score, gender, and hs-TnT). For comparisons between models, empirical equivalence tests of the AUCs, non-inferiority tests, as well as integrated discrimination improvement (IDI) were performed, and the performance of the two models illustrated as predictiveness curves.

Results

Baseline characteristics

Baseline characteristics of 377 patients stratified according to the occurrence of CE within 30 days are summarized in table 1. Urgent coronary angiography was performed in 165 (44%) patients with subsequent PCI in 123 (33%) patients, and CABG in 5 (1%) patients, respectively. From the 377 patients presenting with suspected ACS, 132 (35%) were finally diagnosed with coronary artery disease including 66 patients with acute STEMI, and 66 patients with acute NSTEMI/UA, respectively. Median time of symptom duration was 253 [148–496] minutes. Final diagnoses of the patients are summarized in table 2.

In 6 patients, heparin was administered before the first blood analysis. In 12 patients, no information about heparin administration was available. The remaining 359 were treated with heparin at the emergency room or during revascularization, or received no heparin at all due to the clinical course.

Cardiac events (CE) in ST-elevation and Non-ST-elevation patients

Of all patients, 69 (18%) presented with and 308 (82%) without ST-elevations. Cardiac events within 30 days were observed in 131 (35%) and an uneventful course was noted in the remaining 246 (65%) patients. In ST-elevation patients, 66 (96%) underwent coronary revascularization, 64 (93%) by PCI, and 2 (3%) by CABG. One patient (1%) died without intervention and another 2 (2%) patients presenting with ST-elevations were diagnosed as having Takotsubo cardiomyopathy with essentially normal coronaries and an uneventful 30-day course. In Non-ST-elevation patients, 66 were diagnosed with coronary artery disease. CE included revascularization in 62 (20%) patients with PCI in 59 (19%) and CABG in 3 (1%), cardiovascular death in 2 (1%), and subsequent acute myocardial infarction in 1 (0.3%) patient, respectively.

Biomarkers in patients with and without cardiac events (CE) within 30 days

Levels of biomarkers in patients presenting with and without CE are summarized in table 3. Patients with CE showed significantly elevated levels of 11 out of 15 biomarkers compared to those without, including all markers of myocardial ischemia/necrosis ($p<0.001$ for CK, CK-MB, H-FABP, myoglobin, c-cTnT, and hs-cTnT), 3 out of 4 inflammatory markers ($p<0.03$ for hs-CRP, MPO, and MRP 8/14), and PAPP-A, a marker of atherosclerosis ($p<0.0001$), as well as NT-proBNP ($p = 0.04$). No differences in serum levels between patients with and without CE were observed for IL-6, IGF-1, D-dimer, and fibrinogen, respectively.

Single biomarkers for the prediction of cardiac events (CE) within 30 days in the total cohort of patients and in Non-ST-elevation patients

Results from univariate analysis of biomarkers for the prediction of CE within 30 days are summarized in table 4. In the total cohort of patients presenting with suspected ACS, hs-cTnT was the best single biomarker for the prediction of CE within 30 days (AUC = 0.83, sensitivity = 76%, and negative predictive value [NPV] = 86% at a cut-off level of 16.2 pg/mL). Best specificity (92%) resulting in the highest positive predictive value (PPV = 75%) at a cut-off level of 0.02 μg/L was noted for c-cTnT, which overall was less predictive (AUC = 0.69) than hs-cTnT. Similarly, the predictive value of MRP 8/14 (AUC = 0.65) for CE within 30 days in patients with suspected ACS was inferior to hs-cTnT.

In Non-ST-elevation patients, univariate analysis again revealed hs-cTnT as the biomarker with the best performance in predicting CE within 30 days (AUC = 0.80, sensitivity = 86%, and NPV = 84% at a cut-off level 9.26 pg/mL). As for the total cohort, specificity for detecting CE within 30 days by a single marker in Non-ST-elevation patients was highest for c-cTnT, with a specificity of 93% and a PPV of 55% at a cut-off level of 0.02 μg/L. Altogether, predictive values of single biomarkers for CE within 30 days decreased in Non-ST-elevation compared to the total population of patients with suspected ACS. This was evidenced by smaller AUCs for all biomarkers except for NT-proBNP, fibrinogen, D-dimer, and IGF-1, which showed an increase in AUC.

Univariate decision tree analysis (CRT) in Non-ST-elevation patients confirmed hs-cTnT as the best biomarker for the prediction of CE within 30 days (classification = 84.7%), however, with only minor incremental value over c-cTnT (classification = 82.5%), and only if continuous values instead of the manufacturer's pre-defined cut-off level (13 pg/ml) were utilized. The CE-rate increased highly significantly ($p<0.001$) with hs-cTnT (hs-cTnT<9: 5.8%; 9≤hs-cTNT<28: 22.6%; hs-cTNT≥28: 55.7%).

Clinical TIMI risk score for the prediction of cardiac events (CE) in Non-ST-elevation patients

At presentation, in Non-ST-elevation patients, 66 (21%) patients had a clinical TIMI risk score of 0, 69 (22%) patients of 1, 73 (24%) patients of 2, 60 (20%) patients of 3, 29 (9%) patients of 4, 10 (3%) patients of 5, and 1 (0.3%) patient of 6, respectively. The observed CE rate at 30 days was 100% (1/1) in patients with a score of 6, 50% (5/10) in patients with a score of 5, 69% (20/29) in patients with a score of 4, 35% (21/60) in patients with a score

Table 1. Baseline characteristics.

Characteristics	All patients (n = 377)	Patients with cardiac events (n = 131)	Patients free from cardiac events (n = 246)	P value
Demographics				
Age, years	60 [51–71]	62 [53–72]	59 [48–71]	0.10
Male gender, n (%)	275 (73)	111 (85)	164 (67)	<0.001
Risk factors				
Family history of CAD, n (%)	105 (28)	40 (31)	65 (26)	0.26
Hypercholesterolemia, n (%)	173 (46)	70 (53)	103 (42)	0.03
Diabetes, n (%)	63 (18)	26 (20)	37 (15)	0.23
Hypertension, n (%)	214 (57)	89 (68)	125 (51)	0.001
Current smoker, n (%)	110 (29)	42 (32)	68 (28)	0.007
Previous history				
Previous MI, n (%)	78 (21)	26 (20)	52 (21)	0.77
Previous CABG, n (%)	28 (7)	10 (8)	18 (7)	0.91
Previous PCI, n (%)	82 (22)	26 (20)	56 (23)	0.51
PVD, n (%)	26 (10)	16 (12)	20 (8)	0.20
CVD, n (%)	31 (8)	11 (8)	20 (8)	0.93
Previous medication				
Aspirin, n (%)	147 (39)	51 (39)	96 (39)	0.99
Clopidogrel, n (%)	36 (10)	12 (8)	24 (10)	0.12
ACE-inhibitor, n (%)	83 (22)	20 (15)	63 (26)	0.02
Beta-blocker, n (%)	149 (40)	44 (34)	105 (43)	0.09
CCB, n (%)	52 (14)	22 (17)	30 (12)	0.22
Statin, n (%)	130 (35)	44 (34)	86 (35)	0.79
Clinical presentation				
BMI, kg/m^2	26.5 [24.0–29.4]	26.6 [24.4–26.7]	26.5 [23.7–29.4]	0.33
Systolic blood pressure, mmHg	140 [121–156]	138 [117–156]	142 [123–157]	0.15
Heart rate, beats/min	77 [64–90]	74 [60–87]	79 [66–91]	0.006
Serum creatinine, µmol/L	83 [72–97]	84 [73–98]	83 [71–95]	0.23
Time from symptom onset, min	253 [148–496]	282 [172–516]	245 [136–488]	0.14
Chest pain, n (%)	332 (88)	128 (98)	204 (83)	<0.001
ST-segment elevation, n (%)	69 (18)	67 (51)	2 (1)	<0.001
Coronary angiography, n (%)	165 (44)	128 (98)	37 (15)	<0.001

Abbreviations: CAD, coronary artery disease; MI, myocardial infarction; PCI, percutaneous coronary intervention; CABG, coronary artery bypass grafting, PVD, peripheral vascular disease; CVD, cerebrovascular disease; ACE, angiotensin converting enzyme; CCB, calcium channel blocker; BMI, body mass index.

of 3, 14% (10/73) in patients with a score of 2, 9% (6/69) in those with a score of 1, and 2% (1/66) in those with 0 points, respectively. Hs-cTnT was not better than the clinical TIMI risk score in predicting CE within 30 days, as substantiated both by univariate ROC and decision tree analysis [AUC = 0.80 (standard error 0.03, 95% CI 0.74–0.86; p<0.001), vs. AUC = 0.82 (standard error 0.03, 95% CI 0.76–0.87; p<0.001); p = 0.69].

Clinical GRACE risk score for the prediction of cardiac events (CE) in Non-ST-elevation patients

At presentation, in Non-ST-elevation patients, the clinical GRACE risk score was 92 (70–120). The observed CE rate at 30 days was 15% in patients with a score ≤100, and 29% in those with a score >100, respectively (p = 0.003). The AUC was 0.62 (95% CI 0.54–0.69) for the clinical GRACE score in predicting CE within 30 days.

Combination of the clinical TIMI risk score and biomarkers for individual risk prediction and decision making in Non-ST-elevation patients

For the clinical TIMI risk score, the AUC was 0.82 (95% CI 0.76–0.87) alone and 0.86 (95% CI 0.82–0.91) when combined with hs-cTnT (p<0.001). The clinical TIMI risk score alone as well as hs-cTnT (AUC = 0.80, 95% CI 0.74–0.86) alone are not inferior at the 5% significance level to the combination of the clinical TIMI risk score with hs-cTnT.

Most remarkably, performance of single biomarkers – notably of hs-cTnT, MPO, MRP 8/14, and c-cTnT – in predicting CE within 30 days, depended on the clinical pretest probability of ACS. Figure 2 illustrates ROC curves of hs-cTnT, MPO, MRP 8/14, and c-cTnT for the prediction of CE within 30 days in patients with low, intermediate, and high clinical TIMI risk scores, respectively. In patients with low (≤2) and intermediate (= 3)

Table 2. Final diagnoses.

Final diagnoses	All patients	Patients with cardiac events	Patients free from cardiac events
	(n = 377)	(n = 131)	(n = 246)
Patients with ST-segment elevations			
CAD	66 (96)	66 (50)	0
Cardiovascular death	1 (0.3)	1 (1)	0
Takotsubo cardiomyopathy	2 (0.6)	0	2 (1)
Patients without ST-segment elevations			
CAD (NSTEMI, UA)	66 (18)	58 (44)	8 (3)
Arrhythmia	39 (10)	1 (1)	38 (15)
Musculoskeletal	55 (15)	0	55 (22)
Syncopal event	18 (5)	1 (1)	17 (7)
Hypertension	21 (6)	1 (1)	20 8)
Gastrointestinal	14 (4)	0	14 (6)
Panic attack	6 (1.6)	1 (1)	6 (2)
Pulmonary	5 (1.3)	0	5 (2)
Myocarditis	4 (1.1)	1 (1)	3 (1)
Congestive heart failure	2 (0.5)	0	2 (1)
Other	14 (3.7)	0	14 (6)
Unclear	64 (17)	0	64 (26)

Abbreviations: CAD, coronary artery disease; NSTEMI, non-ST-elevation myocardial infarction; UA, unstable angina.

Table 3. Biomarker levels in patients with and without cardiac events (CE).

Biomarker	All patients	Patients with cardiac events	Patients free from cardiac events	P value
	(n = 377)	(n = 131)	(n = 246)	
Myocardial necrosis				
CK	115 [76–183] U/L	139 [81–290] U/L	105 [71–155] U/L	0.001
CK-MB	18 [13–27] U/L	20 [14–42] U/L	17 [12–24] U/L	<0.001
H-FABP	2.4 [1.4–6.1] ng/mL	5.0 [1.9–18.7] ng/mL	2.0 [1.2–3.2] ng/mL	<0.001
Myoglobin	46 [32–77] µg/L	71 [42–209] µg/L	40 [31–58] µg/L	<0.001
c-cTnT	0.01 [0.01–0.01] µg/L	0.01 [0.01–0.19] µg/L	0.01 [0.01–0.01] µg/L	<0.001
hs-cTnT	11.6 [4.7–33.0] pg/mL	34.9 [16.3–235.3] pg/mL	7.4 [3.2–15.4] pg/mL	<0.001
Myocardial function				
NT-proBNP	134 [48–674] ng/L	186 [51–940] ng/L	121 [45–406] ng/L	0.04
Inflammation				
hs-CRP	2.4 [0.9–5.9] mg/L	3.0 [1.1–7.3] mg/L	2.2 [0.9–4.9] mg/L	0.02
IL-6	3.4 [1.9–7.5] ng/L	3.9 [1.9–6.4] ng/L	3.3 [1.9–8.1] ng/L	0.4
MPO	41 [26–68] ng/mL	57 [32–97] ng/mL	36 [24–104] ng/mL	<0.001
MRP 8/14	2.9 [2.0–4.5] µg/mL	3.6 [2.3–5.7] µg/mL	2.6 [1.8–3.7] µg/mL	<0.001
Atherosclerosis				
PAPP-A	9 [7–13] mIU/L	11 [8–22] mIU/L	9 [7–11] mIU/L	<0.001
IGF-I	126 [98–157] µg/L	122 [95–150] µg/L	129 [100–163] µg/L	0.2
Coagulation				
D-dimer	0.19 [0.19–0.39] mg/L	0.21 [0.19–0.45] mg/L	0.19 [0.19–0.37] mg/L	0.5
Fibrinogen	3.4 [2.8–4.3] g/L	3.4 [2.8–4.6] g/L	3.4 [2.7–4.2] g/L	0.3

Abbreviations: CK, creatine kinase; CK-MB, creatine kinase-myocardial band; H-FABP, heart-type fatty acid-binding protein; c-cTnT, conventional cardiac troponin T; hs-cTnT, high-sensitive cardiac troponin T; NT-proBNP, N-terminal pro-brain natriuretic peptide; hs-CRP, high-sensitive C-reactive protein; Il-6, interleukin-6; MPO, myeloperoxidase; MRP 8/14, myeloid-related protein 8/14; PAPP-A, pregnancy-associated protein A; IGF-1, insulin-like growth factor 1.

Table 4. ROC-analysis for cardiac events (CE) at 30 days.

Biomarker	AUC	SE	Asymptotic 95% CI	Asymptotic P value	Best cut-off	Sensitivity	Specificity	PPV	NPV
All patients (n = 377)									
hs-cTnT	0.83	0.02	0.78–0.87	<0.0001	16.2 pg/mL	0.76	0.78	0.64	0.86
c-cTnT	0.69	0.03	0.63–0.75	<0.0001	0.02 µg/L	0.44	0.92	0.75	0.76
H-FABP	0.72	0.03	0.66–0.78	<0.0001	3.2 ng/mL	0.62	0.76	0.59	0.78
Myoglobin	0.71	0.03	0.65–0.76	<0.0001	75 µg/L	0.49	0.85	0.63	0.76
MRP 8/14	0.65	0.03	0.59–0.71	<0.0001	3.7 µg/mL	0.49	0.76	0.52	0.74
PAPP-A	0.64	0.03	0.58–0.70	<0.0001	17 mIU/L	0.32	0.93	0.70	0.72
MPO	0.63	0.03	0.57–0.68	<0.0001	55 ng/mL	0.56	0.68	0.48	0.75
CK-MB	0.62	0.03	0.56–0.68	<0.0001	34 U/L	0.34	0.86	0.57	0.71
CK	0.61	0.03	0.55–0.68	0.001	137 U/L	0.52	0.70	0.48	0.73
hs-CRP	0.57	0.04	0.50–0.63	0.039	5.2 mg/L	0.38	0.77	0.47	0.70
NT-proBNP	0.55	0.03	0.49–0.61	0.109	17 ng/L	0.11	0.93	0.44	0.66
Fibrinogen	0.52	0.03	0.46–0.59	0.386	2.8 g/L	0.81	0.27	0.37	0.73
D-dimer	0.52	0.03	0.45–0.58	0.610	0.23 mg/L	0.95	0.09	0.36	0.75
IL-6	0.52	0.03	0.45–0.58	0.652	12.7 ng/L	0.91	0.17	0.37	0.77
IGF-1	0.47	0.03	0.40–0.53	0.298	132 µg/L	0.63	0.48	0.39	0.71
Patients without ST-segment elevations (n = 308)									
Clinical GRACE score	0.61	0.04	0.53–0.68	0.009	100	0.55	0.64	0.28	0.84
Clinical TIMI risk score	0.82	0.03	0.76–0.87	<0.0001	3.00	0.73	0.78	0.47	0.92
Clinical TIMI risk score + hs-cTnT	0.86	0.01	0.82–0.91	<0.001	−1.66	0.83	0.76	0.47	0.94
hs-cTnT	0.80	0.03	0.74–0.86	<0.0001	9.26 pg/mL	0.86	0.61	0.37	0.84
c-cTnT	0.64	0.04	0.55–0.73	<0.001	0.02 µg/L	0.34	0.93	0.55	0.84
H-FABP	0.60	0.04	0.52–0.69	0.014	3.2 ng/mL	0.44	0.77	0.34	0.84
Myoglobin	0.61	0.04	0.54–0.69	0.007	43 µg/L	0.63	0.55	0.27	0.85
MRP 8/14	0.63	0.04	0.55–0.71	0.003	3.7 µg/mL	0.45	0.75	0.33	0.84
PAPP-A	0.61	0.04	0.54–0.69	0.009	11.0 mIU/L	0.52	0.70	0.31	0.85
MPO	0.60	0.04	0.52–0.68	0.015	54.9 ng/mL	0.51	0.69	0.30	0.84
CK-MB	0.56	0.04	0.47–0.64	0.172	34 U/L	0.28	0.86	0.35	0.82
CK	0.49	0.04	0.41–0.58	0.858	57 U/L	0.22	0.87	0.31	0.81
hs-CRP	0.56	0.04	0.48–0.64	0.148	5.2 mg/L	0.41	0.77	0.32	0.83
NT-proBNP	0.62	0.04	0.54–0.70	0.004	738 ng/L	0.39	0.84	0.38	0.84
Fibrinogen	0.56	0.04	0.48–0.64	0.141	2.9 g/L	0.81	0.30	0.23	0.86
D-dimer	0.57	0.04	0.48–0.65	0.114	3.1 mg/L	0.44	0.69	0.27	0.82
IL-6	0.48	0.04	0.41–0.56	0.678	5.2 ng/L	0.75	0.36	0.24	0.85
IGF-1	0.49	0.04	0.41–0.57	0.749	163 µg/L	0.84	0.25	0.23	0.86

Abbreviations: AUC, area under the curve; SE, standard error; CI, confidence intervall; PPV, positive predictive value; NPV, negative predictive value; hs-cTnT, high-sensitive cardiac troponin T; c-cTnT, conventional cardiac troponin T; H-FABP, heart-type fatty acid-binding protein; MRP 8/14, myeloid-related protein 8/14; PAPP-A, pregnancy-associated protein A; MPO, myeloperoxidase; CK-MB, creatine kinase-myocardial band; CK, creatine kinase; hs-CRP, high-sensitive C-reactive protein; NT-proBNP, N-terminal pro-brain natriuretic peptide; IL-6, interleukin-6; and IGF-1, insulin-like growth factor 1. The clinical TIMI risk score is the sum of 6 clinical factors without the biomarker variable of the 7 originally described risk predictors of the TIMI unstable angina/Non-ST myocardial infarction risk score.

clinical TIMI risk scores, hs-cTnT significantly predicted CE within 30 days ($p<0.001$ and $p=0.005$), while it did not add to risk prediction in patients with high (>3) clinical TIMI risk scores ($p=0.35$). To the contrary, MPO accurately predicted CE within 30 days in patients with high (>3) clinical TIMI risk scores ($p=0.006$), while ROC-analyses were not significant in patients with low (≤2) and intermediate (=3) clinical TIMI risk scores ($p=0.23$ and $p=0.35$, respectively). ROC-analyses revealed no significant AUC curves for MRP 8/14 independent of the clinical TIMI risk group, and only significant values for low (≤2) clinical TIMI risk scores for c-cTnT ($p=0.013$).

In Non-ST-elevation patients, multivariate decision tree analysis incorporating clinical data and information of all 15 biomarkers identified a model primarily based on clinical TIMI risk score complemented by serum values of hs-cTnT as most predictive for CE within 30 days (classification accuracy = 85.1%; figure 3). Age, gender, and renal function did not affect classification tree analyses. Using best cutoff-points for the clinical GRACE risk score, no significant classification with regard to CE at 30 days was possible in classification tree analysis ($p=0.37$; figure 4).

Comparison of two risk models for the prediction of cardiac events (CE) in Non-ST-elevation patients

In a binary logistic regression model to predict CE including all biomarkers, the clinical TIMI and GRACE risk scores, as well as age and gender, the clinical TIMI risk score, hs-TnT, and gender were the only significant predictor variables. While both gender ($p=0.03$) and the clinical TIMI risk score ($p=0.002$) remained significant predictors, hs-cTnT was no longer significant ($p=0.30$) after bootstrapping.

To further elucidate the impact of hs-TnT on risk prediction based on the clinical TIMI risk score, two risk models were established, i.e. clinical TIMI risk score and gender alone (model I) and combined with hs-TnT (model II). Female gender negatively predicted CE in binary logistic regression analysis. The AUC was 0.84 (95% CI 0.78–0.89; $p<0.001$) for model I, and 0.87 (95% CI 0.83–0.92; $p<0.001$) for model II, respectively. We could neither conclude equality (test of (AUC(model I)-AUC(model II)) = 0; diff value = 0.067; $p=0.002$) nor equivalence of the AUCs at the 5% significance level ($p=0.087$). An empirical non-inferiority test for AUCs showed that model I is no worse than model II with a non-inferiority bound of 5% ($p<0.001$), i.e. that the AUC for model I is no less than the AUC for model II at the 5% significance level. The addition of hs-TnT to base model I with an IDI of 0.054 indicates that the difference in average predicted risks between the individuals with and without CE increased by 5.4% in model II compared to model I. The performance of the two risk models is illustrated by predictiveness curves (figure 5).

Discussion

This study assessed novel sensitive biomarkers along with established clinical parameters on admission of patients with suspected ACS, for the prediction of CE defined as a composite of early coronary revascularization, myocardial infarction, and cardiovascular death within 30 days. At variance with other biomarker studies, in this analysis CE were prespecified to include immediate revascularization therapy, since in the contemporary setting of primary PCI for ACS, emergency room triage firstly aims at identifying patients in need of PCI or CABG. Acute coronary syndromes presenting as myocardial infarction may be suspected or diagnosed by ECG already at admittance, and diagnosis may be corroborated or not with biomarker testing. Most likely, those patients will undergo cardiac catheterization immediately. But in all patients with suspected ACS, identification and therapy of a culprit lesion nowadays is paramount and complementary to the clinical endpoints of myocardial infarction and cardiovascular death within 30 days, which in turn may reflect both success or failure of therapy, or a missed diagnosis in patients not having undergone coronary angiography.

Importantly, this study showed that performance of single biomarkers – notably of hs-cTnT and MPO – depend on the clinical pretest probability of ACS, with hs-cTnT adding to the sensitivity in patients with low and MPO improving the specificity of patients with high clinical risk scores, respectively. Accordingly, identification of those prone to CE was best based on clinical criteria complemented by hs-cTnT based on decision tree analysis. Interestingly, prediction of CE based on the clinical TIMI risk score alone was not improved by adding hs-cTnT to the risk prediction model. Although this study was originally designed also to assess the diagnostic value of MRP 8/14 for early diagnosis of ACS [16], in the current setting this marker of phagocyte activation did not show sufficient discriminatory performance, notwithstanding its significant elevation in ACS.

Scoring systems predicting the patients' risk of ischemic events and cardiovascular death have been established such as the TIMI risk score for unstable angina/NSTEMI [23]. The TIMI risk score is a simple, well-validated score for which prediction of cardiac ischemic events and cardiovascular death has been shown in patients with unstable angina or NSTEMI [26,27], and in patients presenting with acute chest pain to the emergency department [28]. The TIMI risk score offers clinical applications as it categorizes patients with a wide, about 5- to 10-fold, range of major adverse clinical events risk into different risk groups [23]. Indeed, patients with intermediate (score 3–4) and high-risk (score 5–7) scores, in particular those with prior history of PCI and CABG, have been shown to benefit most from an early invasive strategy as compared to low-risk patients. Therefore, a modified TIMI risk score devoid of the biomarker component was used in this study for comprehensive clinical risk assessment at patient admission to the emergency department.

In this patient cohort, the clinical TIMI risk score outranged the clinical GRACE risk score in predicting CE at 30 days. These findings might at least in part be due to the different clinical criteria incorporated in the two risk scores and the different weighting of each criterion. While the GRACE risk score focuses more on clinical parameters on admission such as heart rate and systolic blood pressure, the TIMI risk score incorporates patient history including risk factors for coronary artery disease, known coronary artery disease, the use of antiplatelet therapy, and severe episodes of angina [23,24]. Moreover, the endpoint definition of this study varies from the ones used to validate these risk scoring systems, and limited predictive value of the GRACE risk score has previously been described [29]. However, this study was not designed to allow a comparison between different risk scoring systems, and further studies are needed to compare predictive values of risk scores in different subsets of patients.

In ST-elevation patients, distinctive ECG patterns usually determine an early invasive strategy with rare contraindications. However, the heterogenous population of Non-ST-elevation patients requires an appropriate patient selection for early revascularization. Although the combination of clinical parameters or risk scores, respectively with several conventional markers such as c-cTnT and NT-proBNP have occasionally been suggested [30,31], our findings show for the first time that integrating clinical and novel cardiac biomarker data including continuous hs-cTnT levels best predicted CE at 30 days in Non-ST-elevation patients. Stand-alone, cardiac biomarkers including hs-cTnT were not

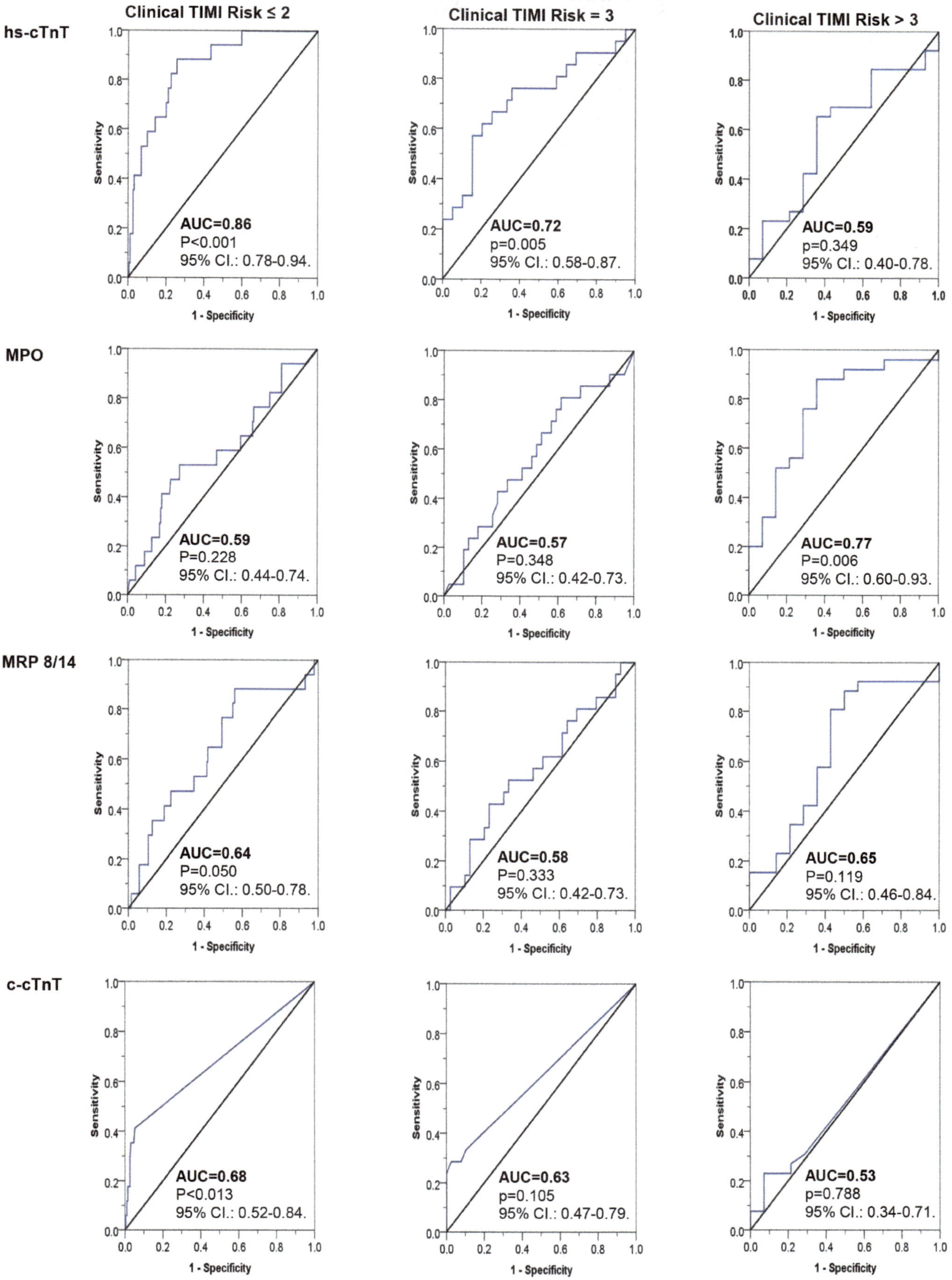
Clinical TIMI Risk ≤ 2
Clinical TIMI Risk = 3
Clinical TIMI Risk > 3
hs-cTnT
AUC=0.86
P<0.001
95% CI.: 0.78-0.94.
AUC=0.72
p=0.005
95% CI.: 0.58-0.87.
AUC=0.59
p=0.349
95% CI.: 0.40-0.78.
MPO
AUC=0.59
P=0.228
95% CI.: 0.44-0.74.
AUC=0.57
P=0.348
95% CI.: 0.42-0.73.
AUC=0.77
P=0.006
95% CI.: 0.60-0.93.
MRP 8/14
AUC=0.64
P=0.050
95% CI.: 0.50-0.78.
AUC=0.58
P=0.333
95% CI.: 0.42-0.73.
AUC=0.65
P=0.119
95% CI.: 0.46-0.84.
c-cTnT
AUC=0.68
P<0.013
95% CI.: 0.52-0.84.
AUC=0.63
p=0.105
95% CI.: 0.47-0.79.
AUC=0.53
p=0.788
95% CI.: 0.34-0.71.
Sensitivity
1 - Specificity

Figure 2. Diagnostic performance of high-sensitive cardiac troponin T (hs-cTnT), myeloperoxidase (MPO), myeloid-related protein 8/14 (MRP 8/14), and conventional cardiac troponin T (c-cTnT) in relation to the clinical TIMI risk score of patients with suspected ACS and no obvious ST-segment elevations at presentation (Non-ST-elevation patients). AUC indicates area under the curve. The clinical TIMI risk score is the sum of 6 clinical factors without the biomarker variable of the 7 originally described risk predictors of the TIMI unstable angina/Non-ST myocardial infarction risk score.

better predictors of CE compared to clinical judgment using the modified TIMI risk score. These findings further strengthen the value of traditional clinical practice in assessing the probability that the symptoms represent cardiac ischemia. Both safety issues and limitations of health care resources demand the effective targeting of therapy to those who are likely to benefit most in the heterogeneous population of Non-ST-elevation patients.

Observed	Predicted		
	no	yes	**Percent Correct**
No-CE	224	20	**91.8%**
CE	26	38	**59.4%**
Overall Percentage	81.2%	18.8%	**85.1%**

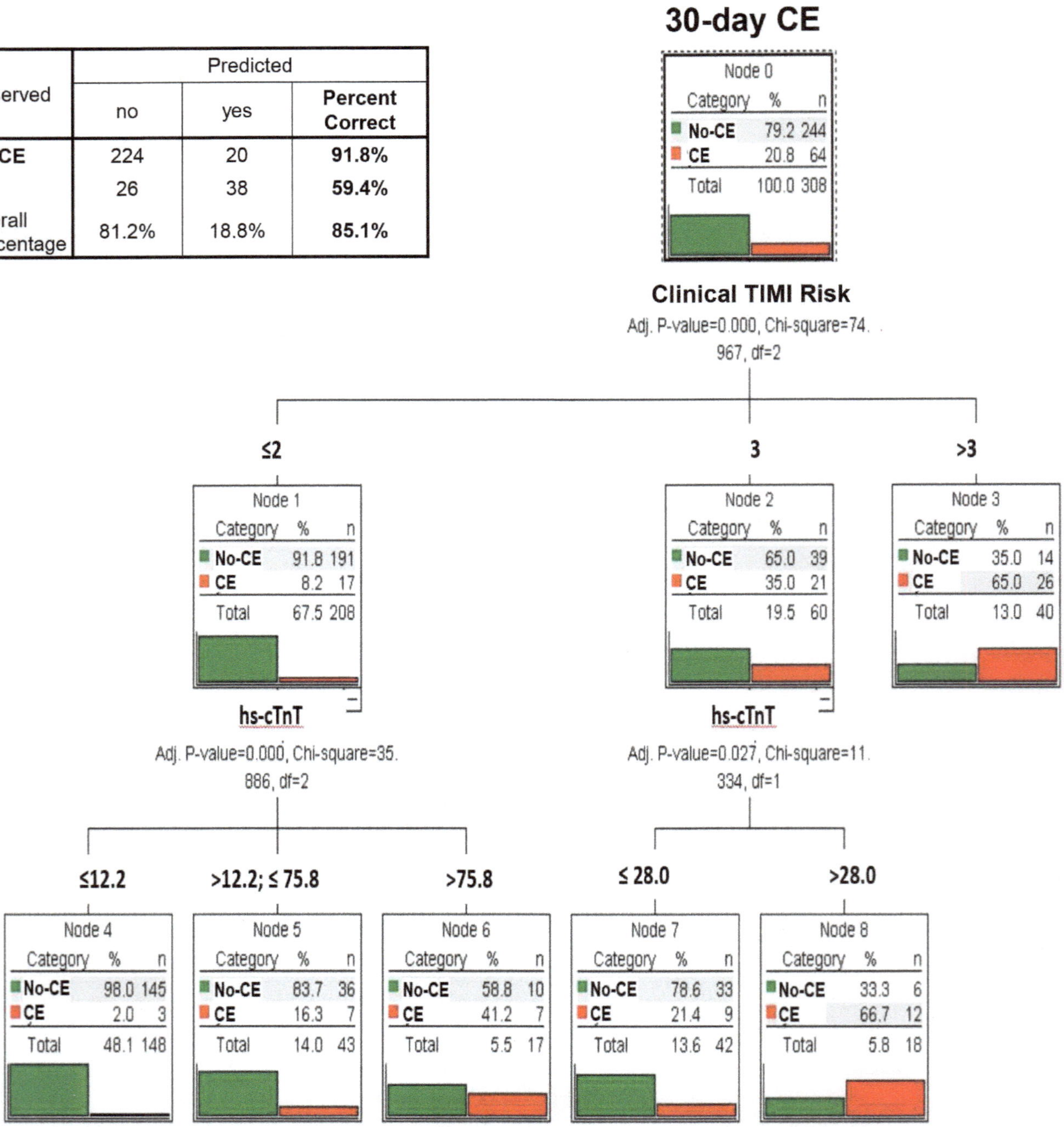

Figure 3. Multivariate classification tree analysis of clinical and multiple biomarker information and the resulting algorithm for the identification of those at risk of cardiac events (CE) within 30 days among patients presenting with suspected ACS and no apparent ST-segment elevations (Non-ST-elevation patients). Hs-cTnT indicates high-sensitive cardiac troponin T (pg/mL), no-CE denotes patients free from cardiac events (CE) within 30 days. The clinical TIMI score is the sum of 6 clinical factors without the biomarker variable of the 7 originally described risk predictors of the TIMI unstable angina/Non-ST myocardial infarction risk score.

Classification

Observed	Predicted no	Predicted yes	Percent Correct
No-CE	244	0	**100.0%**
CE	64	0	**0.0%**
Overall Percentage	100.0%	0.0%	**79.2%**

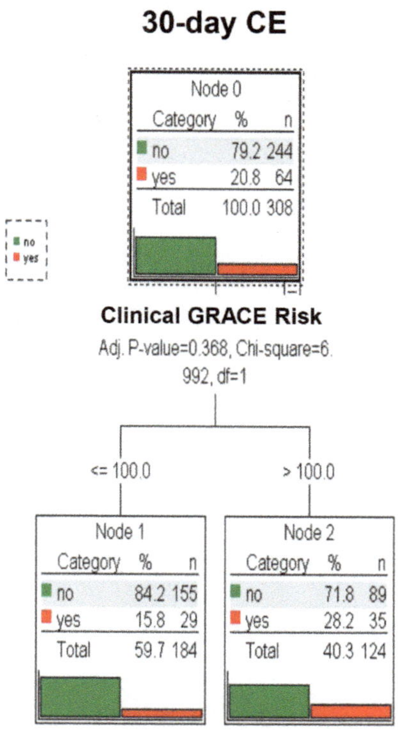

Figure 4. Multivariate classification tree analysis of clinical and multiple biomarker information and the resulting algorithm for the identification of those at risk of cardiac events (CE) within 30 days among patients presenting with suspected ACS and no apparent ST-segment elevations (Non-ST-elevation patients). No significant classification with regard to 30-day CE was possible using the clinical GRACE risk score (Bonferroni-adjusted p-value = 0.368).

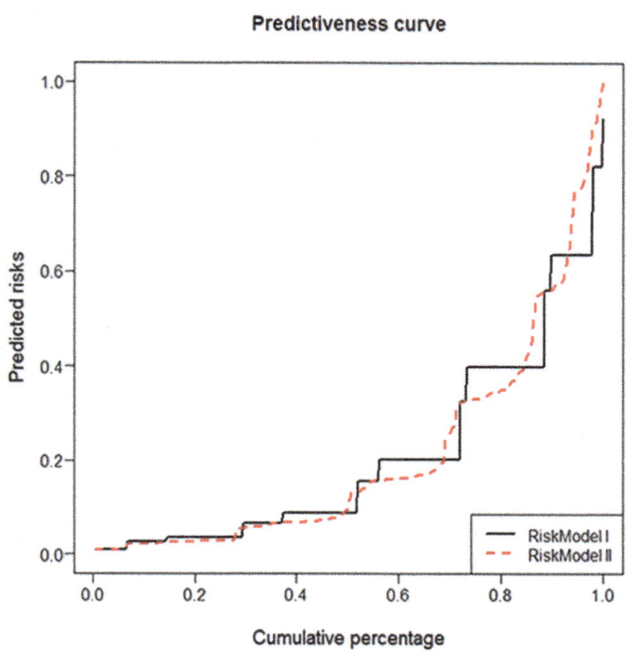

Figure 5. Predictiveness curves illustrating the prognostic performance of two different risk models in predicting cardiac events (CE). Risk model I: clinical TIMI risk score and gender; Risk model II: clinical TIMI risk score, gender, and hs-cTnT, respectively.

The use of the highly sensitive troponin assays has substantially increased the number of chest pain patients tested troponin positive [32]. This bears the potential of setting off an avalanche of ischemia-related diagnostics. However, in patient with Non-ST-elevation ACS, also low increases in troponin levels detected by highly sensitive assays were reported to be associated with a higher risk of cardiovascular death and myocardial infarction at 30 days and at 1 year [33]. It is well known, that hs-cTnT is superior to MPO for rapid and accurate diagnosis of acute myocardial infarction among patients presenting with chest pain at the emergency department [18,34,35]. Interestingly, MPO was not predictive for CE in patients with clinical TIMI risk score ≤ 3, whereas it was predictive in patients with higher risk scores. On the contrary, with increasing clinical TIMI risk scores, c-cTnT and hs-cTnT showed a gradual decline of the AUC for the prediction of CE within 30 days. Hence, risk prediction of biomarkers such as hs-cTnT and MPO clearly depends on the pretest probability. Further studies are needed to understand the different risk prediction profiles of hs-cTnT and MPO in low- and high-risk patients with suspected ACS.

Interestingly, no improvement in risk prediction was observed with the combination of the clinical TIMI risk score and hs-cTnT with the pre-specified cut-off value of 13 pg/mL. Hence, in line with previous data [33], the recommended and arbitrary defined hs-cTnT decision limit seems to be less important for CE risk prediction than continuous hs-cTnT levels including also low-level increases. Furthermore, cut-off values of hs-cTnT may differ in various patient populations as has been suggested for other biomarkers such as NT-proBNP which shows dependency on age, gender, and body mass index [36,37].

Limitations of this study are the single-centre design and the fact that risk assessment was only performed at time of presentation to the emergency department. However, this approach is in accordance with the original design of the TIMI risk score for prognostication at time of presentation [23]. The rather high rate of patients presenting with ST-elevation myocardial infarction observed might at least in part be due to the fact that the study was performed at a tertiary referral center. However, the high rate of coronary angiographies associated with this constellation allowed for confirming or ruling out the diagnosis of coronary artery disease based on current gold standard. Nevertheless, the fact that decision making relied on c-cTnT measurements might have led to an underestimation of true ACS needing validation. As binary data whether events occurred or not were recorded in the study, time-to-event analyses could not be included.

In conclusion, the combination of the patients' clinical condition as represented in the clinical TIMI risk score, and a biomarker approach involving levels of continuous hs-cTnT, best predicted 30-day CE rate in Non-ST-elevation patients; thus, in this heterogeneous patient population the traditional but nevertheless sustainable clinical assessment remains fundamental for risk stratification.

Acknowledgments

The authors are grateful to the patients who participated in the study, as well as the staff of the emergency department, the cath lab staff, and the laboratory technicians for their most valuable efforts. We further acknowledge the contribution of Dr. R. Kientsch-Engel and Dr. H. Hüdig, Roche Diagnostics GmbH, 82377 Penzberg, Germany. All authors take responsibility for all aspects of the reliability and freedom from bias of the data presented and their discussed interpretation.

Author Contributions

Conceived and designed the experiments: LA KY GS WM. Performed the experiments: LA KY BS CW DH PF AB GS PK MH AvE MN TL WM. Analyzed the data: BS LA KY DH IN RW MF MW WM. Contributed reagents/materials/analysis tools: KY DH AvE MH MN. Wrote the paper: BS LA KY SG TL WM.

References

1. Go AS, Mozaffarian D, Roger VL, Benjamin EJ, Berry JD, et al. (2014) Heart disease and stroke statistics—2014 update: a report from the American Heart Association. Circulation 129: e28–e292.
2. Goodacre S, Cross E, Arnold J, Angelini K, Capewell S, et al. (2005) The health care burden of acute chest pain. Heart 91: 229–230.
3. James SK, Lindback J, Tilly J, Siegbahn A, Venge P, et al. (2006) Troponin-T and N-terminal pro-B-type natriuretic peptide predict mortality benefit from coronary revascularization in acute coronary syndromes: a GUSTO-IV substudy. J Am Coll Cardiol 48: 1146–1154.
4. Ohman EM, Armstrong PW, Christenson RH, Granger CB, Katus HA, et al. (1996) Cardiac troponin T levels for risk stratification in acute myocardial ischemia. GUSTO IIA Investigators. The New England journal of medicine 335: 1333–1341.
5. Morrow DA, Cannon CP, Jesse RL, Newby LK, Ravkilde J, et al. (2007) National Academy of Clinical Biochemistry Laboratory Medicine Practice Guidelines: Clinical characteristics and utilization of biochemical markers in acute coronary syndromes. Circulation 115: e356–375.
6. Antman EM, Tanasijevic MJ, Thompson B, Schactman M, McCabe CH, et al. (1996) Cardiac-specific troponin I levels to predict the risk of mortality in patients with acute coronary syndromes. The New England journal of medicine 335: 1342–1349.
7. Hamm CW, Ravkilde J, Gerhardt W, Jorgensen P, Peheim E, et al. (1992) The prognostic value of serum troponin T in unstable angina. The New England journal of medicine 327: 146–150.
8. Reichlin T, Hochholzer W, Bassetti S, Steuer S, Stelzig C, et al. (2009) Early diagnosis of myocardial infarction with sensitive cardiac troponin assays. N Engl J Med 361: 858–867.
9. Reichlin T, Irfan A, Twerenbold R, Reiter M, Hochholzer W, et al. (2011) Utility of absolute and relative changes in cardiac troponin concentrations in the early diagnosis of acute myocardial infarction. Circulation 124: 136–145.
10. Thygesen K, Mair J, Katus H, Plebani M, Venge P, et al. (2010) Recommendations for the use of cardiac troponin measurement in acute cardiac care. European heart journal 31: 2197–2204.
11. de Lemos JA, Drazner MH, Omland T, Ayers CR, Khera A, et al. (2010) Association of troponin T detected with a highly sensitive assay and cardiac structure and mortality risk in the general population. JAMA : the journal of the American Medical Association 304: 2503–2512.
12. Saunders JT, Nambi V, de Lemos JA, Chambless LE, Virani SS, et al. (2011) Cardiac troponin T measured by a highly sensitive assay predicts coronary heart disease, heart failure, and mortality in the Atherosclerosis Risk in Communities Study. Circulation 123: 1367–1376.
13. Shand JA, McEneaney DJ, Menown IB (2011) Heart-type fatty acid-binding protein in the early diagnosis of acute myocardial infarction: a systematic review and meta-analysis. Heart 97: 605; author reply 605.
14. Seino Y, Ogata K, Takano T, Ishii J, Hishida H, et al. (2003) Use of a whole blood rapid panel test for heart-type fatty acid-binding protein in patients with acute chest pain: comparison with rapid troponin T and myoglobin tests. The American journal of medicine 115: 185–190.
15. Healy AM, Pickard MD, Pradhan AD, Wang Y, Chen Z, et al. (2006) Platelet expression profiling and clinical validation of myeloid-related protein-14 as a novel determinant of cardiovascular events. Circulation 113: 2278–2284.
16. Altwegg LA, Neidhart M, Hersberger M, Muller S, Eberli FR, et al. (2007) Myeloid-related protein 8/14 complex is released by monocytes and granulocytes at the site of coronary occlusion: a novel, early, and sensitive marker of acute coronary syndromes. Eur Heart J 28: 941–948.
17. Vora AN, Bonaca MP, Ruff CT, Jarolim P, Murphy S, et al. (2012) Diagnostic evaluation of the MRP-8/14 for the emergency assessment of chest pain. Journal of thrombosis and thrombolysis.
18. Brennan ML, Penn MS, Van Lente F, Nambi V, Shishehbor MH, et al. (2003) Prognostic value of myeloperoxidase in patients with chest pain. The New England journal of medicine 349: 1595–1604.
19. Bayes-Genis A, Conover CA, Overgaard MT, Bailey KR, Christiansen M, et al. (2001) Pregnancy-associated plasma protein A as a marker of acute coronary syndromes. The New England journal of medicine 345: 1022–1029.
20. Sabatine MS, Morrow DA, de Lemos JA, Gibson CM, Murphy SA, et al. (2002) Multimarker approach to risk stratification in non-ST elevation acute coronary syndromes: simultaneous assessment of troponin I, C-reactive protein, and B-type natriuretic peptide. Circulation 105: 1760–1763.
21. McCann CJ, Glover BM, Menown IB, Moore MJ, McEneny J, et al. (2009) Prognostic value of a multimarker approach for patients presenting to hospital with acute chest pain. The American journal of cardiology 103: 22–28.
22. Oemrawsingh RM, Lenderink T, Akkerhuis KM, Heeschen C, Baldus S, et al. (2011) Multimarker risk model containing troponin-T, interleukin 10, myeloperoxidase and placental growth factor predicts long-term cardiovascular risk after non-ST-segment elevation acute coronary syndrome. Heart 97: 1061–1066.
23. Antman EM, Cohen M, Bernink PJ, McCabe CH, Horacek T, et al. (2000) The TIMI risk score for unstable angina/non-ST elevation MI: A method for prognostication and therapeutic decision making. JAMA : the journal of the American Medical Association 284: 835–842.
24. Granger CB, Goldberg RJ, Dabbous O, Pieper KS, Eagle KA, et al. (2003) Predictors of hospital mortality in the global registry of acute coronary events. Arch Intern Med 163: 2345–2353.
25. Alpert JS, Thygesen K, Antman E, Bassand JP (2000) Myocardial infarction redefined—a consensus document of The Joint European Society of Cardiology/American College of Cardiology Committee for the redefinition of myocardial infarction. Journal of the American College of Cardiology 36: 959–969.
26. Bijsterveld NR, Peters RJ, Murphy SA, Bernink PJ, Tijssen JG, et al. (2003) Recurrent cardiac ischemic events early after discontinuation of short-term heparin treatment in acute coronary syndromes: results from the Thrombolysis in Myocardial Infarction (TIMI) 11B and Efficacy and Safety of Subcutaneous Enoxaparin in Non-Q-Wave Coronary Events (ESSENCE) studies. Journal of the American College of Cardiology 42: 2083–2089.
27. Scirica BM, Cannon CP, Antman EM, Murphy SA, Morrow DA, et al. (2002) Validation of the thrombolysis in myocardial infarction (TIMI) risk score for unstable angina pectoris and non-ST-elevation myocardial infarction in the TIMI III registry. The American journal of cardiology 90: 303–305.
28. Conway Morris A, Caesar D, Gray S, Gray A (2006) TIMI risk score accurately risk stratifies patients with undifferentiated chest pain presenting to an emergency department. Heart 92: 1333–1334.
29. Wang L, Hu XB, Zhang W, Wu LD, Liu YS, et al. (2013) Dickkopf-1 as a novel predictor is associated with risk stratification by GRACE risk scores for predictive value in patients with acute coronary syndrome: a retrospective research. PLoS One 8: e54731.
30. Manenti ER, Bodanese LC, Camey SA, Polanczyk CA (2006) Prognostic value of serum biomarkers in association with TIMI risk score for acute coronary syndromes. Clinical cardiology 29: 405–410.
31. Tello-Montoliu A, Marin F, Roldan V, Mainar L, Lopez MT, et al. (2007) A multimarker risk stratification approach to non-ST elevation acute coronary

syndrome: implications of troponin T, CRP, NT pro-BNP and fibrin D-dimer levels. Journal of internal medicine 262: 651–658.
32. Hochholzer W, Reichlin T, Twerenbold R, Stelzig C, Hochholzer K, et al. (2011) Incremental value of high-sensitivity cardiac troponin T for risk prediction in patients with suspected acute myocardial infarction. Clinical chemistry 57: 1318–1326.
33. Bonaca M, Scirica B, Sabatine M, Dalby A, Spinar J, et al. (2010) Prospective evaluation of the prognostic implications of improved assay performance with a sensitive assay for cardiac troponin I. Journal of the American College of Cardiology 55: 2118–2124.
34. Schaub N, Reichlin T, Meune C, Twerenbold R, Haaf P, et al. (2011) Markers of Plaque Instability in the Early Diagnosis and Risk Stratification of Acute Myocardial Infarction. Clinical chemistry.
35. Khan DA, Sharif MS, Khan FA (2011) Diagnostic performance of high-sensitivity troponin T, myeloperoxidase, and pregnancy-associated plasma protein a assays for triage of patients with acute myocardial infarction. The Korean journal of laboratory medicine 31: 172–178.
36. Krauser DG, Lloyd-Jones DM, Chae CU, Cameron R, Anwaruddin S, et al. (2005) Effect of body mass index on natriuretic peptide levels in patients with acute congestive heart failure: a ProBNP Investigation of Dyspnea in the Emergency Department (PRIDE) substudy. American heart journal 149: 744–750.
37. Wang TJ, Larson MG, Levy D, Leip EP, Benjamin EJ, et al. (2002) Impact of age and sex on plasma natriuretic peptide levels in healthy adults. The American journal of cardiology 90: 254–258.

2

Soluble ST2 and Interleukin-33 Levels in Coronary Artery Disease: Relation to Disease Activity and Adverse Outcome

Svitlana Demyanets[1,2], Walter S. Speidl[1], Ioannis Tentzeris[3], Rudolf Jarai[3], Katharina M. Katsaros[1,5], Serdar Farhan[3], Konstantin A. Krychtiuk[1,5], Anna Wonnerth[1,5], Thomas W. Weiss[3], Kurt Huber[3], Johann Wojta[1,4,5]*

1 Department of Internal Medicine II, Medical University of Vienna, Vienna, Austria, **2** Department of Laboratory Medicine, Medical University of Vienna, Vienna, Austria, **3** 3rd Medical Department for Cardiology and Emergency Medicine, Wilhelminenhospital, Vienna, Austria, **4** Core Facilities, Medical University of Vienna, Vienna, Austria, **5** Ludwig Boltzmann Cluster for Cardiovascular Research, Vienna, Austria

Abstract

Objectives: ST2 is a receptor for interleukin (IL)-33. We investigated an association of soluble ST2 (sST2) and IL-33 serum levels with different clinical stages of coronary artery disease. We assessed the predictive value of sST2 and IL-33 in patients with stable angina, non-ST elevation myocardial infarction (NSTEMI) and ST elevation myocardial infarction (STEMI).

Methods: We included 373 patients of whom 178 had stable angina, 97 had NSTEMI, and 98 had STEMI. Patients were followed for a mean of 43 months. The control group consisted of 65 individuals without significant stenosis on coronary angiography. Serum levels of sST2 and IL-33 were measured by ELISAs.

Results: sST2 levels were significantly increased in patients with STEMI as compared to patients with NSTEMI and stable angina as well as with controls. IL-33 levels did not differ between the four groups. During follow-up, 37 (10%) patients died and the combined endpoint (all cause death, MI and rehospitalisation for cardiac causes) occurred in 66 (17.6%) patients. sST2 serum levels significantly predicted mortality in the total cohort. When patients were stratified according to their clinical presentation, the highest quintile of sST2 significantly predicted mortality in patients with STEMI, but not with NSTEMI or stable coronary artery disease. sST2 was a significant predictor for the combined endpoint in STEMI patients and in patients with stable angina. Serum levels of IL-33 were not associated with clinical outcome in the total cohort, but the highest quintile of IL-33 predicted mortality in patients with STEMI.

Conclusions: Serum levels of sST2 are increased in patients with acute coronary syndromes as compared to levels in patients with stable coronary artery disease and in individuals without coronary artery disease. sST2 and IL-33 were associated with mortality in patients with STEMI but not in patients with NSTEMI or stable angina.

Editor: Ingo Ahrens, University Hospital Medical Centre, Germany

Funding: This work was supported by the Austrian Science Fund (FWF-Project number T445-B11 to SD), Ludwig Boltzmann Cluster for Cardiovascular Research (Vienna, Austria), and Association for the Promotion of Research in Arteriosclerosis, Thrombosis and Vascular Biology (Vienna, Austria). The funders had no role in study design, data collection and analysis, decision to publish, or preparation of the manuscript.

Competing Interests: The authors have declared that no competing interests exist.

* E-mail: johann.wojta@meduniwien.ac.at

Introduction

ST2 (also known as T1 or interleukin (IL)-1 receptor-like-1 (IL1RL1)) is a member of the Toll-like/IL-1-receptor superfamily [1,2]. ST2 was known for more than 15 years as an orphan receptor before its ligand cytokine IL-33 was discovered in 2005 [3]. The soluble ST2 (sST2) and the transmembrane ST2 (ST2L) isoforms arise from a dual promoter system to drive differential mRNA expression [4]. ST2 is established as a selective marker of T helper type 2 (Th2) lymphocytes [1]. In addition, ST2 is also expressed on mast cells, epithelial, endothelial and smooth muscle cells, rat neonatal cardiac fibroblasts and cardiac myocytes [2,5–8]. IL-33 is a dual-function cytokine, which is either expressed in the nucleus or activates cells via the receptor complex consisting of ST2L and IL-1 receptor accessory protein (IL-1RaP) [2,3]. IL-33 is a multifunctional immunomodulatory cytokine that acts both pro- and anti-inflammatory depending on the disease state or experimental conditions [9,10]. sST2 acts as a decoy receptor by binding free IL-33 and preventing its signaling through ST2L [7].

Weinberg et al. were the first who showed increased sST2 levels in patients after myocardial infarction, which correlated positively with peak creatine kinase and negatively with left ventricle ejection fraction [6]. The same group revealed a predictive value of sST2 in patients with ST-elevation myocardial infarction (STEMI) by showing that baseline levels of sST2 were significantly higher in those patients who died or developed new congestive heart failure during short-term follow-up (30 days) [11]. Multi-marker approach revealed that the combination of sST2 and N-terminal prohormone B-type natriuretic peptide (NT-proBNP) significantly improves risk stratification in STEMI patients during 30-day follow-up [12]. A possible pathophysiological importance of sST2 in infarct remodeling was further confirmed by a study of Weir et al. who found relationships between sST2 and infarct magnitude/evolution over 24 weeks of observation in patients with acute myocardial infarction with resultant left ventricle systolic dysfunction [13].

In non-ST elevation myocardial infarction (NSTEMI), sST2 was related to 1-year mortality, to cardiovascular death/heart failure at 30 days and 1 year as well as to death, heart failure readmission, and reinfarction during the long term, respectively [14–16]. Until now there is no data on the predictive value of sST2 in stable coronary artery disease (CAD).

Thus, increased levels of the soluble receptor for IL-33, sST2, are recognized as a marker of poor prognosis in patients with myocardial infarction and heart failure [9,11,17]. However, the prognostic value of circulating IL-33 in cardiovascular disease is not clear. Recently, Dhillon et al. showed that elevated sST2 and IL-33 were both associated with increased mortality in STEMI patients [18], but in patients with NSTEMI only sST2 and not IL-33 levels were related to adverse events such as all-cause mortality, heart failure hospitalization, and reinfarction [16]. Our group found recently that an increase of IL-33 serum levels after coronary stent implantation is associated with coronary in-stent restenosis in patients with both stable and unstable CAD [19].

Although increased levels of sST2 in patients with STEMI and NSTEMI were shown over different periods of time [6,11,13,14], a comparison of sST2 and IL-33 concentrations in patients with stable angina and acute coronary syndromes and individuals without CAD was not studied before and was the aim of our study. Additionally, we determined the long-term predictive value of sST2 and IL-33 levels in the examined groups of patients. It should be emphasized, however, that it was not the main objective of this work to identify yet another clinical biomarker or point of care test for the diagnosis of acute coronary syndrome or for the clinical risk prediction in stable coronary artery disease. Rather it was the aim of this study to gain additional insights in the pathophysiological role of the ST2/IL-33 system in atherosclerotic disease and myocardial infarction.

Methods

Ethics Statement

The study protocol conforms to the ethical guidelines of the Declaration of Helsinki as reflected in a priori approval by the ethics committee of the city of Vienna, Austria. All subjects provided written consent.

Study Population

Blood samples were taken from 373 consecutive patients with angiographically proven CAD. From these patients 178 had stable angina (SA), 97 NSTEMI, and 98 STEMI, respectively. In addition we included 65 subjects without evidence of coronary stenosis on coronary angiogram. Exclusion criteria were presence of autoimmune diseases, chronic infections, hepatic or renal disorders. Aspirin and unfractionated heparin were administered per standard practice. Clopidogrel therapy was started either on the day before angiography or immediately after stent implantation with 300 mg. Other medications such as beta-blockers and angiotensin-converting-enzyme inhibitors were given as appropriate. Statin therapy was routinely administered to all patients according to international guidelines. At inclusion time new antiplatelet drugs like ticagrelor and prasugrel were not yet available.

Blood Samples

Blood samples were taken under fasting conditions directly before coronary angiography. Venous blood was drawn from the antecubital vein with minimal tourniquet pressure into serum separator tubes. Samples were allowed to clot for 30 minutes (min) before centrifugation (4°C; 3,000 g for 15 min) and stored at −80°C until use.

Laboratory Measurements

sST2 and IL-33 were measured with specific enzyme-linked immunosorbent assays (ELISAs; both from R&D Systems, Minneapolis, MN, USA). Minimum detection limit for sST2 was 31.3 pg/mL; for IL-33 minimum detection limit was 23.4 pg/mL. Laboratory determinations were performed by investigators that were blinded to clinical characteristics and patients' outcome.

Follow-up

Patients were followed for a mean of 43 months for the occurrence of death and a combined clinical endpoint (all cause death, myocardial infarction and rehospitalisation for cardiac causes).

Statistical Analysis

We estimated a mortality of 10% in this cohort of patients with STEMI, NSTEMI and SA. Therefore, calculation of sample size revealed that we would need at least 320 patients to detect a difference in sST2 serum levels of 50% with a power of 80% and significance level (two-tailed) of 0.05 [20]. Variables were tested for normal distribution using the Kolmogorov-Smirnov test. Continuous variables were expressed as mean ± SD or as median, interquartile range according their distribution. Categorical variables were summarized as counts and percentages and were compared by the chi-square or by Fisher exact test as appropriate. Continuous variables were compared using Student's t-test when normally distributed and by Mann-Whitney-U test when not normally distributed. ANOVA followed by Bonferroni-Holm multiple comparisons correction was carried out in case when more than 2 groups were compared. Spearman correlation was used to determine the correlation between level of sST2 and cardiovascular risk factors or level of IL-33 and cardiovascular risk factors. Multivariate analysis was performed with the Cox proportional hazard model in which mortality was used as dependent variable and potentially confounding baseline variables were used as independent variables. Baseline variables were selected for the model if they appeared to be imbalanced between patients with and without survival indicated by a univariate p-value <0.20 or if they were correlated with ST2 or IL-33, respectively. A value of $p<0.05$ (two-tailed) was considered statistically significant. All statistical analyses were performed with the statistical software package SPSS version 18.0 (SPSS, Inc., Chicago, Illinois).

Results

Study Population Characteristics

Demographic data of the entire cohort, controls and patients with SA, NSTEMI and STEMI, respectively are shown in the Table 1. There were no differences in regard to gender, age, diabetes, and kidney function between the four study groups. Although controls had a higher body mass index (BMI), they were

Table 1. Baseline characteristics of study population.

	Total (n = 438)	Controls (n = 65)	SA (n = 178)	NSTEMI (n = 97)	STEMI (n = 98)	P-value
Age (yrs)	64.4±12.1	62.6±8.9	65.9±11.5	64.6±13.5	62.9±13.7	0.14
Male sex, N (%)	279 (63.7)	32 (49.2)	122 (68.5)	60 (61.9)	65 (66.3)	0.06
Hypertension, N (%)	328 (74.9)	46 (70.8)	142 (79.8)	80 (82.5)	60 (61.2)	0.001
Smoker, N (%)	130 (29.7)	20 (30.8)	43 (24.2)	26 (26.8)	41 (41.8)	0.02
Hyperlipidaemia, N (%)	324 (74.0)	35 (53.8)	140 (78.7)	76 (78.4)	73 (74.5)	0.001
Diabetes, N (%)	95 (21.7)	18 (27.7)	39 (21.9)	15 (15.5)	23 (23.5)	0.29
BMI (kg/m^2)	27.9±4.6	28.7±6.0	27.4±4.1	27.9±4.2	27.6±4.6	0.005
Serum creatinine (mg/dL)	1.04±0.64	1.02±0.28	1.08±0.93	1.01±0.31	1.03±0.33	0.80

SA denotes stable angina, NSTEMI denotes non-ST-elevation myocardial infarction, STEMI denotes ST-elevation myocardial infarction, CAD denotes coronary artery disease, BMI denotes body mass index.

less likely to have hyperlipidemia as compared to patients with CAD. Patients with STEMI were more likely to be smokers (p = 0.02) but less likely to be hypertensive (p = 0.001) (Table 1).

Serum Levels of sST2 and IL-33 in Relation to Cardiovascular Risk Factors

IL-33 was detectable in 46.1% of study participants and was below detection limit in 53.9%. IL-33 levels were significantly higher in females (p<0.05) and in non-smokers (p<0.05). Serum levels of sST2 and IL-33 showed a significant correlation (r = 0.38, p<0.000001). sST2 levels correlated positively with creatinine levels (r = 0.126; p = 0.009) but were not associated with classic cardiovascular risk factors.

sST2 and IL-33 Concentrations in Persons without CAD and Patients with Different Clinical Stages of CAD

Study participants showed significantly different sST2 serum levels according to their clinical presentation (Figure 1A). Controls (163, IQR 114–260 pg/mL) showed similar sST2 levels as compared to patients with SA (169, IQR 79–260 pg/mL; p = 0.34). Patients with STEMI showed the highest serum levels of sST2 (453, IQR 313–688 pg/mL) as compared to patients with NSTEMI (269, IQR 157–496 pg/mL; p<0.0001), patients with SA (p<0.000001) and controls (p<0.000001). In addition, patients with NSTEMI showed significantly higher levels of sST2 as compared to patients with stable CAD (p<0.0001) and controls (p<0.0001, Figure 1A). In contrast, IL-33 was detectable in 58.5%, 42.4%, 46.8% and 43.6% of individuals without CAD, patients with SA, NSTEMI and STEMI, respectively (p = NS) and IL-33 serum levels did not differ between the respective groups (p = NS, Figure 1B).

Relation of sST2 and IL-33 Serum Levels to Outcome

Mean follow-up time was 43 months. During follow-up, 37 (10%) patients died and the combined endpoint occurred in 66 (17.6%) patients. Patients who died during follow-up showed significantly higher serum levels of sST2 as compared to survivors (415, IQR 136–1158 pg/mL vs. 241, IQR 129–426 pg/mL; p< 0.05). The highest quintile of sST2 serum levels significantly predicted mortality in the total cohort (p<0.05, Figure 2A). When the total cohort was stratified according clinical presentation, sST2 was a strong predictor of mortality in patients with STEMI (p< 0.001, Figure 2B) but not in patients with NSTEMI (p = NS, Figure 2C) or SA (p = NS, Figure 2D), respectively. sST2 serum levels significantly predicted the occurrence of the combined endpoint in patients with STEMI (p<0.005) and patients with SA (p<0.05), but not in patients with NSTEMI (p = NS, data not shown). The rate of IL-33 above detection limit was 44.1% in survivors vs. 41.7% in non-survivors (p = NS), and IL-33 serum levels were not associated with mortality in the total cohort of patients with CAD (p = NS, Figure 3A). However, when patients were stratified for their clinical presentation, the highest quintile of IL-33 was a significant predictor of mortality in patients with STEMI (p<0.05, Figure 3B) but not in patients with NSTEMI (p = NS, Figure 3C) and SA (p = NS, Figure 3D). Serum levels of IL-33 did not predict the combined endpoint in the total cohort (p = NS) and in the subgroups with SA (p = NS), NSTEMI (p = NS) and STEMI (p = NS, data not shown), respectively.

Multivariate Analysis

Patients in the highest quintile of sST2 serum levels had a 2.1-fold risk for mortality as compared to patients in the lower quintiles (p<0.05). Multivariate analysis revealed that the fifth quintile of sST2 serum levels was a significant predictor of mortality after adjustment for clinical risk factors including creatinine levels (Table 2).

Discussion

In the present study we found that sST2 levels are significantly increased in patients with acute coronary syndrome as compared to patients with stable coronary artery disease and as a control in individuals without significant stenosis on coronary angiography. Moreover we could demonstrate that patients with STEMI show higher levels of sST2 than patients with NSTEMI. However, sST2 levels were not significantly different between the control group and patients with stable angina. In addition, sST2 significantly predicted death in the total cohort over 43 months, which is mainly driven by the STEMI group. sST2 also significantly predicts the combined endpoint in the STEMI group and in the SA group. sST2 levels independently predicted mortality in these patients. IL-33 levels were not different between the patients with stable coronary artery disease and acute coronary syndrome and the control group. IL-33 levels predicted mortality only in patients with STEMI. sST2 and IL-33 levels positively correlated in this study population.

A predictive value for sST2 was shown previously in patients with NSTEMI, STEMI, as well as in apparently healthy individuals [11,12,14,15,21,22]. We confirm the data about long-term prognostic value of sST2 in acute coronary syndrome, and showed for the first time that in addition to that, sST2 levels

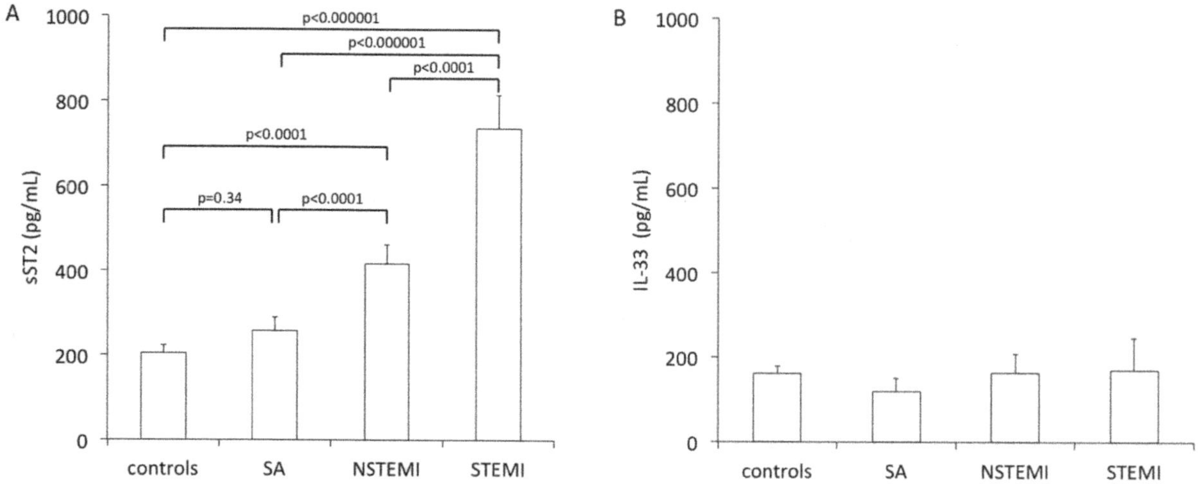

Figure 1. sST2 and IL-33 serum levels in controls and according clinical presentation of coronary artery disease. sST2 (A) and IL-33 (B) serum levels were measured as described under "Methods". SA denotes stable angina, NSTEMI denotes non-ST-elevation myocardial infarction, STEMI denotes ST-elevation myocardial infarction. Mean ± standard error of mean.

predicted the combined endpoint also in patients with stable coronary artery disease. Combined measurements of sST2 and IL-33 were performed recently by Dhillon et al. in patients with NSTEMI and STEMI, who revealed that sST2 levels predicted adverse outcomes in both cohorts, however, IL-33 levels were associated with increased mortality at 30-days and 1-year only in STEMI patients [18], and was not different across any endpoint in the NSTEMI cohort [16]. According with the findings of Dhillon et al. [18], we demonstrated in this study that circulating IL-33 levels predict mortality only in the patients with STEMI, but not in the patients with NSTEMI or stable angina. It should be noted that this predictive value of IL-33 was observed over a period of time of more than 3.5 years in our study.

Furthermore, we showed here for the first time that the level of circulating sST2, but not that of IL-33, is associated with the stage of disease and is increased continuously from stable CAD to NSTEMI and STEMI. Previously, genetic variability of the distal promoter of the ST2 gene was shown to be associated with angiographic severity of CAD [23]. Interestingly, we found no differences in sST2 levels between patients with stable angina and individuals without significant stenosis on coronary angiography, although both STEMI and NSTEMI patients demonstrated significantly higher sST2 serum levels than the control group. Therefore, our findings highlight increased levels of circulating sST2 specifically under destabilization of coronary artery disease.

In a community-based cohort of Framingham Heart Study, values for sST2 differ between men and women, increase with age, and are associated with diabetes and hypertension [24]. However, sST2 did not correlate with classic markers linked to CAD risk, including cholesterol, blood pressure, smoking, common carotid intima-media thickness or plaque presence in the cross-sectional pSoBid study [25]. In our cohort here, sST2 levels were not associated with classic cardiovascular risk factors such as age, sex, hypertension, family history of CAD, smoking, hyperlipidaemia or diabetes but correlated positively with creatinine levels. IL-33 levels were significantly higher in females and in non-smokers.

The IL-33/ST2 system attracted special attention of cardiologists after ST2 was identified to be inducible by mechanical strain in neonatal rat cardiac myocytes in 2002 [6], and after the identification of IL-33 as a ligand for the ST2 receptor in 2005 [3]. Two main isoforms of ST2 are known – the soluble form sST2 and the transmembrane form ST2L. The sST2 isoform lacks the transmembrane and cytoplasmic domains contained within the structure of ST2L [2,4]. Despite its similarity to the IL-1 receptor (IL-1R), ST2 does not bind IL-1α, IL-1β, or IL-1R antagonist [1]. sST2 in the extracellular environment might bind free IL-33, thereby decreasing the concentration of IL-33 that is available for ST2L binding and reducing the biological effects of IL-33 [2,3,7].

Data on possible cellular sources of circulating sST2 and IL-33 as well as their regulation in cardiac cells are controversial. Rat neonatal cardiac myocytes and fibroblasts were shown to increase sST2 mRNA as well as IL-33 mRNA expression upon mechanical strain [6,7]. Recently, IL-33 was revealed to be released by murine fibroblasts undergoing mechanical strain in the absence of cellular necrosis [26]. However, release of sST2 and/or IL-33 by human cardiac cells under the same conditions was not demonstrated before.

Data published by Bartuneck et al. showed no difference in arterial and coronary sinus levels of sST2 and thus argues against myocardial production of sST2 [27]. Those authors found IL-33 protein to be localized to endothelial cells in the human coronary artery [27]. According with these findings, we recently showed that both human macrovascular (aortic and coronary artery) and heart microvascular endothelial cells secrete sST2 protein, whereas human adult cardiac myocytes, cardiac fibroblasts and vascular smooth muscle cells do not secrete detectable amounts of sST2 antigen *in vitro* [8].

The regulation of sST2 and IL-33 seems to be development-dependent and cell- and species-specific. In neonatal rat cardiac myocytes and fibroblasts, sST2 expression is increased by IL-1β, phorbol ester, uridine triphosphate and endothelin-1, but not by TNF-α, angiotensin II, hydrogen peroxide, IL-4 or lipopolysaccharide (LPS) [6,28,29]. However, in human endothelial cells, sST2 was shown to be upregulated by the inflammatory cytokines IL-1β, TNF-α and by phorbol ester [27]. Additionally, proinflammatory mediators IL-1α, IL-1β, and TNF-α as well as supernatants of LPS-stimulated peripheral blood mononuclear cells led to an enhanced secretion of sST2 in cultured human adult cardiac myocytes, but not in cardiac fibroblasts [30]. IL-33 expression is increased upon treatment with phorbol 12-myristate 13-acetate and angiotensin II, but not TNF-α or IL-1β in rat neonatal cardiomyocytes and cardiac fibroblasts [7], and upon

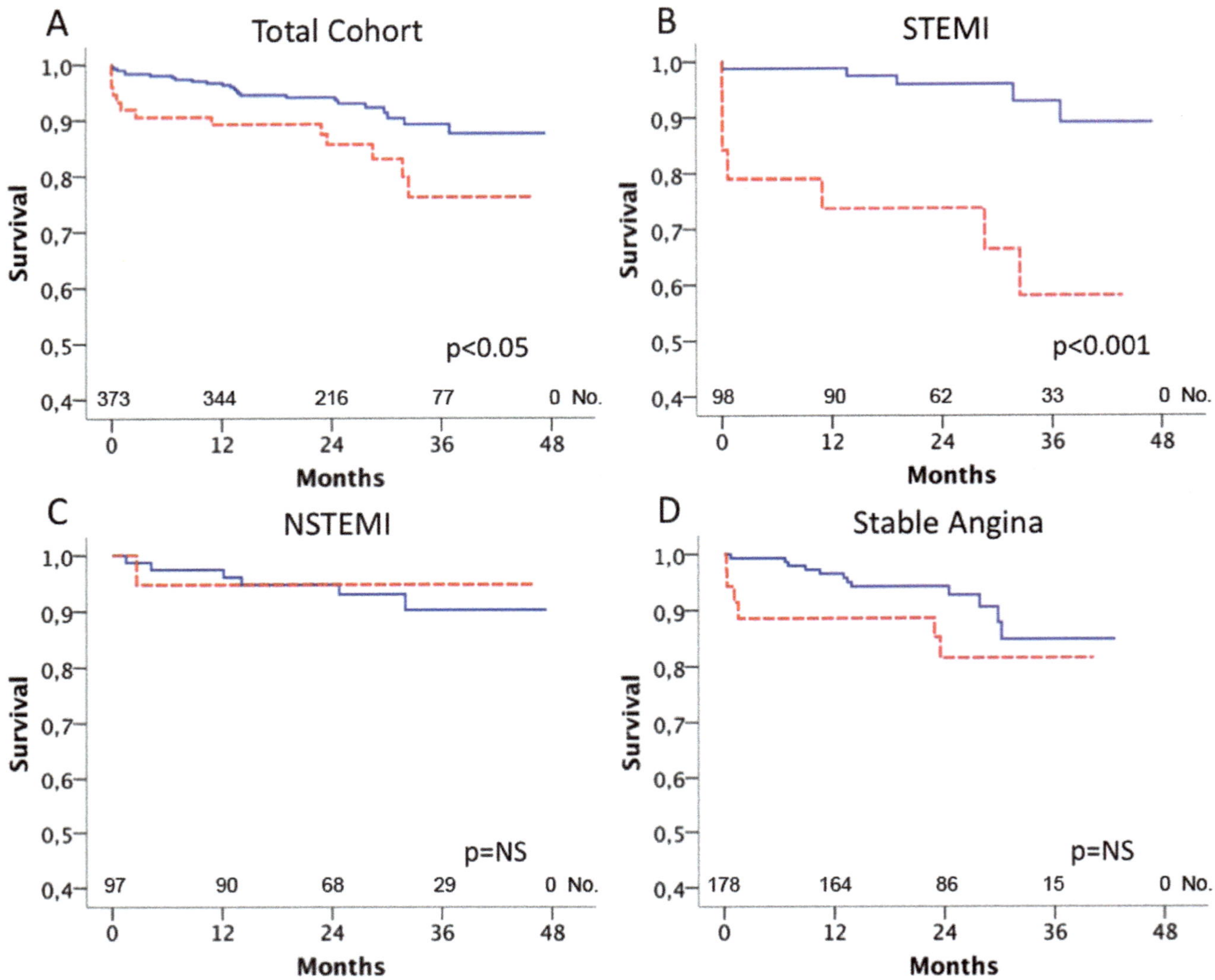

Figure 2. Relation of sST2 serum levels to mortality. sST2 serum levels were measured as described under "Methods". Kaplan Meier survival curves for the highest quintile of sST2 serum levels (red, dashed line) vs. the lower four quintiles of sST2 (blue, full line) in all patients (A), patients with ST-elevation myocardial infarction (B), non-ST-elevation myocardial infarction (C) and stable angina (D).

treatment with TNF-α, IL-1β, and IFN-γ in human adult cardiac myocytes and fibroblasts [8].

IL-33 and ST2 were proposed to comprise a cardioprotective signaling system because IL-33 was found to antagonize cardiac hypertrophy as well as hypoxia-induced apoptosis *in vitro* and *in vivo* and was thereby shown to protect mice from experimental pressure overload and myocardial infarction [7,31]. Exogenous IL-33 also attenuated ischaemia/reperfusion injuries in the diabetic myocardium in mice [32]. A cardioprotective role of this system was confirmed in ST2-deficient mice [7,31]. However, in a model of autoimmune heart disease treatment with IL-33 induced eosinophilic pericarditis and cardiac dilation, whereas sST2 prevents eosinophilia and improves systolic function [33]. Therefore, caution should be taken to transfer results from animal experiments into the clinical setting.

Data about expression of the components of IL-33/ST2 system in human heart under different pathologies are still scarce. Left ventricular (LV) ST2 mRNA levels were not significantly different in patients with aortic stenosis, congestive cardiomyopathy and stable angina pectoris with normal LV function (control group), however, IL-33 mRNA levels were lower in LV biopsies from aortic stenosis patients compared to control [27]. Our group found IL-33 mRNA expression to be positively correlated with IFN-γ and TNF-α mRNA expression in human myocardial tissue from patients undergoing heart transplantation [8]. Moreover, we demonstrated that both IL-33 and ST2 protein are expressed predominantly by endothelial cells in human heart [8].

Some limitations of the present study have to be acknowledged. First, our study is of observational nature. Accordingly, our results may be explained by unmeasured confounding factors. Therefore, we tried to control for baseline imbalances by multivariate modeling. However, the possibility of residual or undetected confounding is small but cannot be ruled out completely. In addition, IL-33 was not detectable in 54% of the study participants. Similar to our findings, Dhillon et al. found that in more than half of the patients with NSTEMI and STEMI IL-33 levels were below the lower detection limit of the assay used [16,18]. However, IL-33 in the last quintile was statistically associated with an adverse outcome in patients with STEMI. It should also be pointed out, that the study was not undertaken and

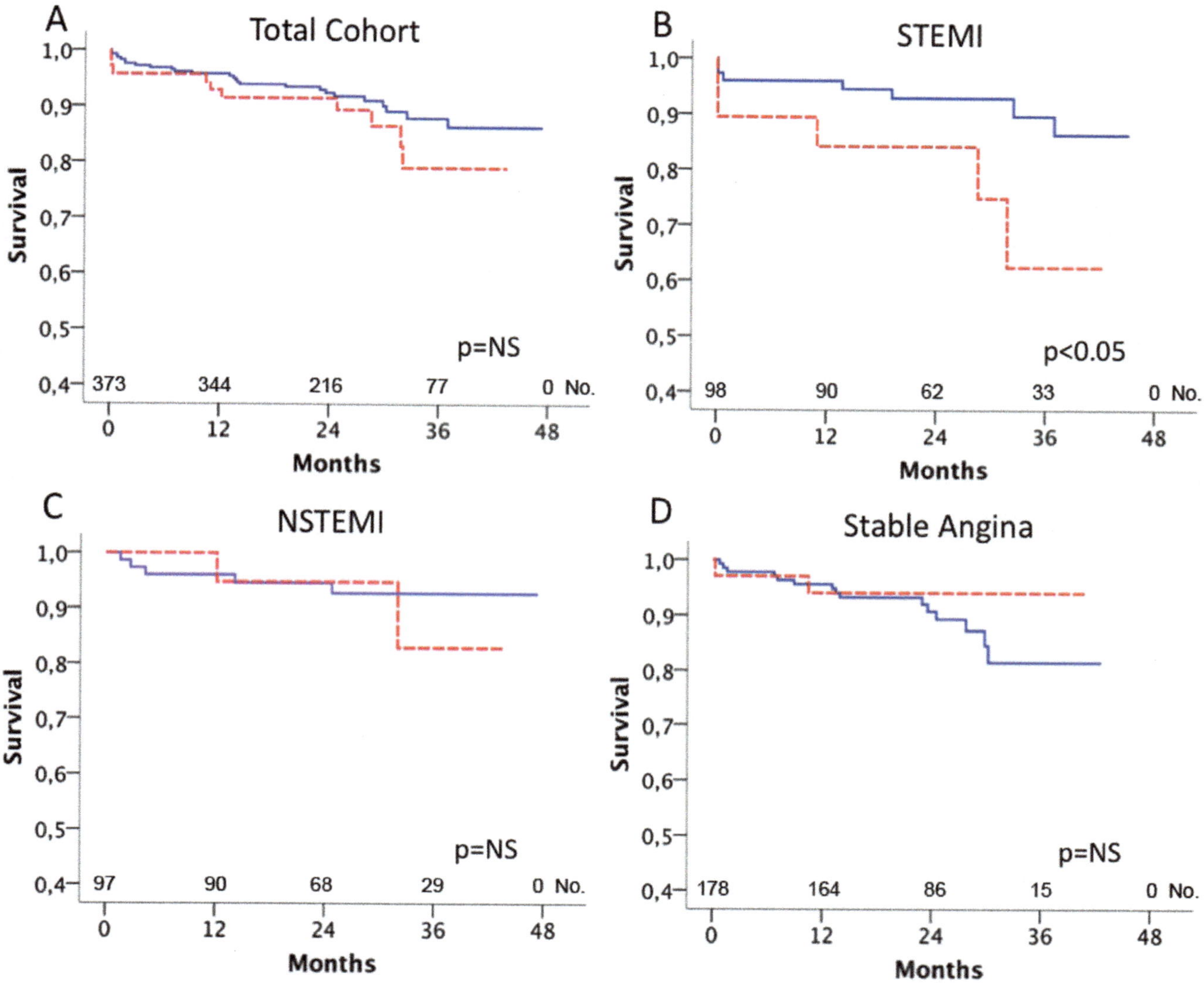

Figure 3. Relation of IL-33 serum levels to mortality. IL-33 serum levels were measured as described under "Methods". Kaplan Meier survival curves for the highest quintile of IL-33 serum levels (red, dashed line) vs. the lower four quintiles of IL-33 (blue, full line) in all patients (A), patients with ST-elevation myocardial infarction (B), non-ST-elevation myocardial infarction (C) and stable angina (D).

thus not designed to identify yet another clinical biomarker or point of care test for the diagnosis of acute coronary syndrome or for the clinical risk prediction in stable coronary artery disease. Our study aimed to gain additional insights in a possible pathophysiological role of the ST2/IL-33 system in atherosclerotic disease and myocardial infarction.

Table 2. Cox proportional hazard model assessing the risk for mortality according to sST2 levels.

	Odds ratio	95% confidence interval	P-value
univariate			
Patients with sST2 serum levels in quintile 1–4 (5–538 pg/mL)	1		
Patients with sST2 serum levels in quintile 5 (539–3618 pg/mL)	2.1	1.1–4.2	0.029
adjusted for age, gender, hyperlipidemia, hypertension, smoking, BMI, serum creatinine			
Patients with sST2 serum levels in quintile 1–4 (5–538 pg/mL)	1		
Patients with sST2 serum levels in quintile 5 (539–3618 pg/mL)	2.2	1.1–4.4	0.03

sST2 denotes soluble ST2, CAD denotes coronary artery disease, BMI denotes body mass index.

Conclusions

In conclusion, we identified for the first time circulating sST2 levels to be associated with disease activity in coronary artery disease, and to be increased in patients with acute coronary syndrome as compared to patients with stable CAD and persons without CAD. Both sST2 and IL-33 were associated with mortality in patients with STEMI but not in patients with NSTEMI or stable angina over a period of time of more than 3.5 years. sST2 also significantly predicts the combined endpoint in the STEMI group and in the stable angina group. Further studies on the role of IL-33/ST2 system in cardiovascular pathologies are warranted.

Author Contributions

Conceived and designed the experiments: SD WSS IT RJ KMK SF KAK AW TWW KH JW. Performed the experiments: SD RJ KMK SF AW. Analyzed the data: SD WSS RJ KMK. Contributed reagents/materials/analysis tools: SD WSS RJ KMK. Wrote the paper: SD WSS RJ KMK SF AW TWW KH JW.

References

1. Trajkovic V, Sweet MJ, Xu D (2004) T1/ST2–an IL-1 receptor-like modulator of immune responses. Cytokine Growth Factor Rev 15: 87–95.
2. Kakkar R, Lee RT (2008) The IL-33/ST2 pathway: therapeutic target and novel biomarker. Nat Rev Drug Discov 7: 827–840.
3. Schmitz J, Owyang A, Oldham E, Song Y, Murphy E, et al. (2005) IL-33, an interleukin-1-like cytokine that signals via the IL-1 receptor-related protein ST2 and induces T helper type 2-associated cytokines. Immunity 23: 479–490.
4. Iwahana H, Yanagisawa K, Ito-Kosaka A, Kuroiwa K, Tago K, et al. (1999) Different promoter usage and multiple transcription initiation sites of the interleukin-1 receptor-related human ST2 gene in UT-7 and TM12 cells. Eur J Biochem 264: 397–406.
5. Miller AM, Xu D, Asquith DL, Denby L, Li Y, et al. (2008) IL-33 reduces the development of atherosclerosis. J Exp Med 205: 339–346.
6. Weinberg EO, Shimpo M, De Keulenaer GW, MacGillivray C, Tominaga S, et al. (2002) Expression and regulation of ST2, an interleukin-1 receptor family member, in cardiomyocytes and myocardial infarction. Circulation 106: 2961–2966.
7. Sanada S, Hakuno D, Higgins LJ, Schreiter ER, McKenzie AN, et al. (2007) IL-33 and ST2 comprise a critical biomechanically induced and cardioprotective signaling system. J Clin Invest 117: 1538–1549.
8. Demyanets S, Kaun C, Pentz R, Krychtiuk KA, Rauscher S, et al. (2013) Components of the interleukin-33/ST2 system are differentially expressed and regulated in human cardiac cells and in cells of the cardiac vasculature. J Mol Cell Cardiol 60: 16–26.
9. Miller AM (2011) Role of IL-33 in inflammation and disease. J Inflamm (Lond) 8: 22.
10. Demyanets S, Konya V, Kastl SP, Kaun C, Rauscher S, et al. (2011) Interleukin-33 induces expression of adhesion molecules and inflammatory activation in human endothelial cells and in human atherosclerotic plaques. Arterioscler Thromb Vasc Biol 31: 2080–2089.
11. Shimpo M, Morrow DA, Weinberg EO, Sabatine MS, Murphy SA, et al. (2004) Serum levels of the interleukin-1 receptor family member ST2 predict mortality and clinical outcome in acute myocardial infarction. Circulation 109: 2186–2190.
12. Sabatine MS, Morrow DA, Higgins LJ, MacGillivray C, Guo W, et al. (2008) Complementary roles for biomarkers of biomechanical strain ST2 and N-terminal prohormone B-type natriuretic peptide in patients with ST-elevation myocardial infarction. Circulation 117: 1936–1944.
13. Weir RA, Miller AM, Murphy GE, Clements S, Steedman T, et al. (2010) Serum soluble ST2: a potential novel mediator in left ventricular and infarct remodeling after acute myocardial infarction. J Am Coll Cardiol 55: 243–250.
14. Eggers KM, Armstrong PW, Califf RM, Simoons ML, Venge P, et al. (2010) ST2 and mortality in non-ST-segment elevation acute coronary syndrome. Am Heart J 159: 788–794.
15. Kohli P, Bonaca MP, Kakkar R, Kudinova AY, Scirica BM, et al. (2012) Role of ST2 in non-ST-elevation acute coronary syndrome in the MERLIN-TIMI 36 trial. Clin Chem 58: 257–266.
16. Dhillon OS, Narayan HK, Quinn PA, Squire IB, Davies JE, et al. (2011) Interleukin 33 and ST2 in non-ST-elevation myocardial infarction: comparison with Global Registry of Acute Coronary Events Risk Scoring and NT-proBNP. Am Heart J 161: 1163–1170.
17. Weinberg EO, Shimpo M, Hurwitz S, Tominaga S, Rouleau JL, et al. (2003) Identification of serum soluble ST2 receptor as a novel heart failure biomarker. Circulation 107: 721–726.
18. Dhillon OS, Narayan HK, Khan SQ, Kelly D, Quinn PA, et al. (2013) Pre-discharge risk stratification in unselected STEMI: is there a role for ST2 or its natural ligand IL-33 when compared with contemporary risk markers? Int J Cardiol 167: 2182–2188.
19. Demyanets S, Tentzeris I, Jarai R, Katsaros KM, Farhan S, et al. (2014) An increase of interleukin-33 serum levels after coronary stent implantation is associated with coronary in-stent restenosis. Cytokine.
20. Dupont WD, Plummer WD Jr (1990) Power and sample size calculations. A review and computer program. Control Clin Trials 11: 116–128.
21. Wang TJ, Wollert KC, Larson MG, Coglianese E, McCabe EL, et al. (2012) Prognostic utility of novel biomarkers of cardiovascular stress: the framingham heart study. Circulation 126: 1596–1604.
22. Zhang K, Zhang XC, Mi YH, Liu J (2013) Predicting value of serum soluble ST2 and interleukin-33 for risk stratification and prognosis in patients with acute myocardial infarction. Chin Med J (Engl) 126: 3628–3631.
23. Tsapaki A, Zaravinos A, Apostolakis S, Voudris K, Vogiatzi K, et al. (2010) Genetic variability of the distal promoter of the ST2 gene is associated with angiographic severity of coronary artery disease. J Thromb Thrombolysis 30: 365–371.
24. Coglianese EE, Larson MG, Vasan RS, Ho JE, Ghorbani A, et al. (2012) Distribution and clinical correlates of the interleukin receptor family member soluble ST2 in the Framingham Heart Study. Clin Chem 58: 1673–1681.
25. Miller AM, Purves D, McConnachie A, Asquith DL, Batty GD, et al. (2012) Soluble ST2 Associates with Diabetes but Not Established Cardiovascular Risk Factors: A New Inflammatory Pathway of Relevance to Diabetes? PLoS One 7: e47830.
26. Kakkar R, Hei H, Dobner S, Lee RT (2012) Interleukin 33 as a mechanically responsive cytokine secreted by living cells. J Biol Chem 287: 6941–6948.
27. Bartunek J, Delrue L, Van Durme F, Muller O, Casselman F, et al. (2008) Nonmyocardial production of ST2 protein in human hypertrophy and failure is related to diastolic load. J Am Coll Cardiol 52: 2166–2174.
28. Braun OO, Lu D, Aroonsakool N, Insel PA (2010) Uridine triphosphate (UTP) induces profibrotic responses in cardiac fibroblasts by activation of P2Y2 receptors. J Mol Cell Cardiol 49: 362–369.
29. Yndestad A, Marshall AK, Hodgkinson JD, Tham el L, Sugden PH, et al. (2010) Modulation of interleukin signalling and gene expression in cardiac myocytes by endothelin-1. Int J Biochem Cell Biol 42: 263–272.
30. Mildner M, Storka A, Lichtenauer M, Mlitz V, Ghannadan M, et al. (2010) Primary sources and immunological prerequisites for sST2 secretion in humans. Cardiovasc Res 87: 769–777.
31. Seki K, Sanada S, Kudinova AY, Steinhauser ML, Handa V, et al. (2009) Interleukin-33 prevents apoptosis and improves survival after experimental myocardial infarction through ST2 signaling. Circ Heart Fail 2: 684–691.
32. Rui T, Zhang J, Xu X, Yao Y, Kao R, et al. (2012) Reduction in IL-33 expression exaggerates ischaemia/reperfusion-induced myocardial injury in mice with diabetes mellitus. Cardiovasc Res 94: 370–378.
33. Abston ED, Barin JG, Cihakova D, Bucek A, Coronado MJ, et al. (2012) IL-33 Independently Induces Eosinophilic Pericarditis and Cardiac Dilation: ST2 Improves Cardiac Function. Circ Heart Fail 5: 366–375.

Quantitative Analysis of Coronary Vessels with Optimized Intracoronary CT Number

Sei Komatsu[1]*, Teruaki Kamata[2], Atsuko Imai[1,3], Tomoki Ohara[1], Kazuaki Miyaji[2], Yasuhiko Kobayashi[1], Kazuhisa Kodama[1]

1 Cardiovascular Center, Amagasaki Central Hospital, Hyogo, Japan, **2** Department of Diagnostic Imaging, Amagasaki Central Hospital, Hyogo, Japan, **3** Department of Cardiology, Osaka University School of Medicine, Osaka, Japan

Abstract

Background: Variability in intracoronary computed tomography (CT) number may influence vessel quantification. We confirmed the feasibility of a novel method for measuring vessel diameter and area using coronary CT angiography (CCTA) with an optimized intracoronary CT number, 350 HU.

Methods: We performed intravascular ultrasound (IVUS) imaging in 52 patients with significant stenosis detected by coronary CT angiography targeting 350 HU using a CT number-controlling system. We measured 0-to-0 HU distances in the cross-sectional coronary images of 32 patients. We analyzed the ratio of 0-to-0 HU distances in CT images to media-to-media distances in IVUS images (C:I ratio). The area of ≥0 HU for 103 representative points in the remaining 20 patients was compared to the area of the traced external elastic membrane (EEM) in IVUS images.

Results: There was a strong correlation between 0-to-0 HU distance in CT images and media-to-media diameter in IVUS images ($r = 0.97$, $p < 0.001$). The C:I ratio was 1.1. EEM area was estimated by dividing the area of ≥0 HU by the square of C:I. There was also a strong correlation between the estimated EEM area and the EEM area in IVUS images ($r = 0.95$, $p < 0.001$).

Conclusions: Media-to-media diameter and EEM area can be estimated by CCTA targeting the optimized intracoronary CT number when blood vessel borders are defined at 0 HU.

Editor: Toru Hosoda, Tokai University, Japan

Funding: Dr Komatsu is a technical consultant for Nemoto Kyorindo Co., Ltd. This funding source had no role in study design, data collection and analysis, decision to publish or preparation of the manuscript. No other current external funding sources for this study.

Competing Interests: Dr Komatsu is a technical consultant for Nemoto Kyorindo Co., Ltd.

* E-mail: plaquemap@yahoo.co.jp

Introduction

The diagnostic accuracy of coronary computed tomography angiography (CCTA) for coronary artery stenosis is now as good as that of invasive coronary angiography [1]. The ability to perform quantitative analysis of coronary arteries with CCTA may alter diagnostic and treatment strategies for coronary artery disease. For example, stent size may be decided on the basis of CT instead of intravascular ultrasound (IVUS) images.

The quantification of vessel diameters has been attempted [2,3]. However, the visual determination of vessel borders is plagued by poor reproducibility and inter-observer variability [4]. Marwan et al. [5] reported that the bias in vessel area determinations varied between 65% and 155% for different window widths/levels. Additionally, the visual determination of vessel borders was inaccurate even with the same window widths/levels. Fig. 1A and Fig. 1B are examples of 2 independent visual determinations of the same cross-sectional image of a normal coronary artery with different window widths/levels. Showing the threshold of the image in a different color by Image J software after visual determination of the vessel border, the thresholds of Fig. 1A and Fig. 1B were found to be between −16 HU and 62 HU (Fig. 1C and Fig. 1D) and between −14 HU and 47 HU (Fig. 1E and Fig. 1F), respectively.

Media-to-media distance and external elastic membrane (EEM) area are measurable in cross-sectional IVUS images. However, cross-sectional CT images include 3 vessel layers and extra-adventitial tissue that is not distinguishable. On CT images, there is no vessel boundary point or inflection point in the profile curve [6]. Methods for vessel measurement in commercially available workstations have not been published, and there seems to be no universal method of measuring structures in CT images.

A high intracoronary CT number may cause misdiagnosis of coronary stenosis because of a partial volume effect [7]. Thus, an optimized CT number is required to measure vessels. An intracoronary CT number of 350 Hounsfield units (HU) is desirable to achieve a precise diagnosis of coronary stenosis and plaque [7]. However, the optimized CT number has been difficult to obtain. We established a CT number-controlling system [8] that controls the intracoronary CT number for CCTA.

In our study, CCTA targeted 350 HU, the optimized intracoronary CT number for analyzing coronary stenosis and plaque [8]. We set the optimal border as 0 HU for CT imaging and calculated

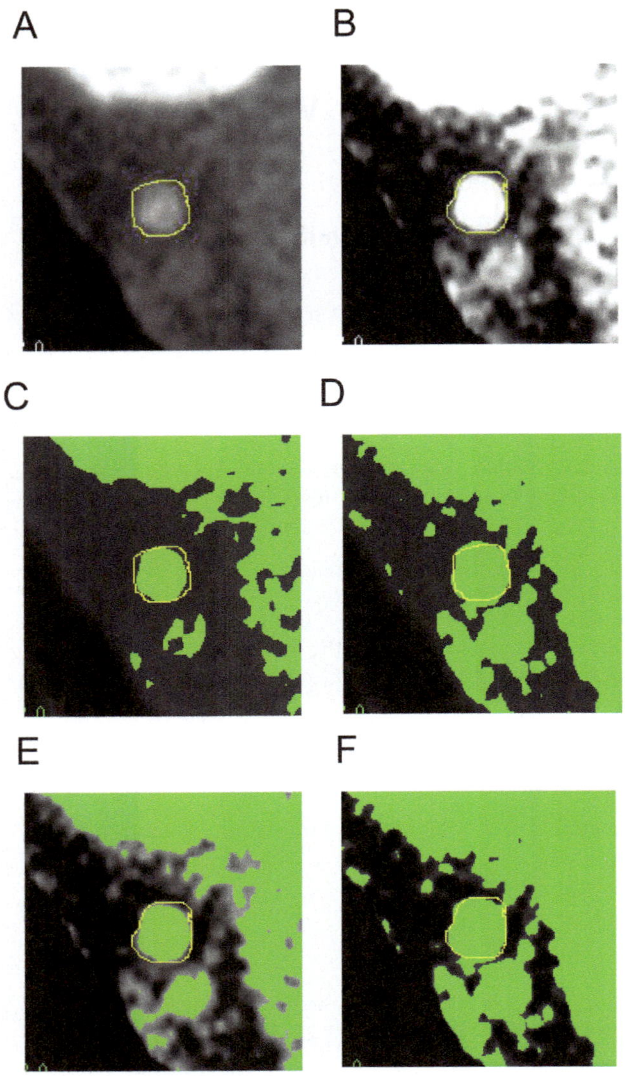

Figure 1. Independent visual determinations of the same cross-sectional image of coronary artery with different window widths/levels.

the ratio of the 0-to-0 HU distance in CT images to the media-to-media distance in IVUS images. The feasibility of the ratio was confirmed by comparing the estimated EEM area obtained by dividing the area of ≥0 HU by the square of the ratio with the EEM area in IVUS images.

Methods

Study Sample

We prospectively enrolled 56 patients (age, 64±15 years; range, 42–85 years) with significant coronary stenosis and ischemia who underwent percutaneous coronary intervention (PCI) using IVUS. CCTA indications were consistent with the guidelines of the Society of Cardiovascular Computed Tomography [9]. CCTA was performed 1 day to 4 weeks before the PCI.

Patients were randomly divided into the following 2 groups in a 6:4 ratio: the diameter comparison group and the area verification group. The diameter comparison group comprised 34 patients for whom we calculated the ratio of 0-to-0 HU distance (in CT images) to media-to-media distance (in IVUS images), defined as the C:I ratio. The area verification group comprised 22 patients, whose data we used to evaluate the feasibility of the C:I ratio for correcting the ≥0 HU area to estimate the EEM area.

This study was approved by the ethics committee of Amagasaki Central Hospital, and all patients provided written informed consent. Clinical exclusion criteria for CCTA were contrast media (CM) allergy, renal insufficiency (glomerular filtration rate <60 mL/min/1.73 mm^2), pregnancy, congenital heart disease, and coronary artery bypass graft.

Patients were administered an oral beta-blocker (25 mg Atenolol, AstraZeneca, Osaka, Japan) 120 min before CCTA and 0.3 mg of sublingual nitroglycerin 5 min before CCTA. Heart rate was maintained between 55 and 65 bpm through the administration of additional intravenous beta-blocker (2–10 mg Propranolol, AstraZeneca).

Scanning Protocol

We used a 64-detector CT scanner (Lightspeed VCT; GE Healthcare; Milwaukee, USA) with electrocardiogram (ECG) gating and Advantage Workstation 4.3 software. The scan sequence was as follows: scanogram, scout, test scan, and coronary angiography.

Patients underwent CCTA with a prospective ECG-triggered axial scan (Snapshot Pulse) with the following parameters: slice acquisition, 64×0.625 mm (40-mm volume coverage); 75% of the RR interval with 0–100 ms of padding; rotation time, 350 ms; temporal resolution, 175 ms; tube voltage, 120 kV; and tube current, 450–680 mA. Retrospectively ECG triggered CCTA was selected if difficulties were encountered in maintaining the heart rate at 55–65 bpm or if blurring was detected by the ECG-triggered scanogram. ECG modulation of 40–80% of the RR interval was used. The pitch was approximately 0.2–0.3.

Contrast medium (CM) (350 mg I/mL; Omnipaque 350; Daiichi Pharmaceutical Co, Ltd, Japan) was injected into an antecubital vein at 4 mL/s with a saline chaser using a dual-headed injector system (Dual Shot GX, Nemoto Kyorindo Co, Ltd, Tokyo, Japan) during the timing bolus and CCTA. The amount of CM was determined with a CT number-controlling system, as described elsewhere [7]. CM (5 mL) with 40 mL of a saline chaser was used as a timing bolus for determining the circulation time for the enhanced scan. Sequential scans were obtained every 2 s, from 10 to 40 s after the timing bolus. The region of interest (ROI) was located in the ascending aorta, and a time-density curve (TDC) was determined. The peak time was identified, and the absolute value of the CT number of the ascending aorta at the peak time was measured at the ROI. A scan delay was defined as 2 s after peak enhancement. The determined amount of CM with 40 mL of a saline chaser was administered for CCTA.

The TDC was considered valid if it was a unimodal curve with a measurable peak time and peak CT number. The TDC was invalid if it was flat or a multimodal curve, or if the peak time and peak CT number could not be determined.

Data Selection

One reader enrolled vessel lesions of different sizes from each patient. The 0-to-0 HU distances on the enrolled CT images were determined by 2 readers who had evaluated the cardiovascular CT images of at least 500 cases to examine inter-observer variability. Curved multiplanar reformation images were used to determine the candidates. Lesions with stents or with a calcified plaque size measuring less than half the diameter of the vessel were excluded owing to the possible presence of a hypershooting artifact. Lesions with blurring artifacts or motion artifacts were excluded. Lesions with a myocardial bridge or those in contact with the myocardium, branches, or veins were excluded because the border of a vessel with the myocardium, branches, or veins showed more than 0 HU. Lesions with 1.5 mm of 0–0 HU distance were excluded.

The Border-0 Method

Cross-sectional images (256×256 pixels) were constructed using commercial software (Advantage Workstation 4.6, GE Healthcare; Milwaukee, USA). The field of view was magnified between 22 and 30 mm for recognizing the shape of the image, depending on the software. Changing the size of the image does not influence the measurements (data not shown). Because there is no inflection point indicating the border of a vessel on CT images, we established the border-0 method: we set the optimal border as 0 HU and measured the C:I ratio, which is the ratio of the 0-to-0 HU distance in CT images to media-to-media distance in IVUS images. We manually compared cross-sectional images of the long axis and short axis of the vessel (Fig. 2A) with a Plaque Map [10] (Fig. 2B) and analyzed the 0-to-0 HU distance in the long axis and short axis by profile curve of perpendicular straight line a (left) and line b (right) with ImageJ software 1.43u (US National Institutes of Health) (Fig. 2C). The 0-to-0 HU distance was 5.5×4.9 mm, and the media-to-media diameter in the IVUS image was 5.0×4.4 mm. (Fig. 2D).

We performed IVUS with a 40-MHz, 2.9-Fr IVUS catheter (Atlantis, Boston Scientific; Natick, MA, USA) with 0.5 mm/s automatic pullback. Media-to-media distances were analyzed by 2 readers with at least 5 years of IVUS experience to examine inter-observer variability.

Anatomic cross-correlation between MDCT and IVUS images was achieved by using the nearest bifurcation points as reference markers and by taking plaque shape into account (Fig. 2D). We rotated either the CT image or the corresponding IVUS image until the location of the plaque components matched. A line was drawn for the 0-to-0 HU distance such that it did not penetrate the calcification and surrounding area, because the quite high CT number of the calcification enhances the CT number of the surrounding area. We excluded CT images containing calcifications of more than 90° or motion artifacts. IVUS images with nonuniform rotational distortion or catheter artifacts and those with calcification-generated shadows were also excluded. Media-to-media distances on IVUS images were traced manually on IVUS images displayed with Image J software. Correspondences between CT and IVUS images were initially determined by 1 reader. If anatomical discordance was present between them following evaluation by the second reader, the readers continued to individually evaluate the images until consensus was reached.

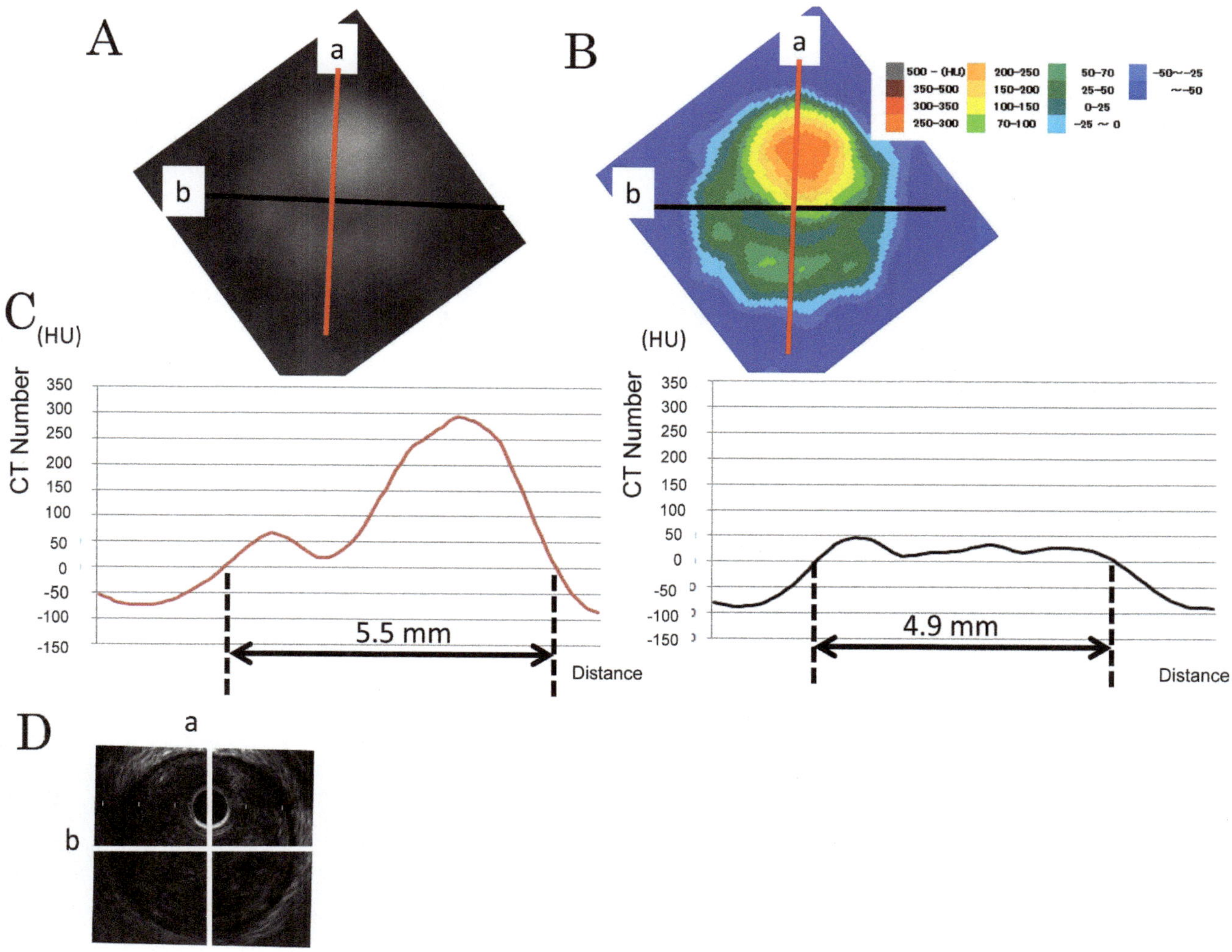

Figure 2. Quantitative analysis of grayscale image (A), Plaque Map (B), Profile curve (C) and IVUS image (D).

We calculated the ratio of the 0-to-0 HU distance in cross-sectional vessel images (Fig. 2C) to the media-to-media diameter in IVUS images (Fig. 2D).

The Feasibility of the C:I Ratio for Estimating EEM Area

If the ratio of the 0-to-0 HU distance on CT image to the media-to-media distance on IVUS image is constant, the EEM area in IVUS images can be estimated by the ≥0 HU area in CT images by correcting with the C:I ratio. The estimated EEM was defined as the ≥0 HU area on CT image divided by the square of the C:I ratio. The estimated EEM areas determined by CT were compared to the EEM areas determined by IVUS in the area verification group.

The region that included the vessel was manually traced wider than the outside of the vessel, as shown in Fig. 3. The analysis of the ≥0 HU area for estimated external elastic membrane by the Border-0 method. The region including the vessel was manually traced wider than the outside of the vessel. (A, B) Two independent manual traces (yellow lines) wider than the outside of the vessel. (C, D) Profile curves of white dotted lines in Fig. 3A, 3B. The ≥0 HU areas (shown in blue) are the same. The ≥0 HU areas of Fig. 3A, 3B are 27.0 mm^2 and 27.3 mm^2, respectively. (E) The threshold of 0 HU of Fig. 3A was shown in a different color. If the trace does not include stained myocardium, the ≥0 HU areas of any manual traces may have good reproducibility. A custom macro in Excel 2007 for Windows 7 calculated the ≥0 HU area in the selected area exported as text data from Image J.

Statistical Analysis

Statistical analysis was performed using SPSS 17.0 (SPSS Inc.; Chicago, Illinois). Data are expressed as means ± SD. We used linear regression analysis and Bland and Altman's analysis of agreement method to assess the association between 0-to-0 HU distance in cross-sectional images and media-to-media distance in IVUS images. We used the same methods to assess the association between estimated EEM area in CT images and EEM area in IVUS images.

Results

Patient Characteristics

Table 1 summarizes patient characteristics and CCTA conditions. Two patients in the diameter comparison group and 2 from the area verification group had invalid TDCs and were excluded from the analysis, because our system cannot control the intracoronary CT number in such cases. The amount of contrast media averaged 36±5 mL in the diameter comparison group and 34±6 mL in the area verification group. The average intracoronary CT number was 349±38 HU in the diameter comparison group and 352±36 HU in the area verification group.

Correlation between 0-to-0 HU Distance and Media-to-media (IVUS) Distance

We enrolled 238 slices from 32 patients in the diameter comparison group. Thirty-three slices were excluded. We examined 205 slices (86%) and found a strong correlation between 0-to-0 HU distance (x) and media-to-media (IVUS) distance (y) (Fig. 4A) ($y = 0.90x+0.01$, $r = 0.97$, $p<0.001$). A Bland–Altman plot is shown in Fig. 4B. Mean difference was −0.48, limits of agreement was −0.08 to 1.04. Inter-observer variability was 0.88±2.45% for 0-to-0 HU distance and 0.75±3.00% for media-to-media distance. The 0-to-0 HU distance was 10±5.3% larger than the media-to-media distance. Thus, the media-to-media distance in

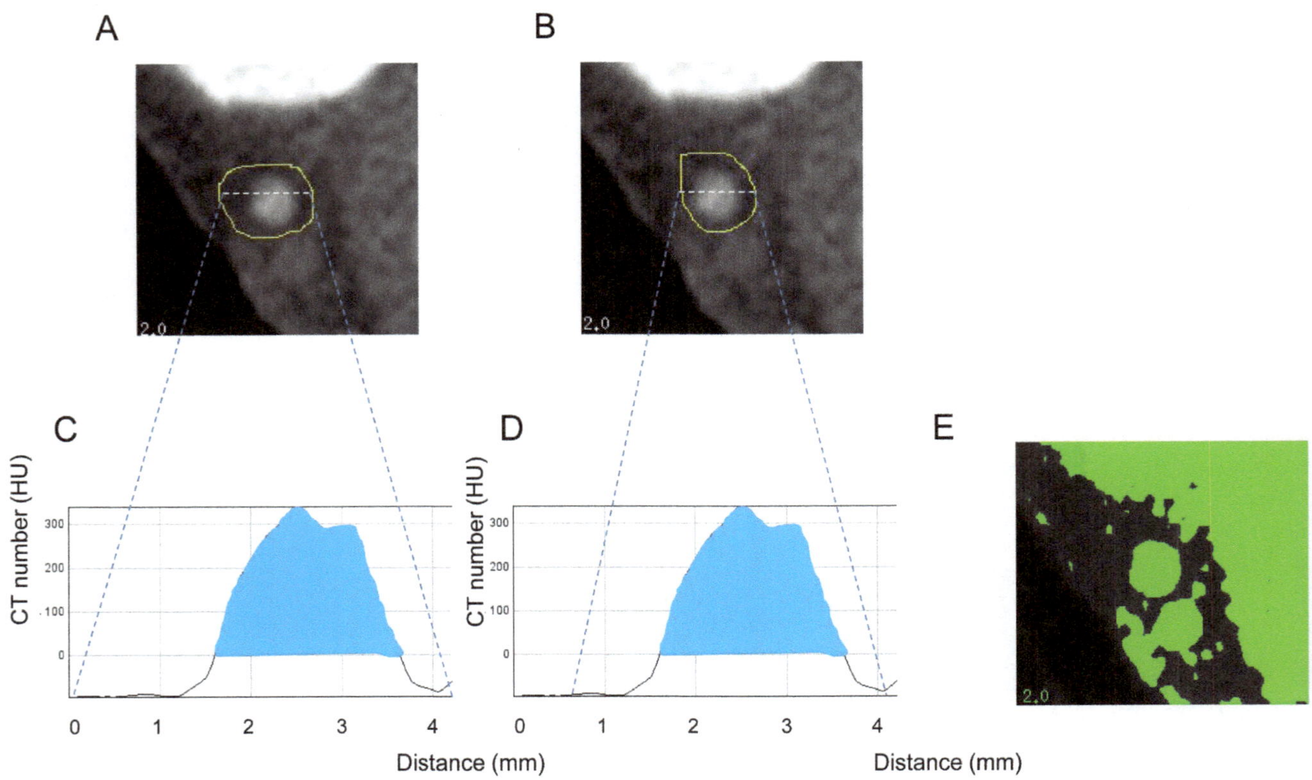

Figure 3. Different traces (A, B), the region (C, D) and the image (E) of of the ≥0 HU.

Table 1. Patient Characteristics and Coronary Computed Tomography Angiography Conditions.

	Diameter comparing group	Area verification group
N	34	22
Gender (M%)	7 (21%)	4 (18%)
Age	68±14	66±15
Hypertension	16 (47%)	12 (54%)
Hyperlipidemia	26 (76%)	14 (63%)
Diabetes	2 (6%)	2 (9%)
Smokers	14 (41%)	8 (36%)
Stable angina pectoris	21 (62%)	14 (64%)
Unstable angina	13 (38%)	8 (36%)
Valid time-density curve at timing bolus	32 (94%)	20 (91%)
Amount of contrast media (mean ± SD, mL)	36±5	34±6
Intracoronary CT number (mean ± SD, HU)	349±38	352±36

SD: standard deviation; HU: Hounsfield unit.

IVUS images can be estimated by dividing the 0-to-0 HU distance in MDCT images by 1.1, and EEM area in IVUS can be estimated by dividing the ≥0 HU area in CT images by the square of 1.1.

Correlation between Estimated EEM Area and EEM Area in IVUS Images

We examined 126 slices from 20 patients from the area verification group. Twenty-three slices were excluded. We examined 103 slices (82%) to assess the correlation between estimated EEM area in CT images and EEM area in IVUS images (Fig. 5A). The C:I ratio was 1.1, and the square of the ratio was 1.21. There was a strong correlation between the estimated EEM area (x) and the EEM area in IVUS images (y) (y = 0.95x+0.19). A Bland–Altman plot is shown in Fig. 5B. Mean difference was 1.00, limits of agreement was −3.01 to 5.01. The difference between the estimated EEM area in CT images and the EEM area in IVUS images was 9.0±14%.

Discussion

The ability to quantify vessels with MDCT is valuable, for example, for deciding on stent size and evaluating the change of

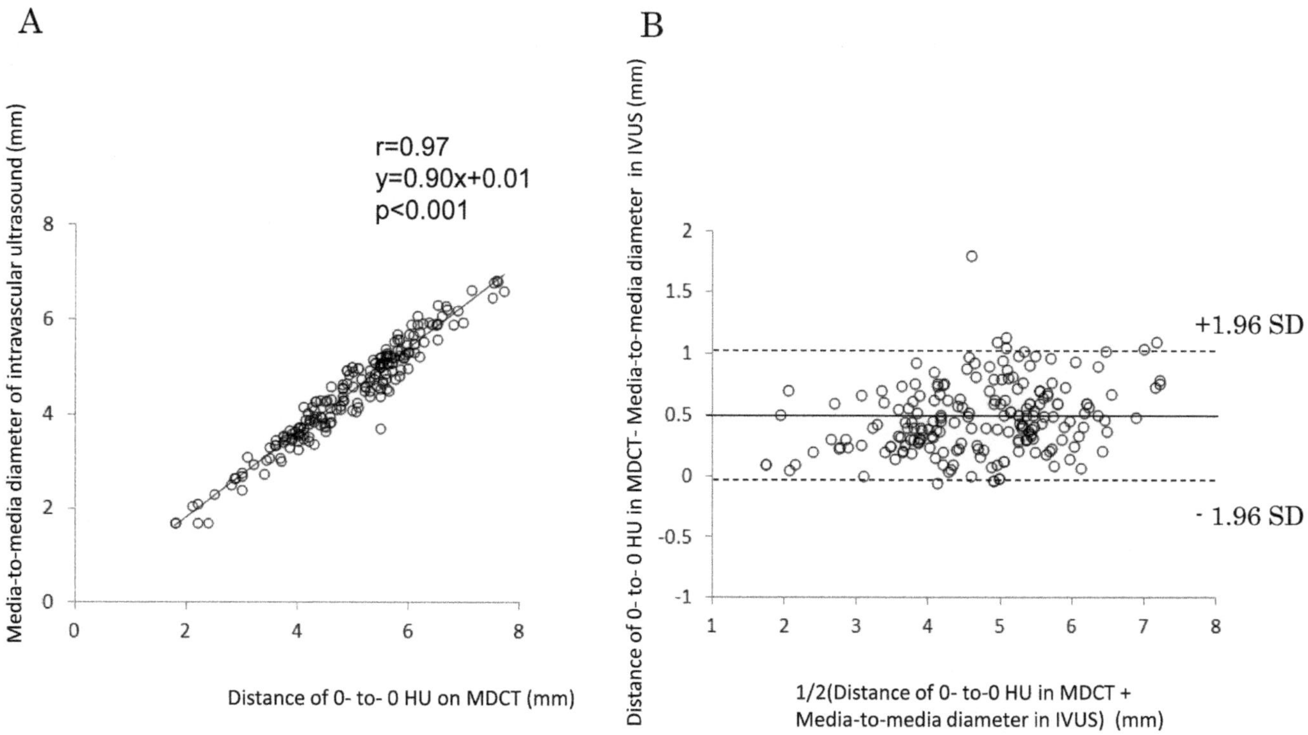

Figure 4. The correlation between 0-to-0 HU distance on MDCT (x) and media-to-media (IVUS) distance (y).

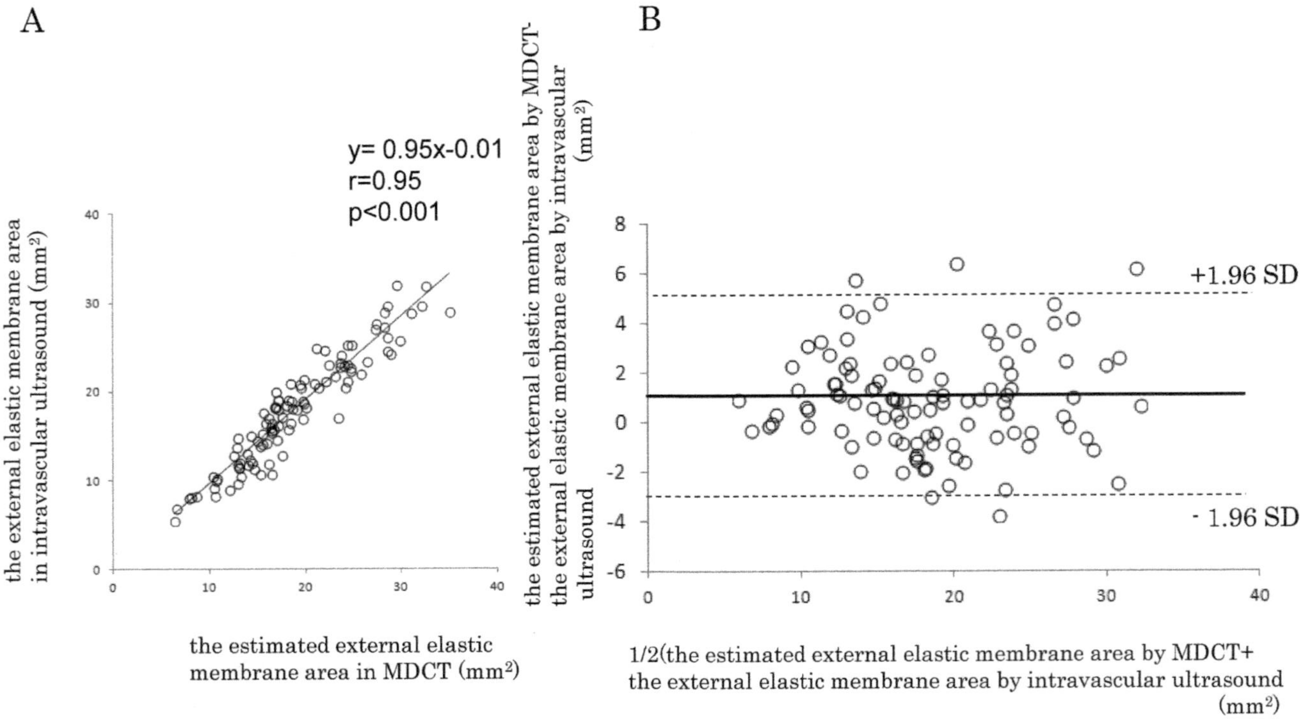

Figure 5. The correlation between the estimated and the measured EEM area (A), and Bland-Altman plot (B).

positive or negative remodeling. Three problems seem to prevent precise measurement with MDCT images: variability of quantitative measurements according to the cardiac cycle, variable intracoronary CT number, and lack of standard methods for measurement with CT images.

The diastolic cardiac cycle was used for CT images, but every cardiac cycle was used for IVUS images in our study. The difference does not seem to be significant because only a 2.0% to 5.7% difference in luminal area was observed between the systolic and diastolic phases in diseased coronary artery segments, and the difference was not statistically significant in other studies [11,12]. Moreover, variability of quantitative measurements according to the cardiac cycle is not considered to determine stent size in the clinical setting.

CT number and diameter were thought to be unreliable because CT numbers and spatial resolutions vary [6]. The CT number of the coronary lumen is influenced the most. A high intracoronary CT number may amplify the plaque CT number [13]. Recent reports have proposed that the amount of CM should be adapted to body surface area [14] or body mass index [15] rather than to body weight for better prediction. However, the coronary CT number for a specific amount of CM differed by more than 200 HU with these methods. The SD of a CT number targeting 350 HU by the CT number-controlling system decreased; in 2 groups, it was only 38 HU and 36 HU, respectively. Using the CT number-controlling system, the difference of intracoronary CT numbers between the second and first CCTAs was the smallest when compared to CCTAs using the same contrast volumes or constant volumes per body weight [16].

Owing to the partial volume effect and extra-adventitial tissue, determining the border of the coronary artery from CT images has been difficult. An additional disadvantage of IVUS is that the borders of media and adventitia are measurable, but the actual vessel diameter is not because adventitia and adventitial tissues are indistinguishable [17]. Therefore, we set 0 HU as the marker for borders on CT images and calculated the ratio of 0-to-0 HU distance to media-to-media distance. The ≥0 HU areas of any manual traces wider than the outside of the vessel may have good reproducibility if the trace does not include stained myocardium.

The tentative available border might be −10 HU or −50 HU instead of 0 HU. The C:I ratio might be greater than 1.1. If the border is defined at 50 HU or 100 HU for obtaining a C:I ratio close to 1, most of the area of lipid-rich plaque might be truncated. The border 0 HU has the advantage of accuracy because 0 HU is one of the standards of a CT image. Measurements that are manually traced on CT images are fundamentally inaccurate because the CT number of the borders is not fixed, and such measurements are inflated compared to those made with IVUS. It is difficult to set the fixed border between the vessel and plaques, which shows varied CT numbers of approximately 60 to 80 HU (Fig. 1). Therefore, measuring plaque area has been difficult so far.

Using a ratio of 1.1 and targeting an intracoronary CT number of 350 HU, we found a strong correlation between estimated EEM area and EEM area measured with IVUS, which differed by 9.0±14%. The difference, for instance, between a vessel diameter of 0.09 mm and a vessel diameter of 3 mm is not clinically significant. The slight computational error may be due to the conditional difference in vessel dilatation between CT and IVUS.

Study Limitations

We excluded invalid TDCs at the timing bolus. In such cases, our CT number-controlling system cannot predict the intracoronary CT number because of a lack of data. We quantified plaque in a small subset of the patients because only patients with both significant stenosis detected by MDCT and evidence of ischemia had been enrolled. More studies are needed in other subtypes of patients in order to identify the optimal intracoronary CT number.

We had few data of less than 2 mm in diameter for 2 reasons. One is that small coronary arteries were excluded because small coronary arteries are often in contact with the myocardium. The other is that the measurement of a vessel less than 2 mm in diameter has little clinical significance because diseased lesions with 2 mm of diameter are treated by medication instead of percutaneous coronary intervention. Measurement by CT and IVUS was performed to avoid the calcification and surrounding area. The calcified area with shadowing is also immeasurable by CT and IVUS. The number of measurable lesions may depend on the extent of calcium deposition or the number of stents. In clinical settings, that the location of measurement is limited may be inevitable with both IVUS and CT.

Conclusions

Media-to-media distance and EEM area in IVUS images can be estimated by CCTA targeting the optimized intracoronary CT number when blood vessel boundaries are defined at 0 HU.

Author Contributions

Conceived and designed the experiments: SK TK KK. Performed the experiments: SK TK. Analyzed the data: AI TK KM YK. Contributed reagents/materials/analysis tools: SK AI. Wrote the paper: SK TO KK.

References

1. Budoff MJ, Achenbach S, Blumenthal RS, Carr JJ, Goldin JG, et al. (2006) Assessment of coronary artery disease by cardiac computed tomography. Circulation 114: 1761–91.
2. Leber AW, Becker A, Knez A, von Ziegler F, Sirol M, et al. (2006) Accuracy of 64-slice computed tomography to classify and quantify plaque volumes in the proximal coronary system. J Am Coll Cardiol 47: 672–7.
3. Voros S, Rinehart S, Qian Z, Vazquez G, Anderson H, et al. (2011) Prospective validation of standardized, 3-dimensional, quantitative coronary computed tomographic plaque measurements using radiofrequency backscatter intravascular ultrasound as reference standard in intermediate coronary arterial lesions: results from the ATLANTA I study. JACC Cardiovasc Interv 4: 198–208.
4. Petranovic M, Soni A, Bezzera H, Loureiro R, Sarwar A, et al. (2009) Assessment of nonstenotic coronary lesions by 64-slice multidetector computed tomography in comparison to intravascular ultrasound. J Cardiovasc Comput Tomogr 3: 24–31.
5. Marwan M, Pflederer T, Schepis T, Seltmann M, Ropers D, et al. (2011) Coronary vessel and luminal area measurement using dual-source computed tomography in comparison with intravascular ultrasound: effect of window settings on measurement accuracy.J Comput Assist Tomogr. 35: 113–8.
6. Komatsu S, Imai A, Kodama K (2011) Multidetector row computed tomography may accurately estimate plaque vulnerability. Circ J 75: 1515–21.
7. Fei X, Du X, Yang Q, Shen Y, Li P, et al. (2008) 64-MDCT coronary angiography: phantom study of effects of vascular attenuation on detection of coronary stenosis.AJR Am J Roentgenol. 191: 43–9.
8. Komatsu S, Kamata T, Imai A, Ohara T, Takewa M, et al. (2013) Controlling Intracoronary CT Number for Coronary CT Angiography. J Cardiol 61: 155–61.
9. Abbara S, Arbab-Zadeh A, Callister TQ, Desai MY, Mamuya W, et al. (2009) SCCT guidelines for performance of coronary computed tomographic angiography: a report of the Society of Cardiovascular Computed Tomography Guidelines Committee. J Cardiovasc Comput Tomogr 3: 190–204.
10. Komatsu S, Hirayama A, Omori Y, Ueda Y, Mizote I, et al. (2005) Detection of coronary plaque by computed tomography with a novel plaque analysis system, 'Plaque Map', and comparison with intravascular ultrasound and angioscopy. Circ J.69: 72–7.
11. Peters RJ, Kok WE, Rijsterborgh H, van Dijk M, Koch KT, et al. (1996) Reproducibility of quantitative measurements from intracoronary ultrasound images. Beat-to-beat variability and influence of the cardiac cycle.Eur Heart J. 17: 1593–9.
12. Alfonso F, Macaya C, Goicolea J, Hernandez R, Segovia J, et al. (1994) Determinants of coronary compliance in patients with coronary artery disease: an intravascular ultrasound study. J Am Coll Cardiol23: 879–84.
13. Cademartiri F, Mollet NR, Runza G, Bruining N, Hamers R, et al. (2005) Influence of intracoronary attenuation on coronary plaque measurements using multislice computed tomography. Eur Radiol. 15: 1426–31.
14. Pazhenkottil AP, Husmann L, Buechel RR, Herzog BA, Nkoulou R, et al. (2010) Validation of a new contrast material protocol adapted to body surface area for optimized low-dose CT coronary angiography with prospective ECG-triggering. Int J Cardiovasc Imaging 26: 591–7.
15. Herzog BA, Husmann L, Valenta I, Tay FM, Burkhard N, et al. (2009) Determinants of vessel contrast in BMI-adapted low dose CT coronary angiography with prospective ECG-triggering. Int J Cardiovasc Imaging 25: 625–30.
16. Komatsu S, Imai A, Kamata T, Ohara T, Takewa M, et al. (2013) A CT number-controlling system for reproducibility of intracoronary CT number on follow-up coronary CT angiography. J Cardiol. 62: 82–6.
17. Mintz GS, Nissen SE, Anderson WD, Bailey SR, Erbel R, et al. (2001) American College of Cardiology Clinical Expert Consensus Document on Standards for Acquisition, Measurement and Reporting of Intravascular Ultrasound Studies (IVUS). A report of the American College of Cardiology Task Force on Clinical Expert Consensus Documents.J Am Coll Cardiol. 37: 1478–92.

Coronary Collateral Circulation in Patients of Coronary Ectasia with Significant Coronary Artery Disease

Po-Chao Hsu[1,2,6], Ho-Ming Su[1,6,7], Hsiang-Chun Lee[1,2], Suh-Hang Juo[3,4,5], Tsung-Hsien Lin[1,6*], Wen-Chol Voon[1,6], Wen-Ter Lai[1,6], Sheng-Hsiung Sheu[1,6]

1 Division of Cardiology, Department of Internal Medicine, Kaohsiung Medical University Hospital, Kaohsiung Medical University, Kaohsiung, Taiwan, **2** Graduate Institute of Medicine, College of Medicine, Kaohsiung Medical University, Kaohsiung, Taiwan, **3** Department of Medical Research, Kaohsiung Medical University Hospital, Kaohsiung Medical University, Kaohsiung, Taiwan, **4** Medical Genetics, Kaohsiung Medical University, Kaohsiung, Taiwan, **5** Center of Excellence for Environmental Medicine, Kaohsiung Medical University, Kaohsiung, Taiwan, **6** Faculty of Medicine, College of Medicine, Kaohsiung Medical University, Kaohsiung, Taiwan, **7** Department of Internal Medicine, Kaohsiung Municipal Hsiao-Kang Hospital, Kaohsiung, Taiwan

Abstract

Objectives: Patients with coronary ectasia (CE) usually have coexisting coronary stenosis resulting in myoischemia. Coronary collateral plays an important role in protecting myocardium from ischemia and reducing cardiovascular events. However, limited studies investigate the role of CE in coronary collaterals development.

Methods: We evaluated 1020 consecutive patients undergoing coronary angiography and 552 patients with significant coronary artery disease (SCAD), defined as diameter stenosis more than 70%, were finally analyzed. CE is defined as the ectatic diameter 1.5 times larger than adjacent reference segment. Rentrop collateral score was used to classify patients into poor (grades 0 and 1) or good (grades 2 and 3) collateral group.

Results: 73 patients (13.2%) had CE lesions which were most located in the right coronary artery (53.4%). Patients with CE had a lower incidence of diabetes (43.8% vs 30.1%, $p = 0.03$), higher body mass index (25.4 ± 3.5 vs 26.7 ± 4.6, $p = 0.027$) and poorer coronary collateral (58.2% vs 71.2%, $p = 0.040$). Patients with poor collateral ($n = 331$) had a higher incidence of CE (15.7% vs 9.5%, $p = 0.040$) and fewer diseased vessels numbers (1.96 ± 0.84 vs 2.48 ± 0.69, $p < 0.001$). Multivariate analysis showed diabetes (odd ratio (OR) 0.630, $p = 0.026$), CE ($OR = 0.544$, $p = 0.048$), and number of diseased vessels ($OR = 2.488$, $p < 0.001$) were significant predictors of coronary collaterals development.

Conclusion: The presence of CE was associated with poorer coronary collateral development in patients with SCAD.

Editor: Claudio Moretti, S.G.Battista Hospital, Italy

Funding: The authors have no support or funding to report.

Competing Interests: The authors have declared that no competing interests exist.

* E-mail: lth@kmu.edu.tw

Introduction

Coronary ectasia (CE) is an uncommon disease and its incidence has been reported as between 0.3 and 5% in different studies despite some exception [1–5]. It is defined as the diameter of the ectatic segment being more than 1.5 times larger compared with an adjacent healthy reference segment [2]. Most cases of CE are considered as a variant of coronary artery disease (CAD) [6]. The pathogenesis of CE is not completely illustrated. However, it is likely to involve the destruction of the arterial media, increased wall stress, thinning of the arterial wall, and progressive dilatation of the coronary artery segment [7].

The development of coronary collaterals is an adaptive response to chronic myoischemia and serves as a conduit bridging the significantly stenotic coronary vessels [8–10]. Collateral circulation can hence protect and preserve myocardium from episodes of ischemia, enhance residual myocardial contractility, and reduce angina symptoms and cardiovascular events [11–13]. However, there is inter-individual difference of coronary collateral formation and the mechanisms for the different individual ability to develop collateral circulation are still unclear.

Because CE are usually associated with atherosclerosis and even obstructive CAD resulting coronary ischemia, whether the presence of good coronary collateral or not is a very important issue for the CE population [2,6]. However, there were limited literatures discussing the coronary collateral formation in the CE population. Therefore we designed this study to investigate the role of CE in patients with obstructive CAD.

Patients and Methods

Study subjects

We evaluated 1020 patients scheduled for diagnostic coronary angiography from the Kaohsiung Medical University Hospital (KMUH) in Taiwan. Patients with coronary artery lumen diameter stenosis <70%, history of coronary artery bypass surgery (CABG), history of percutaneous coronary intervention (PCI), inadequate angiograms for CE evaluation were excluded. Finally

552 patients were recruited in our study. We collected patients' demographic and baseline information including sex, age, body mass index (BMI), duration of chest pain, history of diabetes, hypertension, hypercholesterolemia, and cigarette smoking.

Ethics Statement

The research protocol was approved and registered by the Institutional Review Board of the Kaohsiung Medical University Hospital (KMUH-IRB). Informed consents were obtained in written form from patients and all clinical investigation was conducted according to the principles expressed in the Declaration of Helsinki. The patients gave consent for the publication of the clinical details.

Coronary angiography

The coronary artery angiography films were reviewed by two experienced cardiologists blind to patients' clinical characteristics. A third reviewer blinded to the readings of the first two reviewers served as arbitrator of differences. Coronary angiography was performed by the femoral or radial approach with 6Fr diagnostic catheters. Images were recorded in multiple projections for left and right coronary arteries. Coronary artery stenosis was determined by quantitative coronary angiography. The presence of significant coronary artery disease (SCAD) is defined as coronary diameter stenosis more than 70%. CE is defined as the diameter of the ectatic segment being more than 1.5 times larger compared with an adjacent healthy reference segment [2]. The classification of CE developed by Markis et al. and based on the extent of ectatic involvement was used [14]. In decreasing order of severity, diffuse CE of two or three vessels was classified as Type I, diffuse disease in one vessel and localized disease in another vessel as Type II, diffuse CE of one vessel only as Type III and localized or segmental ectasia as Type IV. The recorded data also included the location, number of CAD and CE, percentage of stenosis of diseased vessels, the vessel to which the collaterals were connected, the grade of coronary collateral circulation, and the coronary artery disease severity scoring.

Collateral scoring and pathways evaluation by coronary angiography

In subjects with more than one SCAD vessel, the vessel with the highest collateral grade was chosen for analysis. The collateral scoring system developed by Rentrop and Cohen was used [15]. Grades of collateral filling from the contralateral vessel were: 0 = none; 1 = filling of side branches of the artery to be dilated via collateral channels without visualization of the epicardial segment; 2 = partial filling of the epicardial segment via collateral channels; 3 = complete filling of the epicardial segment of the artery being dilated via collateral channels. In subjects with more than one collateral vessel supplying the distal aspect of the diseased artery, the highest collateral grade was recorded. Patients were then classified according to their collateral grades as either poor (grade 0 or grade 1 collateral) or good (grade 2 or grade 3 collateral). In addition, the size of the collateral connection (CC) diameter was assessed by 3 grades: CC grade 0, no continuous connection between donor and recipient artery; CC grade 1, continuous, threadlike connection, and CC grade 2, continuous, small side branch-like size of the collateral throughout its course [16]. In the case of coexisting collateral connections, the prominent one was defined as the principal. The anatomic pathways were categorized according to Levin's pathways and summarized in 4 categories: septal, intra-arterial (bridging), epicardial with proximal takeoff (atrial branches), and epicardial with distal takeoff [10,17]. In the case of coexisting collateral pathways, the principal pathway was defined as the one that was the first to opacify the stenotic epicardial segments.

Statistical analysis

All data were expressed as means ± standard deviation. Independent t test was used to compare continuous variables between the two groups. Chi-square test was used to compare categorical data. Subsequently, significantly correlated variables in the univariate analysis or relevant variables were further analyzed by binary logistic regression analysis to predict the collateral development (good vs. poor). All p values were two-sided with a significance level of $p<.05$. The Statistical Package for the Social Sciences 11.0 for Windows (SPSS Inc.,Chicago, IL) was used for statistical analysis.

Results

Clinical characteristics

Among the 1020 subjects initially evaluated, 468 patients were excluded for the following reasons: coronary artery lumen diameter stenosis <70%, history of CABG or PCI, or inadequate angiograms for collateral evaluation. The final study population was 552 subjects (443 male and 109 female; average age, 62.5±12.5 years old). Regarding numbers of diseased vessels, 148 patients (26.8%) were 1 vessel disease (VD), 163 patients (29.5%) were 2VD, and 241 patients (43.7%) were 3VD.

Coronary ectasia and collaterals

There were 73 patients (13.2%) with CE with 24 patients (32.9%) 1VD, 26 (35.6%) 2VD, and 23 (31.5%) 3VD. Table 1 summarizes the angiographic characteristics of the patients with CE. 55 (75.3%) patients had CE involving one major vessel (right coronary artery: 39 patients, left anterior descending artery: 3 patient, left circumflex artery: 13 patients); 13 (17.8%) patients had CE involving two major vessel (right coronary artery and left anterior descending artery: 5 patients, right coronary artery and left circumflex artery: 7 patients, left anterior descending artery and left circumflex artery: 1 patients); 5 (6.8%) patients had CE involving all three vessels. For type of CE, 14 (19.2%) patients were type 1, 4 (5.5%) patients were type 2, 50 (68.5%) patients were type 3, and 5 (6.8%) patients were type 4. For coronary collateral grade and pathway evaluation, the 2 collaterals readers obtained a 96% agreement in the collateral classifications. Of the 73 patients with CE, the Rentrop coronary grade was distributed as follows: 40 (54.8%) patients with grade 0, 12 (16.4%) patients with grade 1, 13 (17.8%) patients with grade 2, and 8 (11%) patients with grade 3. The CC grade was distributed as follows: 49 (67.1%) patients with CC grade 0, 19 (26%) patients with CC grade 1, and 5 (6.8%) patients with CC grade 2. Furthermore, for the collateral pathways: the principal pathways was through septal connections in 57.6%, atrial-epicardial connections in 27.3%, bridging connections in 9.1%, and distal inter-arterial connections in 6.1%.

Baseline characteristics in patients with and without CE were shown in the Table 2. The patients with CE (n = 73) had a lower incidence of DM (30.1% vs 43.8%, $p=0.030$), higher BMI (26.7±4.6 vs 25.4±3.5, $p=0.027$), and poor coronary collateral (71.2% vs 58.2%, $p=0.040$). The multivariate regression analysis of coronary collateral formation (good vs poor collateral) in CE population with SCAD and found that only number of diseased vessels (OR = 2.358, 95% CI = 1.148–4.843, $p=0.02$) was a significant independent predictor of coronary collaterals development (Table 3).

Table 1. Angiographic Characteristics of the Patients With Coronary Ectasia.

Ectasia(s) location	N (%)
Right coronary artery	39 (53.4%)
Left anterior descending artery	3 (4.1%)
Left circumflex artery	13 (17.8%)
Right coronary artery + left anterior descending artery	5 (6.8%)
Right coronary artery + left circumflex artery	7 (9.6%)
Left anterior descending artery + left circumflex artery	1 (1.4%)
All three vessels	5 (6.8%)
Number of vessel(s) with coronary ectasia(s)	
1	55 (75.3%)
2	13 (17.8%)
3	5 (6.8%)
Type of coronary ectasia	
Type 1	14 (19.2%)
Type 2	4 (5.5%)
Type 3	50 (68.5%)
Type 4	5 (6.8%)
Rentrop collateral grade	
Grade 0	40 (54.8%)
Grade 1	12 (16.4%)
Grade 2	13 (17.8%)
Grade 3	8 (11%)
Collateral connection grades	
CC0	49 (67.1%)
CC1	19 (26%)
CC2	5 (6.8%)
Collateral pathway	
Septal	19 (57.6%)
Atrial-epicardial	9 (27.3%)
Bridging	3 (9.1%)
Distal inter-arterial	2 (6.1%)

CC, collateral connection

Coronary collaterals development in the whole population

Baseline characteristics in patients with poor and good collateral were shown in the Table 4, the patients with poor collateral (n = 331) had a higher incidence of CE (15.7% vs 9.5%, p = 0.040), and a fewer diseased vessels numbers (1.96±0.84 vs 2.48±0.69, p<0.001). Table 5 showed the multivariate analysis of coronary collateral formation (good vs poor collateral) in whole population with SCAD. We found diabetes (OR = 0.619, 95% CI = 0.410–0.934, p = 0.022), coronary ectasia (OR = 0.544, 95% CI = 0.297–0.996, p = 0.048), and number of diseased vessels (OR = 2.488, 95% CI = 1.917–3.228, p<0.001) were significant independent predictors of coronary collaterals development.

Treatment strategies in CE patients

Among the 73 patients with CE, 58 patients (79.5%) received PCI, 8 patients (11%) received CABG, and 7 patients (9.6%) only received medical treatment for the coronary lesions. There was no significant association between treatment strategies and presence of good or poor coronary collaterals (p = 0.284).

Table 2. Baseline Characteristics between Patients without and with Coronary Ectasia.

	Control	Ectasia	
Parameters N (%)	**(n = 479)**	**(n = 73)**	**p Value**
Sex (male)	379 (79.1)	64 (87.7)	0.113
Age (years)	62.8±12.1	60.3±14.8	0.174
DM	210 (43.8)	22 (30.1)	0.030
Hypertension	312 (65.1)	47 (64.4)	0.896
Smoking	280 (58.6)	50 (68.5)	0.124
Family history	16 (3.4)	2 (2.7)	1.000
Hypercholesterolemia (%)	264 (56.3)	36 (49.3)	0.311
CAD number			0.080
1-vessel disease	124 (25.9)	24 (32.9)	
2-vessel disease	137 (28.6)	26 (35.6)	
3-vessel disease	218 (45.5)	23 (31.5)	
BMI	25.4±3.5	26.7±4.6	0.027
Poor Collateral, n (%)	279 (58.2%)	52 (71.2%)	0.040

Data are presented as mean ± standard deviation or number (%); CAD, coronary artery disease; DM, diabetes mellitus; BMI, body mass index;

Discussion

There were three major findings in the present study. First, most CE lesion were located in the right coronary artery. Second, CE patients with significant coronary artery disease have poor coronary collateral development compared with non-CE patients. Third, CE is a significantly independent predictor of poor coronary collaterals in patients with SCAD.

The association between CE and coronary collaterals

CE is a variant of coronary artery abnormality [6]. It may be congenital or acquired. Acquired causes include atherosclerosis, Kawasaki disease, various inflammatory and infectious diseases, and so on [2–6]. However, most cases of CE are associated with atherosclerosis and had coexistence of obstructive CAD [2,6]. It

Table 3. Multivariate logistic regression analysis of collateral circulation in CE population (poor collateral group as reference group).

	OR	95% CI	p Value
Sex (male vs female)	-	-	0.896
Age	-	-	0.110
Hypertension	-	-	0.881
DM	-	-	0.178
Smoking	-	-	0.330
Hypercholesterolemia	-	-	0.291
BMI	-	-	0.652
Number of diseased vessels	2.358	1.148–4.843	0.020

BMI, body mass index; CE, coronary ectasia; DM, diabetes mellitus

Table 4. Baseline Characteristics between good and poor collaterals.

	Poor	Good	
Parameters N (%)	(n = 331)	(n = 221)	p Value
Sex (male)	263 (79.5%)	180 (81.4%)	0.587
Age (years)	62.6±13.0	62.4±11.8	0.815
DM	143 (43.2%)	89 (40.3%)	0.538
Hypertension	214 (64.7%)	145 (65.6%)	0.856
Smoking	201 (60.7%)	129 (58.6%)	0.658
Family history	7 (2.1%)	11 (5.0%)	0.086
Hypercholesterolemia (%)	169 (52.3%)	131 (59.8%)	0.095
CAD number	1.96±0.84	2.48±0.69	<0.001
1-vessel disease	123 (37.2)	25 (11.3)	
2-vessel disease	97 (29.3)	66 (29.9)	
3-vessel disease	111 (33.5)	130 (58.8)	
BMI	25.5±3.74	25.7±3.6	0.553
Coronary ectasia, n (%)	52 (15.7%)	21 (9.5%)	0.040

Data are presented as mean ± standard deviation or number (%); CAD, coronary artery disease; DM, diabetes mellitus; BMI, body mass index

Table 5. Multivariate logistic regression analysis of collateral circulation in whole population (poor collateral group as reference group).

	OR	95% CI	p Value
Sex (male vs female)	-	-	0.395
Age	-	-	0.675
Hypertension	-	-	0.879
DM	0.619	0.410–0.934	0.022
Hypercholesterolemia	-	-	0.361
Smoking	-	-	0.270
BMI	-	-	0.318
Coronary ectasia	0.544	0.297–0.996	0.048
Number of diseased vessels	2.488	1.917–3.228	<0.001

BMI, body mass index; DM, diabetes mellitus

was considered to be a variant of CAD and is associated with the similar risk as the patients with CAD [2,14,18–19]. The clinical presentation and the long-term cardiac complications are associated with the severity of coexisting CAD [20]. Even in patients with isolated CE without coronary stenosis, there is still higher incidence of adverse events in this population compared to people with normal coronary arteries. The pathogenesis of CE is not completely understood, however, it is likely to involve the destruction of the arterial media, increased wall stress, thinning of the arterial wall, and progressive dilatation of the coronary artery segment[7]. The presence of ectatic segments produces sluggish blood flow, with exercise-induced angina and myocardial infarction, regardless of the severity of coexisting obstructive CAD [14. 18–19]. The possible causes of higher adverse events might be related to the repeated dissemination of microemboli to distal segments, or thrombotic occlusion of the dilated vessel. In addition, slow blood flow in the ectatic coronary arteries might be another cause which predisposes to the occurrence of AMI. Disturbances in blood flow filling and washout in the ectatic vessels were due to inappropriate coronary dilatation and were clearly associated with the severity of CE [21]. The turbulent and stagnant blood flow could induce endothelial damage, increase wall stress, and even cause extensive thrombosis. In past literature, all three coronary arteries can be affected by CE, but most patients had single-vessel involvement [22.23]. Furthermore, In CE patients with coexistent CAD, the right coronary artery is the most frequently involved. These findings were also similar with our current study.

The development of coronary collaterals can reduce angina and infarct size, preserve left ventricular ejection fraction, decrease aneurysmal dilatation, and provide a survival benefit in patients with SCAD [11–13]. However, there are limited studies discussing about the coronary collateral formation in the CE population and most of the studies were focused on the young patients with Kawasaki disease [24–25]. In children with Kawasaki disease, Onouchi Z et al. reported that coronary collaterals did not develop in the presence of localized stenosis regardless of the occurrence of myocardial ischemia, but total occluded vessels had collateral development regardless of the presence of myocardial infarction [24]. Tatara K et al. also indicated that collateral circulation cannot be seen angiographically unless there is total occlusion and the presence of collateral circulation cannot provide protection against stress-induced myocardial ischemia [25]. These findings all suggest that relative poor collateral formation in the patients with etiology of Kawasaki disease. Despite of the etiologies different from previous studies, our study showed that CE is significantly associated with poor coronary collateral formation both in univariate and multivariate analysis. Although CE is reported to be associated with increased plasma levels of inflammatory markers, cytokines, and oxidative stress, the detailed mechanism of poor coronary collateral development is not well understood nowadays and may need further investigation in the future [26–28].

In addition, number of diseased vessels was not only a significant predictor of coronary collateral formation in the patients with SCAD, but also the only significant predictor in the CE population with SCAD. It is well known that coronary collateral formation is mainly dependent on the CAD severity [29–31]. Patients with good coronary collaterals appear to have a more extensive CAD. In previous studies, number of diseased vessels is a significant predictor of good collateral formation [32,33]. Hence, extent of coronary atherosclerosis significantly plays an important role in coronary collateral formation.

Limitations of the present study

First, the collateral formation was assessed by coronary angiography in this study. Measuring collateral flow index by intravascular Doppler guidewire may provide a more objective physiological measurement of collateral grade. However, the invasiveness of intravascular ultrasound limits its use in large-scale studies. Second, since this was only a clinical association study, potential mechanisms were not fully elucidated and long term follow-up of clinical outcome data will be needed to see whether CE patients with poorer coronary collaterals have higher incidence of cardiovascular adverse events in the future.

Conclusions

To our best, our study is the first study to show the poor coronary collateral development in the adult patients with CE and SCAD. Our data might partially explain why patients with CE have higher incidence of cardiovascular adverse events.

Author Contributions

Conceived and designed the experiments: PCH THL. Performed the experiments: PCH HMS THL SHS. Analyzed the data: HCL SHJ WCV WTL. Contributed reagents/materials/analysis tools: PCH HMS THL SHS. Wrote the paper: PCH THL.

References

1. Oliveros RA, Falsetti HL, Carroll RJ, Heinle RA, Ryan GF (1974) Atherosclerotic coronary artery aneurysm: report of five cases and a review of the literature. Arch Intern Med 134: 1072–1076.
2. Swaye PS, Fisher LD, Litwin P, Vignola PA, Judkins MP, et al. (1983) Aneurysmal coronary artery disease. Circulation 67: 134–138.
3. Hartnell GG, Parnell BM, Pridie RB (1985) Coronary artery ectasia. Its prevalence and clinical significance in 4993 patients. Br Heart J 54(4): 392–5.
4. Yilmaz H, Sayar N, Yilmaz M, Tangürek B, Cakmak N, et al. (2008) Coronary artery ectasia: clinical and angiographical evaluation. Turk Kardiyol Dern Ars 36: 530–535.
5. Sharma SN, Kaul U, Sharma S, Wasir HS, Manchanda SC, et al. (1990) Coronary arteriographic profile in young and old Indian patients with ischaemic heart disease: a comparative study. Indian Heart J 42(5): 365–9.
6. Swanton RH, Thomas ML, Coltart DJ, Jenkins BS, Webb-Peploe MM, et al. (1978) Coronary artery ectasia—a variant of occlusive coronary arteriosclerosis. Br Heart J 40(4): 393–400.
7. Rodbars S, Ikeda K, Montes M (1967) An analysis of mechanisms of poststenotic dilatation. Angiology 18: 349–353.
8. Fujita M, Sasayama S, Ohno A, Nakajima H, Asanoi H (1987) Importance of angina for development of collateral circulation. Br Heart J 57: 139.
9. Tayebjee MH, Lip GY, MacFadyen RJ (2004) Collateralization and the response to obstruction of epicardial coronary arteries. QJM 97: 259.
10. Levin DC (1974) Pathways and functional significance of the coronary collateral circulation. Circulation 50: 831–7.
11. Cohen M, Rentrop KP (1986) Limitation of myocardial ischemia by collateral circulation during sudden controlled coronary artery occlusion in human subjects: a prospective study. Circulation 74(3): 469–76.
12. Meier P, Gloekler S, Zbinden R, Beckh S, de Marchi SF, et al. (2007) Beneficial effect of recruitable collaterals: a 10-year follow-up study in patients with stable coronary artery disease undergoing quantitative collateral measurements. Circulation 116(9): 975–83.
13. Regieli JJ, Jukema JW, Nathoe HM, Zwinderman AH, Ng S, et al. (2009) Coronary collaterals improve prognosis in patients with ischemic heart disease. Int J Cardiol 132(2): 257–62.
14. Markis JE, Joffe CD, Cohn PF, Fen DJ, Herman MV, et al. (1976) Clinical significance of coronary artery ectasia. Am J Cardiol 37: 217–222.
15. Rentrop KP, Cohen M, Blanke H, Phillips RA (1985) Changes in collateral channel filling immediately after controlled coronary artery occlusion by an angioplasty balloon in human subjects. J Am Coll Cardiol 5(3): 587–92.
16. Werner GS, Ferrari M, Heinke S, Kuethe F, Surber R, et al. (2003) Angiographic assessment of collateral connections in comparison with invasively determined collateral function in chronic coronary occlusions. Circulation 107: 1972–7.
17. Brown G, Rockstroh J (2002) Coronary collateral size, flow capacity, and growth estimates from the angiogram in patients with obstructive coronary disease. Circulation 105: 168–73.
18. Befeler B, Aranda JM, Embi A, Mullin F, Ei-Sherif N, et al. (1977) Coronary artery aneurysms: Study of their etiology, clinical course and effect on left ventricular function and prognosis. Am J Cardiol 62: 597–607.
19. Demopoulos VP, Olympios CD, Fakiolas CN, Pissimissis EG, Economides NM, et al. (1997) The natural history of aneurysmal coronary artery disease. Heart 78: 136–141.
20. Manginas A, Cokkinos DV (2006) Coronary artery ectasias: imaging, functional assessment and clinical implications. Eur Heart J 27(9): 1026–31.
21. Mavrogeni S (2010) Coronary artery ectasia: from diagnosis to treatment. Hellenic J Cardiol 51(2): 158–63.
22. Daoud AS, Pankin D, Tulgan H, Florentin RA (1963) Aneurysms of the coronary artery. Report of ten cases and review of literature. Am J Cardiol 11: 228–237.
23. al-Harthi SS, Nouh MS, Arafa M, al-Nozha M (1991) Aneurysmal dilatation of the coronary arteries: diagnostic patterns and clinical significance. Int J Cardiol 30: 191–194.
24. Onouchi Z, Hamaoka K, Kamiya Y, Hayashi S, Ohmochi Y, et al. (1993) Transformation of coronary artery aneurysm to obstructive lesion and the role of collateral vessels in myocardial perfusion in patients with Kawasaki disease. J Am Coll Cardiol 21(1): 158–62.
25. Tatara K, Kusakawa S, Itoh K, Honma S, Hashimoto K, et al. (1991) Collateral circulation in Kawasaki disease with coronary occlusion or severe stenosis. Am Heart J 121: 797–802.
26. Ozbay Y, Akbulut M, Balin M, Kayancicek H, Baydas A, et al. (2007) The level of hs-CRP in coronary artery ectasia and its response to statin and angiotensin-converting enzyme inhibitor treatment. Mediators Inflamm 89649.
27. Li JJ, Nie SP, Qian XW, Zeng HS, Zhang CY (2009) Chronic inflammatory status in patients with coronary artery ectasia. Cytokine 46(1): 61–4.
28. Sezen Y, Bas M, Polat M, Yildiz A, Buyukhatipoglu H, et al. (2010) The relationship between oxidative stress and coronary artery ectasia. Cardiol J 17(5): 488–94.
29. Abaci A, Oğuzhan A, Kahraman S, Eryol NK, Unal S, et al. (1999) Effect of diabetes mellitus on formation of coronary collateral vessels. Circulation 99(17): 2239–2242.
30. Helfant RH, Kemp HG, Gorlin R (1970) Coronary atherosclerosis, coronary collaterals, and their relation to cardiac function. Ann Intern Med 73: 189–193.
31. Sezer M, Ozcan M, Okcular I, Elitok A, Umman S, et al. (2007) A potential evidence to explain the reason behind the devastating prognosis of coronary artery disease in uraemic patients: renal insufficiency is associated with poor coronary collateral vessel development. Int J Cardiol 115(3): 366–372.
32. Gulec S, Ozdemir AO, Maradit-Kremers H, Dincer I, Atmaca Y, et al. (2006) Elevated levels of C-reactive protein are associated with impaired coronary collateral development. Eur J Clin Invest 36(6): 369–75.
33. Resar JR, Roguin A, Voner J, Nasir K, Hennebry TA, et al. (2005) Hypoxia-inducible factor 1alpha polymorphism and coronary collaterals in patients with ischemic heart disease. Chest 128(2): 787–91.

5

Impaired Dynamic Cerebral Autoregulation and Cerebrovascular Reactivity in Middle Cerebral Artery Stenosis

Jie Chen[1], Jia Liu[2]*, Wei-Hai Xu[1], Ren Xu[2], Bo Hou[3], Li-Ying Cui[1], Shan Gao[1]*

1 Department of Neurology, Peking Union Medical College Hospital, Chinese Academy of Medical Sciences and Peking Union Medical College, Beijing, China, **2** Shenzhen Institutes of Advanced Technology, Chinese Academy of Sciences, Shenzhen, China, **3** Department of Radiology, Peking Union Medical College Hospital, Chinese Academy of Medical Sciences and Peking Union Medical College, Beijing, China

Abstract

Purpose: We sought to investigate the capacity of cerebral autoregulation and cerebrovascular reactivity (CVR) in patients with middle cerebral artery (MCA) stenosis.

Methods: Twenty-one patients with MCA stenosis diagnosed by magnetic resonance angiography and 15 healthy controls were enrolled. Cerebral autoregulation was assessed by autoregulatory parameters (rate of recovery/phase/gain) derived from transfer function from spontaneous oscillations of cerebral blood flow velocity and blood pressure. CVR was tested by a rebreathing maneuver.

Results: Rate of recovery, phase and CVR estimated from moderate MCA stenosis (rate of recovery $=17.76\pm8.21$%/s, phase $=26.93\pm15.67°$, and CVR $=1.53\pm0.84$%/mmHg, respectively) were significantly different ($p<0.05$) from controls (rate of recovery $=39.62\pm27.99$%/s, phase $=55.66\pm22.10°$, and CVR $=2.18\pm0.80$%/mmHg, respectively). Rate of recovery ($r=-0.698$, $p<0.001$), phase ($r=-0.738$, $p<0.001$)) and CVR ($r=-0.690$, $p<0.001$) were all significantly correlated with the degree of stenosis.

Conclusion: Cerebral autoregulation and CVR were impaired in patients with $\geq$ 50% MCA stenosis. The measures of both hemodynamic properties were inversely correlated with the stenotic degree.

Editor: Jeroen Hendrikse, University Medical Center (UMC) Utrecht, Netherlands

Funding: This study was funded by Innovation Fund of the Chinese Academy of Medical Sciences and Peking Union Medical College (No. 20121002039), (http://graduate.pumc.edu.cn/). Dr Jia Liu's work was supported by the Natural Science Foundation of China (No. 81000644), (http://www.nsfc.gov.cn/Portal0/default152.htm). The funders had no role in study design, data collection and analysis, decision to publish, or preparation of the manuscript.

Competing Interests: The authors have declared that no competing interests exist.

* E-mail: jia.liu@siat.ac.cn (JL); dr.sgao@gmail.com (SG)

Introduction

Intracranial artery occlusive diseases, especially middle cerebral artery (MCA) stenosis, are major causes of ischemic stroke in Asian, Black, and Hispanic populations [1]. In Chinese populations, they account for approximately 33–50% of stroke and 45% of transient ischemic attack (TIA) [1].

A number of studies reported that stenosis in internal carotid artery (ICA) may impair cerebral hemodynamics, including cerebral autoregulation and cerebrovascular reactivity (CVR), which increases the risk of cerebral ischemic events [2–8]. It is however unknown how these cerebral hemodynamic parameters alter with respect to the stenotic degree in MCA. One would expect that both physiological mechanisms become affected interactively, as stenosis is likely to cause vasodilation which reduces CVR and, at the meantime, also decreases the effectiveness of autoregulation. Nevertheless, according to the previous studies on ICA stenosis, autoregulation is much vulnerable to the stenotic changes yet with almost immediate restoration after carotid endarterectomy or stenting, whereas the status of CVR varies in patients and the response to carotid recanalization is not as sensitive as autoregulation [9]. This is sensible as they are intrinsically controlled by different mechanisms. Cerebral autoregulation can be affected by a number of physiological parameters, such as transmural pressure, carbon dioxide (CO_2), autonomic function, intracranial pressure, and etc., whereas CVR is solely in connection with vasodilation or vasoconstriction. It hence necessary to investigate these two mechanisms in patients with MCA stenosis.

With the advent of transcranial Doppler (TCD) and continuous blood pressure measurement techniques, dynamic cerebral autoregulation, considering short term dynamics between cerebral blood flow velocity (CBFV) and arterial blood pressure (ABP), has been widely studied using transfer function analysis (TFA), providing information both in frequency and time domain [2–4,10–14]. We thus assessed dynamic cerebral autoregulation using this technique. Autoregulatory parameters (rate of recovery (RoRc)/phase/gain) can then be derived from TFA to indicate the status of cerebral autoregulation. The test of CVR is rather standardized by inducing hypercapnia and calculating the increment of CBFV with respect to the inspired CO_2.

Applying TFA, Haubrich et al. demonstrated that the phase shift between ABP and CBFV oscillations were reduced with increasing degree of MCA stenosis compared with controls [15]. Gong et al. also reported the impaired cerebral autoregulation in patients with MCA stenosis, using the parameter of autoregulatory index evaluated using thigh cuff method [16]. Both studies, however, did not exclude patients with either acute stroke or white matter disease (WMD), which may affect the effectiveness of autoregulation [17–19]. Cerebral autoregulation may become impaired after stroke, even in the unaffected hemispheres, though it might recover within the next 3 months [17]. And the impaired autoregulation and CVR have also been demonstrated in patients with WMD [18,19]. The present study excluded these confounding factors (stroke and WMD) and attempt to show if MCA stenosis is an independent factor affecting cerebral autoregulation and CVR and how these hemodynamic parameters change with respect to the degree of stenosis in MCA.

Methods

Subjects

The study was approved by the Peking Union Medical College Hospital Research Ethics Committee and each participant gave written informed consent.

Twenty-one patients with stenosis in M1 segment of MCA diagnosed by magnetic resonance angiography were recruited from March to April, 2012. Patients were excluded from the study, if they had coexistent ≥50% ipsilateral ICA stenosis, stroke or TIA onset within 3 months, or severe WMD (≥3 grades for either periventricular hyperintensity or deep white matter hyperintensity based on the Fazekas visual scale) [20]. All patients received careful evaluations of vascular risk factors and history of stroke.

Fifteen age-matched healthy individuals were recruited as control subjects. Controls who were found to have carotid artery and intracranial stenosis by TCD were excluded [21].

Image Acquisition, Degree of Stenosis, and WMD Severity Scales

All patients were imaged using a 3T scanner (Signa VH/i, GE Medical Systems, Milwaukee, WI, USA). The typical magnetic resonance image (MRI) protocol included at least T1 and T2-weighted images, fluid- attenuated inversion recovery (FLAIR), and 3-dimensional time-of-flight magnetic resonance angiography (MRA). The FLAIR parameters were as follows: repetition time/echo time, 8000/165 ms; number of excitations, 1; flip angle, 90°; field of view, 24 cm × 24 cm; matrix size, 288×192; slice thickness, 6 mm; and slice gap, 1 mm. MRA was performed using the following parameters: repetition time/echo time, 27/6.9 ms; number of excitations, 1; flip angle, 20°; field of view, 24 cm × 16 cm; matrix size, 320×256; and slice thickness, 1.6 mm.

The degree of MCA stenosis was graded as mild (<50%), moderate (50%–69%), or severe stenosis (70%–99%, but with apparent distal segment) [22].

The severity of white matter lesion was assessed by using FLAIR images, except for one patient using T2-weighted images, whose motion artifact was severe on FLAIR. Both the periventricular hyperintensity and deep white matter hyperintensity of each side were graded into 3 stages (grade 0-I, grade II, grade III) by a radiologist, according to the Fazekas rating scale [20].

Measurement of Dynamic Autoregulation and Cerebrovascular Reactivity

Bilateral flow velocity of MCAs was measured via TCD (mutidop-X2, DWL, Sipplingen, Germany) by using 2 MHz transducers fixed to the head with the headframe (Spencer Technologies, Seattle, WA, USA). The distal segment of the affected MCA was insonated, at the depth of 45 to 50 mm. Continuous beat-to-beat ABP was registered by a servo-controlled finger plethysmograph (Nexfin-cc, BMEYE, Amsterdam, Netherlands) in the right hand positioned at the heart level. End-tidal partial pressure of carbon dioxide ($PETCO_2$) was measured with an infrared capnometer (OEM-Module, Envitec, Wismar, Germany) connected via a breathing mask cover the nose during nasal expiration. All the subjects breathed spontaneously in supine position. After a resting time of 10 minutes, the CBFV of bilateral MCAs, ABP, and $PETCO_2$ were recorded for at least 5 minutes. And then a half blocked long tube (1 meter, 600 mL) was connected with the mask for 2 minutes, which composed a semi-closed system for the accumulation of exhaled CO_2 [23]. With the increasing of the concentration of CO_2 in the semi-closed tube, the CO_2 inhalation of the subject was increased (Fig. 1). All the data (including CBFV, ABP, and $PETCO_2$) were recorded online in a sample rate of 100 Hz and stored on a hard disk for further analysis.

Autoregulation Analysis

The dynamic cerebral autoregulation was evaluated using TFA [12,13]. The recorded ABP and CBFV were filtered by an anti-aliasing filter (a 3rd order Butterworth low-pass filter) with cut-off frequency at 0.5 Hz and then down-sampled to 1 Hz. The auto-spectrum, S_{xx}, of ABP and the oss-spectrum, S_{xy}, between ABP and CBFV were estimated using Welch's method, a modified periodogram method. The transfer function was then calculated as:

$$H(f) = S_{xy}/S_{xx} \tag{1}$$

Phase and gain were then computed as:

$$\phi(f) = \tan^{-1}(H_I(f)/H_R(f)) \tag{2}$$

$$|H(f)| = \sqrt{[H_I(f)]^2 + [H_R(f)]^2} \tag{3}$$

where $\phi(f)$ is the phase response and $|H(f)|$ is the gain of the transfer function, respectively. $H_I(f)$ and $H_R(f)$ denote the image and real part of the transfer function, respectively.

The magnitude squared coherence function, C_{xy}, was then estimated also using Welch's method. The coherence function is a function of frequency with values between 0 to 1, indicating how well ABP corresponds to CBFV in frequency, which is formulated as:

$$C_{xy} = \frac{|S_{xy}|^2}{S_{xx}S_{yy}} \tag{4}$$

where S_{yy} is the auto-spectrum of CBFV. The impulse and frequency responses can then be derived from $H(f)$ by inverse Fourier transform. The step response of CBFV can then be calculated by the convolution between the impulse response and a

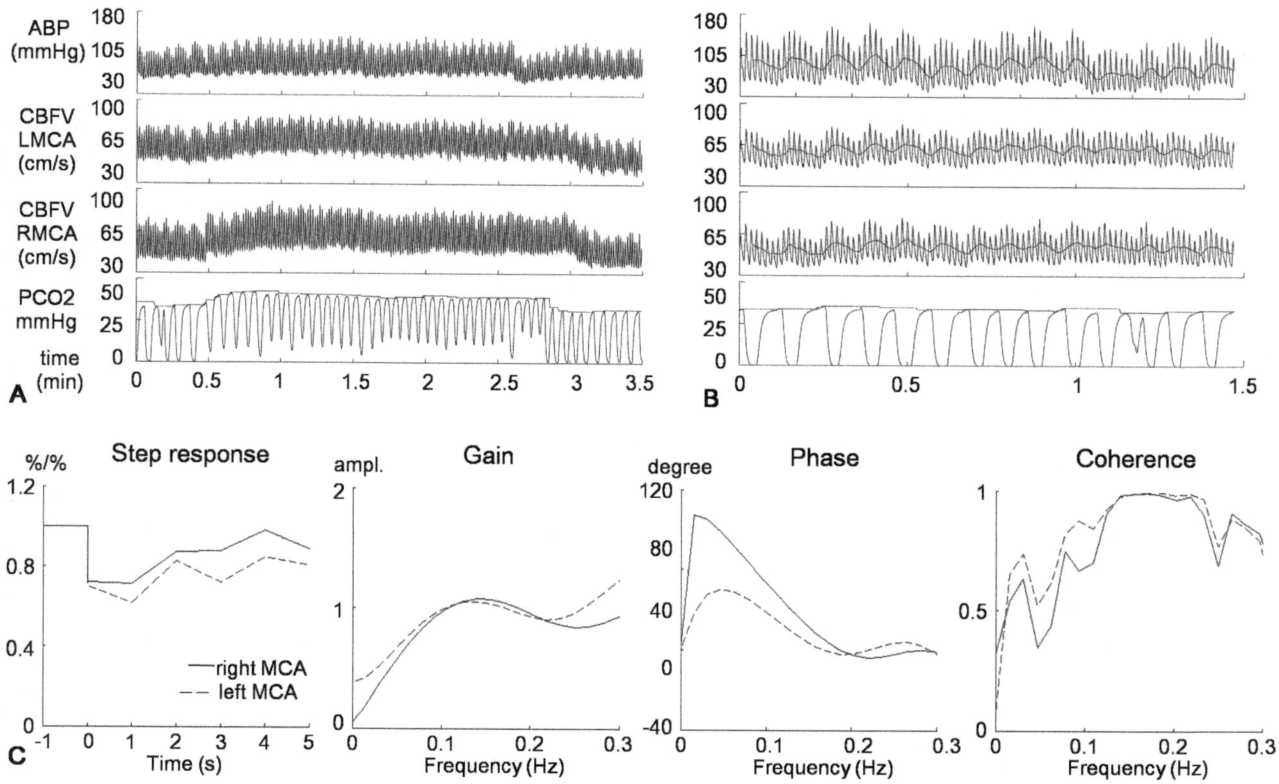

Figure 1. Illustrative recording of cerebrovascular reactivity testing and dynamic cerebral autoregulation analysis. A 52-yr-old patient with severe stenosis of the left MCA and mild stenosis of the right MCA. (A) A rebreathing test for cerebrovascular reactivity. Values were 1.30%/mmHg on the left and 2.21%/mmHg on the right side. (B) Raw data of spontaneously breathing, showing the oscillations of the blood pressure and cerebral blood flow velocity. (C) Transfer function analysis shows, compared with the right side, the recovery of the blood flow of the left side was slower, the phase shift was lower, and the coherence was higher.

normalized step change of ABP from 1 to 0, which shows the recovery of cerebral blood flow after a step-wise change of ABP. In order to quantify the speed of the recovery, we applied a previously defined parameter, the RoRc of CBFV ($RoRc = \frac{\Delta CBFV}{\Delta t} \times 100\%$), where the first 3 seconds of the step response were used for the calculation [14]. The step response was normalized by the first value to reduce the effect of under- or overshoot of the step response. In frequency domain, we only used the parameters (phase, gain, and coherence function) within 0.06–0.12 Hz to evaluate cerebral autoregulation.

Cerebrovascular reactivity Analysis

The CVR was calculated as the maximum percentage increase of CBFV during hypercapnia per unit increase in $PETCO_2$ (in mmHg) [5].

Statistical Analysis

In statistical analysis, Student's t-test, Analysis of variance (ANOVA) and SNK-q test were performed to compare the continuous variables across groups, and Pearson χ^2 was used to compare categorical variables between groups. The correlation between autoregulatory parameters and degree of MCA stenosis, was analyzed by Spearman's method. The correlation between phase shift and CVR was analyzed by Pearson's method. A p value less than 0.05 was considered statistically significant. All statistical analysis was done with SPSS 16.0 (SPSS Inc, Chicago, IL, USA).

Results

Among all the 21 patients recruited, six could be classified as symptomatic (four experienced ischemic stroke and two had TIA). More patients had history of hypertension compared with controls, but there were no significant difference between cases and controls in age, sex, history of diabetes, and previous or current smoking (Table 1).

All subjects were examined bilaterally except for 2 patients with inadequate temporal window of the unaffected side. Thus, a total of 70 MCAs were investigated including 32 stenotic MCAs and 38 normal MCAs (bilateral stenosis was found in 11 patients). The

Table 1. Clinical characteristics of subjects with MCA stenosis and controls.

	MCA stenosis	Controls	P
	(n = 21)	(n = 15)	
Age, years	56.72±15.24	49.8±11.88	0.152
Female, n(%)	13 (61.9)	9 (60.0)	0.908
Hypertension, n (%)	14 (66.7)	3 (20.0)	0.028
Diabetes mellitus, n (%)	4 (19.0)	3 (20.0)	0.943
previous or current smoking, n (%)	7 (33.3)	7 (46.7)	0.418

MCA, middle cerebral artery.

Table 2. Results of RoRc, phase shift, magnitude, coherence and CVR in controls and different degree of MCA stenosis.

		Degree of MCA Stenosis		
	Controls	Mild	Moderate	Severe
	(n = 38)	(n = 8)	(n = 11)	(n = 13)
RoRc(%/s)	39.62±27.99	29.81±16.10	17.76±8.21*	1.16±13.22*
Gain (ampl.)	0.58±0.35	1.30±1.34*	0.70±0.42	0.42±0.20
Phase (degree)	55.66±22.10	42.37±13.10	26.93±15.67*	6.88±14.14*
Coherence	0.51±0.18	0.51±0.15	0.56±0.20	0.52±0.23
CVR(%/mmHg)	2.18±0.80	2.76±0.85	1.53±0.84*	0.98±0.67*

MCA, middle cerebral artery; RoRc, rate of recovery, CVR: cerebrovascular reactivity;
*p<0.05, compared with normal controls.

distribution of the 32 stenotic MCAs was as follows: mild stenosis, 8 hemispheres; moderate stenosis, 11 hemispheres; and severe stenosis, 13 hemispheres.

The average $PETCO_2$ was 33.10±5.06 mmHg during normocapnia, and 46.21±4.15 mmHg during hypercapnia. And the rebreathing procedure induced an increase of ABP about 3.98±4.23 mmHg.

Time and frequency analysis of cerebral autoregulation using transfer function were shown in Fig. 1 and the corresponded statistical analysis was given in Table 2 and Fig. 2. In the time domain, the averaged step response estimated from the controls was evidently steeper than hemispheres with mild stenosis (Fig. 2A,E). The step response could rapidly reach the baseline level within approximately 3 seconds for the controls, whilst it took 4 seconds for the hemispheres with mild stenosis, indicating a slower recovery of blood flow for the mild stenotic hemispheres, if ABP changed in a step-wise manner. The situation became even worse as stenosis develops, where, in moderate to severe stenosis, the averaged step responses were almost flat, implying cerebral blood flow could not be regulated to the baseline level within 5 seconds. The autoregulatory parameter, RoRc, showed a trend towards poorer value, but only moderate to severe stenosis reached statistic significance (Fig. 3A). The decrease of the RoRc was significantly correlated with the degree of stenosis (correlation coefficients $= -0.70$, $p<0.001$).

In the frequency domain, the gain estimated from the controls and the patients all showed the shape of a high-pass filter, suggesting autoregulation was active (Fig. 2B). However, the shape showed a trend towards flat from mild to severe stenosis (Fig. 2F). The mean values (see Table 2) of gain at 0.06–0.12 Hz was decreased gradually when the stenosis became more severe, which was significantly correlated (correlation coefficients $= -0.41$, $p = 0.02$) with the degree of stenosis. In Fig. 1C, D, we observed that the phase at 0.06–0.12 Hz reduced as stenosis towards severe degree. ANOVA indicated that compared with controls, MCAs with moderate to severe stenosis showed pronounced reduction of phase shift (Fig. 3B). And Decrement of Phase shift was highly correlated with the degree of stenosis (correlation coefficient $= -0.74$, $p<0.001$). But there was no significant difference between cases and controls in coherence (Table 2).

With respect to CVR, the value was also significantly reduced in hemispheres with moderate to severe stenosis compared with controls (Table 2, Fig. 3C). The decrement of CVR was well correlated with the degree of stenosis (correlation coefficient $= -0.69$, $p<0.001$).

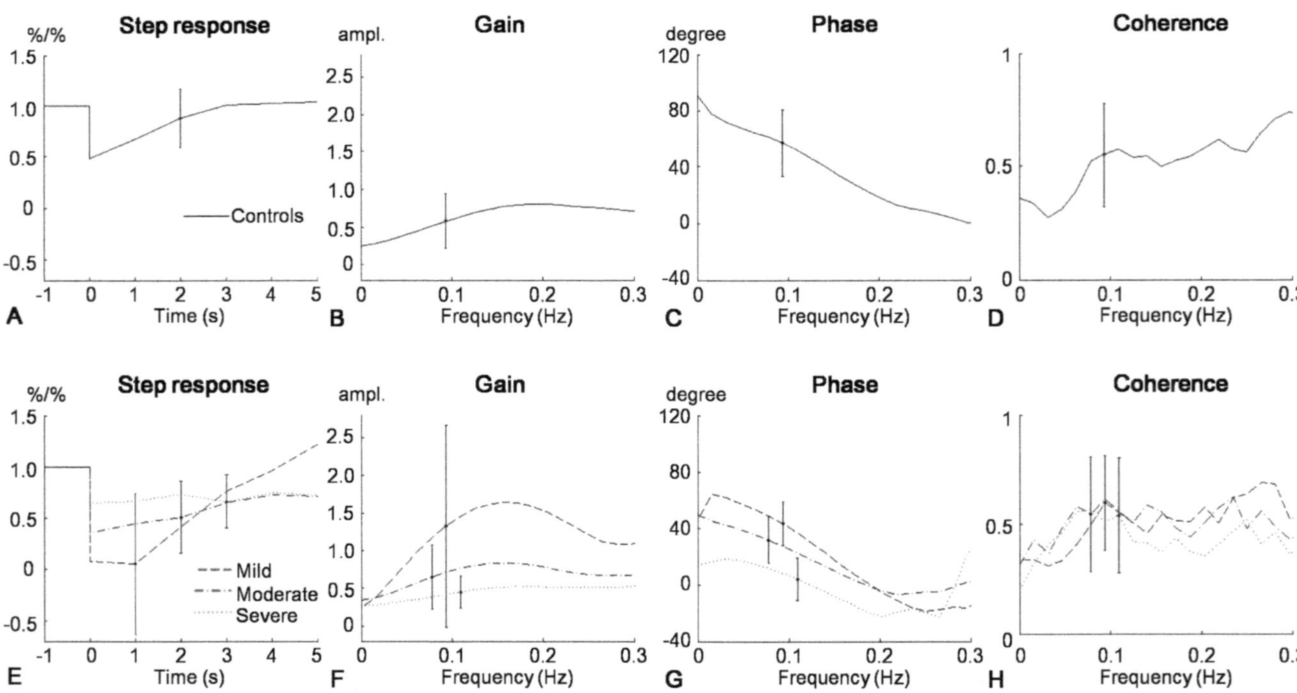

Figure 2. Time and frequency domain analysis of cerebral autoregulation using transfer function. The figures in rows are the averaged step response, gain, phase, and coherence function, respectively for the controls (**A–D**) and patients with middle cerebral artery stenosis (**E–H**), derived from the transfer function. As defined in (**E**), different line styles in the patients' row denote the stages, where mild, moderate, severe stenosis are the dashed, dashed-dotted, dotted, respectively. Each vertical bar shows the averaged standard deviation of the plotted parameter.

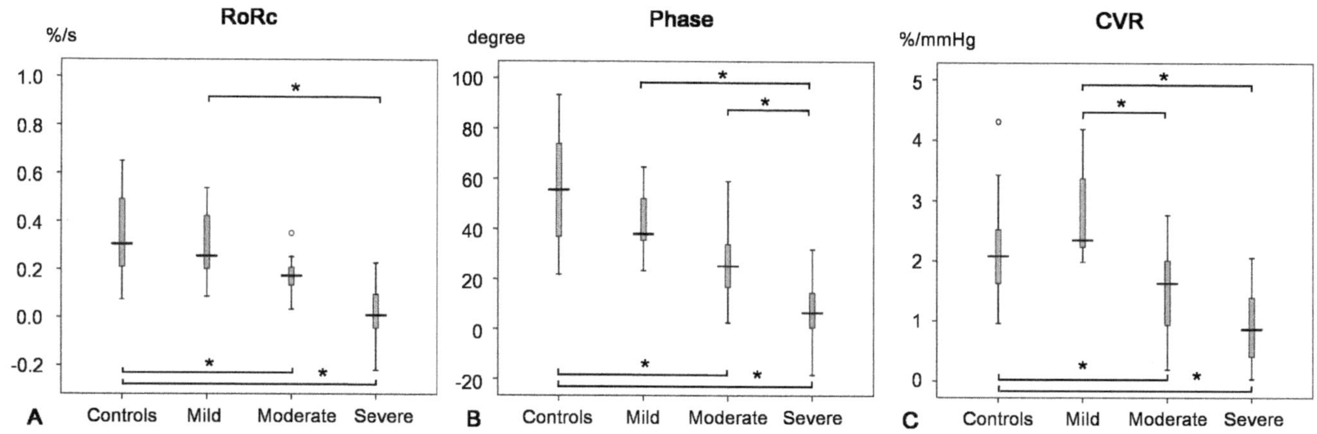

Figure 3. Box plots of cerebral autoregulation and cerebrovascular reactivity (CVR). The figures in rows are the rate of recovery (RoRc) (**A**), phase (**B**), and CVR (**C**) according to the degree of middle cerebral artery (MCA) stenosis. * denotes $p<0.05$ between the groups. ○ denotes exceeding values (>1.5 box length).

The CVR was significantly correlated with phase shift and RoRc, with the correlation coefficient of 0.44 and 0.38 ($p<0.001$), pooling all hemisphere ($n = 71$).

Discussion

In general, the autoregulatory parameters (phase/RoRc) derived from transfer function showed that the effectiveness of cerebral autoregulation is inversely correlated with the degree of stenosis. CVR is also significantly decreased with respect to the degree of stenosis. We also found that the measures of both mechanisms were significantly correlated. These major findings are in line with previous studies on cerebral autoregulation and CVR [15,16,23].

It is however worth noting that the transfer function gain estimated in the patients with mild stenosis is higher than that in the controls. Though it is expected that impaired autoregulation results in higher gain as it indicates a less dampening effect, this finding, however, disagrees with previous studies on ICA and MCA stenosis [3,11,15]. One possible reason for this is that we defined mild stenosis with lower degree of stenosis (<50%) which may merely cause subtle dilation of arterioles, allowing more passive changes of CBFV in amplitude with respect to the changes of ABP. However, in the previous studies, authors reported decreased gain when mild stenosis was defined with higher degree of stenosis [3,11,15]. The decreased gain in their studies was attributed to the inability to achieve active diameter changes in fully (or almost fully) dilated arterioles, resulting in decreased CBFV amplitude oscillations [3,11].The higher gain also led to amplified changes of the step response when comparing with other stages. Furthermore, this can also explain the slightly 'better' CVR than the controls as we observed in Fig. 3C, as impaired autoregulation may trigger 'passive autoregulation' due to a possible rise in ABP associated with inspiration of increased levels of inspired CO_2 [24]. However, further investigation on this is required to confirm.

We found significant but relatively low correlation coefficients between CVR and the autoregulatory parameters – the phase shift and RoRc (0.44 and 0.38 for phase and RoRc, respectively). This is in consistent with previous study in ICA stenosis [2]. We consider that the relatively low correlation might indicate that the impairment of cerebral autoregulation is only partially attributed to the vasodilation caused by stenosis, as cerebral autoregulation and CVR are intrinsically two different mechanisms [25,26]. Indeed, we did observe evident increase of CBFV and ABP (more than 10 mmHg increment in ABP in two cases) in response to the rebreathing test, which imposes a multivariate process of the hemodynamics. The current TFA assuming cerebral autoregulation as a univariate process may therefore fail to interpret it. Multivariate modeling techniques developed by a number of recent studies might be helpful in the future study of this interactive dynamics [27–30].

Although artery-to-artery embolism is considered as the major mechanism causing ischemia in intracranial atherosclerotic disease, hypo-perfusion with impaired embolism clearance may also play a role [31]. In patients with intracranial occlusive disease, only pial or menigeal collaterals are available to maintain the cerebral perfusion pressure [32]. When collaterals are not adequate, decreases in perfusion pressure may lead to vasodilation of cerebral arterioles and potential impairment of cerebral reserve capacity. Using TCD to test CVR is a non-invasive and non-pharmacologic technique to access the cerebral reserve capacity after intracranial stenosis. And our study showed that both autoregulation and CVR reduction are linearly correlated with degree of MCA stenosis. Thus the assessment of these two hemodynamic mechanisms might thus be helpful in monitoring the progress of MCA stenosis.

According to our results, cerebral autoregulation was significantly impaired in patients with moderate to severe MCA stenosis. Therefore, it should be cautious when considering antihypertensive therapy for these patients, as cerebral blood flow may become 'vulnerable' to the changes of ABP. For instance, drops in ABP might result in hypo-perfusion, that may impair the clearance of emboli and thereby increase the risk of ischemia. Thus assessment of cerebral hemodynamics in patients with intracranial stenosis should be considered, especially for the guidance of hypertensive therapy.

In summary, this study shows that cerebral autoregulation and CVR are impaired in patients with moderate to severe MCA stenosis. Furthermore, with increasing degree of stenosis, the impairment of autoregulation and CVR tend to be worsened. The assessment of these two hemodynamic mechanisms might thus be helpful in monitoring the progress of MCA stenosis.

Acknowledgments

The authors would like to thank the participants who gave their time to the study.

Author Contributions

Conceived and designed the experiments: JC JL WHX SG LYC. Performed the experiments: JC RX JL BH WHX SG. Analyzed the data: JC JL BH. Wrote the paper: JC JL WHX SG.

References

1. Wong LK (2006) Global burden of intracranial atherosclerosis. Int J Stroke 1: 158–159.
2. Hu HH, Kuo TB, Wong WJ, Luk YO, Chern CM, et al. (1999) Transfer function analysis of cerebral hemodynamics in patients with carotid stenosis. J Cereb Blood Flow Metab 19: 460–465.
3. Diehl RR, Diehl B, Sitzer M, Hennerici M (1991) Spontaneous oscillations in cerebral blood flow velocity in normal humans and in patients with carotid artery disease. Neurosci Lett 127: 5–8.
4. Reinhard M, Gerds TA, Grabiak D, Zimmermann PR, Roth M, et al. (2008) Cerebral dysautoregulation and the risk of ischemic events in occlusive carotid artery disease. J Neurol 255: 1182–1189.
5. Marshall RS, Rundek T, Sproule DM, Fitzsimmons BF, Schwartz S, et al. (2003) Monitoring of cerebral vasodilatory capacity with transcranial Doppler carbon dioxide inhalation in patients with severe carotid artery disease. Stroke 34: 945–949.
6. Ziyeh S, Rick J, Reinhard M, Hetzel A, Mader I, et al. (2005) Blood oxygen level-dependent MRI of cerebral CO2 reactivity in severe carotid stenosis and occlusion. Stroke 36: 751–756.
7. Markus H, Cullinane M (2001) Severely impaired cerebrovascular reactivity predicts stroke and TIA risk in patients with carotid artery stenosis and occlusion. Brain 124: 457–467.
8. King A, Serena J, Bornstein NM, Markus HS (2011) Does impaired cerebrovascular reactivity predict stroke risk in asymptomatic carotid stenosis? A prospective substudy of the asymptomatic carotid emboli study. Stroke 42: 1550–1555.
9. Reinhard M, Roth M, Müller T, Guschlbauer B, Timmer J, et al. (2004) Effect of carotid endarterectomy or stenting on impairment of dynamic cerebral autoregulation. Stroke 35:1381–1387.
10. Panerai RB (2008) Cerebral autoregulation: from models to clinical applications. Cardiovasc Eng 8: 42–59.
11. Reinhard M, Müller T, Guschlbauer B, Timmer J, Hetzel A (2003) Transfer function analysis for clinical evaluation of dynamic cerebral autoregulation—a comparison between spontaneous and respiratory-induced oscillations. Physiol Meas 24: 27–43.
12. Liu J, Simpson DM, Allen R (2005) High spontaneous fluctuation in arterial blood pressure improves the assessment of cerebral autoregulation. Physiol Meas 26: 725–741.
13. Zhang R, Zuckerman JH, Giller CA, Levine BD (1998) Transfer function analysis of dynamic cerebral autoregulation in humans. Am J Physiol 274: H233–H241.
14. Chen J, Liu J, Duan L, Xu R, Han YQ, et al. (2013) Impaired dynamic cerebral autoregulation in moyamoya disease.CNS Neurosci Ther 19: 638–640.
15. Haubrich C, Kruska W, Diehl RR, Möller-Hartmann W, Klötzsch C (2003) Dynamic autoregulation testing in patients with middle cerebral artery stenosis. Stroke 34: 1881–1885.
16. Gong XP, Li Y, Jiang WJ, Wang Y (2006) Impaired dynamic cerebral autoregulation in middle cerebral artery stenosis. Neurol Res 28: 76–81.
17. Aries MJ, Elting JW, De Keyser J, Kremer BP, Vroomen PC (2010) Cerebral autoregulation in stroke: a review of transcranial Doppler studies. Stroke 41: 2697–2704.
18. Matsushita K, Kuriyama Y, Nagatsuka K, Nakamura M, Sawada T, et al. (1994) Periventricular white matter lucency and cerebral blood flow autoregulation in hypertensive patients. Hypertension 23: 565–568.
19. Kozera GM, Dubaniewicz M, Zdrojewski T, Madej-Dmochowska A, Mielczarek M, et al. (2010) Cerebral vasomotor reactivity and extent of white matter lesions in middle-aged men with arterial hypertension: a pilot study. Am J Hypertens 23:1198–1203.
20. Scheltens P, Erkinjunti T, Leys D, Wahlund LO, Inzitari D, et al. (1998) White matter changes on CT and MRI: an overview of visual rating scales. European Task Force on Age-Related White Matter Changes. Eur Neurol 39: 80–99.
21. Sloan MA, Alexandrov AV, Tegeler CH, Spencer MP, Caplan LR, et al. (2004) Assessment: transcranial Doppler ultrasonography: report of the Therapeutics and Technology Assessment Subcommittee of the American Academy of Neurology. Neurology 62: 1468–1481.
22. Wong KS, Lam WW, Liang E, Huang YN, Chan YL, et al. (1996) Variability of magnetic resonance angiography and computed tomography angiography in grading middle cerebral artery stenosis. Stroke 27: 1084–1087.
23. Lee JY, Lee YS (2011) Vasomotor reactivity in middle cerebral artery stenosis. J Neurol Sci 301: 35–37.
24. White RP, Markus HS (1997) Impaired dynamic cerebral autoregulation in carotid artery stenosis. Stroke 28: 1340–1344.
25. Birns J, Jarosz J, Markus HS, Kalra L (2009) Cerebrovascular reactivity and dynamic autoregulation in ischemic subcortical white matter disease. J Neurol Neurosurg Psychiatry 80: 1093–1098.
26. van Lieshout JJ, Wieling W (2003) Perfusion of the human brain: a matter of interactions. J Physiol 551: 402.
27. Marmarelis VZ, Shin DC, Orme ME, Zhang R (2013) Closed-loop dynamic modeling of cerebral hemodynamics. Ann Biomed Eng 41:1029–1048.
28. Kostoglou K, Debert CT, Poulin MJ, Mitsis GD (2013) Nonstationary multivariate modeling of cerebral autoregulation during hypercapnia. Med Eng Phys. In press.
29. Peng T, Rowley AB, Ainslie PN, Poulin MJ, Payne SJ (2008) Multivariate system identification for cerebral autoregulation. Ann Biomed Eng 36:308–320.
30. Liu J, Koochakpour H, Panerai RB, Katsogridakis E, Wang Z, et al. (2013) Tracking instantaneous pressure-to-flow dynamics of cerebral autoregulation induced by CO2 reactivity. Conf Proc IEEE Eng Med Biol Soc. 2013:3929–3932.
31. Caplan LR, Wong KS, Gao S, Hennerici MG (2006) Is hypoperfusion an important cause of strokes? If so, how? Cerebrovasc Dis 21:145–153.
32. Lau AY, Wong EH, Wong A, Mok VC, Leung TW, et al. (2012) Significance of good collateral compensation in symptomatic intracranial atherosclerosis. Cerebrovasc Dis 33:517–524.

Inpatient Coronary Angiography and Revascularisation following Non-ST-Elevation Acute Coronary Syndrome in Patients with Renal Impairment: A Cohort Study Using the Myocardial Ischaemia National Audit Project

Catriona Shaw[1,2]*, Dorothea Nitsch[3], Retha Steenkamp[1], Cornelia Junghans[4], Sapna Shah[5], Donal O'Donoghue[6], Damian Fogarty[7], Clive Weston[8], Claire C. Sharpe[2]

1 UK Renal Registry, Southmead Hospital, Bristol, United Kingdom, **2** Department of Renal Sciences, Division of Transplantation Immunology and Mucosal Biology, Kings College London, London, United Kingdom, **3** London School of Hygiene and Tropical Medicine, London, United Kingdom, **4** Department of Epidemiology and Public Health, University College London, London, United Kingdom, **5** Department of Renal Medicine, Kings College Hospital, London, United Kingdom, **6** Department of Renal Medicine, Salford Royal NHS Foundation Trust, Salford, United Kingdom, **7** Department of Renal Medicine, Belfast Health and Social CareTrust, Belfast, Northern Ireland, United Kingdom, **8** Myocardial Ischaemia National Audit Project, College of Medicine, Swansea University, Swansea, Wales, United Kingdom

Abstract

Background: International guidelines support an early invasive management strategy (including early coronary angiography and revascularisation) for non-ST-elevation acute coronary syndrome (NSTE-ACS) in patients with renal impairment. However, evidence from outside the UK suggests that this approach is underutilised. We aimed to describe practice within the NHS, and to determine whether the severity of renal dysfunction influenced the provision of angiography and modified the association between early revascularisation and survival.

Methods: We performed a cohort study, using multivariable logistic regression and propensity score analyses, of data from the Myocardial Ischaemia National Audit Project for patients presenting with NSTE-ACS to English or Welsh hospitals between 2008 and 2010.

Findings: Of 35 881 patients diagnosed with NSTE-ACS, eGFR of <60 ml/minute/1.73 m^2 was present in 15 680 (43.7%). There was a stepwise decline in the odds of undergoing inpatient angiography with worsening renal dysfunction. Compared with an eGFR>90 ml/minute/1.73 m^2, patients with an eGFR between 45–59 ml/minute/1.73 m^2 were 33% less likely to undergo angiography (adjusted OR 0.67, 95% CI 0.55–0.81); those with an eGFR<30/minute/1.73 m^2 had a 64% reduction in odds of undergoing angiography (adjusted OR 0.36, 95%CI 0.29–0.43). Of 16 646 patients who had inpatient coronary angiography, 58.5% underwent inpatient revascularisation. After adjusting for co-variables, inpatient revascularisation was associated with approximately a 30% reduction in death within 1 year compared with those managed medically after coronary angiography (adjusted OR 0.66, 95%CI 0.57–0.77), with no evidence of modification by renal function (p interaction = 0.744).

Interpretation: Early revascularisation may offer a similar survival benefit in patients with and without renal dysfunction, yet renal impairment is an important determinant of the provision of coronary angiography following NSTE-ACS. A randomised controlled trial is needed to evaluate the efficacy of an early invasive approach in patients with severe renal dysfunction to ensure that all patients who may benefit are offered this treatment option.

Editor: Joshua M. Hare, University of Miami Miller School of Medicine, United States of America

Funding: The authors have no support or funding to report.

Competing Interests: The authors have declared that no competing interests exist.

* E-mail: catriona.shaw@nbt.nhs.uk

Introduction

Thirty to forty percent of patients presenting with NSTE-ACS have renal impairment [1]. Compared with patients with preserved renal function those with impairment have a 2–5 fold greater risk of death after NSTE-ACS; those with most severe renal impairment being at highest risk [2]. The projected annual cost to the National Health Service (NHS) of additional cardiovascular events occurring in patients with chronic kidney disease (12 000 myocardial infarctions and 7 000 strokes per year) is £174–178 million [3].

Generally an 'early invasive' approach after NSTE-ACS – characterised by routine coronary angiography, followed where possible by early percutaneous or surgical revascularisation – has been demonstrated to improve patient survival [4]. Yet patients with renal impairment were under-represented in the clinical trials that showed this benefit [5]. Current European and American guidelines advise early angiography after NSTE-ACS *irrespective* of renal function [6,7]. However, several reports from outside the UK suggest that patients with renal dysfunction are significantly less likely to undergo angiography or subsequent revascularisation [1,8–10]. Reasons for this discrepancy, between guidelines and practice, are likely to be complex. Remaining uncertainty as to whether renal dysfunction negates the benefit associated with early revascularisation may contribute.

We used data from the Myocardial Ischaemia National Audit Project (MINAP) to describe and quantify use of an early invasive approach after NSTE-ACS in those with normal and those with impaired renal function in NHS clinical practice. We investigated the association between inpatient coronary angiography and death. Furthermore, for patients undergoing inpatient angiography, we investigated whether renal dysfunction at the time of presentation modified the association between revascularisation and death within 1 year.

Methods

Study Population

Care of patients presenting with ACS to all acute NHS hospitals in England and Wales are monitored through MINAP [11–13]. Briefly, each patient entry contains prospectively collected information on aspects of diagnosis, investigation and management. The project uses highly secure electronic systems of data entry and transmission, and allows linkage with the NHS Central Register for mortality tracking. Assurance of data quality involves continual monitoring of key fields and an annual validation exercise. MINAP is supported by the British Cardiovascular Society under the auspices of the National Institute for Cardiovascular Outcomes Research (NICOR) and is commissioned and funded by the Healthcare Quality Improvement Partnership.

Anonymised data from an adult population with a diagnosis of NSTE-ACS admitted to hospital between 1st Jan 2008 and 31st March 2010 were used. The diagnosis of NSTE-ACS was made by the local clinician using their judgement of presenting symptoms and requiring elevated blood troponin concentration, with or without electrocardiographic changes consistent with ischaemia. Patients with ST elevation were excluded from this analysis.

Study Exposures

The first single serum creatinine (μmol/l) within 24 hours of admission was used to estimate the glomerular filtration rate (eGFR) in ml/minute/1.73 m^2 using the equation developed by the Chronic Kidney Disease Epidemiology Collaboration (CKD EPI) [14]. All creatinine values were assumed not to have been calibrated by isotope dilution mass spectrometry and therefore were multiplied by a 0.95 standardisation factor. Renal function was initially categorised as eGFR>90 ml/minute/1.73 m^2, eGFR 60–90 ml/minute/1.73 m^2, eGFR 45–59 ml/minute/1.73 m^2, eGFR 30–44 ml/minute/1.73 m^2, eGFR 15–29 ml/minute/1.73 m^2 and <15 ml/minute/1.73 m^2 for the descriptive analysis [15]. As relatively low numbers of patients with an eGFR 15–29 ml/minute/1.73 m^2 and <15 ml/minute/1.73 m^2 underwent inpatient coronary angiography or inpatient revascularisation the two eGFR categories were combined for subsequent analyses (eGFR<30 ml/minute/1.73 m^2].

Inpatient revascularisation was defined as inpatient percutaneous coronary intervention (PCI) or coronary artery bypass grafting (CABG). Patients were categorised as medically managed following inpatient coronary angiography if i) PCI or CABG was planned after discharge, or ii) the patient refused such interventions, or iii) the procedures were neither planned nor performed during the index admission.

Study Outcomes

The primary study outcomes were performance of inpatient coronary angiography – dichotomised as performed or not performed – and all-cause death within one year of presentation. Patients who died on the day of admission were excluded from analyses.

Confounder Variables

Demographic factors included age (10 year categories), sex, ethnicity, hospital of admission and self- reported smoking status. The Index of Multiple Deprivation was included. This index reflects information on the seven domains of income: employment; health and disability; education, skills and training; barriers to housing and services; living environment; and crime [16]. Co-morbidities included a history of hypertension, previous angina, previous myocardial infarction, hyperlipidaemia, peripheral vascular disease, cerebrovascular disease, chronic obstructive airways disease, congestive cardiac failure, diabetes mellitus, previous PCI and previous CABG. Haemoglobin (g/dl) recorded within 24 hours of admission and peak troponin were also used.

We lacked direct measurements of left ventricular function. Surrogates for reduced function included a history of congestive cardiac failure or previous myocardial infarction. Systolic blood pressure (SBP) and heart rate at the time of admission are validated prognostic markers in ACS and thought to be representative of the degree of acute left ventricular dysfunction [17]. The first SBP (mmHg) recorded after admission to hospital was used. If the patient presented with a treatable tachyarrhythmia, the first stable SBP after treatment was used. The heart rate (beats/minute) was recorded from the first ECG after admission to hospital, whilst in a stable cardiac rhythm. The ECG appearances at presentation were included (normal, left bundle branch block, ST segment depression, T wave changes only, other abnormality).

Statistical Analyses

All statistical analyses were done using STATA version 11.2.

Confounder exposure associations were cross-tabulated both in the full study population and in the subgroup of patients undergoing inpatient coronary angiography. The frequency and proportions of missing data within each variable were tabulated and distributions of population characteristics for participants included in the complete case analysis were compared with individuals who were excluded due to incomplete data on the *a priori* variables.

Univariable and then multivariable logistic regression models adjusted for all study covariables were used to estimate the odds ratio for the association between eGFR category and undergoing inpatient coronary angiography. Robust standard errors were used to account for clustering at hospital level.

Logistic regression models were also used to assess the association between inpatient coronary angiography and all-cause death. As it was expected that in some cases those that did not undergo inpatient angiography would vary substantially in their baseline characteristics compared with those that did, a propensity score was estimated to help ensure adequate overlap between the distributions of confounders in the two treatment groups [18]. The analysis was repeated restricting to a sub group of the cohort with improved balance in baseline co-variables. The propensity score was the conditional probability that an individual had inpatient coronary angiography and was obtained for each individual by fitting a logistic regression model with outcome inpatient coronary

Table 1. Selected covariates stratified by eGFR category at time of presentation in 35 881 adults presenting with non-ST-elevation acute coronary syndrome (all data is presented as numbers with column percentage unless otherwise stated).

	eGFR (ml/minute/1.73 m²)					
	>90	60–90	45–59	30–44	15–29	<15
	N=6 482	N=13 719	N=6 990	N=5 452	N=2 665	N=573
Demographic						
Male gender	4781(73.8)	9223(67.2)	4010(57.4)	2749(50.4)	1326(49.8)	336(58.6)
Age, median (IQR)	58(50–66)	72(63–80)	79(72–85)	83(77–88)	84(78–88)	80(73–86)
Past Medical History						
Hypertension	2680(41.4)	7089(51.7)	4161(59.5)	3375(61.9)	1671(62.7)	387(67.5)
Stroke	333(5.1)	1276(9.3)	950(13.6)	883(16.2)	439(16.5)	107(18.7)
PVD	241(3.7)	591(4.3)	442 (6.3)	390(7.2)	235(8.8)	71(12.4)
Treated hyperlipidaemia	2243(34.6)	4805(35.0)	2449(35.0)	1866(34.2)	854(32.1)	177(30.9)
CCF	128(2.0)	723(5.3)	688(9.8)	917(16.8)	584(21.9)	106(18.5)
Previous MI	1382(21.3)	3964(28.9)	2662(38.1)	2394(43.9)	1318(49.5)	256(44.7)
Previous PCI	787(12.1)	1488(10.9)	727(10.4)	549(10.1)	227(8.5)	52(9.1)
Previous CABG	362(5.6)	1121(8.2)	695(9.9)	536(9.8)	256(9.6)	57(10.0)
Diabetes Mellitus	1150(17.7)	2727(19.9)	1748(25.0)	1735 (31.8)	965(36.2)	235(41.0)
Current smoker	2820(43.5)	2948(21.5)	950(13.6)	520(9.5)	237(8.9)	59(10.3)
Diagnostics						
Haemoglobin (g/dl), median (IQR)	14.2(13.0–15.2)	13.8(12.4–15.0)	13.0(11.7–14.1)	12.0(10.9–13.5)	11.3(10.0–12.6)	10.6(9.5–12.0)
Peak Troponin, median(IQR)	0.7(0.2–3.1)	0.7(0.2–3.3)	0.8(0.2–3.9)	0.9(0.2–4.1)	1.2(0.3–5.3)	1.7(0.4–8.2)
Systolic blood pressure (mmHg), mean (sd)	143(26)	144(28)	142(29)	140(30)	135(31)	137(33)
Heart rate (beats/min), median (IQR)	77(66–90)	78(66–93)	82(69–99)	85(71–101)	85(71–100)	86 (71–100)
IP Coronary angiography	4720(72.8)	7445(54.3)	2613(37.4)	1366(25.1)	416(15.6)	86(15.0)
IP revascularisation	2992(46.2)	4422(32.2)	1370(19.6)	697(12.8)	205(7.7)	46(8.0)
IP PCI	2758(42.5)	3977(29.0)	1208(17.3)	609(11.2)	183(6.9)	44(7.7)
IP CABG	234(3.6)	445(3.2)	162(2.3)	88(1.6)	22(0.8)	2(0.3)

Abbreviations: IMD score = score of deprivation; PVD = peripheral vascular disease; CCF = congestive cardiac failure; MI = myocardial infarction; PCI = percutaneous coronary intervention; CABG = coronary artery bypass graft; eGFR = estimated glomerular filtration rate; IP - inpatient; IQR = interquartile range; sd = standard deviation.

angiography with all the pre-specified co-variables included. All of the pre-specified co-variables were considered *a priori* confounders.

Diagnostic coronary angiography is a pre-requisite for being considered for revascularisation. The analysis to evaluate whether renal dysfunction modified patient survival after inpatient coronary revascularisation compared with medical management was therefore limited to individuals who underwent inpatient coronary angiography. Again a propensity score was estimated to help ensure adequate overlap between the distributions of confounders in the two treatment groups. The propensity score was the conditional probability that an individual had inpatient revascularisation, and was obtained for each individual by fitting a logistic regression model with outcome inpatient revascularisation with all the pre-specified co-variables. After estimation of the conditional propensity score one patient from the medically managed group was excluded as they could not be matched due to a very low propensity score. Improved balance in the distribution in the co-variables between the two treatment groups was achieved (Appendix S1). Multivariable logistic regression analysis was subsequently carried out using robust standard errors with outcome death or alive within one year. Evidence of effect modification between eGFR category and inpatient revascularisation or medical management on the odds of death within one year was tested (Wald test). Evidence of effect modification between gender and inpatient revascularisation or medical management was also tested [19]. The interaction terms were maintained in the model at a threshold of $p<0.01$. Results are presented as multivariable adjusted odds ratios with 95% confidence intervals.

Sensitivity Analyses

Logistic regression with the propensity score included as the single co-variable was conducted. Robust standard errors and bootstrapping methods (50 repetitions) were used.

To evaluate possible bias introduced by patients who died early after admission to hospital the analyses were repeated using a cohort limited to individuals who survived five days or more.

Secondary preventative medications including aspirin, clopidogrel, ACE inhibitors, beta-blockers and statins have been shown to influence outcome after NSTE-ACS [20–23]. Whether these medications were prescribed at time of discharge was included in the multivariable model evaluating the association between inpatient revascularisation and death within one year.

Sensitivity analysis using datasets derived using multiple imputation was also conducted [24].

Ethical Approval

Ethics committee (11/L0/0246), Kings College Hospital Research and Development (KCH11-081), and MINAP Academic Group approvals were obtained prior to commencement of the analysis.

Results

Renal Impairment at the Time of Presentation with NSTE-ACS and Subsequent Inpatient Coronary Angiography

GFR could not be estimated for 18.2% (16 632/91 342) due to missing data on creatinine, gender, age or ethnicity (Appendix S2). Data was missing regarding coronary angiography in 4.5%, management strategy (inpatient revascularisation or medical management) in 18.3% and for mortality in <1% of patients. 15.8% of individuals excluded from the complete case analysis due to incomplete data died compared with 19.0% of those included (Appendix S3). Complete data on all co-variables was available in 35 881 cases. Approximately 40% (n = 15 680/35 881) had an eGFR<60 ml/minute/1.73 m^2, and 9.0% (n = 3 238) an eGFR< 30 ml/minute/1.73 m^2 (Table 1). The median age was 75 years, and 22 425 (62.5%) were male. Individuals with impaired renal function tended to be older, with a higher co-morbid profile, and more likely to die within 1 year (Table 1, Figure 1).

Inpatient coronary angiography was performed in 16 646 (46.4%) of the cohort. Patients who had inpatient coronary angiography were more likely to be male, younger and have fewer co-morbid conditions than those who did not (Table 2). Death within 1 year occurred in 30.6% patients who did not undergo inpatient coronary angiography compared with 5.7% in those that did. 72.8% of individuals with normal renal function (an eGFR> 90 ml/minute/1.73 m^2) underwent inpatient coronary angiography compared with 15.5% of those with an eGFR<30 ml/minute/1.73 m^2 (Table 1).

After adjusting for all other comorbidities and covariables, there was a stepwise reduction in the odds of undergoing inpatient coronary angiography with increasing severity of renal impairment; a reduction of 33% in patients with eGFR 45–59 ml/minute/1.73 m^2 (adjusted OR 0.67, 95% CI 0.55–0.81), 42% in those with an eGFR between 30–44 ml/minute/1.73 m^2 (adjusted OR 0.58, 95% CI 0.48–0.70), and 64% in those with eGFR< 30 ml/minute/1.73 m^2 (adjusted OR 0.36, 95% CI 0.29–0.43) compared with patients with an eGFR>90 ml/minute/1.73 m^2 (Table 3).

Renal Impairment at the Time of Presentation with NSTE-ACS and the Association between Inpatient Coronary Angiography and Death within 1 Year

In patient coronary angiography was associated with a survival benefit in each eGFR category (Table 4). In those with an eGFR 60–90 ml/minute/1.73 m^2 inpatient coronary angiography was associated with a reduction in the estimated odds of death of 70% (adjusted OR 0.29, 95% CI 0.25–0.33) and by 54% in those with an eGFR<30 ml/minute/1.73 m^2 (adjusted OR 0.46, 95%CI 0.36–0.58). On restricting the analysis to a subgroup with improved balance in the distribution of baseline characteristics based on estimated propensity score (N = 16 617), the estimated survival benefit observed did not change, except in those with an eGFR<30 ml/minute/1.73 m^2 in whom the estimated survival benefit was more conservative (adjusted OR 0.59, 95% CI 0.37–0.96) (data not shown).

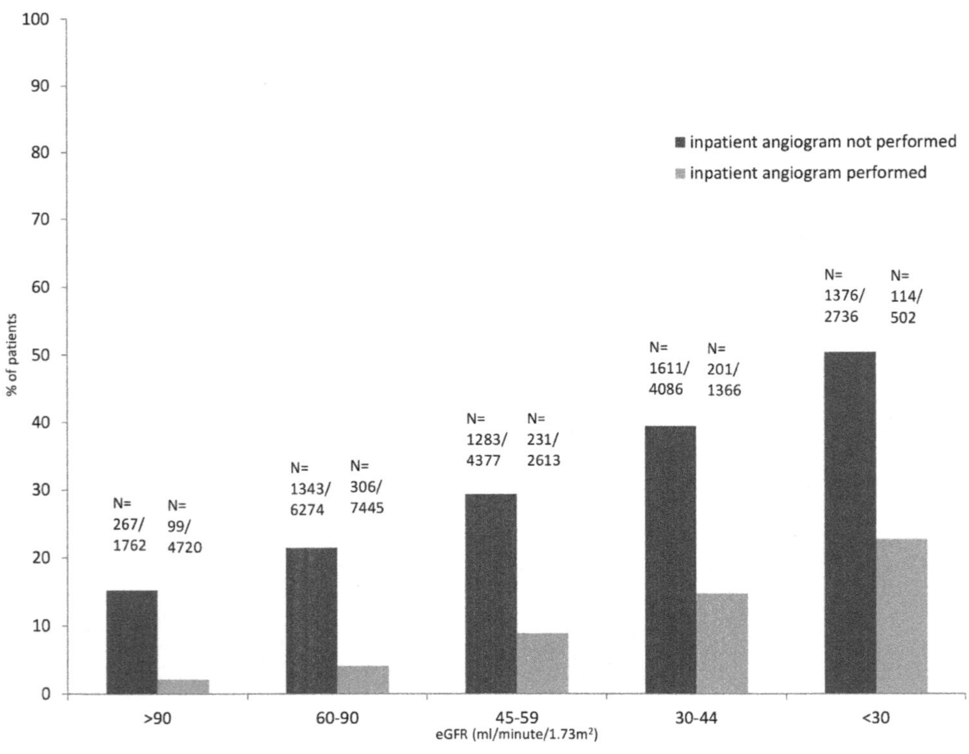

Figure 1. Percentage of patients that died within 1 year after non-ST-elevation acute coronary syndrome. Percentage of patients that died within 1 year after non-ST-elevation acute coronary syndrome stratified by category of estimated glomerular filtration rate at the time of presentation and whether inpatient coronary angiography was performed. *Abbreviations eGFR = estimated glomerular filtration rate; *this analysis included 35 881 patients presenting with NSTE-ACS.

Table 2. Selected covariates stratified by whether inpatient coronary angiography was performed or not, in 35 881 adults presenting with non-ST-elevation acute coronary syndrome (all data is presented as numbers with column percentage unless otherwise stated).

	IP Coronary angiography not performed	IP Coronary angiography performed
	N = 19 235	N = 16 646
Demographic		
Male gender	10 821 (56.3)	11 604 (69.7)
Age in years, median (IQR)	81 (72–87)	68 (56–76)
Past Medical History		
Hypertension	10 631 (55.3)	8 732 (52.5)
Stroke	2 842 (14.8)	1 146 (6.9)
PVD	1 228 (6.4)	7 42 (4.5)
Treated hyperlipidaemia	5 717 (29.7)	6 677 (40.1)
CCF	2 466 (12.8)	680 (4.1)
Previous MI	7 586 (39.4)	4 309 (26.4)
Previous PCI	1 559 (8.3)	2 231 (13.4)
Previous CABG	1 736 (9.0)	1 291 (7.8)
Diabetes Mellitus	5 030 (26.2)	3 530 (21.2)
Current smoker	2 912 (15.1)	46 22 (27.8)
Diagnostics		
Haemoglobin (g/dl), median (IQR)	12.6 (11.0–14.0)	14.0 (12.8–15.0)
Peak Troponin, median (IQR)	0.8 (0.2–3.7)	0.8 (0.2–3.6)
eGFR (ml/minute/1.73 m^2)		
>90	1 762 (9.2)	4 720 (28.4)
60–90	6 274 (32.6)	7 445 (44.7)
45–59	4 377 (22.8)	2 613 (15.7)
30–44	4 086 (21.2)	1 366 (8.2)
15–29	2 249 (11.7)	416 (2.5)
<15	487 (2.5)	86 (0.5)
Systolic blood pressure (mmHg), mean (sd)	140 (29)	145 (27)
Heart rate (beats/min), median (IQR)	84 (70–100)	76 (65–90)

Abbreviations: IP = inpatient; IMD score = score of deprivation; PVD = peripheral vascular disease; CCF = congestive cardiac failure; MI = myocardial infarction; PCI = percutaneous coronary intervention; CABG = coronary artery bypass graft; eGFR = estimated glomerular filtration rate; IQR = interquartile range; sd = standard deviation.

Table 3. Results of the multivariable logistic regression analysis in 35 881 individuals with non-ST-elevation acute coronary syndrome for the association between eGFR and inpatient coronary angiography.

eGFR (ml/minute/1.73 m^2)	Age & gender adjusted OR (95% CI)	P-value (Wald)	Multivariable Adjusted OR (95% CI)*	P-value (Wald)
>90	1		1	
60–90	0.81 (0.71–0.93)	0.003	0.81 (0.70–0.94)	0.006
45–59	0.58 (0.48–0.70)	<0.001	0.67 (0.55–0.81)	<0.001
30–44	0.42 (0.35–0.51)	<0.001	0.58 (0.48–0.70)	<0.001
<30	0.21 (0.18–0.26)	<0.001	0.36 (0.29–0.43)	<0.001

*Multivariable model adjusted for age, ethnicity, gender, IMD score, systolic blood pressure, heart rate, haemoglobin, peak troponin, ECG diagnosis, history of angina, hyperlipidaemia, hypertension, peripheral vascular disease, cerebrovascular disease, chronic obstructive airways disease, congestive cardiac failure, previous percutaneous coronary intervention, previous coronary artery bypass graft, previous myocardial infarction, diabetes, current smoking status and hospital.
Abbreviations: OR = odds ratio; CI = confidence interval; eGFR = estimated glomerular filtration rate.

Table 4. Results of the multivariable logistic regression analysis in 35 881 individuals with non-ST-elevation acute coronary syndrome for the association between inpatient coronary angiography and all-cause death.

eGFR (ml/minute/1·73 m^2)	Inpatient angiography status	Multivariable Adjusted OR (95% CI)*	P-value (Wald)
>90	Inpatient angiography not performed	1	
	Inpatient angiography	0.21 (0.17–0.27)	<0.001
60–90	Inpatient angiography not performed	1	
	Inpatient angiography	0.29 (0.25–0.33)	<0.001
45–59	Inpatient angiography not performed	1	
	Inpatient angiography	0.37 (0.32–0.43)	<0.001
30–44	Inpatient angiography not performed	1	
	Inpatient angiography	0.41 (0.34–0.48)	<0.001
<30	Inpatient angiography not performed	1	
	Inpatient angiography	0.46 (0.36–0.58)	<0.001

*p-interaction (Wald test) between eGFR category and inpatient coronary angiography and mortality: <0.001.
*Multivariable model adjusted for age, ethnicity, gender, IMD score, systolic blood pressure, heart rate, haemoglobin, peak troponin, ECG diagnosis, history of angina, hyperlipidaemia, hypertension, peripheral vascular disease, cerebrovascular disease, chronic obstructive airways disease, congestive cardiac failure, previous percutaneous coronary intervention, previous coronary artery bypass graft, previous myocardial infarction, diabetes, current smoking status and hospital.
Abbreviations: OR = odds ratio; CI = confidence interval; eGFR = estimated glomerular filtration rate.

Renal Impairment at the Time of Presentation with NSTE-ACS and the Association between Inpatient Revascularisation and Death within 1 Year

Of 16 646 patients who had inpatient coronary angiography, 9 732 (58.5%) underwent inpatient revascularisation (Figure 2). On the basis of the propensity score, there was good overlap in the distribution of baseline characteristics between the group that underwent inpatient revascularisation and those who underwent angiography only (Appendix S1). Only 16% of patients with severe renal dysfunction at presentation (eGFR<30 ml/min/1.73 m^2) underwent inpatient coronary angiography and could be considered for early revascularisation. However, of the 502 patients in this renal category that did have diagnostic angiography, nearly 50% underwent subsequent inpatient revascularisation (Table 5). The adjusted odds of undergoing inpatient revascularisation did not vary depending on eGFR category (data not shown).

538 deaths (7.8%) occurred within a year in those patients managed medically after inpatient coronary angiography compared with 413 deaths (4.2%) amongst patients who had inpatient revascularisation. After adjusting for co-variables, inpatient revascularisation was associated with a reduction in the odds of death within 1 year of approximately 30% (adjusted OR 0.66, 95%CI 0.57–0.77) (Table 6). When stratified by eGFR category there was a trend that the relative survival benefit of inpatient revascularisation may be less in those with an eGFR<30 ml/minute/1.73 m^2 (adjusted OR 0.80, 95% CI 0.52–1.24) compared with the other eGFR categories (eGFR 60–90 ml/minute/1.73 m^2 adjusted OR 0.63, 95% CI 0.49–0.81). However the confidence intervals between eGFR categories overlapped and there was no statistical evidence of modification by severity of renal dysfunction on the association between inpatient revascularisation and death (p-interaction = 0.744) (Table 6 and 7). There was weak evidence of effect modification by gender on this association with a trend to a lower adjusted odds of death in women (p-interaction = 0.060).

Sensitivity Analysis

Results of the logistic regression model adjusted for the propensity score as a single co-variable demonstrated a similar reduction in the odds for death within 1 year associated with inpatient revascularisation (adjusted OR 0.68, 95% CI 0.58–0.80, Table 6).

Limiting the analysis to 5-day survivors did not alter the associations observed (Appendix S4a, 4b and 4c).

We repeated the analysis excluding 116 patients who had declined revascularisation. No change in the associations found in our main analysis was observed (data not shown).

Inclusion of aspirin, clopidogrel, ACE inhibitors, beta-blockers or statins prescribed at discharge in the model did not change the adjusted odds for death associated with inpatient revascularisation within 1 year (adjusted OR 0.68, 95% CI 0.57–0.80), with no evidence of modification by severity of renal dysfunction (p-interaction = 0.711).

After multiple imputation, the adjusted odds ratios were marginally more conservative (Appendix S5a and 5b; data not shown for the analysis of the association between inpatient coronary angiography and death).

Discussion

In this study of over 35 000 individuals with NSTE-ACS in England and Wales, admitted to NHS hospitals between 2008 and 2010, we have demonstrated that renal dysfunction is common and that patients with renal impairment are much less likely to undergo inpatient diagnostic coronary angiography than patients with normal renal function. This association was maintained after adjusting for differences in numerous baseline characteristics and comorbidities and was observed across the range of renal impairment, including those patients with moderate renal dysfunction (eGFR 30–59 ml/minute/1.73 m^2). Inpatient coronary angiography was associated with an improved survival. In those patients with moderate renal dysfunction that did undergo inpatient angiography, nearly 50% of patients then underwent

Table 5. Selected covariates stratified by management strategy in 16 646 adults who underwent inpatient coronary angiography presenting with non-ST-elevation acute coronary syndrome.

	In patient Medical Management	In Patient Revascularisation
	N = 6 914	N = 9 732
Demographic		
Male gender	4 552 (65.8)	7 052 (72.5)
Age in years, median (IQR)	69 (60–77)	66 (57–75)
Past Medical History		
Hypertension	3 784 (54.7)	4 948 (50.8)
Stroke	563 (8.1)	583 (6.0)
PVD	359 (5.2)	383 (3.9)
Treated hyperlipidaemia	2 709 (39.2)	3 968 (40.8)
CCF	369 (5.3)	311 (3.2)
Previous MI	2 050 (29.7)	2 340 (24.0)
Previous PCI	912 (13.2)	1 319 (13.6)
Previous CABG	618 (8.9)	673 (6.9)
Diabetes Mellitus	1 594 (23.1)	1 936 (19.9)
Current smoker	1 656 (24.0)	2 966 (30.5)
Diagnostics		
Haemoglobin (g/dl), median (IQR)	13.8 (12.5–15.0)	14.0 (13.0–15.0)
Peak Troponin, median(IQR)	0.9 (0.2–4.0)	0.8 (0.2–3.3)
eGFR (ml/minute/1.73 m^2)		
>90	1 728 (25.0)	2 992 (30.7)
60–90	3 023 (43.7)	4 422 (45.4)
45–59	1 243 (18.0)	1 370 (14.1)
30–44	669 (9.7)	697 (7.2)
15–29	211 (3.1)	205 (2.1)
<15	40 (0.6)	46 (0.5)
Systolic blood pressure (mmHg), mean (sd)	144 (27)	145 (28)
Heart rate (beats/min), median (IQR)	79 (67–93)	76 (65–88)

Abbreviations: PVD = peripheral vascular disease; CCF = congestive cardiac failure; MI = myocardial infarction; PCI = percutaneous coronary intervention; CABG = coronary artery bypass graft; eGFR = estimated glomerular filtration rate; IQR = interquartile range; sd = standard deviation.
All data is presented as numbers with column percentage unless otherwise stated. Where percentages do not equal 100% this is due to rounding.

revascularisation with a similar survival benefit as seen in patients with preserved renal function.

The majority of patients (84%) with severe renal dysfunction (eGFR<30 ml/min/1.73 m^2) did not undergo inpatient diagnostic angiography. Therefore it is unclear whether, amongst this large group without inpatient diagnostic angiography, early revascularisation in those with suitable coronary lesions would have imparted a survival benefit.

Our finding that patients with renal dysfunction are less likely to undergo early coronary angiography than patients with preserved renal function is supported by several other analyses from different health care systems [1,8–10,25]. We suspect that the reasons are complex, reflecting both individual patient and clinician level factors as well as organisational factors spanning community and hospital level care. Patients with renal dysfunction are more likely to present with atypical clinical features [25,26] and not necessarily directly to cardiologists. Clinical uncertainty as to the interpretation of troponin measurements in patients with renal impairment can compound diagnostic difficulties [27]. Concerns regarding the risk of acute kidney injury (AKI), in particular related to contrast-induced AKI, or a presumed increased risk of bleeding complications are also likely to influence management decisions [6,28]. However, recent work suggests the risks of AKI associated with coronary angiography after ACS are overstated [9]. In addition, routine coronary angiography as part of renal transplant work-up in patients with advanced renal impairment is not associated with an accelerated decline in renal function [29]. As many patients with NSTE-ACS undergo angiography on a semi-urgent basis there are opportunities for clinicians to ensure adequate hydration and optimal angiographic practices that reduce the risk of AKI. In a previous study from the GRACE collaboration the most commonly reported reason for foregoing an early-invasive management strategy in those with renal impairment was insufficient risk (37.7%), while concerns over comorbidity (12.5%) and bleeding (7.2%) were minor in comparison [30]. However, the median GRACE score of those patients deemed 'low risk' was paradoxically high. Misrepresentation of risk and resultant denial of early-invasive management may contribute to worse outcomes in patients with renal dysfunction

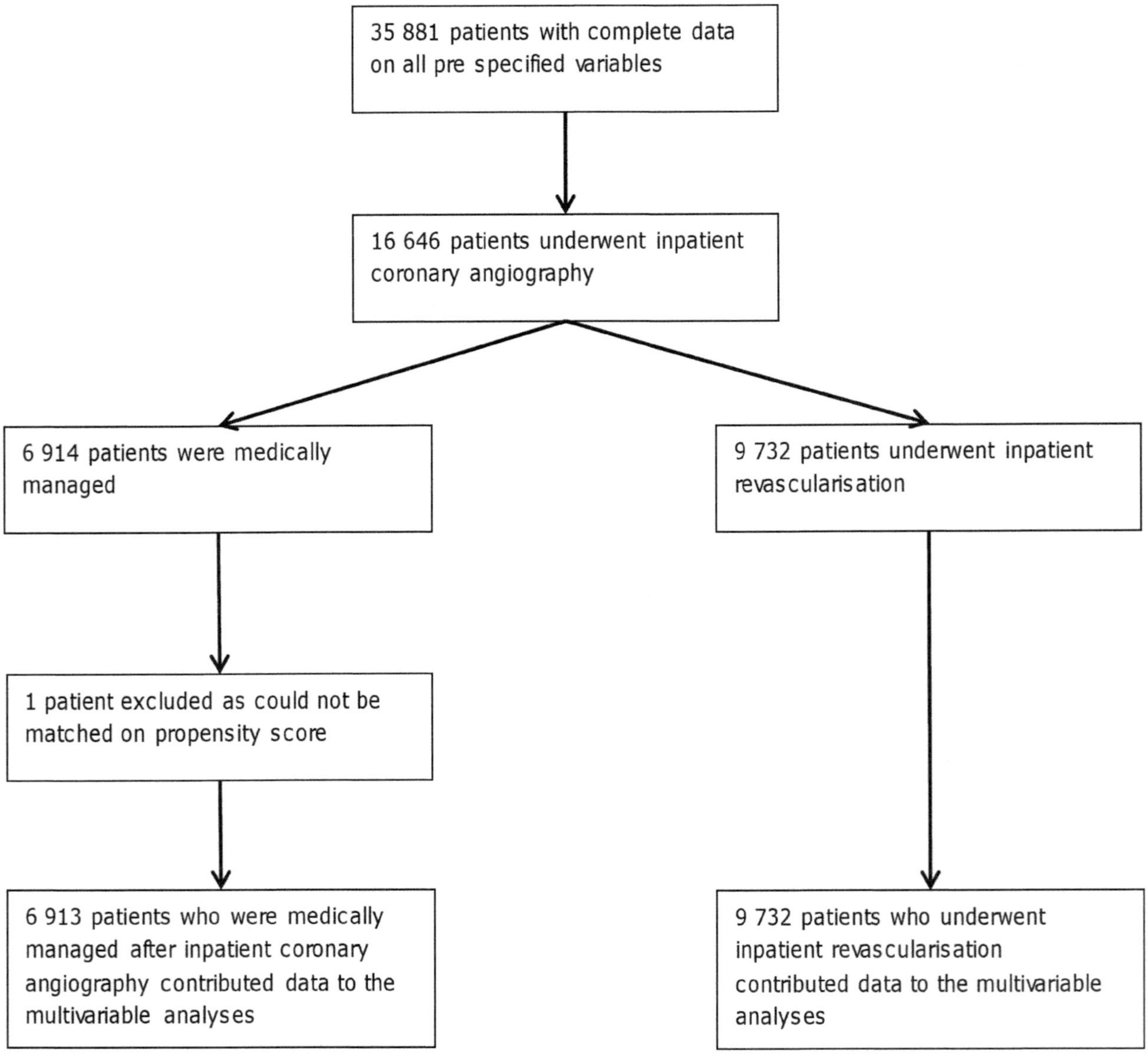

Figure 2. Number of patients in the complete case analysis contributing to various stages of the analysis.

Table 6. Results of the adjusted logistic regression analysis in 16 645 individuals with non-ST-elevation acute coronary syndrome for the association between inpatient revascularisation and mortality compared with individuals who were medically managed after inpatient coronary angiography.

Management Strategy	Age & gender adjusted OR (95% CI)	P-value (Wald)	Multivariable Adjusted OR (95% CI)*	P-value (Wald)	Propensity score adjusted OR (95% CI)	P-value (Wald)
Medical Mx	1		1		1	
In patient Revascularisation	0.60(0.52–0.70)	<0.001	0.66(0.57–0.77)	<0.001	0.68(0.58–0.80)	<0.001

*p-interaction (Wald test) between eGFR category and inpatient revascularisation and mortality: 0.744.
Multivariable Model adjusted for age, ethnicity, gender, IMD score, eGFR, systolic blood pressure, heart rate, haemoglobin, peak troponin, ECG diagnosis, history of angina, hyperlipidaemia, hypertension, peripheral vascular disease, cerebrovascular disease, chronic obstructive airways disease, congestive cardiac failure, previous percutaneous coronary intervention, previous coronary artery bypass graft, previous myocardial infarction, diabetes, current smoking status and hospital.
Propensity Score estimated using age, ethnicity, gender, IMD score, eGFR, systolic blood pressure, heart rate, haemoglobin, peak troponin ECG diagnosis, history of angina, hyperlipidaemia, hypertension, peripheral vascular disease, cerebrovascular disease, chronic obstructive airways disease, congestive cardiac failure, previous percutaneous coronary intervention, previous coronary artery bypass graft, previous myocardial infarction, diabetes, current smoking status.
Abbreviations: Medical Mx = medical management; OR = odds ratio; CI = confidence interval; eGFR = estimated glomerular filtration rate.

Table 7. Results of the adjusted logistic regression analysis in 16 645 individuals with non-ST-elevation acute coronary syndrome for the association between inpatient revascularisation and mortality compared with individuals who were medically managed after inpatient coronary angiography stratified by category of renal dysfunction.

eGFR (ml/minute/1.73 m^2)	Management Strategy	Multivariable Adjusted OR (95% CI)*	P-value (Wald)
>90	Medical Mx	1	
	In patient Revascularisation	0.55(0.36–0.85)	0.008
60–90	Medical Mx	1	
	In patient Revascularisation	0.63(0.49–0.81)	<0.001
45–60	Medical Mx	1	
	In patient Revascularisation	0.69(0.51–0.95)	0.020
30–45	Medical Mx	1	
	In patient Revascularisation	0.68(0.49–0.94)	0.021
<30	Medical Mx	1	
	In patient Revascularisation	0.80(0.52–1.24)	0.320

*p-interaction (Wald test) between eGFR category and inpatient revascularisation and mortality: 0.744.
Multivariable Model adjusted for age, ethnicity, gender, IMD score, eGFR, systolic blood pressure, heart rate, haemoglobin, peak troponin, ECG diagnosis, history of angina, hyperlipidaemia, hypertension, peripheral vascular disease, cerebrovascular disease, chronic obstructive airways disease, congestive cardiac failure, previous percutaneous coronary intervention, previous coronary artery bypass graft, previous myocardial infarction, diabetes, current smoking status and hospital.
Propensity Score estimated using age, ethnicity, gender, IMD score, eGFR, systolic blood pressure, heart rate, haemoglobin, peak troponin ECG diagnosis, history of angina, hyperlipidaemia, hypertension, peripheral vascular disease, cerebrovascular disease, chronic obstructive airways disease, congestive cardiac failure, previous percutaneous coronary intervention, previous coronary artery bypass graft, previous myocardial infarction, diabetes, current smoking status.
Abbreviations: Medical Mx = medical management; OR = odds ratio; CI = confidence interval; eGFR = estimated glomerular filtration rate.

[30], and in other high risk groups in whom the same treatment paradox has been observed [31–33].

Earlier major clinical trials have compared a routine early invasive strategy with a selective invasive strategy after NSTE-ACS, rather than outcomes after revascularisation specifically [4,34–36]. Patients with renal impairment have been under-represented in these studies [5] and no direct RCT evidence regarding an early invasive strategy, or specifically outcomes after revascularisation, are available in patients with renal impairment. A systematic review and meta-analysis of individual level data from five RCTs that had recorded information on renal function suggested that the benefits of an early invasive strategy are preserved in patients with renal impairment, with a trend in reduction of risk of death and non-fatal re-infarction at one year (in patients with chronic kidney disease (CKD) stages 3–5 i.e. an eGFR<60 ml/minute/1.73 m^2, a pooled estimate risk ratio 0.76 (95% CI 0.49–1.17) was reported) [37]. Among the studies included in that meta-analysis the mean age ranged from 59–66 years, 14–28% had diabetes and mortality rates in the 'conservative' arms were 2.5–10%. Patients with CKD accounted for 19.4% (1 453/7 481) with the majority having an eGFR 30–60 ml/minute/1.73 m^2 (80%). Our real world ACS cohort was quite different to those in the RCTs. In our study, the median age was 75 years, 40% had an eGFR at time of presentation of <60 ml/minute/1.73 m^2 and at one year 30% of those who did not undergo inpatient coronary angiography had died.

Our analysis of the outcomes associated with inpatient coronary angiography will have included people in the comparison group (those that did not have inpatient coronary angiography) that would have been excluded from the randomised trials, and would therefore not have been considered for revascularisation, thus suggesting a possibly overoptimistic benefit of an early invasive approach. Some of the benefit observed in our comparison of those receiving and those not receiving inpatient angiography may also reflect other management differences between the groups, such as more aggressive antiplatelet or adjunctive medical therapies in the group in our cohort who underwent inpatient coronary angiography [1]. Thus, to further evaluate whether renal function modified outcomes after inpatient revascularisation we restricted the analysis to those in whom a clinical decision to consider revascularisation had been taken following inpatient coronary angiography.

Previous registry-based analyses have reported varied results. Data from the SWEDEHEART registry suggested that early revascularisation improved 1-year survival in patients with NSTE-ACS and mild-to-moderate renal insufficiency [8]. However, the observed benefit declined with lower renal function, and there was a trend toward harm in those with an eGFR<15 ml/minute/1.73 m^2 or on dialysis (HR 1.61 95% CI 0.84–3.09). The wide confidence interval reflects the low number of patients in this eGFR category (n = 278, with 41 patients undergoing early revascularisation) making it hard to draw firm conclusions. In our study there was no statistical evidence of modification by eGFR category on the survival benefit associated with inpatient revascularisation, a finding supported by a study from the GRACE collaboration [30].

None of our analyses suggest that inpatient angiography or subsequent revascularisation was associated with harm in patients with renal dysfunction, though the fear of this may be influencing clinical judgement and decision making. Consistent with previous studies, the main barrier to revascularisation appears to be the decision to undertake inpatient coronary angiography [30]. The few patients with eGFR<30 ml/min/1.73 m^2 that do undergo diagnostic angiography may represent a highly select subset of patients with severe renal impairment in whom an early invasive approach is likely to be of most benefit. However, the efficacy of a routine early invasive approach in individuals presenting with this severity of renal dysfunction currently remains essentially undefined.

Our cohort from a national ACS registry provides the most comprehensive account of current clinical practice in England and Wales in terms of the relationships between renal function, early angiography and revascularisation and patient outcomes after NSTE-ACS, and adds further contemporary data to the available research in this field. We have taken account of a range of confounders and have conducted multiple sensitivity analyses, including using datasets derived from multiple imputation, the results of which have supported the findings of our main analyses. However, there are limitations. Most importantly, this is an observational study and not a randomised controlled trial. Confounding may be present although we aimed to minimise this by incorporating a propensity score methodology and a wide range of baseline characteristics. We did not have a direct measure of true kidney function and used eGFR based on the CKD-EPI formula. As only a single creatinine was available for each patient we were unable to evaluate the components of chronic kidney disease or acute kidney injury. Our conclusions therefore refer to renal function at the time of presentation. However, given that historical creatinine values may not always be available to practising clinicians when they make decisions regarding angiography or revascularisation we argue that the findings of this analysis are relevant to clinical practice. Currently, identification of patients on dialysis or those with a renal transplant is not possible within the MINAP dataset. Very few individuals with an eGFR<30 ml/minute/1.73 m^2 contributed to the analysis focussed on inpatient revascularisation and survival as so few had an inpatient coronary angiogram, so it is very likely that individuals on dialysis were excluded. We did not have details of coronary anatomy. After coronary angiography some patients will be treated medically because no treatable culprit lesion is present and others because revascularisation carries unacceptable risk or is unlikely to be successful. Having this information would enable a much more detailed description of the differences between patients with various degrees of renal function, and a deeper understanding of management strategies used and patient outcomes. We lacked information on other important characteristics that stratify risk (in patients who are not offered a routine invasive approach), for example the results of stress tests and measurements of left ventricular function. Nor did we have information on clinical events in hospital, such as further myocardial infarction, which may have influenced clinical decision making. While we were able to categorise patients into those with and those without angiography (and subsequent revascularisation) we lacked information regarding delay from admission to intervention. To evaluate the risk of potential survivor bias we undertook sensitivity analyses restricted to those who survived more than five days, but this is an important limitation. Other outcomes such as cardiac specific mortality, in-hospital mortality and length of stay would be valuable additional information. As mentioned above, our analysis may also have lacked power to detect evidence of modification by category of renal dysfunction on outcomes by management strategy due to the relatively low numbers of individuals with severe renal impairment contributing to that analysis.

Our analyses from MINAP provide further evidence that patients with renal dysfunction are much less likely to undergo inpatient coronary angiography than individuals with preserved renal function which is not explained by associated comorbidity. Inpatient coronary angiography was associated with improved survival across all categories of renal dysfunction. After inpatient angiography, relative outcomes following revascularisation were not modified by severity of renal dysfunction. As in previous studies however low patient numbers with severe renal dysfunction limit the ability to draw firm conclusions.

There is a discrepancy between the care advised in clinical guidelines regarding an early invasive strategy in patients with renal dysfunction and NSTE-ACS, and care delivered in clinical practice. Further research is required to understand why this variation exists and determine whether there are missed opportunities for quality improvement. In patients with severe renal impairment or those on dialysis a RCT is required to definitively evaluate the efficacy and optimal timing of early angiography and subsequent revascularisation after NSTE-ACS.

Supporting Information

Appendix S1 Distribution of the conditional propensity scores for undergoing inpatient revascularisation after inpatient coronary angiography.

Appendix S2 Frequency of missing data in the non-ST-elevation acute coronary syndrome dataset.

Appendix S3 Key covariates in the patients included in the complete case analysis and patients that were excluded due to incomplete data.

Appendix S4 Comparison between the results of the complete case analysis and the analysis restricted to patients who survived for 5 days or more.

Appendix S5 Comparison between the results of the complete case analysis and the analysis using 10 datasets derived using multiple imputation.

Author Contributions

Conceived and designed the experiments: C. Shaw JS DN C. Sharpe. Analyzed the data: C. Shaw RS. Wrote the paper: C. Shaw. Commented on drafts and approved the final version of the paper and are in agreement with submission to PLOS ONE: DN RS CJ SS DO'D DF CW C. Sharpe.

References

1. Fox CS, Muntner P, Chen AY, Alexander KP, Roe MT, et al. (2010) Use of Evidence-Based Therapies in Short-Term Outcomes of ST-Segment Elevation Myocardial Infarction and Non–ST-Segment Elevation Myocardial Infarction in Patients With Chronic Kidney Disease: A Report From the National Cardiovascular Data Acute Coronary Treatment and Intervention Outcomes Network Registry. Circulation 121: 357–365.
2. Go AS, Chertow GM, Fan D, McCulloch CE, Hsu C-y (2004) Chronic Kidney Disease and the Risks of Death, Cardiovascular Events, and Hospitalization. New England Journal of Medicine 351: 1296–1305.
3. Kerr M, Bray B, Medcalf J, O'Donoghue DJ, Matthews B (2012) Estimating the financial cost of chronic kidney disease to the NHS in England. Nephrology Dialysis Transplantation 27 (Suppl 3): 373–80.
4. Fox KAA, Clayton TC, Damman P, Pocock SJ, de Winter RJ, et al. (2010) Long-Term Outcome of a Routine Versus Selective Invasive Strategy in Patients With Non–ST-Segment Elevation Acute Coronary SyndromeA Meta-Analysis of Individual Patient Data. Journal of the American College of Cardiology 55: 2435–2445.
5. Coca S, Krumholz HM, Garg AX, Parikh CR (2006) Under representation of renal disease in randomized controlled trials of cardiovascular disease. JAMA 296: 1377–1384.
6. Hamm CW, Bassand JP, Agewall S, Bax J, Boersma E, et al. (2011) ESC Guidelines for the management of acute coronary syndromes in patients presenting without persistent ST-segment elevation: The Task Force for the management of acute coronary syndromes (ACS) in patients presenting without

persistent ST-segment elevation of the European Society of Cardiology (ESC). European Heart Journal 32(23): 2999–3054.
7. Jneid H, Anderson JL, Wright RS, Adams CD, Bridges CR, et al. (2012) ACCF/AHA Focused Update of the Guideline for the Management of Patients With Unstable Angina/Non–ST-Elevation Myocardial Infarction (Updating the 2007 Guideline and Replacing the 2011 Focused Update): A Report of the American College of Cardiology Foundation/American Heart Association Task Force on Practice Guidelines. Circulation 126: 875–910.
8. Szummer K, Lundman P, Jacobson SH, Schön S, Lindbäck J, et al. (2009) Influence of Renal Function on the Effects of Early Revascularization in Non-ST-Elevation Myocardial Infarction: Data From the Swedish Web-System for Enhancement and Development of Evidence-Based Care in Heart Disease Evaluated According to Recommended Therapies (SWEDEHEART). Circulation 120: 851–858.
9. James MT, Tonelli M, Ghali WA, Knudtson ML, Faris P, et al. (2013) Renal outcomes associated with invasive versus conservative management of acute coronary syndrome: propensity matched cohort study. BMJ 347: f4151.
10. Blicher TM, Hommel K, Olesen JB, Torp-Pedersen C, Madsen M, et al. (2013) Less use of standard guideline-based treatment of myocardial infarction in patients with chronic kidney disease: a Danish nation-wide cohort study. European Heart Journal 34: 2916–2923.
11. Herrett E, Smeeth L, Walker L, Weston C (2010) The Myocardial Ischaemia National Audit Project (MINAP). Heart 96: 1264–1267.
12. Birkhead J, Pearson M, Norris RM, Rickards AF, Georgiou A (2002) The National Audit of Myocardial Infarction: a new development in the audit process. Journal of Clinical Excellence 4: 379–385.
13. Birkhead JS (2000) Responding to the requirements of the National Service Framework for coronary disease: a core data set for myocardial infarction. Heart 84: 116–117.
14. Levey AS, Stevens LA, Schmid CH, Zhang Y, Castro F III, et al. (2009) A New Equation to Estimate Glomerular Filtration Rate. Annals of Internal Medicine 150: 604–612.
15. Kidney Disease: Improving Global Outcomes (KDIGO) CKD Work Group (2013) KDIGO Clinical Practice Guideline for the Evaluation and Management of Chronic Kidney Disease. Kidney inter., Suppl.; 3: 1–150.
16. Department for Communities and Local Government (2010) The English Indices of Deprivation.
17. Eagle KA, Lim MJ, Dabbous OH Pieper KS, Goldberg RJ, et al. (2004) A validated prediction model for all forms of acute coronary syndrome: Estimating the risk of 6-month postdischarge death in an international registry. JAMA 291(22): 2727–2733.
18. Rosenbaum PR, Rubin DB (1983) The central role of the propensity score in observational studies for causal effects. Biometrika 70: 41–55.
19. Hoenig MR, Aroney CN, Scott IA (2010) Early invasive versus conservative strategies for unstable angina and non-ST elevation myocardial infarction in the stent era. Cochrane Database of Systematic Reviews.
20. Flather MD, Yusuf S, Køber L, Pfeffer M, Hall A, et al. (2000) Long-term ACE-inhibitor therapy in patients with heart failure or left-ventricular dysfunction: a systematic overview of data from individual patients. The Lancet 355: 1575–1581.
21. Cannon CP, Braunwald E, McCabe CH, Rader DJ, Rouleau JL, et al. (2004) Intensive versus Moderate Lipid Lowering with Statins after Acute Coronary Syndromes. New England Journal of Medicine 350: 1495–1504.
22. López Sendó J, Swedberg K, McMurray J, Tamargo J, Maggioni AP, et al. (2004) Expert consensus document on β-adrenergic receptor blockers: The Task Force on Beta-Blockers of the European Society of Cardiology. European Heart Journal 25: 1341–1362.
23. Antithrombotic Trialists' Collaboration (2002) Collaborative meta-analysis of randomised trials of antiplatelet therapy for prevention of death, myocardial infarction, and stroke in high risk patients. BMJ 324: 71–86.
24. Rubin DB (1987) Multiple Imputation for Nonresponse in Surveys; John Wiley and Sons.
25. Fox KAA, Anderson FA, Dabbous OH, Steg PG, López Sendón J, et al. (2007) Intervention in acute coronary syndromes: do patients undergo intervention on the basis of their risk characteristics? The Global Registry of Acute Coronary Events (GRACE). Heart 93: 177–182.
26. Herzog CA (2003) How to Manage the Renal Patient with Coronary Heart Disease: The Agony and the Ecstasy of Opinion-Based Medicine. Journal of the American Society of Nephrology 14: 2556–2572.
27. Kanderian AS, Francis GS (2006) Cardiac troponins and chronic kidney disease. Kidney Int 69: 1112–1114.
28. Wickenbrock I, Perings C, Maagh P, Quack I, Bracht M, et al. (2009) Contrast medium induced nephropathy in patients undergoing percutaneous coronary intervention for acute coronary syndrome: differences in STEMI and NSTEMI. Clinical Research in Cardiology 98: 765–772.
29. Kumar N, Dahri L, Brown W, Duncan N, Singh S, et al. (2009) Effect of Elective Coronary Angiography on Glomerular Filtration Rate in Patients with Advanced Chronic Kidney Disease. Clinical Journal of the American Society of Nephrology 4: 1907–1913.
30. Wong JA, Goodman SG, Yan RT, Wald R, Bagnall AJ, et al. (2009) Temporal management patterns and outcomes of non-ST elevation acute coronary syndromes in patients with kidney dysfunction. European Heart Journal 30: 549–557.
31. Lee CH, Tan M, Yan AT, Fitchett D, Grima EA, et al. (2008) Use of cardiac catheterization for non–st-segment elevation acute coronary syndromes according to initial risk: Reasons why physicians choose not to refer their patients. Archives of Internal Medicine 168: 291–296.
32. Yan AT, Yan RT, Tan M, Fung A, Cohen EA, et al. (2007) Management patterns in relation to risk stratification among patients with non–st elevation acute coronary syndromes. Archives of Internal Medicine 167: 1009–1016.
33. Chertow GM, Normand SLT, McNeil BJ (2004) "Renalism": Inappropriately Low Rates of Coronary Angiography in Elderly Individuals with Renal Insufficiency. Journal of the American Society of Nephrology 15: 2462–2468.
34. Damman P, Hirsch A, Windhausen F, Tijssen JGP, de Winter RJ (2010) 5-Year Clinical Outcomes in the ICTUS (Invasive versus Conservative Treatment in Unstable coronary Syndromes) Trial: A Randomized Comparison of an Early Invasive Versus Selective Invasive Management in Patients With Non–ST-Segment Elevation Acute Coronary Syndrome. Journal of the American College of Cardiology 55: 858–864.
35. Boden WE, ORourke RA, Crawford MH, Blaustein AS, Deedwania PC, et al. (1998) Outcomes in Patients with Acute Non–Q-Wave Myocardial Infarction Randomly Assigned to an Invasive as Compared with a Conservative Management Strategy. New England Journal of Medicine 338: 1785–1792.
36. Cannon CP, Weintraub WS, Demopoulos LA, Vicari R, Frey MJ, et al. (2001) Comparison of Early Invasive and Conservative Strategies in Patients with Unstable Coronary Syndromes Treated with the Glycoprotein IIb/IIIa Inhibitor Tirofiban. New England Journal of Medicine 344: 1879–1887.
37. Charytan DM, Wallentin L, Lagerqvist B, Spacek R, De Winter RJ, et al. (2009) Early Angiography in Patients with Chronic Kidney Disease: A Collaborative Systematic Review. Clinical Journal of the American Society of Nephrology 4: 1032–1043.

7

Pathological Mechanism for Delayed Hyperenhancement of Chronic Scarred Myocardium in Contrast Agent Enhanced Magnetic Resonance Imaging

Jian Wang[1,2,3,4]*, Bo Xiang[2,3], Hung-Yu Lin[2], Hongyu Liu[4], Darren Freed[2,3,5], Rakesh C. Arora[2,3,5], Ganghong Tian[2,3]

1 Department of Vascular Surgery, Union Hospital, Tongji Medical College, Huazhong University of Science and Technology, Wuhan, Hubei, China, **2** National Research Council, Winnipeg, Manitoba, Canada, **3** Department of Physiology, Faculty of Medicine, University of Manitoba, Winnipeg, Manitoba, Canada, **4** Department of Cardiac Surgery, the First Affiliated Hospital, Harbin Medical University, Harbin, Heilongjiang, China, **5** Cardiac Science Program, Institute of Cardiovascular Sciences, St. Boniface General Hospital, Winnipeg, Manitoba, Canada

Abstract

Objectives: To evaluate possible mechanism for delayed hyperenhancement of scarred myocardium by investigating the relationship of contrast agent (CA) first pass and delayed enhancement patterns with histopathological changes.

Materials and Methods: Eighteen pigs underwent 4 weeks ligation of 1 or 2 diagonal coronary arteries to induce chronic infarction. The hearts were then removed and perfused in a Langendorff apparatus. The hearts firstly experienced phosphorus 31 MR spectroscopy. The hearts in group I ($n = 9$) and II ($n = 9$) then received the bolus injection of Gadolinium diethylenetriamine pentaacetic acid (0.05 mmol/kg) and gadolinium-based macromolecular agent (P792, 15 μmol/kg), respectively. First pass T_2^* MRI was acquired using a gradient echo sequence. Delayed enhanced T_1 MRI was acquired with an inversion recovery sequence. Masson's trichrome and anti- von Willebrand Factor (vWF) staining were performed for infarct characterization.

Results: Wash-in of both kinds of CA caused the sharp and dramatic T_2^* signal decrease of scarred myocardium similar to that of normal myocardium. Myocardial blood flow and microvessel density were significantly recovered in 4-week-old scar tissue. Steady state distribution volume (ΔR_1 relaxation rate) of Gd-DTPA was markedly higher in scarred myocardium than in normal myocardium, whereas ΔR_1 relaxation rate of P792 did not differ significantly between scarred and normal myocardium. The ratio of extracellular volume to the total water volume was significantly greater in scarred myocardium than in normal myocardium. Scarred myocardium contained massive residual capillaries and dilated vessels. Histological stains indicated the extensively discrete matrix deposition and lack of cellular structure in scarred myocardium.

Conclusions: Collateral circulation formation and residual vessel effectively delivered CA into scarred myocardium. However, residual vessel without abnormal hyperpermeability allowed Gd-DTPA rather than P792 to penetrate into extravascular compartment. Discrete collagen fiber meshwork and loss of cellularity enlarged extracellular space accessible to Gd-DTPA, resulting in the delayed hyper-enhanced scar.

Editor: Vincenzo Lionetti, Scuola Superiore Sant'Anna, Italy

Funding: This study was supported by National Natural Sciences Foundation of China (81200105, http://www.nsfc.gov.cn/Portal0/default152.htm) and China Postdoctoral Science Foundation funded Project (20100470050, http://res.chinapostdoctor.org.cn/Program/Main.html). The funders had no role in study design, data collection and analysis, decision to publish, or preparation of the manuscript.

Competing Interests: The authors have declared that no competing interests exist.

* E-mail: jianwang1030@126.com

Introduction

MR delayed hyperenhanement after administration of extracellular contrast agent (CA) such as Gd-DTPA was exclusively associated with scar tissue in chronic myocardial infarction (MI) [1,2]. The accuracy of delayed enhancement imaging in determining scar size was validated with nuclear imaging techniques [3,4]. However, the mechanism for delayed hyperenhancement of scarred MI remains poorly understood. Scar healing after MI is associated with vascular adaption and structural reconfiguration, greatly affecting first pass and delayed distribution of CA. Therefore, to investigate the relationship of CA first pass and delayed enhancement patterns with pathological changes might provide important insight into possible mechanism.

MR delayed enhancement observed after CA injection is affected by the infarct-related artery patency and microvascular obstruction [5,6,7]. After release of prolonged coronary occlusion, restoration of blood flow to infracted regions is heterogeneous and relevant to differential delayed enhancement patterns in acute reperfused MI. Hyperenhanced regions, mainly located in the periphery of acute MI, display definite restoration of regional blood flow [5,6]. After massive CAs enter into MI region with effective reperfusion, loss of cell membrane integrity cannot exclude CA from intracellular space and results in an enlarged distribution volume. Hypoenhancement at the infarct core is closely related to the no-reflow phenomenon, which reveals severe and widespread microvascular obstruction due to erythrocytes stasis, neutrophils accumulation and endothelial cell swelling [7,8]. Consequently, effective delivery of CA into MI regions is the prerequisite for late delayed hyperenhancement. Whether the reestablishment of collateral circulation during scar healing allows for CA into scarred myocardium remains to be clarified.

Equilibrium distribution patterns of CA not only depend on its delivery by blood flow perfusion, but also on the properties of CA, vascular permeability and the size of interstitial space accessible to CA. Myocytes necrosis results in the disruption of cellular membrane, allowing for extracellular CA into intracellular space and creating an increased distribution volume [9,10]. Therefore, myocardial cell injury might be evaluated by extracellular agent. Additionally, myocardial ischemia causes the injury to vasculature and elevates the permeability of capillaries. Intravascular agent is retained within intravascular space in normal myocardium, but leaks into interstitial space and causes a relatively increased distribution volume in MI region [11,12]. Therefore, microvascular damage might be probed by intravascular agent. Scar repairing in chronic MI originates from complete cellular necrosis and ends with marked deposition of collagen matrix. It is unclear whether vascular reconstruction causes hyperpermeability of vessel wall in scar tissue. Therefore, the potential of MRI to provide information about vascular permeability and the accessibility of interstitial space will be determined by the relation of contrast enhancement patterns with the underlying pathophysiology.

Phenylphosphonate (PPA) distributes only into the extracellular compartment, whereas dimethyl methylphosphonate (DMMP) evenly expands into the entire water space. Both phosphorous-containing compounds have the specific and distinct peak position in phosphorous 31 MR spectra, and intensity of corresponding peak reflects the volume of extracellular compartment and the entire water space. Thus, the ratio of PPA to DMMP signal intensity can reflect the percentage of interstitial compartment to the whole space.

Materials and Methods

Ethics statement

This study was carried out in strict accordance with the recommendations in the Guide for the Care and Use of Laboratory Animals of Huazhong University of Science and Technology. The protocol was approved by the Committee on the Ethics of Animal Experiments of Wuhan Union Hospital (Permit Number: 2008037). All surgery were performed under general anesthesia, and all efforts were made to minimize suffering.

Pig model of chronic scarred myocardium

Eighteen domestic pigs weighing 20–25 kg were sedated with an intramuscular injection of diazepam (0.4 mg/kg body wt) and ketamine (20 mg/kg body wt). After the induction of anesthemia, pigs were intubated and ventilated with gas anesthesia comprising 1%–2% isoflurance in a mixture of oxygen and nitrous oxide. Using a sterile technique, a lateral thoracotomy was performed at the fourth left intercostals space to expose the heart, and the pericardium was opened. The first and second diagonal branches of left anterior descending coronary artery (LAD) were permanently ligated at their origin. The presence of occlusion was confirmed by development of regional myocardial cyanosis. The chests were closed and the animals were allowed to recover for 4 weeks for the development of chronic scarred myocardium.

Isolated pig heart preparation

At the end of 4-week recovery period, animal chest was reopened through median sternotomy under a general anesthesia. The pericardium was opened longitudinally along the midline. The aorta and pulmonary artery, inferior and superior vena cava were dissected and clamped. Cold (−4°C) cardioplegia was infused into aortic root to arrest the heart. The heart was quickly excised and immersed in cold saline solution for instrumentation. The brachiocephalic artery and subclavian artery were cannulated for achievement of antegrade perfusion and measurement of antegrade pressure. A mixture of autogenous blood and modified Krebs-Henseleit solution in 1:1 ratio was used to perfuse the hearts. The concentrations of potassium and magnesium in the perfusion medium were each adjusted in 16 mmol/l to keep hearts quiescent throughout the imaging period.

Experimental protocol

Isolated hearts were placed in Langendorff perfusion apparatus positioned in the center of a 7T magnet. The hearts were perfused by mixture of pig blood with K-H solution at perfusion pressure of approximately 60 mmHg. All hearts were subjected to a protocol consisting of 40-min P^{31} MR spectroscopy and 55-min acquisition of MR imaging. Dimenthyl methylphosphonate (DMMP, 20 mmol/L) and phenylphosphonic acid (PPA, 10 mmol/L) were added into perfusion medium. ^{31}P MR spectra were acquired from normal region and scarred myocardium, respectively. DMMP evenly distributes to the entire water space, whereas PPA distributes only into extracellular compartment. Both phosphorous-containing compounds have the specific peak position in ^{31}P MR spectra, and intensity of corresponding peak reflects the volume of extracellular compartment and the entire water space.

In the phase of MR imaging studies, T_1- weighted imaging was firstly performed without CA using T_1-weighted inversion-recovery (IR) turbo fast low-angle shot (turboFLASH) sequence. Afterward, hearts received the bolus injection of either 0.05 mmol/kg of Gd-DTPA (group I; n = 9) or 15 μmol/kg of P792 (group II; n = 9), respectively. To prevent air-tissue interface artifact on T_2^* - weighted imaging, the pig heart was immersed in the perfusate during images study. The effect of CA on T_2^* signal intensity during its first passage through myocardium was monitored using a gradient-recalled echo (GRE) fast low-angle shot (FLASH) sequence. The CA delayed enhanced T_1 imaging was conducted at 5 different time points with 10-minute time interval after CA administration with a T_1-weighted IR turbo-FLASH sequence.

Following the MR imaging studies, perfusion was maintained as during MR imaging and the hearts were injected with colored microsphere to assess regional myocardial blood flow. Hearts were removed from perfusion line and sectioned into slices according to scout imaging to ensure a correlation to MR imaging. The slices were used to perform microsphere analysis and histological examination,

Colored microspheres and histochemical staining procedure

At the end of each experiment, approximately 5×10^6 to 8×10^6 nonradioactive red-colored microspheres (15±1.9 μm diameter, suspended in 2 ml of saline solution) were injected through the aorta. Arterial reference samples were withdrawn simultaneously from the ascending aorta at a constant rate of 5 ml/mm for 3 min, starting 1 min before injection of the microspheres. Hearts were removed and sectioned into short axis slice from base to apex. Alternating sections were used for histochemical staining, with the opposing side used for colored microsphere analysis. Sections for histochemical staining firstly were stained by 2% TTC solution and photographed under room light to determine the infarct region. Following TTC staining, there sections were separated into the infracted scar tissue and normal myocardium, which were frozen by immersion in liquid nitrogen. 5 μm-thick slices from two kinds of myocardium were stained with hematoxylin and eosin. Massion's trichrome stain was used to define scarred myocardium.

Pie – shaped sample was collected from normal regions and infarct scar. Positive TTC staining in the matched, opposing sections and thinning of ventricular wall can be thought to be the index of infarcted region. The average weight of each sample was approximately 0.5 g. After collection, tissue and blood sample were digested. The numbers of microsoheres in the samples were counted using a spectrophotometer at a wavelength of 536 nm. Actual blood flow was calculated based on the microsphere count in the tissue and blood samples and speed of blood collection.

Immunohistochemical staining for von-Willebrand Factor (vWF)

The endothelial cell and angiogenesis were traced by antibody to vWF (Sigma, St. Louis, MO, USA). Tissue sections were fixed with 4% paraformaldehyde for 10 minutes at room temperature, washed three times with PBS containing 0.3% Triton X-100, and blocked with 2% goat serum and 1% bovine serium albumin (BSA) for 30 minutes at room temperature. Slides were then incubated with primary antibodies against vWF for 1 hour at 37°C. After three washes with PBS, slides were incubated with Alexa Fluor 594-conjugated goat anti pig IgG (Invitrogen, Invitrogen, Carlsbad, CA, USA) for 45 minutes at 37°C. After three more washes with PBS, the slides were stained for nuclei with 4′,6-diamidino-2-phenylindole (DAPI, Sigma). The slides were observed by a Carl Zeiss fluorescence microscope. Microvessels were counted in at least three random fields under a fluorescence microscope. The vWF-positive capillaries were counted and the microvessel density was expressed as counts per mm^2.

^{31}P MR spectroscopy

^{31}P MR spectroscopy was performed on a 7-Tesla magnet equipped with a Biospec spectrometer (Bruker, Karlsruhe, Germany). A MR surface coil with 1.5 cm of diameter was firstly positioned over chronic scarred region. Then the surface coil was moved to normal myocardium of LAD region. The P^{31} MR spectra were therefore acquired from normal myocardium and infarcted scar region, respectively.

MR signals (free induction decay, FID) were obtained by use of a hard pulse with a pulse length of 75 μsec and a repetition time of 2 sec. Six FID signals were accumulated for each ^{31}P MR spectrum. Thus each spectrum was averaged over a 2-minute sample time.

The observed phosphorus compounds included DMMP, PPA, inorganic phosphate (Pi), phosphocreatine (PCr), three peaks (α, β, γ) of adenosine triphosphate (ATP).

Magnetic resonance imaging

MR imaging studies were performed on a similar 7T, 40 cm horizontal bore magnet. MR images were acquired with a Helmholtz coil. Scout images were acquired to locate long axis, from which three parallel short-axis slices were prescribed.

Monitoring of T_2^* signal intensity was performed using a FLASH gradient echo sequence during the first pass of CA. Gradient echo sequence parameters were as follows: matrix: 128×128; field of view: 120×120 mm; slice thickness: 3 mm; flip angle: 8°, echo time: 15mesc; acquisition time: 1815.16msec; repetition time: 26msec. All MR images were acquired from the arrested heart to eliminate motion artifact.

Regular T_1-weighted images were acquired with a Turbo-FLASH inversion-recovery sequence. Nine T_1-weighted images were obtained with nine different inversion times (10, 100, 200, 400, 700, 1200, 2000, 5000 and 10,000msec) to measure T1 relaxation time and calculate ΔR_1 relaxation rate. All T_1 images were acquired from a 5 mm thick slice with a 120×120 mm field of view and imager matrix size of 128×128.

Data analysis

^{31}P spectra were analyzed using 1D-WINNER (Bruker, Karlsruhe, Germany). The ratio of extracellular volume to the entire water volume was obtained from dividing DMMP intensity peak by PPA intensity peak. MR imaging data were processed using Marevisi software package (NRC-Institute for Biodiagnostics, Winnipeg, Canada). Round, hand-drawn regions of interest (ROIs) were created by correlating the MR images to the TTC-stained references.

T_2^* time intensity curves were obtained from 50 consecutive perfusion images using the Marevisi software. For one slice, two curves for scarred and normal myocardium were generated to represent the characteristic passage of CA. T_1 relaxation time with or without CA was measured according to T_1 imaging acquired with nine different inversion time in scarred and normal myocardium. Distribution volume of CAs was expressed as ΔR_1 relaxation rate ($1/T_1$ after contrast administration $-1/T_1$ before contrast administration).

Statistical analyses

All numerical results were presented as mean ± standard deviation. Statistical analysis was performed using Statistica (Statsoft Inc, Tulsa, OK). Differences in signal intensity and ΔR_1 relaxation rate between normal and scarred myocardium at specific time points were analyzed by Bonferroni's *t* test. The changes over time of signal intensity and ΔR_1 relaxation rate obtained from scarred myocardium were compared with the patterns obtained from normal myocardium by repeated measures analysis of variance (ANOVA). Moreover, differences in these values determined by histology and spectroscopy were studied by means of a paired *t* test. A value of $p<0.05$ indicates statistical significance.

Results

First pass kinetics and MR perfusion imagings of extravascular or intravascular CA

Baseline T_2^* signal intensity (SI) of scarred and normal myocardium did not differ significantly: 98.2%±2.5% versus 99.2%±3.1% of initial intensity. Wash-in of Gd-DTPA resulted in a great extent of T_2^* signal decrease in scarred myocardium (from 98.2%±2.5% to 23.7%±13.1%) (Figure 1a), even though peak T_2^* SI in scarred myocardium was higher than that in normal myocardium (23.7%±13.1% versus 17.8%±6.8%). Moreover, there wasn't time difference in peak effect or decline of T_2^* SI between scarred and normal myocardium (Figure 1a). Therefore, the extent of T_2^* signal hypoenhancement in scarred myocardium was equivalent to that in normal myocardium at T_2^* wash-in and peak imagings of Gd-DTPA (Upper Panel, Figure 2).

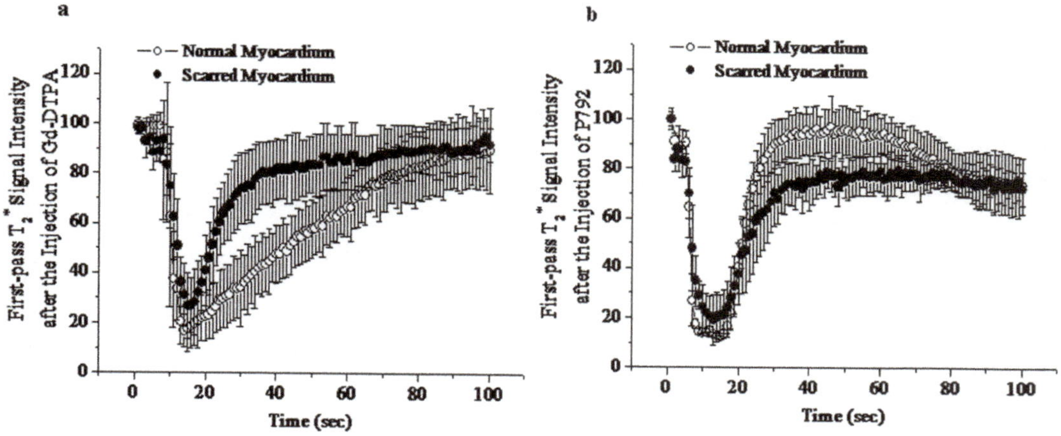

Figure 1. T_2^* time intensity curves obtained during the first pass of Gd-DTPA (a) and P792 (b). Wash-in of both contrast agents caused similar decrease in T_2^* signal intensity of scarred and normal myocardium.

The magnitude of T_2^* signal loss caused by wash-in of P792 in scarred myocardium was comparable to that in normal myocardium (Figure 1b). No delayed transit was observed in scarred myocardium. Thus, there was not difference in T_2^* signal decrement between normal and scarred myocardium at T_2^* wash-in and peak imagines of P792 (Lower Panel, Figure 2). These suggest that low and high molecular weight CAs both can be effectively delivered into scarred myocardium.

The ratio of extracellular volume to the entire water space in normal and scarred myocardium

Normal myocardium was stained brick red, whereas scarred myocardium wasn't completely stained by TTC (Figure 3a). ^{31}P spectra acquired from scarred myocardium displayed a more striking PPA peak and a negligible ATP peak relative to normal myocardium (Figure 3b). The ratio of extracellular volume to the entire water volume was significantly greater in scarred myocardium (0.66±0.03) than in normal myocardium (0.41±0.04) (Figure 3c). These suggest that extracellular volume is significantly enlarged in scarred myocardium. The ATP content was 26.4±3.01 a.u in normal myocardium, whereas scarred myocardium contained almost no ATP (3.71±1.34 a.u) (Figure 3d). This further demonstrates that ^{31}P spectra were exclusively obtained from scarred myocardium.

Distribution volumes and delayed enhanced MR imagings of extravascular and intravascular CA

After the administration of Gd-DTPA, the ΔR_1 relaxation rates of scarred myocardium ranged from 5.4±0.7 to 4.3±0.2 for different time points postinjection of Gd-DTPA and were significantly greater than those of normal myocardium, ranging from 3.6±0.4 to 2.9±0.3 (Figure 4a). Therefore, scarred myocardium exhibited the significant hyperenhancement compared with normal myocardium in Gd-DTPA enhanced T_1

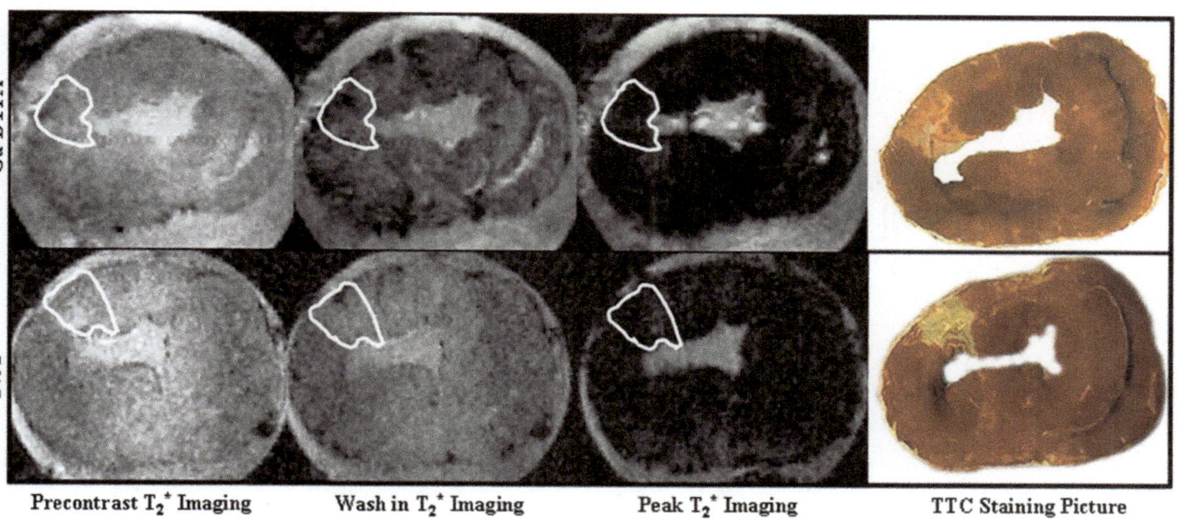

Figure 2. Representative contrast agent first pass T_2^* imagings with a photomicrograph of TTC-stained tissue. The extent of T_2^* signal hypoenhancement caused by entry of Gd-DTPA and P792 in scarred myocardium were comparable to those in normal myocardium. There were no differences in T_2^* signal loss between scarred and normal myocardium at wash-in and peak T_2^* imaging. Upper panel: T_2^* imaging during the first pass of Gd-DTPA; Lower panel: T_2^* imaging during the first pass of P792; First vertical line: precontrast T_2^* imaging; Second vertical line: wash-in T_2^* imaging; Third vertical line: peak T_2^* imaging; Fourth vertical line: TTC stained section.

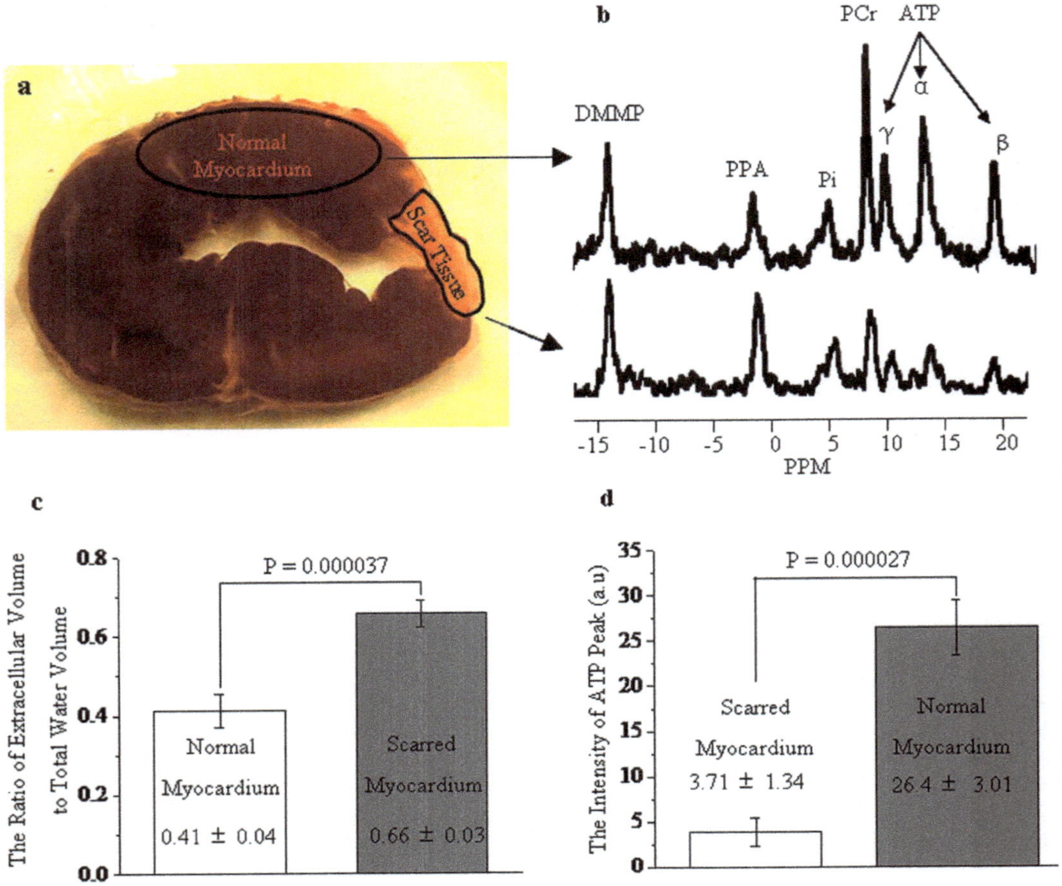

Figure 3. Representative ^{31}P spectra acquired from scarred and normal myocardium. ^{31}P spectra from scarred myocardium exhibited a more striking PPA peak (the extracellular compartment) as compared with normal myocardium (a and b). The ratio of extracellular volume to the entire space was significantly greater in scarred myocardium than in normal myocardium (c). The ATP content was substantially lower in scarred myocardium than in normal myocardium (d).

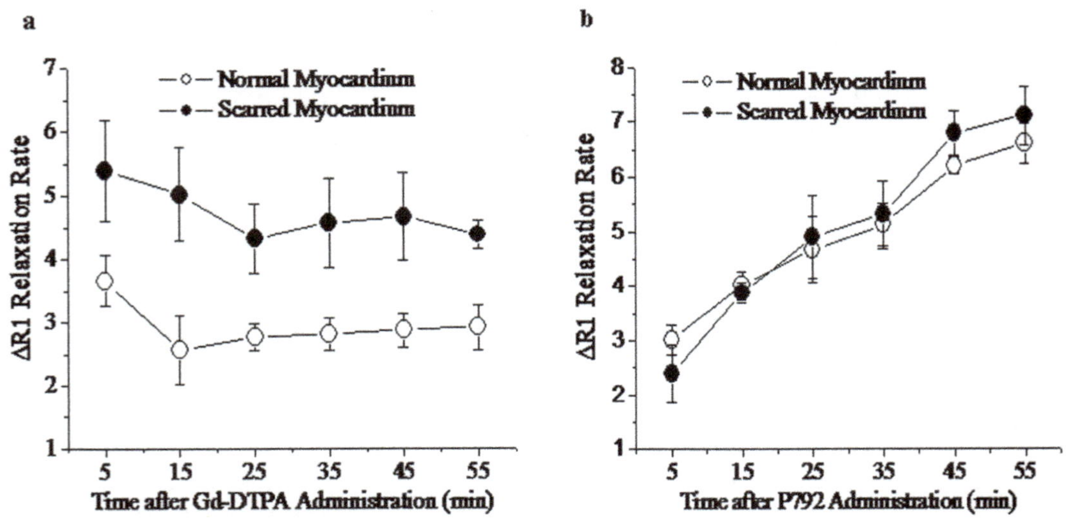

Figure 4. ΔR1 relaxation times measured after the administration of Gd-DTPA (a) and P792 (b). Administration of Gd-DTPA was associated with a higher ΔR1 relaxation time of scarred myocardium compared to normal myocardium, whereas there was not difference in ΔR1 relaxation time between scarred and normal myocardium post injection of P792.

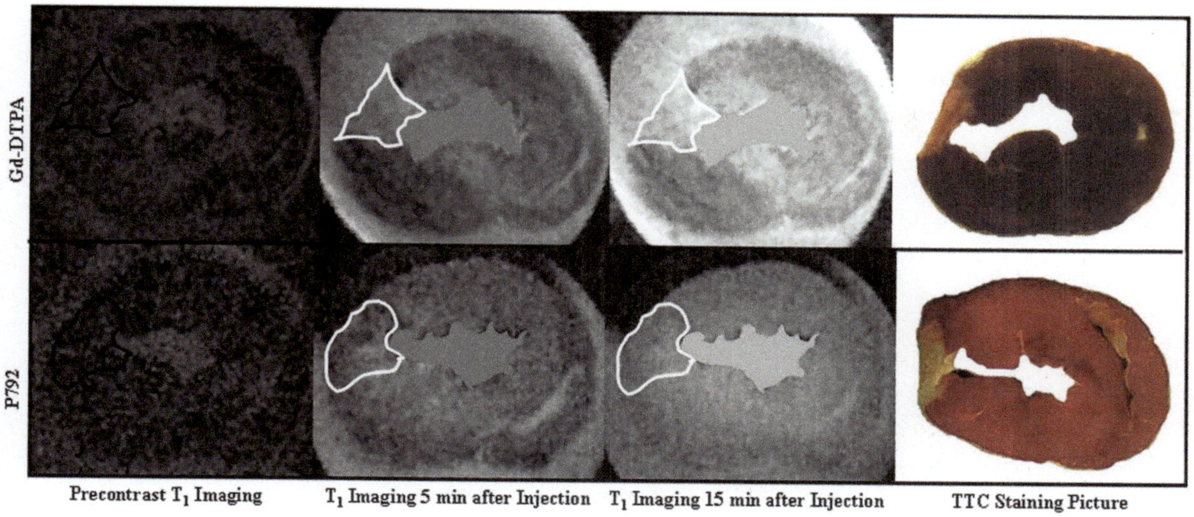

Figure 5. Representative contrast agent delayed enhanced T_1 imagings with a photomicrograph of TTC-stained tissue. Scarred myocardium exhibited the hyperenhancement at Gd-DTPA enhanced T_1 imaging, whereas homogeneous hyperenhancement was observed in scarred and normal myocardium after the administration of P792. Upper panel: Gd-DTPA enhanced T_1 imaging; Lower panel: P792 enhanced T_1 imaging; First vertical line: precontrast T_1 imaging; Second vertical line: T_1 imaging 5 min post injection; Third vertical line: T_1 imaging 15 min post injection; Fourth vertical line: TTC stained section.

imaging (Upper Panel, Figure 5). These suggest that expanded extravascular compartment is accessible to Gd-DTPA in scarred myocardium.

After the administration of P792, the ΔR_1 relaxation rates of scarred myocardium were not significantly different from those of normal myocardium for different time times post injection of P792 (Figure 4b). Thus, homogeneous hyperenhancement was observed within scarred and normal myocardium in P792-enhanced T_1 imaging (Lower Panel, Figure 5). These suggest that capillary wall integrity in scarred myocardium exclude P792 from enlarged extravascular compartment.

Staining of histological sections

Cardiomyocytes were major structural elements and limited extracellular space was accessible to CA due to intact cell membrane (Figure 6a and 6b). Cardiomyocyes had almost vanished and were displaced by extensively extracellular collagen matrix in scarred myocardium (Figure 6c), while vessels of different sizes were seen frequently (Arrowheads, Figure 6d).

Dilated vessels detected within scar tissue provide important routes by which effective delivery and even distribution are rapidly achieved following the injection of CAs. Formation of fibrosis collagen meshwork and loss of cadiomyocytes enlarge extravascular compartment accessible to extracellular agents, leading to the increased distribution volume in scarred myocardium.

Myocardial blood flow and microvessel density

Anti-vWF staining of scar tissue showed large blood vessels and numerous micorvessels (Figure 7a), which resembled those observed in normal myocardium (Figure 7b). Myocardial microvessel density was substantially recovered to 197.6±55.3 vessels/mm^2, reaching approximately 79.6% of that in normal myocardium (248.1±49.6 vessels/mm^2) (Figure 7c).

The microsphere technique also demonstrated that myocardial blood flow to scarred myocardium was significantly restored to 0.92±0.18 ml/g/min, which was slightly lower than that in normal myocardium (1.18±0.14 ml/g/min) (Figure 7d). Therefore, myocardial blood flow and microvessel density have developed rapidly to a surprising level after 4 weeks post infarction.

Discussion

Extracellular and intravascular CAs have dissimilar molecular weights (562 versus 6473 D) and diameters (0.9 versus 5 nm) determining different distribution volume. Thus, we investigated the first pass and delayed enhancement patterns with both types of CAs in chronic MI. Histoimmunopathological examination was performed to characterize scarred myocardium. The percentage of extracellular compartment to the whole water space was evaluated using ^{31}P MR spectroscopy with DMMP and PPA. Restoration of blood flow and alteration on interstitial space in scarred myocardium were compared with those in normal myocardium to define the differential contrast enhancement patterns. All findings demonstrated that pathological changes of scarred myocardium laid structural foundation for substantial wash-in of CAs during first pass and delayed hyperenhancement during following equilibrium.

Entry of CAs into myocardium creates a heterogeneous gradient across capillary wall, resulting in the loss of T_2^* SI. After the rapid bolus of both kinds of CAs, rapid and dramatic T_2^* signal decline was observed in scarred and normal myocardium. The extent of T_2^* signal loss in scarred myocardium was almost equivalent to that in normal myocardium. There were not differences in time to peak (time interval between preinjection and the peak of bolus injection) between scarred and normal myocardium. No perfusion defect was detected on first-pass MRI in 4-week-old scar infarction, which is consistent with prior study demonstrating that the first-pass perfusion defect is detected 4 hours after permanent coronary occlusion and the perfusion defect disappeared 8 days afterwards [13]. These provide strong evidences that two types of CAs can be effectively delivered into scarred myocardium.

We found that myocardial blood flow and microvessel density of scarred myocardium had developed to a surprising level at 4 week postinfarction. Regional myocardial blood flows were 0.92±0.18

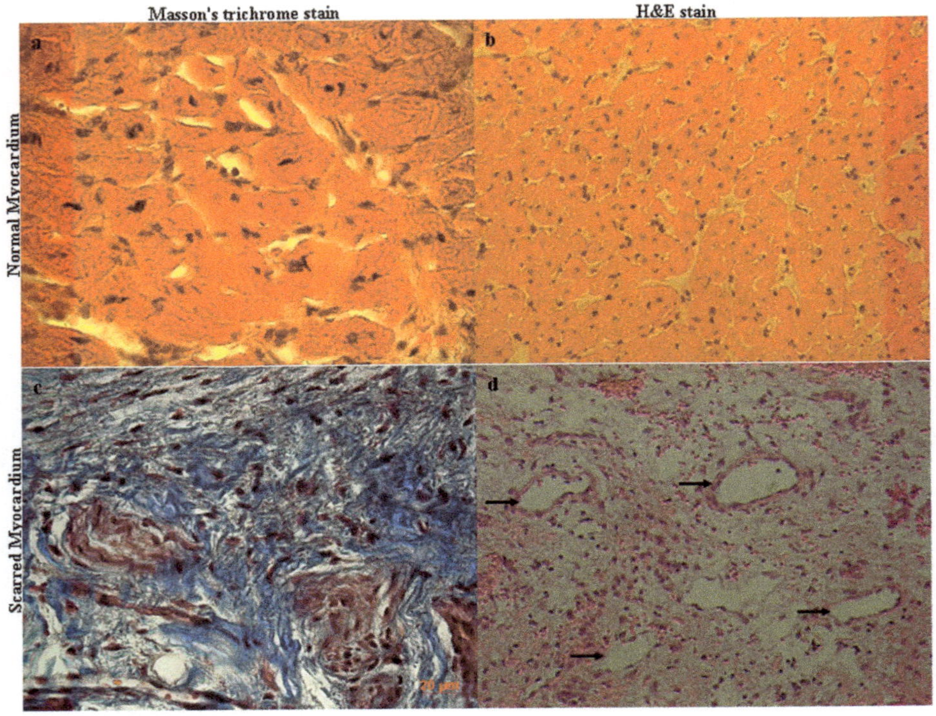

Figure 6. Histological staining sections: normal myocardium (upper panel) and scarred myocardium (lower panel), Masson's trichrome stain (right panel) and H&E stain (left panel). Cadiomyocytes are the major structural elements and interstitial volume only account for a small part of extravascular space of normal myocardium (a and b). The discrete compartment of collagen fiber is major framework of extracellular space in scarred myocardium (c). Cadiomyocytes have almost disappeared and vessels of different sizes were seen frequently (d).

and 1.18±0.14 in scarred and normal myocardium, respectively. Myocardial microvessel densities were 197.6±55.3 and 248.1±49.6 vessels/mm^2 in scarred and normal myocardium, respectively. Other investigators also have demonstrated that the pig develops a significant collateral network and exhibits a substantial increase in collateral blood flow after 3–4 weeks of gradual coronary artery occlusion [14,15,16]. Similar animal model as our study displayed that collateral blood flow was increased dramatically at 4 weeks after permanent coronary occlusion compared to the onset of acute occlusion [17]. Clinical human study also have indicated that well-developed collateral vessels are rarely present at the time of infarction and are manifest with the well visualization of vessel distal to occlusion in angiogram within 2 weeks after permanent occlusion of diseased artery [18]. Therefore, the gradual establishment of collateral circulation might be direct reason for the buck of CAs to flow into scarred myocardium. Coronary collateral vessels originated principally from the branches of other coronary artery or extracardiac artery mainly involving the internal mammary arteries and the bronchial arteries [16]. Maturation and growth of collateral vessel serve as the chief avenue from the other coronary artery to scarred myocardium, typically, bridging across the occluded coronary artery. In addition, our histological staining of scar tissue showed that dilated vessels could be seen frequently within the infracted scar tissue. Although the bulk of capillaries of infracted myocardium disappeared due to ischemic necrosis, many dilated vessels seemed to persist in scarred myocardium [19].

The relative distribution volume of CAs in the tissue can be estimated from the relative change (Δ) in the longitudinal relaxation rate (R_1) ($\Delta R_1 = 1/T_1$ before contrast administration - $1/T_1$ after contrast administration) [11,20]. We found that ΔR_1 relaxation rate of Gd-DTPA (small molecular weight) was significant higher in scarred myocardium than in normal myocardium. This observation is in agreement with several prior studies. Flacke et al demonstrated that the distribution coefficients (λ) of Gd-based contrast in chronic infarction were significantly elevated as compared with those in normal myocardium [21]. Rehwald et al demonstrated that Gd-DTPA concentrations were increased in the infracted scar tissue in comparison with normal myocardium using electron probe x-ray microanalysis [22]. Conversely, there was not a significant difference in ΔR_1 relaxation rate of P792 (large molecular weight) between scarred and normal myocardium. Saeed et al also found that intravascular CA did not produce the delayed hyperenhancement of 8-week-old scar tissue [23]. The absence of delayed enhancement in chronic infarctions after intravascular CA can be attributed to the intact permeability of remodeled vessel which retains intravascular contrast. More importantly, ^{31}P spectra in conjunction with chemical marker of cellular compartment (DMMP and PPA) found that ratio of extracellular volume to the entire water volume was significant higher in scarred myocardium than in normal myocardium. Therefore, delayed enhancement of scar should be attributed to the increased extracellular volume percentage and the enlarged distribution volume of Gd-DTPA.

Striking reduction in cellularity enlarges percentage of the extracellular volume in scarred myocardium. Permanent coronary occlusion produces sudden and total interruption of blood and oxygen supply to cardiomyocytes, resulting in extensive cardiomyocytes necrosis achieved by coagulation necrosis and myocytosis [24]. As a result, histological section of scarred myocardium demonstrated that cardiomyocytes had almost completely vanished at 4 week post infarction. Myocytes density declines abruptly from 98% preinfarction to 9.8% after 1 week and 2.7% after 3 weeks post-infarction in the infracted region [19]. Additionally,

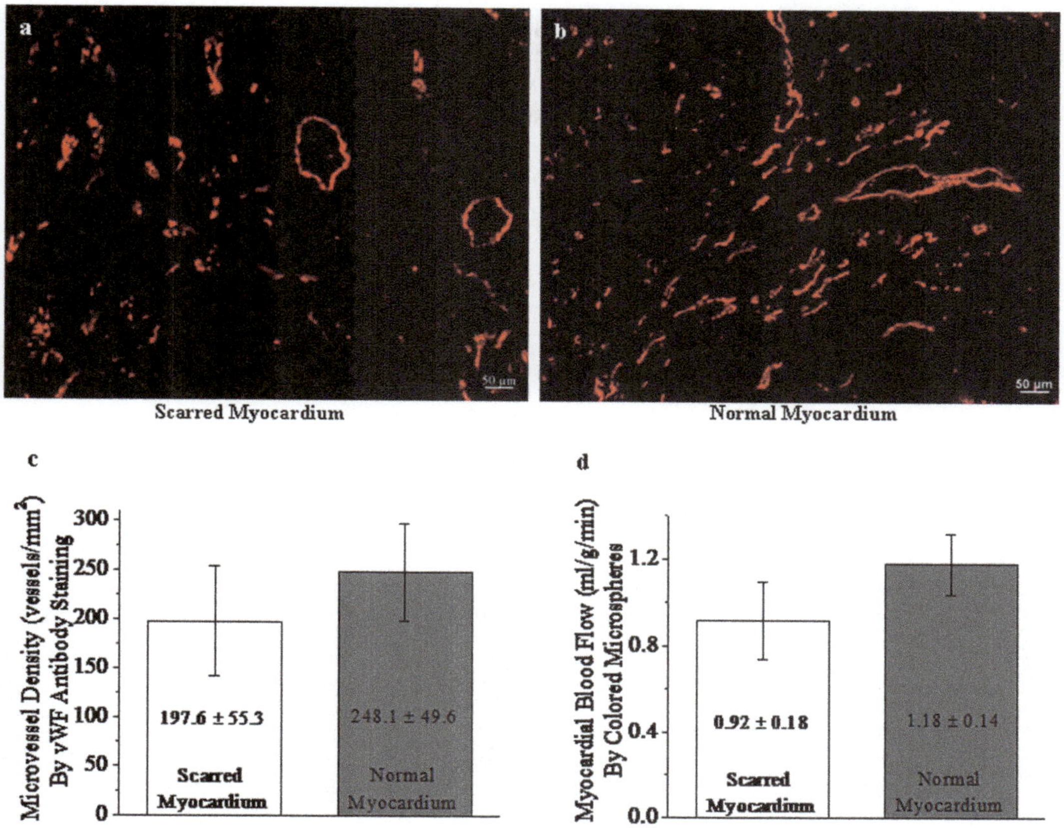

Figure 7. Myocardial blood flow and microvessel density. Scarred myocardium exhibited the dilated vessels and numerous microvessels (a), which resembled those observed in normal myocardium (b). Myocardial blood flow and microvessel density were significantly recovered to 0.92±0.18 ml/g/min (c) and 197.6±55.3 vessels/mm^2 (d) despite slightly lower than these observed measured in normal myocardium.

extensively extracellular matrix deposition is believed to be another critical reason for the increased percentage of extracellular volume. Fibrillar collagen content in the developing scar tissue increases steadily over the first few weeks after myocardial infarction, reaching a plateau after 4 weeks or more post-infarction [25,26]. Subsequently, accumulated collagen gradually deposit into the network of collagen fiber. Most of collagen fibers are typically oriented almost parallel to the longitudinal direction of the original myofiber bundles [27,28]. Other studies have shown that a small amount of collagen fiber is usually aligned at some oblique angle in the longitudinal direction [29]. Consequently, scarred myocardium consists largely of three-dimensional structural framework of fibrosis collagens to which discrete matrix components are attached [30,31]. Our histological staining section clearly indicated that scarred myocardium was deficient in cellularity and mainly comprised discrete matrix deposition. Although increased extracellular volume percentage is mainly responsible for enlarged distribution of CAs, it cannot be neglected that capillary permeability is also the critical factor to affect the distribution of CA. Different from Gd-DTPA, distribution volume of P792 in scarred myocardium didn't differ from that in normal myocardium, indicating that the macromolecular CA was still retained within intravascular space. Therefore, the permeability of vessels within scarred myocardium is comparable to that of normal myocardium, permitting free diffusion of Gd-DTPA rather than P792 into enlarged interstitial space of scarred myocardium.

Delayed enhancement occurs for both acute (necrosis) and chronic (scar) myocardial infarction after the administration of Gd-DTPA [32]. The mechanism responsible for the delayed hyper-enhancement of myocardial infarction has been widely and extensively studied in prior investigations. However, most prior studies have focused more on acute infarction than chronic infarction. Delayed enhancement in acute infarction can be attributed to the increased extracellular space consequent to the loss of cell membrane integrity, which allows the contrast molecule to enter the myocyte intracellular space [33]. As infarction evolves, the necrotic myocytes were replaced by a dense fibrous scar with remodelled vessels. The pathological alterations of acute and chronic infarction differ considerably, thus the enhancement patterns in acute and chronic infarction might also be different. The delayed hyper-enhancement of chronic infarction is mostly due to remodelled microvessels supporting contrast transportation and the relatively large extracellular matrix of the developed scar allowing contrast accumulation.

In summary, MR contrast agents are able to enter the scarred myocardium as a consequence of newly formed collateral flow and remaining vessels of dilation within scar tissue. Microvascular permeability within scarred myocardium allows extracellular rather than intravascular CAs to leak into interstitial compartment. The striking decrease in cellularity and extensively discrete matrix deposition provide the enlarged extravascular space for extracellular CAs. Therefore, scarred myocardium exhibits hyperenhancement in Gd-DTPA enhanced T_1 imaging, whereas administration of P792 causes the homogeneous enhancement in regions of scarred and normal myocardium.

Author Contributions

Conceived and designed the experiments: JW GT. Performed the experiments: JW BX HL. Analyzed the data: H-YL. Contributed reagents/materials/analysis tools: DF RCA. Wrote the paper: JW.

References

1. Ramani K, Judd RM, Holly TA, Parrish TB, Rigolin VH, et al. (1998) Contrast magnetic resonance imaging in the assessment of myocardial viability in patients with stable coronary artery disease and left ventricular dysfunction. Circulation 98:2687–94.
2. Bulow H, Klein C, Kuehn I, Hollweck R, Nekolla SG, et al. (2005) Cardiac magnetic resonance imaging: long term reproducibility of the late enhancement signal in patients with chronic coronary artery disease. Heart 91:1158–63.
3. Klein C, Nekolla SG, Bengel FM, Momose M, Sammer A, et al. (2002) Assessment of myocardial viability with contrast-enhanced magnetic resonance imaging: comparison with positron emission tomography. Circulation 105:162–7.
4. Mahrholdt H, Wagner A, Holly TA, Elliott MD, Bonow RO, et al. (2002) Reproducibility of chronic infarct size measurement by contrast-enhanced magnetic resonance imaging. Circulation 106:2322–7.
5. Lima JA, Judd RM, Bazille A, Schulman SP, Atalar E, et al. (1995) Regional heterogeneity of human myocardial infarcts demonstrated by contrast-enhanced MRI. Potential mechanisms. Circulation 92:1117–25.
6. Saeed M, Wendland MF, Yu KK, Lauerma K, Li HT, et al. (1994) Identification of myocardial reperfusion with echo planar magnetic resonance imaging. Discrimination between occlusive and reperfused infarctions. Circulation 90:1492–501.
7. Judd RM, Lugo-Olivieri CH, Arai M, Kondo T, Croisille P, et al. (1995) Physiological basis of myocardial contrast enhancement in fast magnetic resonance images of 2-day-old reperfused canine infarcts. Circulation 92:1902–10.
8. Ambrosio G, Weisman HF, Mannisi JA, Becker LC (1989) Progressive impairment of regional myocardial perfusion after initial restoration of postischemic blood flow. Circulation 80:1846–61.
9. Pereira RS, Prato FS, Wisenberg G, Sykes J (1996) The determination of myocardial viability using Gd-DTPA in a canine model of acute myocardial ischemia and reperfusion. Magn Reson Med 36:684–93.
10. Tong CY, Prato FS, Wisenberg G, Lee TY, Carroll E, et al. (1993) Measurement of the extraction efficiency and distribution volume for Gd-DTPA in normal and diseased canine myocardium. Magn Reson Med 30:337–46.
11. Schwitter J, Saeed M, Wendland MF, Derugin N, Canet E, et al. (1997) Influence of severity of myocardial injury on distribution of macromolecules: extravascular versus intravascular gadolinium-based magnetic resonance contrast agents. J Am Coll Cardiol 30:1086–94.
12. Saeed M, van Dijke CF, Mann JS, Wendland MF, Rosenau W, et al. (1998) Histologic confirmation of microvascular hyperpermeability to macromolecular MR contrast medium in reperfused myocardial infarction. J Magn Reson Imaging 8:561–7.
13. Wang Y, Sun W, Cao G, Meng L, Song L, et al. (2006) Delayed hyperenhancement patterns in occlusive and reperfused myocardial infarcts during different healing stages. J Magn Reson Imaging 24:851–7.
14. Roth DM, Maruoka Y, Rogers J, White FC, Longhurst JC, et al. (1987) Development of coronary collateral circulation in left circumflex Ameroid-occluded swine myocardium. Am J Physiol 253:H1279–88.
15. Gorge G, Schmidt T, Ito BR, Pantely GA, Schaper W (1989) Microvascular and collateral adaptation in swine hearts following progressive coronary artery stenosis. Basic Res Cardiol 84:524–35.
16. White FC, Carroll SM, Magnet A, Bloor CM (1992) Coronary collateral development in swine after coronary artery occlusion. Circ Res 71:1490–500.
17. Johnston DL, Homma S, Liu P, Weilbaecher DG, Rokey R, et al. (1988) Serial changes in nuclear magnetic resonance relaxation times after myocardial infarction in the rabbit: relationship to water content, severity of ischemia, and histopathology over a six-month period. Magn Reson Med 8:363–79.
18. Schwartz H, Leiboff RH, Bren GB, Wasserman AG, Katz RJ, et al. (1984) Temporal evolution of the human coronary collateral circulation after myocardial infarction. J Am Coll Cardiol 4:1088–93.
19. Kramer MF, Kinscherf R, Aidonidis I, Metz J (1998) Occurrence of a terminal vascularisation after experimental myocardial infarction. Cell Tissue Res 291:97–105.
20. Donahue KM, Burstein D, Manning WJ, Gray ML (1994) Studies of Gd-DTPA relaxivity and proton exchange rates in tissue. Magn Reson Med 32:66–76.
21. Flacke SJ, Fischer SE, Lorenz CH (2001) Measurement of the gadopentetate dimeglumine partition coefficient in human myocardium in vivo: normal distribution and elevation in acute and chronic infarction. Radiology 218:703–10.
22. Rehwald WG, Fieno DS, Chen EL, Kim RJ, Judd RM (2002) Myocardial magnetic resonance imaging contrast agent concentrations after reversible and irreversible ischemic injury. Circulation 105:224–9.
23. Saeed M, Weber O, Lee R, Do L, Martin A, et al. (2006) Discrimination of myocardial acute and chronic (scar) infarctions on delayed contrast enhanced magnetic resonance imaging with intravascular magnetic resonance contrast media. J Am Coll Cardiol 48:1961–8.
24. Morales C, Gonzalez GE, Rodriguez M, Bertolasi CA, Gelpi RJ (2002) Histopathologic time course of myocardial infarct in rabbit hearts. Cardiovasc Pathol 11:339–45.
25. Sun Y, Zhang JQ, Zhang J, Lamparter S (2000) Cardiac remodeling by fibrous tissue after infarction in rats. J Lab Clin Med 135:316–23.
26. Cleutjens JP, Verluyten MJ, Smiths JF, Daemen MJ (1995) Collagen remodeling after myocardial infarction in the rat heart. Am J Pathol 147:325–38.
27. Holmes JW, Yamashita H, Waldman LK, Covell JW (1994) Scar remodeling and transmural deformation after infarction in the pig. Circulation 90:411–20.
28. Vracko R, Thorning D, Frederickson RG (1989) Connective tissue cells in healing rat myocardium. A study of cell reactions in rhythmically contracting environment. Am J Pathol 134:993–1006.
29. Whittaker P, Boughner DR, Kloner RA (1989) Analysis of healing after myocardial infarction using polarized light microscopy. Am J Pathol 134:879–93.
30. Cleutjens JP, Creemers EE (2002) Integration of concepts: cardiac extracellular matrix remodeling after myocardial infarction. J Card Fail 8:S344–8
31. Murry CE, Giachelli CM, Schwartz SM, Vracko R (1994) Macrophages express osteopontin during repair of myocardial necrosis. Am J Pathol 145:1450–62.
32. Kim RJ, Fieno DS, Parrish TB, Harris K, Chen EL, et al. (1999) Relationship of MRI delayed contrast enhancement to irreversible injury, infarct age, and contractile function. Circulation 100:1992–2002.
33. Klein C, Schmal TR, Nekolla SG, Schnackenburg B, Fleck E, et al. (2007) Mechanism of late gadolinium enhancement in patients with acute myocardial infarction. J Cardiovasc Magn Reson 9:653–8.

Abdominal Aortic Intimal Flap Motion Characterization in Acute Aortic Dissection: Assessed with Retrospective ECG-Gated Thoracoabdominal Aorta Dual-Source CT Angiography

Shifeng Yang[1], Xia Li[2], Baoting Chao[1], Lebin Wu[1], Zhaoping Cheng[1], Yanhua Duan[1], Dawei Wu[1], Yiqiang Zhan[3], Jiuhong Chen[4], Bo Liu[5], Xiaopeng Ji[1], Pei Nie[1], Ximing Wang[1]*

1 Shandong Medical Imaging Research Institute, Shandong University, Jinan, Shandong, P.R. China, **2** Departments of Ultrasound, Shandong Provincial Hospital, Jinan, Shandong, P. R. China, **3** Unit of Periodontology, University of Greifswald, Greifswald, Germany, **4** CT Research Collaboration, Siemens Ltd., China, Beijing, P.R. China, **5** Healthcare Sector, Siemens Ltd., China, Shanghai, P.R. China

Abstract

Objectives: To evaluate the feasibility of dose-modulated retrospective ECG-gated thoracoabdominal aorta CT angiography (CTA) assessing abdominal aortic intimal flap motion and investigate the motion characteristics of intimal flap in acute aortic dissection (AAD).

Materials and Methods: 49 patients who had thoracoabdominal aorta retrospective ECG-gated CTA scan were enrolled. 20 datasets were reconstructed in 5% steps between 0 and 95% of the R-R interval in each case. The aortic intimal flap motion was assessed by measuring the short axis diameters of the true lumen and false lumen 2 cm above of celiac trunk ostium in different R-R intervals. Intimal flap motion and configuration was assessed by two independent observers.

Results: In these 49 patients, 37 had AAD, 7 had intramural hematoma, and 5 had negative result for acute aortic disorder. 620 datasets of 31 patients who showed double lumens in abdominal aorta were enrolled in evaluating intimal flap motion. The maximum and minimum true lumen diameter were 12.2±4.1 mm (range 2.6~17.4) and 6.7±4.1 mm (range 0~15.3) respectively. The range of intimal flap motion in all patients was 5.5±2.6 mm (range 1.8~10.2). The extent of maximum true lumen diameter decreased during a cardiac cycle was 49.5%±23.5% (range 12%~100%). The maximum motion phase of true lumen diameter was in systolic phase (5%~40% of R-R interval). Maximum and minimum intimal flap motion was at 15% and 75% of the R-R interval respectively. Intimal flap configuration had correlation with the phase of cardiac cycle.

Conclusions: Abdominal intimal flap position and configuration varied greatly during a cardiac cycle. Retrospective ECG-gated thoracoabdominal aorta CTA can reflect the actual status of the true lumen and provide more information about true lumen collapse. This information may be helpful to diagnosis and differential diagnosis of dynamic abstraction.

Editor: Rudolf Kirchmair, Medical University Innsbruck, Austria

Funding: The authors have no support or funding to report.

Competing Interests: Jiuhong Chen and Bo Liu are employed by the Siemens. Ltd. China. There are no patents, products in development or marketed products to declare.

* E-mail: wxming369@163.com

Introduction

Acute aortic dissection (AAD) is a catastrophic disease with fatal outcomes. The overall in-hospital mortality of AAD was 27.4% [1]. The abdominal aortic branch obstruction is the key risk factor for AAD of both type A and type B [2,3,4]. Branch obstruction is classified as either "static" or "dynamic" with anatomical features [5]. Treatment decision of AAD has to be made depending on the branch obstruction mechanisms [6]. In the type of dynamic obstruction, the intimal flap spared the origin of the vessel, whereas compressed the true lumen at or above the origin of the aortic branch like a curtain [7]. Previous studies have demonstrated that the position and configuration of intimal flap were correlated with dynamic obstruction [5,8]. Furthermore, the aorta is a dynamic structure and the intimal flap often oscillates as a result of changing flow conditions [9]. Therefore the diagnostic information of intimal flap dynamics is important.

Conventional CT angiography (CTA) without ECG-gated only can capture the static images of intimal flap and reflect the conformation of the intimal flap at an arbitrary time point. Retrospective ECG-gated CTA allows the phase-resolved cine imaging and visualization. The "four dimension" images can assess the dynamics of the intimal flap movement within a cardiac cycle [9,10,11]. In addition, the artifacts of the ascending aorta caused by the cardiac pulsation can be eliminated by this technique. And the accurate anatomical information on entire aorta can lead to a higher diagnostic confidence [12].

However, comparing to the conventional CTA, the retrospective ECG-gated CTA is accompanied by higher radiation dose and longer acquisition time [13]. These disadvantages limit the application of the thoracoabdominal retrospective ECG-gated aorta CTA [14]. As a result, the tailored protocols of the combination of retrospective ECG-gated acquisition of the thoracic aorta with standard protocol for the abdominal aorta were used in the clinical practice [9,15,16]. Whereas data acquired from the modified protocols cannot provide the dynamic information on the intimal flap of the abdominal aorta.

With the increased spatial and temporal resolution and tube power of latest CT scanners, the data acquisition of retrospective ECG-gated thoracoabdominal aorta CTA within a single breath hold could be feasible [12,17]. Furthermore, new technologies on radiation dose reduction have been applied, especially in cardiovascular CTA. These strategies include tube voltage optimization, automatic tube current modulation, ECG-controlled tube current modulation and iterative reconstruction [18,19,20,21,22]. These integrated technologies have improved the efficiency for radiation dose reduction, and there are some studies on retrospective ECG-gated thoracoabdominal aortic CTA recently [12,23]. However, to our knowledge, how to evaluate abdominal aortic intimal flap motion with ECG-gated CTA in AAD is still unclear.

The purpose of this study is to evaluate the feasibility of dose-modulated retrospective ECG-gated thoracoabdominal aorta CT angiography (CTA) assessing abdominal aortic intimal flap motion and investigate the motion characteristics of intimal flap in acute aortic dissection (AAD).

Materials and Methods

Study Population

This retrospective study was approved by local institutional review board of Shandong Medical Imaging Research Institute, Shandong University, and written informed consent was obtained from each patient before examinations. Patients with suspected or known AAD were referred for retrospective ECG-gated thoraco-abdominal aortic CTA. From January 2012 to November 2012, a total of 49 consecutive patients(33 men, 16 women; age range, 30–73 years, mean age ± standard deviation, 49.25±10.4 years)were enrolled in the study. No β-blockers or heart-rate-lowering agents were administered before CT data acquisition.

Retrospective ECG-gated CTA Data Acquisition and Dose Estimation

Retrospective ECG-gated contrast enhanced CTA was performed by dual-source CT (Definition Flash; Siemens Healthcare,

Table 1. Data acquisition characteristics and radiation exposure estimates.

Characteristic	Result
BMI (kg/m^2)	24.64±3.36(18.20~35.33)
Heart rate (beats/min)	75.5±13.3(50~105)
Pitch	0.30±0.05(0.19~0.45)
Kv* 120	23
100	26
Scanning duration (sec)	15.8±2.8 (9.3~22.8)
Scanning range (mm)	578.8±36.2 (499~706)
$CTDI_{vol}$ (mGy)	16.1±6.8(7.6~33.6)
Dose-length product(mGy · cm)	896.4±373.4(450.1~1850.1)
Estimated effective radiation(mSv)	12.73±5.3(6.4~26.3)

Note.–Data are means ± standard deviations. Ranges are in parentheses.
*The tube voltage was 100 kV for patients with a BMI of less than 25 kg/m ^{2} and 120 kV for those with a BMI of at least 25 kg/m ^{2}. ***BMI***= Body Mass Index, ***$CTDI_{vol}$***= volume CT Dose Index.

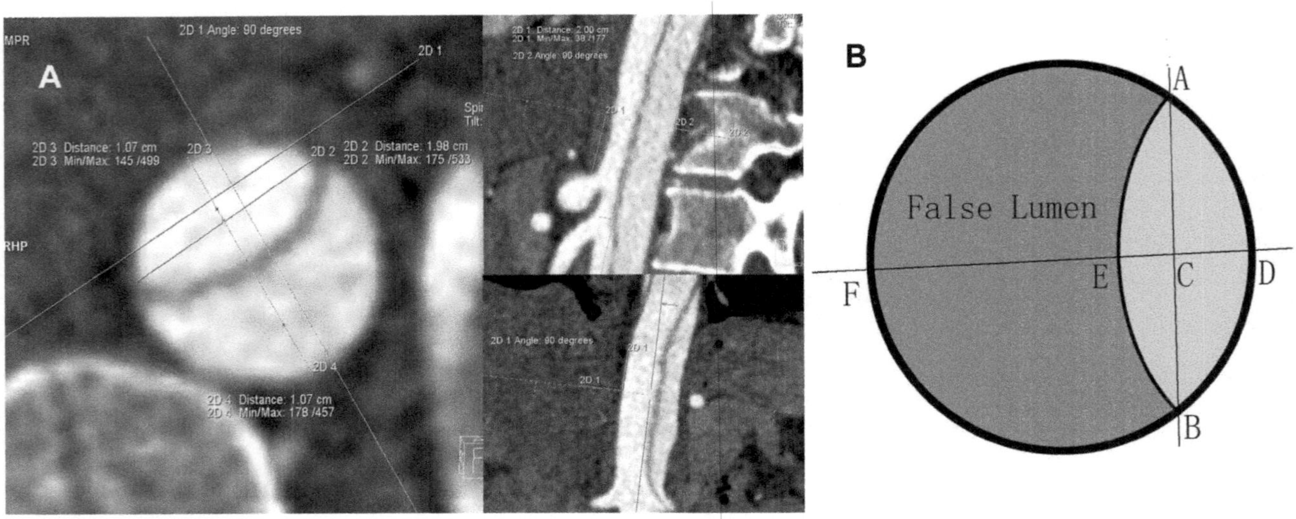

Figure 1. Measurement of lumen short axis diameters A. Double-oblique multiplanar reformations were adjusted perpendicularly to the longitudinal axis of aortic vessel course, at the level of 2 cm distal to the celiac trunk ostium. Outline the true and false lumen short axis diameter manually with the tool of distance measurement. **B.** Schematic illustration of short axis diameter measurement. Connecting the end points A and B of the dissected flap can get the segment AB. The perpendicular line through the mid point C intersects with true lumen wall, dissected flap and false lumen wall at point D, E and F respectively. Segment DE and EF are true lumen and false lumen short axis diameters respectively.

Forchheim, Germany) with 2×64×0.6 mm collimation, section acquisition of 2×64×0.6 mm, and a z-flying focal spot technique. The rotation time was 280 milliseconds. The data was acquired in a craniocaudal direction, with the full scanning range extending from the thoracic inlet to the femoral head. All patients were asked to elevate and place arms on the table and hold their breath after deep inspiration during the examination. Tube voltage was adjusted to body mass index ($\leqq$25.0 kg/m^2, 100 kv, n = 26; >25.0 kg/m^2, 120 kV, n = 23) as previous study [24]. Automatic tube current modulation (Caredose 4D: Siemens Healthcare) [19] was applied using reference mAs setting of 250. ECG-based tube current modulation technique (Adaptive ECG-Pulsing: Siemens Healthcare) [20] was applied using the following parameters. The "phase of interest" was centered at 70% of the R-R cycle. Outside the ECG-pulsing window, tube current was reduced to 20% of the peak tube current. Pitch values were adapted automatically by the lowest expected heart rate on the basis of the longest R-R interval of the last 10 heart beats before the start of data acquisition [25]. The minimum and maximum of pitch values were 0.19 and 0.45, respectively.

Iodinated contrast material (Omnipaque350, GE Healthcare, USA) was injected intravenously through an 18-gauge needle into the upper extremity peripheral vein at a flow rate of 4–4.5 ml/sec (total injected, 100–120 ml), followed by a saline chaser of 30 ml at the same flow rate. This was accomplished by using an electronic power dual injector (Stellant; Medrad, Indianola, PA, USA). Data acquisition was started 5 seconds after the contrast media reached a threshold of 100 Hounsfied unit with a region of interest (ROI) placed in the ascending aorta.

The age, height, and weight of the patients were recorded before the examination,and the average heart rate,scan range, scanning duration, volume CT dose index (CTDIvol), dose length product (DLP) were provided by the scanner. The effective dose estimate was determined by using DLP and appropriate normalized coefficients found in previous report ($k = 0.0145$ mSv·mGy^{-1}.cm^{-1} for chest CT, and $k = 0.0153$ mSv.mGy^{-1}.cm^{-1} for abdominal CT, $k = 0.0129$ mSv.mGy^{-1}.cm^{-1} for pelvic CT) [26]. Because a combination of chest, abdominal, and pelvic acquisitions was performed for thoracoabdominal CTA, the mean conversion coefficients ($k = 0.0142$ mSv.mGy^{-1}.cm^{-1}) was used, as previously described [23].

CT Data Reconstruction

From the ECG-synchronized CT raw datasets, morphological images were generally reconstructed through the entire chest and abdomen at 70% of the R-R interval with 1-mm slice thickness, 0.7-mm increments, I26f reconstruction kernel and 32 cm FOV. Functional imaging was then reconstructed in 5% steps between 0 and 95% of the R-R interval from the ECG with 1-mm slice thickness, 0.7-mm increments, I26f reconstruction kernel and 24 cm FOV. All datasets were reconstructed with sinogram affirmed iterative reconstruction (SAFIRE, Siemens Healthcare, Forchheim, Germany) and a medium strength level of 3 was used in all patients. All datasets were transferred to a Siemens Workstation (Syngo Workplace; Siemens Medical Solutions) for image analysis.

Assessment of Image Quality and Intimal Flap Movement

Aortic intraluminal attenuation and image noise were assessed as objective image quality parameters. Datasets acquired with full tube current and 20% of the peak tube current was analyzed. Images acquired with 20% of the peak tube current had the similar image quality, so datasets acquired at 25% of R-R interval were chosen randomly for objective image quality analyzed. Then datasets acquired at 25% (acquired with 20% of the peak tube current) and 70% (acquired with full tube current) of R-R interval were assessed. The ROIs were placed in the ascending aorta, descending aorta at the level of the right pulmonary trunk plane and at the level of 2 cm above the celiac trunk ostium. In case of aortic dissection, the ROIs were placed in the true lumen. ROIs used for measure were set as large as possible due to the high variation of the true lumen area during a cardiac cycle. In case of true lumen collapsed completely, the ROIs were placed in the false lumen at the same level. Image noise was assessed as the standard deviation of the mean attenuation in all respective ROIs.

Motion artifact of intimal flap of each phase was assessed as subjective image quality parameters. The criteria for the present of motion artifacts is intimal flap blurred outlines or double range. It was assessed by a consensus reading of two radiologists.

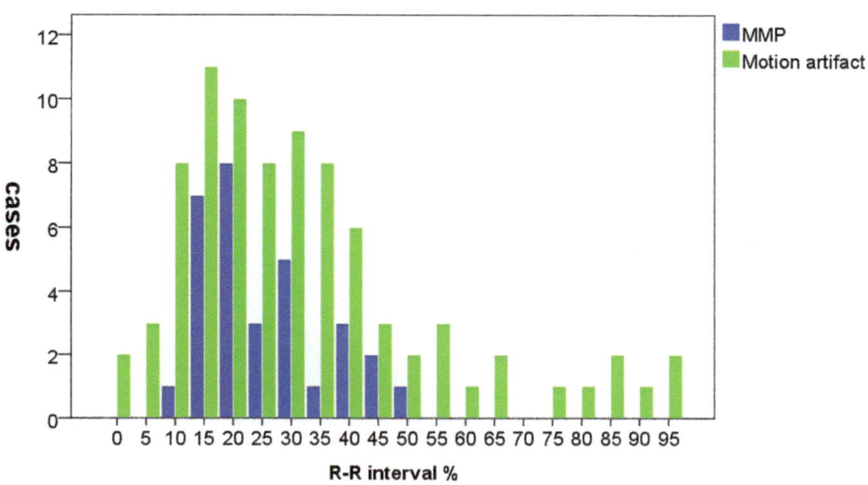

Figure 2. The frequency distributions of MMP and intimal flap motion artifacts during a cardiac cycle. The MMP of all cases was at systolic phase (5%~40% of R-R interval) and the peak was found at 15% of the R-R interval. Most intimal flap motion artifacts were founded at systolic phase. Datasets acquired at 70% R-R interval had no intimal flap motion artifacts.

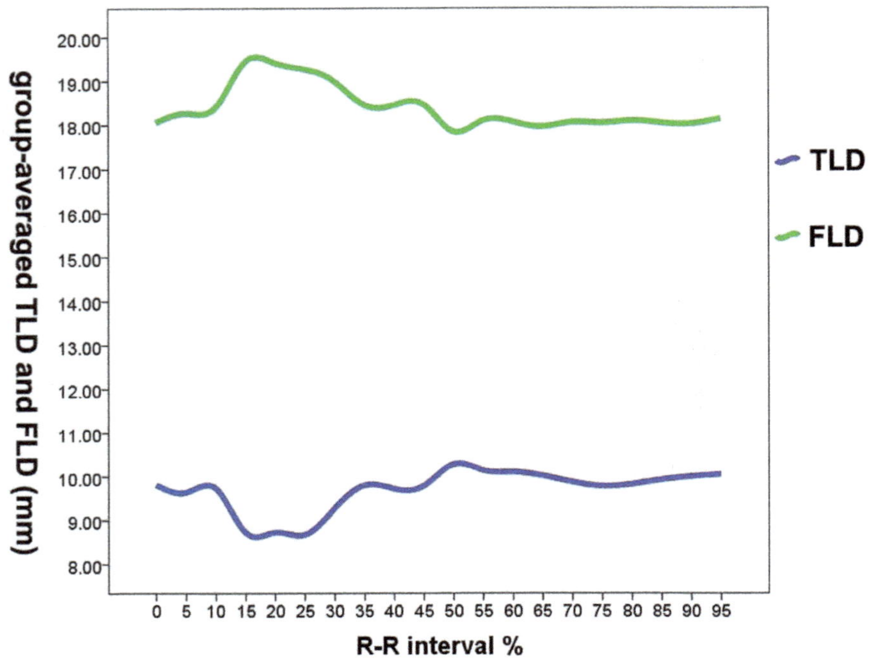

Figure 3. Time courses of TLD and FLD during the R-R interval. Group-averaged TLD, FLD of each phase were plotted against time in percentages of R-R interval. Group-averaged FLD was larger than group-averaged TLD in every phase. Although there was no statistically significant difference in R-R intervals, a peak for group-averaged FLD and a trough for group-averaged TLD were found in 15% of R-R interval.

To assess the dynamic changes of intimal flap related to the phase of cardiac cycle, the true lumen short axis diameter (TLD) and the false lumen short axis diameter (FLD) were measured at different phases of a cardiac cycle. TLD and FLD were measured at the level of 2 cm above the celiac trunk ostium by two independent observers with 4 years and 7 years of experience in CTA. To assess the aortic diameter, multiplanar reformation images were taken in a strictly transverse orientation through the abdominal aorta. How TLD was measured was represented in **Fig. 1**. The configuration of the intimal flap was classified as curved toward the false lumen, curved toward the true lumen and flat, as previously described [27]. It was assessed independently by the two observers. In case of disagreement in classifying between the observers, a final decision was obtained by consensus.

Data Analysis

The method developed by Husmann L et al. [28] was applied in our study, in which all time instances were expressed as percentages of the R-R interval to enable comparisons of intimal flap motion amplitude for all patients. The motion amplitude of intimal flap was quantified by the change of the TLD at every 5% R-R interval. It was expressed as the absolute value of relative change between the TLD (RCTLD) of adjacent phases of R-R interval. With this approach, for example, intimal flap motion amplitude of the time interval 20% refers to the absolute difference of TLD between 15% and 20% of the R-R interval. On the basis of measurements, the following variables were obtained:

(1) The maximum change of TLD (MCTLD) and relative decrease of TLD (RDTLD) during a cardiac cycle: MCTLD was defined as the difference between individual maximum TLD (TLDmax) and minimum TLD (TLDmin) over a cardiac cycle; RDTLD was defined as the ratios of MCTLD to TLDmax. MCTLD reflect the range of intimal flap motion and RDTLD reflect the extent of TLDmax decreased during a cardiac cycle. (2) RCTLD and maximum motion phase (MMP) of TLD over a cardiac cycle: RCTLD defined as the absolute difference between the TLD of adjacent time intervals, which reflects the change of TLD at a given percentage of time intervals. MMP was defined as the phase of R-R interval where the maximum RCTLD was at. The design formulas were as follow:

$$\mathrm{MCTLD} = \mathrm{TLDmax} - \mathrm{TLDmin};$$

$$\mathrm{RDTLD} = (\mathrm{MCTLD}/\mathrm{TLDmax}) \times 100\%;$$

$$\mathrm{RCTLDn} = |\mathrm{TLDn} - \mathrm{TLD(n-1)}|.$$

Where "n" represents a given phase of the R-R interval and "(n−1)" represents the previous phase.

Table 2. True lumen diameter characteristics.

characteristic	median	range
TLDmax(mm)	12.2±4.1	2.6~17.4
TLDmin(mm)	6.7±4.1	0~15.3
MCTLD(mm)	5.5±2.6	1.8~10.2
RDTLD	49.5%±23.5%	12%~100%

Note.- ***TLDmax***= maximum True Lumen Diameter, ***TLDmin***= minimum True Lumen Diameter, ***MCTLD***= Maximum Change of True Lumen Diameter, ***RDTLD***= Relative Decrease of maximum True Lumen Diameter.

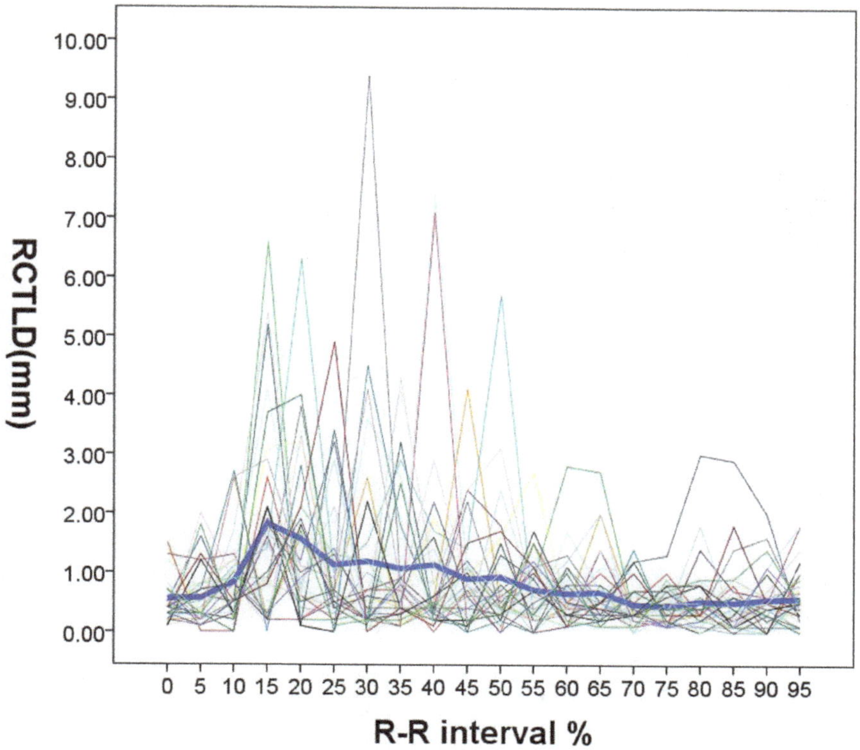

Figure 4. Time courses of RCTLD during the R-R interval. Individual (light line) and group-averaged (dark line) RCTLD were plotted against time in percentages of R-R interval. Despite high inter-individual variation, group-averaged RCTLD showed clear biphasic pulsatility in 10%–25% of R-R intervals.

Statistical Analysis

Quantitative variables were presented as the mean ± standard deviation (ranges). Objective image quality of datasets acquired at 25% and 70% of R-R interval display normal distribution. They were compared with the paired two-tailed Student's t-test. A value of $p<0.05$ was considered statistically significant. Interobserver variation of diameter measurement was evaluated by using the Bland-Altman analysis [29]. Interobserver agreement on classifying the intimal flap configuration was calculated before consensus reading by using Kappa statistics. A kappa value of more than 0.81 corresponded to excellent interobserver agreement, with values of 0.61–0.80 corresponding to good agreement [24]. TLD, FLD measurements were averaged for both observers. TLD, FLD displayed normal distribution, but the RCTLD did not. Therefore, RCTLD was log transformed before analysis to meet assumptions of normality. Bonferroni post-hoc tests were used for multiple pair wise comparisons of FLD, TLD and RCTLD within time intervals. A value of $p<0.05$ was considered statistically significant.

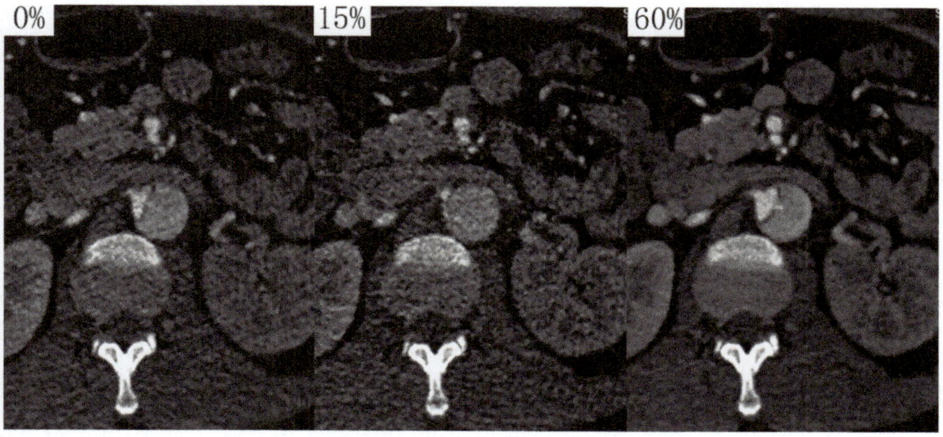

Figure 5. Images in different phases demonstrated different anatomical features. At the right renal artery origin, 0% and 15% datasets could not demonstrate reentry tear, but 60% datasets can demonstrate reentry tear clearly. It was worthy to note that true lumen was completely collapsed and the flap nearly was invisible in 15% R-R interval. However, it was of reasonable caliber in 60% R-R interval.

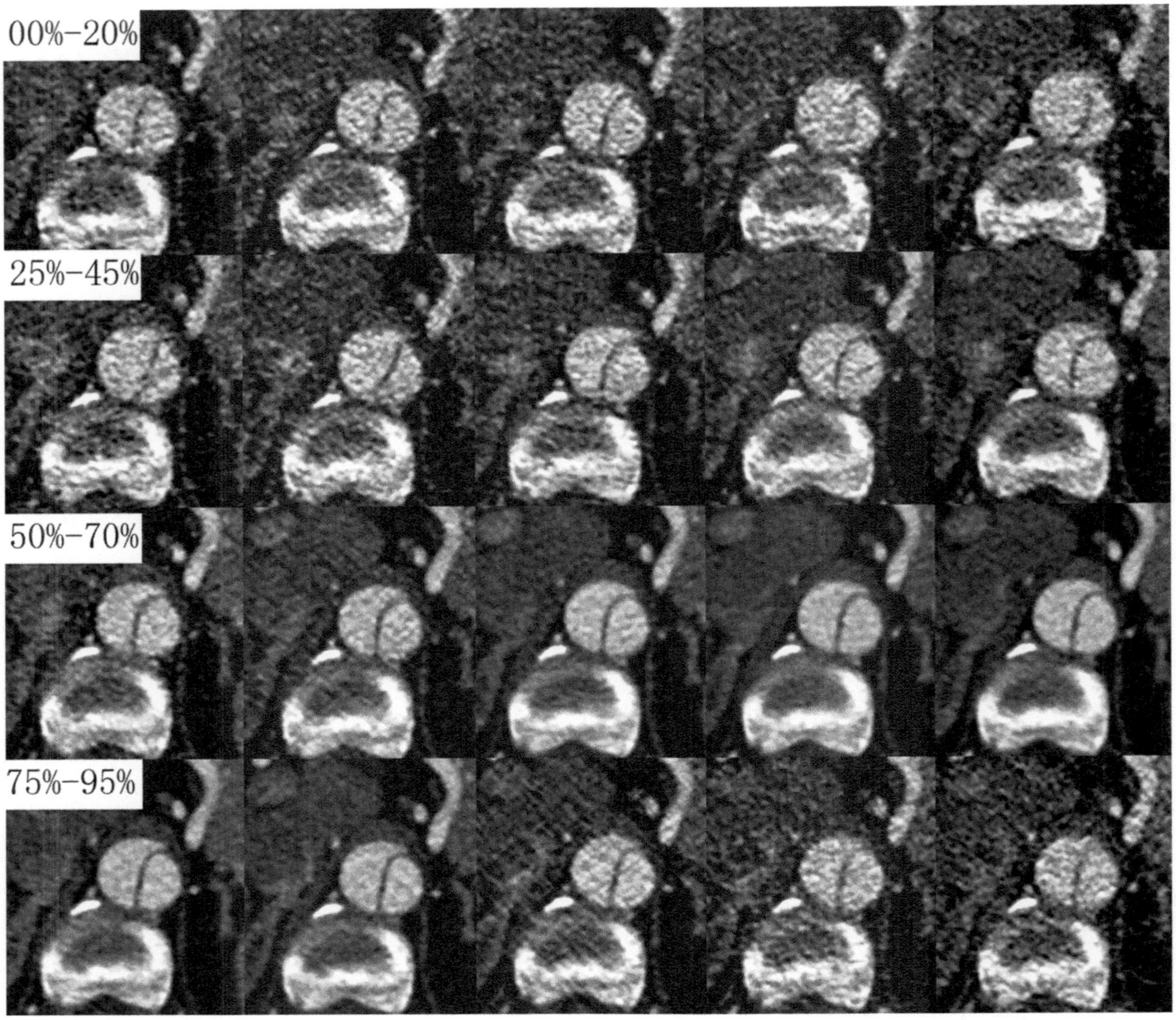

Figure 6. Transverse CT images of different phases at the same level. The intimal flap configuration, position and area of the true and false lumens were extremely variable during a cardiac cycle at the same level.

All statistical analyses were performed with statistical software SPSS 17.0 (SPSS, Chicago, IL, USA).

Results

All retrospective ECG-gated thoracoabdominal aortic CTA examinations were successful. In these 49 patients, 37 had AAD, 7 had intramural hematoma, and 5 had negative result for acute aortic disorder. Onset time of AAD was from 2 hours to 12 days. According to DeBakey classification [30], 20 of the 37 (54.1%) patients were type I, 3 of the 37 (8.1%) patients were type II, and 14 of the 37 (37.8%) were type III. 620 datasets of 31 patients (both type I and type III) who showed double lumens in abdominal aorta were enrolled in evaluating intimal flap motion. The data acquisition characteristics and radiation doses of 49 patients were listed in **Table 1.** The CTDIvol, DLP, and effective dose were 16.1±6.8 (7.6~33.6) mGy, 896.4±373.4 (450.1~1850.1) mGy.cm, and 12.7±5.3 (6.4~26.3) mSv respectively.

Objective and Subjective Image Quality

Datasets acquired at 70% R-R interval had preferable image quality due to its lower image noise and less intimal flap motion artifacts. Image noise was significantly lower in datasets of 70% R-R interval compared with datasets of 25% R-R interval in all measurements (ascending aorta, 26.8±6.4 vs 48.9±5.2, $p<0.01$; descending aorta, 23.2±5.5 vs 46.2±5.8, $p<0.01$; abdomen aorta, 24.4±5.1 vs 47.3±5.4, $p<0.01$). There were no statistically significant differences in intraluminal contrast attenuation between both datasets in all measurements (ascending aorta, 386.9±63.6 Hu vs 382.4±65.1 Hu, $p>0.05$; descending aorta, 381.4±55.3 Hu vs 371.9±58.8 Hu, $p>0.05$; abdomen aorta, 377.6±60.0 Hu vs 376.0±62.4 Hu, $p>0.05$).

The frequency distributions of intimal flap motion artifacts during a cardiac cycle were represented in **Fig. 2**. 83 of 620 (13.4%) intimal flaps had motion artifacts. 65 of 83(78.3%) intimal flaps motion artifacts were at systolic phase (0%~40% of R-R interval) and there was a peak at 15% of the R-R interval. Datasets acquired at 70% R-R interval had no intimal flap motion artifacts.

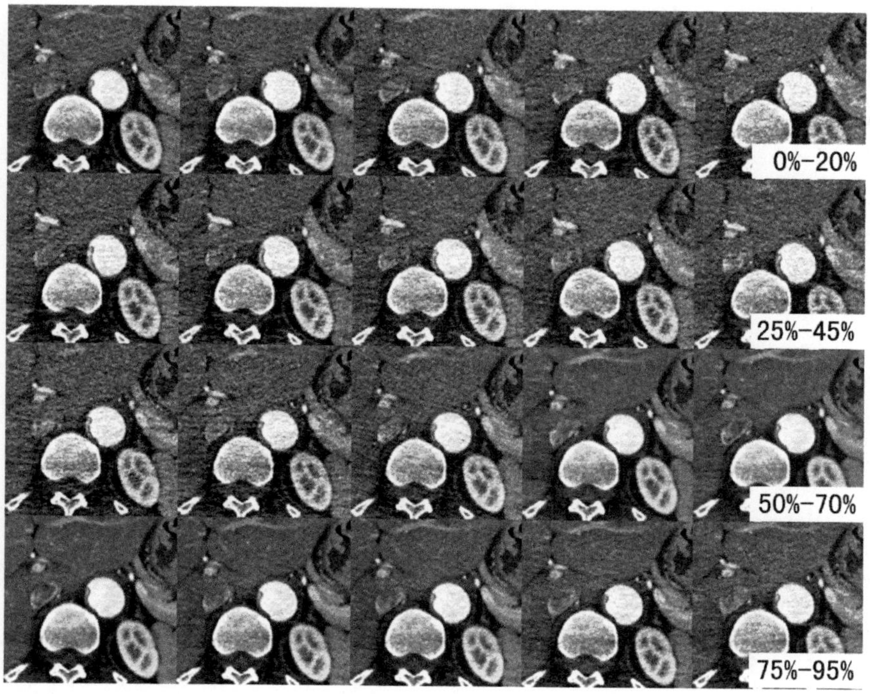

Figure 7. True lumen completely collapses during the cardiac cycle. 0–95% datasets showed that the true lumen was completely collapsed. The position of internal flap was changed mildly, but the configuration of intimal flap was not changed in different R-R intervals.

Interobserver Variation Assessment

The Bland-Altman analysis of interobserver variation of diameter measurements demonstrated good results. The measurement error of TLD and FLD were 0.085 and 0.078 respectively, whereas the 95% limits of agreement were1.630 to −1.460 and 1.410 to −1.254 mm respectively. Overall interobserver agreement on intimal flap configuration classifying was excellent (k = 0.93).

Motion Characterization of Intimal Flap

Time courses of group-averaged TLD and FLD were represented in **Fig. 3**. Both TLD and FLD changed during the cardiac cycle and their dynamic behaviors were highly variable for each patient. Peak of group-averaged FLD (19.44±4.07 mm) and trough of group-averaged TLD (8.67±5.16 mm) were found at 15% of the R-R interval. However, there were no significant statistical differences comparing to other R-R intervals ($p > 0.05$).

The range and means ± standard deviations of the TLDmax, TLDmin, MCTLD and RDTLD in all patients were listed in **Table 2.** The range of intimal flap motion in all patients was 1.8~10.2 mm, means ± standard deviations was 5.5±2.6 mm. TLDmax can decrease up to 100% (mean: 49.5%) during a cardiac cycle. The frequency distributions of MMP during a cardiac cycle were represented in **Fig. 2**. All of the MMP were at systolic phase (5%~40% of R-R interval) and there was a peak at 15% of the R-R interval.

Time courses for individual and group-averaged RCTLD were represented in **Fig. 4**. Although the dynamic behaviors of intimal flap varied greatly in each patient, the group-averaged intimal flap motion was synchronized to the heart pulsation. Peak intimal flap motion amplitude (1.82±1.69 mm) was found at 15% of the R-R interval; group-averaged intimal flap motion amplitude in this interval was higher than those at any other time intervals (0%–10% and 55%–95%: $p < 0.05$; 20%–50%: $p > 0.05$). The minimum intimal flap motion amplitude was found at 75% (0.440±0.31 mm) of the R-R interval, and second minimum (0.464±0.31 mm) was found at 70% of the R-R interval. Intimal flap motion amplitude in these two R-R intervals was less than that in other R-R intervals (15%, 20%: $p < 0.05$; 0%–10% and 25%–95%: $p > 0.05$).

Intimal Flap Configuration

3 types of intimal flap configurations were found in every R-R intervals. 312 of 620(50.3%) intimal flaps curved toward the false lumen, 226 of 620(36.5%) intimal flaps curved toward the true lumen, and 82 of 620(13.2%) intimal flaps were flat**.** However their distribution within the time interval was different. Initial flap curved toward the false lumen at 0%~5% and 35%~95% of the R-R interval in over half the samples. This tendency was reversed at 10~30% of R-R interval. Intimal flap curved toward the true lumen (64.5%) or were flat (22.6%) at 15% and 20% of the R-R interval. Only 4 of 31 (12.9%) intimal flap curved toward the false lumen at 15% and 20% of the R-R interval.

Discussion

By exploiting the currently available options for dose reduction, our retrospective ECG-gated CTA protocol of the whole aorta could maintain radiation doses within acceptable limits, according to the reference values of the International Commission on Radiological Protection [31] (DLP of 650, 780, 570 mGy.cm and CTDIvol of 30, 35, 35 given for routine thorax, abdominal and pelvic scan protocols, respectively). The estimated median effective dose was 12.73±5.30(rang, 6.39~26.27) mSv, which was similar with normal whole chest retrospective ECG-gated CTA (triple-rule-out CTA) [32] and prospective ECG-gated whole aorta CTA [33]. However, both the latter cannot be used for dynamic abdominal aortic intimal flap assessment and may suffer from motion artifacts in abdominal aorta.

Other ECG-gating techniques were recently introduced in whole aorta CTA with lower radiation dose. Prospective ECG-gating sequential data acquisition was introduced for the thoracic aorta or whole aorta CTA, resulting in further dose reduction [24,33]. In these studies, data acquisition time during a cardiac phase was set to a narrow window without additional padding time for further reconstructions. Then it could not reconstruct datasets of whole cardiac phase and assess the aortic intimal flap oscillation. If we expand the acquisition time window to the whole cardiac phase to assess intimal flap motion, the radiation dose will increase significantly. In addition, longer acquisition time is another defect of prospective ECG-gating sequential data acquisition. It will increase the contrast load [34], and the patients may be unable to hold their breath due to the large scan range in our study. High-pitch technique combined with prospective ECG triggering can provide volumetric data at a prespecified phase in the cardiac cycle and reduce radiation dose significantly [35]. However, data acquired by ECG-gated high-pitch CTA can not evaluate the motion of intimal flap because no slice overlap is used.

The ECG-controlled tube current modulation technique plays an important role in the radiation dose reduction while allowing the full phases data acquisition to analyze the aortic flap movement and determine the optimal phase in our study. It has been described in previous studies that the aortic root and ascending thoracic aorta have the greatest motion during systole and have the least motion at mid to late diastole [36]. To acquire motion-free images of ascending aorta, we centered the "phase of interest" at 70% of the R-R cycle. To maintain radiation doses "as low as reasonably achievable", the pulsing window was strictly chosen to a tailored level with the full tube current exposure whilst the outside pulsing window with 20% of the full tube current which allowed for further image reconstructions in the study. Compared with full tube current datasets, images acquired with 20% of the peak tube current had inferior image quality for the increase image noise. But it could meet the requirements for the measurement of lumen diameter and assessment of configuration. Because in the interobserver analysis, both the Bland-Altman analysis of lumen diameter and *k* test of classifying initial flap configuration demonstrated excellent interobserver agreement. Moreover, these datasets were able to provide additional information. For instance they were helpful for demonstrating entry tears and reentry tears because both tears might not be identified clearly in some phases due to motion artifacts or shrinking of the intimal flap (**Fig. 5**).

Our study demonstrated peak intimal flap motion was at 15% of the R-R interval. Centering the "interest phase" at 70% of the R-R cycle not only eliminates the ascending aorta motion artifact,but also avoids the MMP of intimal flap, allowing for motion-free images of the abdominal intimal flap in most cases. Thus, centering the "interest phase" at 70% or 75% of the R-R cycle may be the optimal ECG pulsing window for retrospective thoracoabdominal aorta CTA in AAD.

The intimal flap motion was related to blood pressure change of the two channels. Our study demonstrated the MMP was at systolic phase and maximum intimal flap motion was found at 15% of the R-R interval. This indicated that the transmural pressure gradient on the intimal flap was the highest at systolic phase. The flap would always curve to the lumen with lower pressure. So the direction of flap curvature was pivotal in estimating transmural pressure gradient on the intimal flap. Our study showed that transmural pressure gradient on the intimal flap varied and the variation was related to the phase of cardiac cycle. During middle and later systolic phase, the false lumen pressure was higher than or equivalent to true lumen pressure in most patients. However, during diastolic phase and early systolic phase, the false lumen pressure was lower than true lumen pressure in more than half patients. Only 4 of 31 (12.9%) intimal flap curved toward the false lumen at 15% and 20% of the R-R interval during middle and later systolic phase. This variation may be related to the different anatomic configurations of tear size, number and location [37,38].

Previous studies demonstrated that the position and configuration of intimal flap were correlated with dynamic obstruction [5,8]. Our study demonstrated that the intimal flap oscillated to a large extent during a cardiac cycle. The intimal flap's configuration, position, and then the area of the true and false lumens varied extremely at the same level (**Fig. 6 and Movie S1**). In some cases, the true lumen even collapsed partially. A false lumen could completely fill the aorta and obliterate the true lumen in some certain R-R intervals, whereas in other R-R intervals both lumens were of reasonable calibers (**Fig. 5**). In such cases, the estimation of the true lumen collapse will conflict with images reconstructed from different R-R intervals. However, in other cases, the true lumen collapsed completely (**Fig. 7**). In such cases, the position of internal flap was changed mildly, but the configuration of intimal flap was not changed in different R-R intervals. Conventional static images acquired by non-gated CT often provide anatomical features (such as the position of intimal flap) at an arbitrary location across the cardiac cycle. Then potential errors may occur when we use static images to assess whether the true lumen collapses or not.

Different from static CT images, "four dimension" images acquired with prospective ECG-gated can provide dynamic information of abdominal aortic intimal flap. They can tell whether complete or partial collapse existed in the true lumen. According to the definition of dynamic abstraction, true lumen collapse is the key factor to diagnose dynamic abstraction [5]. Then this information may be helpful to diagnosis and differential diagnosis of dynamic abstraction.

Limitations

In this feasible study, we only assessed the intimal flap motion at the level of top 2 cm to celiac trunk ostium. Because intraaortic hemodynamic is greatly variable in different regions of the aorta [11,38], the intimal flap motion in different regions may have different details. In consequence, more levels should be analyzed in future studies, such as at every branch origin plane.

Conclusions

Dose-modulated retrospective ECG-gated thoracoabdominal aorta CTA can assess the abdominal intimal flap motion in acute AAD in addition to the primary diagnostic question. Abdominal intimal flap position and configuration varied greatly during a cardiac cycle and the variation was related to the phase of cardiac cycle. Retrospective ECG-gated thoracoabdominal aorta CTA can reflect the actual status of the true lumen and provide more information about true lumen collapse. This information may be helpful to diagnosis and differential diagnosis of dynamic abstraction.

Supporting Information

Movie S1 Intimal flap configuration, position changed during a cardiac cycle. The intimal flap configuration, position and area of the true and false lumens were extremely variable during a cardiac cycle at the same level and the motion of intimal flap in different regions had different details.

Author Contributions

Conceived and designed the experiments: XW LW SY XL. Performed the experiments: SY XW BC ZC YD DW XJ PN. Analyzed the data: SY YZ XL BC XW ZC YD. Contributed reagents/materials/analysis tools: SY XL XW. Wrote the paper: SY XL XW JC BL PN.

References

1. Hagan PG, Nienaber CA, Isselbacher EM, Bruckman D, Karavite DJ, et al. (2000) The International Registry of Acute Aortic Dissection (IRAD): new insights into an old disease. JAMA 283: 897–903.
2. Deeb GM, Patel HJ, Williams DM (2010) Treatment for malperfusion syndrome in acute type A and B aortic dissection: A long-term analysis. J Thorac Cardiovasc Surg 140: S98–S100.
3. Yagdi T, Atay Y, Engin C, Mahmudov R, Tetik O, et al. (2006) Impact of organ malperfusion on mortality and morbidity in acute type A aortic dissections. J Card Surg. 2006 21: 363–369.
4. Patel HJ, Williams DM, Dasika NL, Suzuki Y, Deeb GM (2008) Operative delay for peripheral malperfusion syndrome in acute type A aortic dissection: a long-term analysis. J Thorac Cardiovasc Surg 135: 1288–1295.
5. Williams DM, Lee DY, Hamilton BH, Marx MV, Narasimham DL, et al. (1997) The dissected aorta: part III, Anatomy and radiologic diagnosis of branch-vessel compromise. Radiology 203: 37–44.
6. Midulla M, Fattori R, Beregi JP, Dake M, Rousseau H (2013) Aortic dissection and malperfusion syndrome: a when, what and how-to guide. Radiol Med 118: 74–88.
7. Williams DM, Lee DY, Hamilton BH, Marx MV, Narasimham DL, et al. (1997) The dissected aorta: percutaneous treatment of ischemic complications-principles and results. J Vasc Interv Radiol 8: 605–625.
8. Gaxotte V, Cocheteux B, Haulon S, Vincentelli A, Lions C, et al. (2003) Relationship of intimal flap position to endovascular treatment of malperfusion syndromes in aortic dissection. J Endovasc Ther 10: 719–727.
9. Ganten MK, Weber TF, von Tengg-Kobligk H, Böckler D, Stiller W, et al. (2009) Motion characterization of aortic wall and intimal flap by ECG-gated CT in patients with chronic B-dissection. Eur J Radiol 72: 146–153.
10. Murayama T, Funabashi N, Uehara M, Takaoka H, Komuro I (2010) New classification of aortic dissection during the cardiac cycle as pulsating type and static type evaluated by electrocardiogram-gated multislice CT. Int J Cardiol 142: 177–186.
11. Weber TF, Ganten MK, Böckler D, Geisbüsch P, Kopp-Schneider A, et al. (2009) Assessment of thoracic aortic conformational changes by four-dimensional computed tomography angiography in patients with chronic aortic dissection type b. Eur Radiol 19: 245–53.
12. Schernthaner RE, Stadler A, Beitzke D, Homolka P, Weber M, et al (2012) Dose modulated retrospective ECG-gated versus non-gated 64-row CT angiography of the aorta at the same radiation dose: comparison of motion artifacts, diagnostic confidence and signal-to-noise-ratios. Eur J Radiol 81: e585–590.
13. Primak AN, McCollough CH, Bruesewitz MR, Zhang J, Fletcher JG (2006) Relationship between noise, dose, and pitch in cardiac multi-detector row CT. Radiographics 26: 1785–1794.
14. Seung M, Yoo, White CS (2010) MDCT Evaluation of Acute Aortic Syndrome. Radiol Clin N Am 48: 67–83.
15. Fleischmann D, Mitchell RS, Miller DC (2008) Acute aortic syndromes: new insights from electrocardiographically gated computed tomography. Semin Thorac Cardiovasc Surg 20: 340–347.
16. McMahon MA, Squirrell CA (2010) Multidetector CT of Aortic Dissection: A Pictorial Review. Radiographics 30: 445–460.
17. Budde RP, Huo F, Cramer MJ, Doevendans PA, Bots ML, et al. (2010) Simultaneous aortic and coronary assessment in abdominal aortic aneurysm patients by thoraco-abdominal 64-detector-row CT angiography: estimate of the impact on preoperative management: a pilot study. Eur J Vasc Endovasc Surg 40: 196–201.
18. Schindera ST, Graca P, Patak MA, Abderhalden S, von Allmen G, et al. (2009) Thoracoabdominal-aortoiliac multidetector-row CT angiography at 80 and 100 kVp: assessment of image quality and radiation dose. Invest Radiol 44: 650–655.
19. Mulkens TH, Bellinck P, Baeyaert M, Ghysen D, Van Dijck X, et al. (2005) Use of an automatic exposure control mechanism for dose optimization in multi-detector row CT examinations: clinical evaluation. Radiology 237: 213–223.
20. Jakobs TF, Becker CR, Ohnesorge B, Flohr T, Suess C, et al. (2002) Multislice helical CT of the heart with retrospective ECG gating: reduction of radiation exposure by ECG-controlled tube current modulation. Eur Radiol 12: 1081–1086.
21. Alkadhi H, Schindera ST (2011) State of the art low-dose CT angiography of the body. Eur J Radiol 80: 36–40.
22. Cornfeld D, Israel G, Detroy E, Bokhari J, Mojibian H (2011) Impact of Adaptive Statistical Iterative Reconstruction (ASIR) on radiation dose and image quality in aortic dissection studies: a qualitative and quantitative analysis. AJR196: W336–340.
23. Willemink MJ, Habets J, de Jong PA, Schilham AM, Mali WP, et al.(2013) Iterative reconstruction improves evaluation of native aortic and mitral valves by retrospectively ECG-gated thoracoabdominal CTA. Eur Radiol 23: 968–974.
24. Blanke P, Bulla S, Baumann T, Siepe M, Winterer JT, et al. (2010) Thoracic aorta: prospective electrocardiographically triggered CT angiography with dual-source CT–feasibility, image quality, and dose reduction. Radiology 255: 207–217.
25. McCollough CH, Primak AN, Saba O, Bruder H, Stierstorfer K, et al. (2007) Dose performance of a 64-channel dual-source CT scanner. Radiology 243: 775–784.
26. Deak PD, Smal Y, Kalender WA (2010) Multisection CT protocols: sex- and age-specific conversion factors used to determine effective dose from dose-length product. Radiology 257: 158–166.
27. LePage MA, Quint LE, Sonnad SS, Deeb GM, Williams DM (2001) Aortic dissection: CT features that distinguish true lumen from false lumen. AJR177: 207–211.
28. Husmann L, Leschka S, Desbiolles L, Schepis T, Gaemperli O, et al. (2007) Coronary artery motion and cardiac phases: dependency on heart rate-implications for CT image reconstruction. Radiology 245: 567–76.
29. Bland JM, Altman DG (1986) Statistical methods for assessing agreement between two methods of clinical measurement. Lancet 1: 307–310.
30. DeBakey ME, Henly WS, Cooley DA, Morris GC Jr, Crawford ES, et al. (1965) Surgical management of dissecting aneurysms of the aorta. J Thorac Cardiovasc Surg 49: 130–149.
31. International Commission on Radiological Protection (2001) Diagnostic reference levels in medical imaging: review and additional advice. Ann ICRP 31: 33–52.
32. Krissak R, Henzler T, Prechel A, Reichert M, Gruettner J, et al. (2010) Triple-rule-out dualsource CT angiography of patients with acute chest pain: dose reduction potential of 100 kV scanning. Eur J Radiol 81: 3691–3696.
33. Li Y, Fan Z, Xu L, Yang L, Xin H, et al. (2012) Prospective ECG-gated 320-row CT angiography of the whole aorta and coronary arteries. Eur Radiol 22: 2432–2440.
34. Wu W, Budovec J, Foley WD (2009) Prospective and retrospective ECG gating for thoracic CT angiography: a comparative study. Am J Roentgenol 193: 955–963.
35. Goetti R, Baumüller S, Feuchtner G, Stolzmann P, Karlo C, et al. 2010 High-pitch dual-source CT angiography of the thoracic and abdominal aorta: is simultaneous coronary artery assessment possible? Am J Roentgenol. Apr; 194(4): 938–44.
36. Morgan-Hughes GJ, Owens PE, Marshall AJ, Roobottom CA (2003) Thoracic aorta at multi-detector row CT: motion artifact with various reconstruction windows. Radiology 228: 583–588.
37. Tsai TT, Schlicht MS, Khanafer K, Bull JL, Valassis DT, et al. (2008) Tear size and location impacts false lumen pressure in an ex vivo model of chronic type B aortic dissection. J Vasc Surg 47: 844–851.
38. Karmonik C, Bismuth J, Shah DJ, Davies MG, Purdy D, et al. (2011) Computational study of haemodynamic effects of entry- and exit-tear coverage in a DeBakey type III aortic dissection: technical report. Eur J Vasc Endovasc Surg 42: 172–177.

TIMI Frame Count and Adverse Events in Women with No Obstructive Coronary Disease: A Pilot Study from the NHLBI-Sponsored Women's Ischemia Syndrome Evaluation (WISE)

John W. Petersen[1]*, B. Delia Johnson[2], Kevin E. Kip[3], R. David Anderson[1], Eileen M. Handberg[1], Barry Sharaf[4], Puja K. Mehta[5], Sheryl F. Kelsey[2], C. Noel Bairey Merz[5], Carl J. Pepine[1]

1 Division of Cardiovascular Medicine, University of Florida, Gainesville, Florida, United States of America, **2** Graduate School of Public Health, University of Pittsburgh, Pittsburgh, Pennsylvania, United States of America, **3** College of Nursing, University of South Florida, Tampa, Florida, United States of America, **4** Division of Cardiology, Brown University, Providence, Rhode Island, United States of America, **5** Division of Cardiology, Barbra Streisand Women's Heart Center, Heart Institute, Cedars-Sinai Medical Center, Los Angeles, California, United States of America

Abstract

Background: TIMI frame count (TFC) predicts outcomes in patients with obstructive coronary artery disease (CAD); it remains unclear whether TFC predicts outcomes in patients without obstructive CAD.

Methods: TFC was determined in a sample of women with no obstructive CAD enrolled in the Women's Ischemia Syndrome Evaluation (WISE) study. Because TFC is known to be higher in the left anterior descending artery (LAD), TFC determined in the LAD was divided by 1.7 to provide a corrected TFC (cTFC).

Results: A total of 298 women, with angiograms suitable for TFC analysis and long-term (6–10 year) follow up data, were included in this sub-study. Their age was 55±11 years, most were white (86%), half had a history of smoking, and half had a history of hypertension. Higher resting cTFC was associated with a higher rate of hospitalization for angina (34% in women with a cTFC >35, 15% in women with a cTFC ≤35, P<0.001). cTFC provided independent prediction of hospitalization for angina after adjusting for many baseline characteristics. In this cohort, resting cTFC was not predictive of major events (myocardial infarction, heart failure, stroke, or all-cause death), cardiovascular events, all-cause mortality, or cardiovascular mortality.

Conclusions: In women with signs and symptoms of ischemia but no obstructive CAD, resting cTFC provides independent prediction of hospitalization for angina. Larger studies are required to determine if resting TFC is predictive of major events in patients without obstructive coronary artery disease.

Editor: Alexander G Obukhov, Indiana University School of Medicine, United States of America

Funding: This work was supported by contracts from the National Heart, Lung and Blood Institutes, nos. N01-HV-68161, N01-HV-68162, N01-HV-68163, N01-HV-68164, grants U0164829, U01 HL649141, U01 HL649241, T32HL69751, 1R03AG032631 from the National Institute on Aging, GCRC grant MO1-RR00425 from the National Center for Research Resources and grants from the Gustavus and Louis Pfeiffer Research Foundation, Danville, NJ, The Women's Guild of Cedars-Sinai Medical Center, Los Angeles, CA, The Ladies Hospital Aid Society of Western Pennsylvania, Pittsburgh, PA, and QMED, Inc., Laurence Harbor, NJ, the Edythe L. Broad Women's Heart Research Fellowship, Cedars-Sinai Medical Center, Los Angeles, California, the Barbra Streisand Women's Cardiovascular Research and Education Program, Cedars-Sinai Medical Center, Los Angeles and The Society for Women's Health Research (SWHR), Washington, D.C. Dr. Carl Pepine receives support from the NIH and NCRR CTSA grant UL1 TR000064. The funders had no role in study design, data collection and analysis, decision to publish, or preparation of the manuscript.

Competing Interests: Drs. Noel Bairey Merz, Eileen Handberg, and Carl Pepine declare that they worked with QMED, Inc., Laurence Harbour, NJ, a commercial funder for this study, in the context of receiving digital Holter monitors free of charge for several other Women's Ischemic Syndrome Evaluation (WISE) studies.

* E-mail: john.petersen@medicine.ufl.edu

Introduction

Women with symptoms and signs of ischemia, referred for invasive coronary evaluation, often have no evidence of obstructive coronary artery disease (CAD) [1]. We and others have identified that symptomatic patients with non-obstructive CAD have an elevated risk of adverse outcomes and all-cause mortality compared with cohorts without symptoms and/or signs of ischemic heart disease [2,3]. About 45% to 60% of such patients have coronary vascular dysregulation (endothelial or non-endothelial dependent macro- or microvascular dysfunction) capable of causing ischemia with invasive provocative testing [1,4]. Additionally, we and others have linked coronary vascular dysregulation with adverse outcomes. Thus, additional indices of coronary vasomotor function, beyond standard anatomy from angiography, would be useful to improve risk stratification of these patients [5–9].

The Thrombolysis in Myocardial Infarction (TIMI) frame count (TFC) provides a simple angiographic index of coronary blood flow that does not require additional coronary artery instrumentation [10]. The intra- and inter-observer reproducibility of TFC is good, and dye injection rate and catheter size do not affect its measurement [11,12]. The TFC has correlated with other invasive and non-invasive measures of coronary blood flow [13–16]. Further, TFC estimates of coronary flow after reperfusion for acute myocardial infarction predict short- and long-term clinical outcomes [17–19]. However, the prognostic implication of an abnormal TFC in patients without acute myocardial infarction or obstructive CAD and with suspected microvascular dysfunction remains unclear. Accordingly, we aimed to determine if TFC at rest is predictive of adverse outcomes in patients without obstructive CAD.

Methods

Patients

The Women's Ischemia Syndrome Evaluation (WISE) study (clinicaltrials.gov Identifier NCT00000554) is a National Heart, Lung and Blood Institute–sponsored study aimed at improving diagnostic evaluation and understanding of pathological mechanisms of ischemic heart disease in women. The WISE protocol was approved by the relevant institutional review boards (IRB) (University of Florida IRB, Allegany General Hospital IRB, University of Pittsburgh IRB, University of Alabama at Birmingham IRB), and has previously been described [20]. All participants provided written informed consent to participate in this study. The consent procedure and form were approved by the local IRBs listed. Briefly, women older than 18 years of age with symptoms and signs of ischemia undergoing clinically indicated angiograms were followed for clinical outcomes. Major exclusion criteria included comorbidities likely to compromise follow up. Initial evaluation in addition to coronary angiography included collection of demographics, medical history, symptom data, physical examination, and blood sampling for lipids, reproductive hormones, and inflammatory markers.

Coronary Angiography and TIMI frame counts

Coronary angiography was performed at the clinical sites according to standard methods. Qualitative and quantitative coronary angiographic analyses were conducted by a core laboratory masked to patient data [21]. As previously described, the TFC was determined as the number of cine frames required for contrast to reach standardized distal coronary landmarks [10]. The first frame used for TFC is the frame in which dye fully enters the artery of interest. The last frame that is counted is the frame when dye enters the distal landmark branch (Figure 1). The distal landmark branch of the left anterior descending (LAD) artery was the distal bifurcation. In normal coronaries, the TFC in the LAD is on average 1.7 times longer than the TFC in the other coronary arteries. Therefore, the LAD frame counts were divided by 1.7 to provide a corrected TFC (cTFC) [10]. Those patients who had an angiogram recorded in a way that allowed the determination of TFC by the core lab and were found not to have obstructive CAD are included in this analysis.

Follow-up for adverse events

After the baseline angiogram and coronary reactivity testing, the WISE women had protocol-directed yearly follow-up. During telephone contact, a scripted interview was completed by an experienced nurse or physician at the respective center. Each patient or family member was queried for occurrence of major adverse cardiac events or hospitalizations. Telephone follow-up was terminated at a maximum of 8 years, with a median follow-up of 6 years. Additionally, after the phone follow-up period, a second phase of follow-up was performed with a search of the National Death Index for those patients still alive at last contact who had not withdrawn consent. This extended the follow-up for mortality to approximately 10 years. In the event of death, a death certificate and/or physician narrative was obtained. All deaths were adjudicated as cardiovascular (CV) or non-CV by a committee of senior WISE investigators blinded to angiographic findings. Women sustaining multiple events were counted only once and by the initial event.

Statistical Analysis

Baseline characteristics are described by mean and standard deviation for continuous variables and percentages for categorical variables. The Kaplan-Meier method was used to estimate 10-year CV events rates by tertiles of cTFC, and compared by use of the log-rank statistic. To determine the cTFC cutpoint for predicting hospitalization for angina, we generated a receiver-operator characteristic (ROC) curve using logistic regression. The cTFC value corresponding to the point of the curve closest to 100% sensitivity and specificity was selected and verified in subsequent runs of incremental cut-points near that value. Multivariate Cox proportional hazards regression was used to examine the relationship between baseline characteristics and adverse outcomes. Baseline characteristics were chosen for entry into multivariable Cox models on the basis of their discrimination between those patients above and below the optimal cTFC cutpoint, as well as on univariate associations with adverse outcomes of $P<0.20$. A combination of forward and backward selection procedures were used to aid in determining the best model of independent predictors. This was followed by forcing potential confounders into the models and determining their effect on the relationship of interest. The likelihood ratio test was used to compare the incremental goodness of fit of nested models. All tests were 2-sided, and $P\leq0.05$ was considered statistically significant. All analyses were performed with SAS software version 9.3 (SAS Institute). *Sample Size Considerations.* Using previously published data for women in the WISE with non-obstructive coronary disease [9], we assumed a reference 6-year event-free survival rate of 91% for such women without coronary microvascular dysfunction (e.g. normal cTFC). Event-free survival was taken as freedom from first occurrence of death (all-cause), nonfatal MI, non-fatal stroke, or hospitalization for heart failure. We assumed that women with abnormal coronary microvascular function (e.g. high cTFC) would have reduced event-free survival. This was expressed as a hazard ratio of 2.5 (corresponding to a 6-year event free survival rate of approximately 79%) with proportional hazard assumption. Assuming 5% censoring, we would need 300 women to achieve 80% power and need 500 women to achieve 95% power, using a two-sided log-rank test with alpha level of 0.05. SAS procedure PROC POWER was used to perform the power analysis. We suspected we were underpowered in our comparison of the incidence of the binary outcome of major events between TFC groups, and we used the Kaplan-Meier estimated rates of major events between our two TFC groups in this pilot study (20% vs. 13%) to determine the sample size necessary to detect a statistically significant difference at a power of 80% and an alpha of 0.05 using the SAS procedure PROC POWER with two-sided Pearson's chi square test.

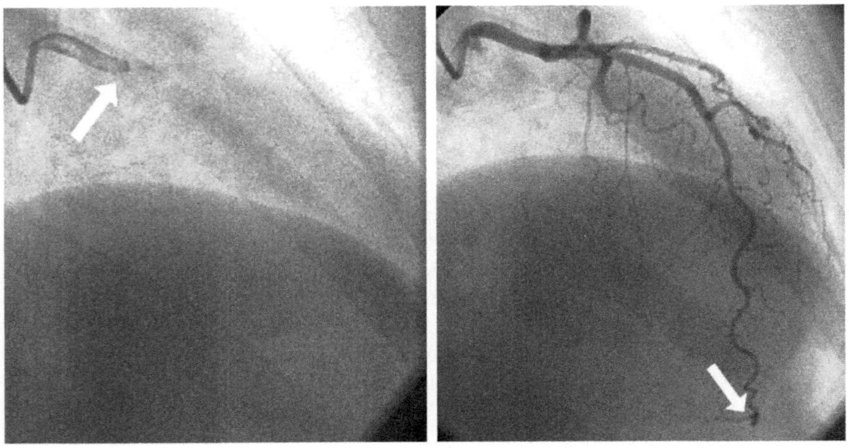

Figure 1. TIMI Frame Count. The first frame used to determine the TIMI Frame Count is the frame in which dye fully enters the artery of interest (left, arrow). The last frame that is counted is the frame when dye enters the distal landmark branch (right, arrow).

Results

Baseline Characteristics

We report on a subgroup of 298 women without obstructive CAD (no stenosis ≥50% diameter reduction), whose angiograms could be retrieved and were suitable for analysis by TFC, and for whom clinical outcome data were available. Their baseline demographics are shown in Table 1. Their mean age was 55±11 years, most were white (86%), nearly half had a history of smoking, and half had a history of hypertension.

Angiography and TFC

These women, in aggregate, had normal overall left ventricular systolic function with a mean ejection fraction of 66±10%. The mean cTFC was 33.9±10.0 with a range of 18 to 91.

Adverse Outcomes

Adverse event rates were compared between patients in the various cTFC tertiles (cTFC ≤28, 29–37, and >37). During a median follow up of 6 years, the Kaplan-Meier event rate for angina hospitalization was highest for those women in the highest cTFC tertile (35%, vs. 24% in the middle cTFC tertile, and 19% in the lowest cTFC tertile, P = 0.022). However, the rates of major events (myocardial infarction, heart failure, stroke, or all-cause death), CV events (myocardial infarction, heart failure, stroke, or CV death), all-cause mortality, or CV mortality were not statistically different between women in the various cTFC tertiles.

By ROC analysis, a cTFC of >35 provided the best cut-point for predicting hospitalization for angina, with a sensitivity of 61% and a specificity of 66%. The area under the curve was 0.63 (95% confidence interval [CI] 0.57 to 0.7). Adverse event rates in those patients above versus at or below a cTFC of 35 are shown in Table 2. Thirty four percent of women with a cTFC >35 were hospitalized for angina, whereas only 15% of women with a cTFC ≤35 were hospitalized for angina (P<0.001) (Figure 2).

Baseline characteristics were examined for their prediction of hospitalization for angina. Patients with white race had a lower risk of hospitalization for angina (age-adjusted HR = 0.43 [95% CI 0.24, 0.76], P = 0.004), whereas a history of unstable angina in the preceding 6 weeks predicted hospitalization for angina (age-adjusted HR 1.79 [95% CI 1.05, 3.03], P = 0.03). Further, the use of various medications at baseline was predictive of angina hospitalization: anti-hypertensives (age-adjusted HR 1.96 [95% CI 1.15, 3.35], P = 0.014); ACE inhibitors (age-adjusted HR 2.17 [95% CI 1.22, 3.86], P = 0.009); and diuretics (age-adjusted HR 2.09 [95% CI 1.2, 3.62], P = 0.009).

When added to a predictive model that included cTFC at cut-point 35, a history of unstable angina and diuretic use were not independently associated with hospitalization for angina. In contrast, when white race was included in a model that contained cTFC at cut-point 35, it did provide an independent predictor of lower risk of hospitalization for angina (HR 0.53 [95% CI 0.3, 0.94], P = 0.03). Additionally, when ACE inhibitor use was included in a model that contained cTFC at cut-point 35, it was associated with a higher risk of hospitalization for angina (HR 2.04 [95% CI 1.15, 3.59], P = 0.014). However, when ACE inhibitor use, white race, and cTFC at cut-point 35 were all included in a predictive model of hospitalization for angina, only cTFC provided independent prediction of hospitalization for angina.

Discussion

Microvascular coronary dysfunction is prevalent in patients presenting with chest pain who have no evidence of obstructive CAD on standard angiography, and is associated with adverse outcomes. Microvascular coronary dysfunction is commonly diagnosed by evaluating coronary blood flow before and after administration of adenosine with a Doppler-tipped guide wire in the coronary. TFC does not require placement of a wire in the coronary artery, and has been shown to correlate with coronary blood flow and prognosis in patients with acute coronary events. The correlation of TFC with adverse outcomes in patients with no obstructive disease but suspected microvascular coronary dysfunction is less clear.

In the 298 women included in this study who had chest pain but no evidence of obstructive CAD, a high cTFC was associated with an increased risk of hospitalization for angina. Moreover, a high cTFC remained the strongest predictor of hospitalization for angina after controlling for baseline characteristics. Interestingly, ACE inhibitor use was also associated with an increased risk of angina hospitalization. We have previously shown that patients randomized to an ACE inhibitor had greater improvement in angina severity as compared to those who received placebo [22]. So these data are biased by WISE investigators likely prescribing

Table 1. Baseline characteristics and risk factors.

Characteristic		All women (n = 298)	cTFC ≤35 n = 179	cTFC >35 n = 119	P (unad-justed)	P (age-adjusted)
Demographics						
	Age (y)	55±11	56±11	54±10	0.20	-
	Postmenopausal (%)**	210/296 (71)	72	69	0.53	-
	White race (%)	257 (86)	90	80	0.009	0.013
	HS educ. or more (%)	243/294 (83)	82	83	0.97	0.94
Body size						
	Waist circumference (in)	36.8±6.8	36.0±5.5	38.2±8.5	0.027	0.020
	BMI	30.3±7.1	29.8±6.6	31.0±7.8	0.17	0.20
	Waist/hip ratio	0.85±0.12	0.85±0.11	0.87±0.14	0.20	0.18
Self-reported risk factors						
	Hx diabetes (%)	42/297 (14)	11	19	0.07	0.053
	Family hx of CAD (%)	181/290 (62)	59	67	0.16	0.18
	Hx hypertension (%)	143/296 (48)	47	51	0.48	0.34
	Hx dyslipidemia (%)	116/275 (42)	43	40	0.65	0.74
	Ever smoker (%)	151/297 (51)	54	47	0.24	0.20
	Current smoker (%)	58/297 (20)	20	19	0.75	0.50
	High stress (%)	117 (39)	40	39	0.86	0.70
Hemodynamic measures						
	Systolic BP (mmHg)	133±20	134±20	131±19	0.21	0.33
	Diastolic BP (mmHg)	76±10	77±11	76±10	0.37	0.34
	Pulse pressure	57±16	58±16	56±16	0.25	0.44
	Mean arterial pressure	95±12	96±12	94±11	0.22	0.28
Lab values						
	LDL-C (mg/dl)	111±37	112±39	109±33	0.52	0.58
	HDL (mg/dl)	53±13	53±13	53±13	0.99	0.82
	Triglycerides (mg/dl) (medians[IQR])*	113 [72, 169]	122 [76, 169]	96 [70, 172]	0.37	0.55*
	Total cholesterol	191±43	192±44	191±41	0.92	0.94
	Fasting blood glucose	104±39	103±38	107±40	0.33	0.31
	Creatinine (mg/dl)	0.79±0.18	0.80±0.19	0.78±0.16	0.48	0.61
	Hemoglobin (g/dl)	13.0±1.4	13.1±1.4	12.9±1.3	0.25	0.21
Medication use						
	Any antihypertensive use (%)	167/283 (59)	60	57	0.62	0.74
	Any lipid lowering meds (%)	52/297 (18)	19	15	0.41	0.45
	Ever HRT use (%)	160/293 (55)	56	52	0.42	0.55
	Current HRT use (%)	116/294 (39)	40	38	0.70	0.83
	Statins (%)	39/297 (13)	13	14	0.86	0.77
	ACE inhibitors (%)	51/269 (19)	18	20	0.66	0.51
	Beta blockers (%)	89/297 (30)	29	31	0.67	0.65
	Aspirin (%)	138/296 (47)	49	42	0.23	0.27
	Diuretics (%)	63/297 (21)	19	24	0.25	0.19
Other variables						
	CAD severity score (medians[IQR])*	5.0 [5.0, 7.5]	5.0 [5.0, 7.5]	5.0 [5.0, 6.2]	0.57	0.72*
	Functional capacity (DASI)	21.4±14.9	22.6±15.3	19.7±14.2	0.11	0.10
	Unstable angina past 6 wks	74/266 (28)	27	29	0.72	0.81

cTFC = corrected TIMI frame count; HS educ = High School education; BMI = body mass index; Hx = history; HRT = hormone replacement therapy; CAD = coronary artery disease.

*Because of skewed distribution, medians [interquartile ranges] are given and Log transformations were used to estimate the age-adjusted p-values.

**For frequencies, where there were missing values, the statistic given is: no. with the condition/no. available (%).

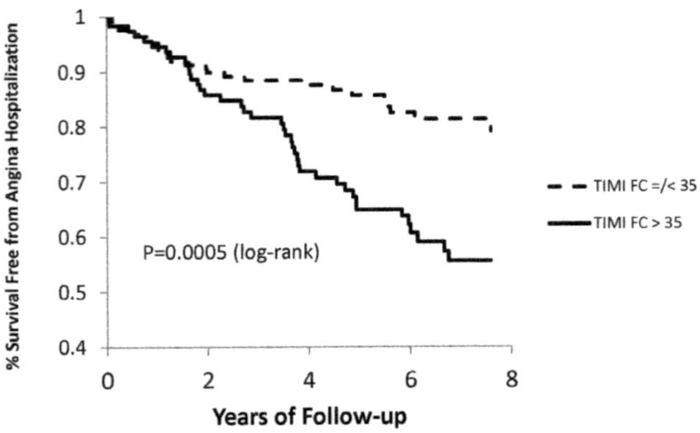

Figure 2. Survival free of hospitalization for angina according to TIMI Frame Count groups. Kaplan-Meier analysis of survival free of hospitalization for angina.

an ACE-I for those with more severe angina. Additionally, follow-up blood pressure for our current cohort was higher than the baseline blood pressure in those patients randomized to an ACE inhibitor in the Pauly et al trial [22]. We suspect that baseline ACE inhibitor use in our current cohort is likely a marker of more advanced vascular disease, which may have contributed to an increased risk of angina hospitalization. In this pilot investigation, cTFC was not associated with a statistically significant increase in risk of major events (myocardial infarction, heart failure, stroke, or all-cause death), CV events, all-cause mortality, or CV mortality.

Studies comparing TFC to more invasive measures of coronary vasomotion (endothelial or non-endothelial dependent macro- or microvascular function) have provided various results. Many studies have shown that TFC does correlate with measures of coronary vasomotion [23–26], whereas others have shown no correlation of TFC and coronary flow reserve [27]. Most of these studies were small. Some of these studies included patients with obstructive CAD and others excluded patients with obstructive CAD. Some of these studies determined the change in TFC from baseline to the TFC at hyperemia, and correlated this change in TFC with measures of coronary vasomotion, whereas some looked at only the correlation of TFC at rest with measures of coronary vasomotion. Therefore, it remains unclear if TFC at rest can replace evaluation of coronary vasomotion with more traditional methods. Because TFC at rest does not require instrumentation of the coronary artery nor vasoactive medication, future study evaluating the correlation of TFC at rest with CFR determined after administration of adenosine and change in coronary artery diameter and coronary blood flow after acetylcholine in patients without obstructive CAD remains warranted.

The major limitation of our study is the relatively small number of major events. Because of the small number of events, the current analysis provides low statistical power to find a relationship between TFC and major events. In order to have appropriate power to determine if there is a significant difference in major event rates between TFC groups, we estimate that we would need approximately 880 patients.

In conclusion, in women with signs and symptoms of ischemia but no obstructive CAD, resting cTFC provides independent prediction of hospitalization for angina. Larger studies are required to determine if resting cTFC is predictive of major events in patients without obstructive coronary artery disease.

Table 2. Adverse Event Rates between TIMI Frame Count Groups.

Event*	All Women (n = 298)		cTFC ≤35 n = 179		cTFC >35 n = 119		P (unadjusted)
	# Events	K-M Rate**	# Events	K-M Rate**	# Events	K-M Rate**	
Major event	38	16%	19	13%	19	20%	0.30
CV event	33	13%	18	12%	15	15%	0.70
All-cause mortality	24	11%	12	10%	12	12%	0.55
CV mortality	13	6%	7	5%	6	7%	0.88
Angina hospitalization	60	26%	24	17.5%	35	38%	0.0005
6-year CV event or angina hospitalization	73	26%	31	19%	42	37%	0.001

cTFC = corrected TIMI Frame Count; K-M = Kaplan-Meier; Major event = MI, heart failure, stroke, or all-cause death; CV (cardiovascular) Event = MI, heart failure, stroke, or CV death.
*Mortality is estimated for up to 10 years of follow up. Non-fatal events are estimated for up to 6 years of follow up.
**Note that the K-M estimated rate is not equivalent to the number of events per n of women.

Author Contributions

Conceived and designed the experiments: JWP KEK RDA EMH BS PKM SFK CNBM CJP. Performed the experiments: JWP KEK RDA EMH BS SFK CNBM. Analyzed the data: JWP BDJ SFK. Wrote the paper: JWP RDA EMH CNBM CJP. Critical revision of paper: JWP BDJ KEK RDA EMH BS PKM SFK CNBM CJP.

References

1. Ong P, Athanasiadis A, Borgulya G, Mahrholdt H, Kaski JC, et al. (2012) High prevalence of a pathological response to acetylcholine testing in patients with stable angina pectoris and unobstructed coronary arteries. The ACOVA Study (Abnormal COronary VAsomotion in patients with stable angina and unobstructed coronary arteries). J Am Coll Cardiol 59: 655–662.
2. Jespersen L, Hvelplund A, Abildstrøm SZ, Pedersen F, Galatius S, et al. (2012) Stable angina pectoris with no obstructive coronary artery disease is associated with increased risks of major adverse cardiovascular events. Eur Heart J 33: 734–744.
3. Gulati M, Cooper-DeHoff RM, McClure C, Johnson BD, Shaw LJ, et al. (2009) Adverse cardiovascular outcomes in women with nonobstructive coronary artery disease: a report from the Women's Ischemia Syndrome Evaluation Study and the St James Women Take Heart Project. Arch Intern Med 169: 843–850.
4. Reis SE, Holubkov R, Conrad Smith AJ, Kelsey SF, Sharaf BL, et al. (2001) Coronary microvascular dysfunction is highly prevalent in women with chest pain in the absence of coronary artery disease: results from the NHLBI WISE study. Am Heart J 141: 735–741.
5. von Mering GO, Arant CB, Wessel TR, McGorray SP, Bairey Merz CN, et al. (2004) Abnormal coronary vasomotion as a prognostic indicator of cardiovascular events in women: results from the National Heart, Lung, and Blood Institute-sponsored Women's Ischemia Syndrome Evaluation (WISE). Circulation 109: 722–725.
6. Halcox JP, Schenke WH, Zalos G, Mincemoyer R, Prasad A, et al. (2002) Prognostic value of coronary vascular endothelial dysfunction. Circulation 106: 653–658.
7. Schächinger V, Britten MB, Zeiher AM (2000) Prognostic impact of coronary vasodilator dysfunction on adverse long-term outcome of coronary heart disease. Circulation 101: 1899–1906.
8. Suwaidi JA, Hamasaki S, Higano ST, Nishimura RA, Holmes DR, et al. (2000) Long-term follow-up of patients with mild coronary artery disease and endothelial dysfunction. Circulation 101: 948–954.
9. Pepine CJ, Anderson RD, Sharaf BL, Reis SE, Smith KM, et al. (2010) Coronary microvascular reactivity to adenosine predicts adverse outcome in women evaluated for suspected ischemia results from the National Heart, Lung and Blood Institute WISE (Women's Ischemia Syndrome Evaluation) study. J Am Coll Cardiol 55: 2825–2832.
10. Gibson CM, Cannon CP, Daley WL, Dodge JT Jr, Alexander B Jr, et al. (1996) TIMI frame count: a quantitative method of assessing coronary artery flow. Circulation 93: 879–888.
11. Abaci A, Oguzhan A, Eryol NK, Ergin A (1999) Effect of potential confounding factors on the thrombolysis in myocardial infarction (TIMI) trial frame count and its reproducibility. Circulation 100: 2219–2223.
12. Dodge JT Jr, Rizzo M, Nykiel M, Altmann J, Hobkirk K, et al. (1998) Impact of injection rate on the Thrombolysis in Myocardial Infarction (TIMI) trial frame count. Am J Cardiol 81: 1268–1270.
13. Umman B, Nisanci Y, Sezer M, Umman S, Yilmaz E, et al. (2002) The relationship between corrected TIMI frame count and myocardial fractional flow reserve. J Invasive Cardiol 14: 125–128.
14. Lee S, Otsuji Y, Minagoe S, Hamasaki S, Toyonaga K, et al. (2005) Correlation between distal left anterior descending artery flow velocity by transthoracic Doppler echocardiography and corrected TIMI frame count before mechanical reperfusion in patients with anterior acute myocardial infarction. Circ J 69: 1022–1028.
15. Mavrogeni SI, Manginas A, Papadakis E, Douskou M, Cokkinos D, et al. (2005) Coronary flow evaluation by TIMI frame count and magnetic resonance flow velocity in patients with coronary artery ectasia. J Cardiovasc Magn Reson 7: 545–550.
16. Ozdemir N, Kaymaz C, Kirma C, Akcay M, Yuce M, et al. (2003) Intravascular ultrasound correlates of corrected TIMI framecount. Jpn Heart J 44: 213–224.
17. Gibson CM, Murphy SA, Rizzo MJ, Ryan KA, Marble SJ, et al. (1999) Relationship between TIMI frame count and clinical outcomes after thrombolytic administration. Thrombolysis In Myocardial Infarction (TIMI) Study Group. Circulation 99: 1945–1950.
18. Gibson CM, Cannon CP, Murphy SA, Marble SJ, Barron HV, et al; TIMI Study Group (2002) Relationship of the TIMI myocardial perfusion grades, flow grades, frame count, and percutaneous coronary intervention to long-term outcomes after thrombolytic administration in acute myocardial infarction. Circulation 105: 1909–1013.
19. French JK, Hyde TA, Straznicky IT, Andrews J, Lund M, et al. (2000) Relationship between corrected TIMI frame counts at three weeks and late survival after myocardial infarction. J Am Coll Cardiol 35: 1516–1524.
20. Merz CN, Kelsey SF, Pepine CJ, Reichek N, Reis SE, et al. (1999) The Women's Ischemia Syndrome Evaluation (WISE) study: protocol design, methodology and feasibility report. J Am Coll Cardiol 33: 1453–1461.
21. Sharaf BL, Pepine CJ, Kerensky RA, Reis SE, Reichek N, et al. (2001) Detailed angiographic analysis of women with suspected ischemic chest pain (pilot phase data from the NHLBI-sponsored Women's Ischemia Syndrome Evaluation [WISE] Study Angiographic Core Laboratory). Am J Cardiol 87: 937–941; A3.
22. Pauly DF, Johnson BD, Anderson RD, Handberg EM, Smith KM, et al. (2011) In women with symptoms of cardiac ischemia, nonobstructive coronary arteries, and microvascular dysfunction, angiotensin-converting enzyme inhibition is associated with improved microvascular function: A double-blind randomized study from the National Heart, Lung and Blood Institute Women's Ischemia Syndrome Evaluation (WISE). Am Heart J 162: 678–684
23. Erdogan D, Caliskan M, Gullu H, Sezqin AT, Yildirir A, et al. (2007) Coronary flow reserve is impaired in patients with slow coronary flow. Atherosclerosis 191: 168–174
24. Manginas A, Gatzov P, Chasikidis C, Voudris V, Pavlides G, et al. (1999) Estimation of coronary flow reserve using the Thrombolysis In Myocardial Infarction (TIMI) frame count method. Am J Cardiol 83: 1562–1565, A7.
25. Barcin C, Denktas AE, Garratt KN, Higano ST, Holmes DR, et al. (2003) Relation of Thrombolysis in Myocardial Infarction (TIMI) frame count to coronary flow parameters. Am J Cardiol 91: 466–469.
26. Sun H, Fukumoto Y, Ito A, Shimokawa H, Sunagawa K (2005) Coronary microvascular dysfunction in patients with microvascular angina: analysis by TIMI frame count. J Cardiovasc Pharmacol 46: 622–626.
27. Chugh SK, Koppel J, Scott M, Shewchuk L, Goodhart D, et al. (2004) Coronary flow velocity reserve does not correlate with TIMI frame count in patients undergoing non-emergency percutaneous coronary intervention. J Am Coll Cardiol 44: 778–782.

Sequence Comparison for Non-Enhanced MRA of the Lower Extremity Arteries at 7 Tesla

Sören Johst[1,2]*, Stephan Orzada[1,2], Anja Fischer[1,2], Lena C. Schäfer[1,2], Kai Nassenstein[2], Lale Umutlu[2], Thomas C. Lauenstein[2], Mark E. Ladd[1,2], Stefan Maderwald[1]

1 Erwin L. Hahn Institute for Magnetic Resonance Imaging, University Duisburg-Essen, Essen, Germany, **2** Department of Diagnostic and Interventional Radiology and Neuroradiology, University Hospital, University Duisburg-Essen, Essen, Germany

Abstract

In this study three sequences for non-contrast-enhanced MRA of the lower extremity arteries at 7T were compared. Cardiac triggering was used with the aim to reduce signal variations in the arteries. Two fast single-shot 2D sequences, a modified Ultrafast Spoiled Gradient Echo (UGRE) sequence and a variant of the Quiescent-Interval Single-Shot (QISS) sequence were triggered via phonocardiogram and compared in volunteer examinations to a non-triggered 2D gradient echo (GRE) sequence. For image acquisition, a 16-channel transmit/receive coil and a manually positionable AngioSURF table were used. To tackle B_1 inhomogeneities at 7T, Time-Interleaved Acquisition of Modes (TIAMO) was integrated in GRE and UGRE. To compare the three sequences quantitatively, a vessel-to-background ratio (VBR) was measured in all volunteers and stations. In conclusion, cardiac triggering was able to suppress flow artifacts satisfactorily. The modified UGRE showed only moderate image artifacts. Averaged over all volunteers and stations, GRE reached a VBR of 4.18 ± 0.05, UGRE 5.20 ± 0.06, and QISS 2.72 ± 0.03. Using cardiac triggering and TIAMO imaging technique was essential to perform non-enhanced MRA of the lower extremities vessels at 7T. The modified UGRE performed best, as observed artifacts were only moderate and the highest average VBR was reached.

Editor: Zhuoli Zhang, Northwestern University Feinberg School of Medicine, United States of America

Funding: The research leading to these results has received funding from the European Research Council under the European Union's Seventh Framework Programme (FP/2007–2013)/ERC Grant Agreement n. 291903. The funders had no role in study design, data collection and analysis, decision to publish, or preparation of the manuscript. The article processing charge was funded by the German Research Foundation (DFG) and the University Duisburg-Essen in the funding programme Open Access Publishing.

Competing Interests: The authors have declared that no competing interests exist.

* E-mail: soeren.johst@uni-duisburg-essen.de

Introduction

For the diagnosis of diseases of the lower extremity vasculature, digital subtraction angiography (DSA) is increasingly performed only in cases where contrast-enhanced MR angiography (CE MRA) has showed positive findings [1]. Recent publications indicate, however, that especially patients with severe renal dysfunction should not be examined with Gadolinium (Gd)-based contrast agents due to reported cases of Nephrogenic Systemic Fibrosis (NSF) after the administration of such contrast agents [2,3]. Accordingly, in recent years several publications have focused on the evaluation of non-enhanced MRA sequences as an alternative to DSA/CE MRA for the diagnosis of lower extremity vascular diseases [1,4–8].

It has been shown that non-enhanced MRA techniques seem to profit from 7T, especially in the head [9,10]. But in order to perform non-contrast-enhanced MRA at 7T, one has to counter challenging issues such as B_0 and B_1 inhomogeneities [11,12], particularly when considering body imaging [13,14]. To tackle the latter issue, a recently published technique, Time-Interleaved Acquisition of Modes (TIAMO) [15,16], was used for this study. The principle is to excite at least two different B_1 transmission modes using static radiofrequency (RF) shimming in an interleaved acquisition. Overall signal homogeneity can be improved by exploiting the complementary radiofrequency patterns of the different transmission modes. Data from e.g. two acquisitions are not just averaged, but reconstructed the same way as if twice the number of coils would have been used. By that considerably more homogeneous images can be created.

Further, for non-enhanced MRA at 7T there is a need for heartbeat triggering due to a periodic variation in the signal intensity of the arteries that was observed in [17]. The most likely reason is interference between image acquisition frequency and heartbeat frequency. Using cardiac triggering combined with single-shot sequences acquiring the center of k-space at approximately the same time point of the cardiac cycle should be possible and thereby reduce the observed signal variations. In clinical routine at lower field strengths, ECG triggering is commonly used. Unfortunately, ECG triggering is severely limited at 7T due to an elevated T wave and other interferences [18]. To avoid this issue, acoustic cardiac triggering can be used [19–21].

In [17] a 2D GRE sequence capable of TIAMO imaging was used. Here, a trigger pulse changes the excitation mode directly after every excitation pulse which means that both modes needed for a complete slice are acquired in an interleaved fashion (Fig. 1 top). Venous saturation pulses were applied every TR. MRA image contrast is created by saturating the background tissue via the excitation RF pulses and by inflowing unsaturated arterial blood spins which provide hyperintense signal. In this study, to avoid the reported blood signal fluctuations, two single-shot sequences were chosen to be combined with cardiac triggering:

(1) An Ultrafast Spoiled Gradient Echo (UGRE) sequence (a modified turboFLASH sequence without T1 contrast preparing inversion RF pulse) where the cardiac trigger starts the acquisition of a complete slice. This is repeated for the second TIAMO mode after the next cardiac trigger event. Venous saturation pulses are applied only sparsely (Fig. 1 middle). Image contrast is created the same way as in GRE, but UGRE is designed for quite fast 2D single-shot acquisitions.

(2) A variant of the Quiescent-Interval Single-Shot (QISS) [22] sequence which is available as vendor-provided work in progress and used at 1.5T. Here, three 90° saturation RF pulses prepare the image contrast. The first one saturates the tissue signal in the imaging slice, the second one suppresses the veins and the third one suppresses fat signals. After the second preparation pulse, a time interval QI is introduced to give the unsaturated arterial blood spins time to enter the imaging slice before one complete slice is acquired (Fig. 1 bottom). As the QISS sequence is a vendor-provided work-in-progress at 7T, no source code was available and TIAMO could not be implemented. Both UGRE and QISS were triggered via phonocardiogram and compared in volunteer examinations to a non-triggered 2D gradient echo (GRE) sequence similar to the one used in [17].

The rationale of choosing UGRE and QISS is that both implementations used here are based on a GRE readout - techniques based on steady-state free precession (SSFP) like [6] are challenging at 7T due to the inherent B_0 inhomogeneities). QISS produces promising results at lower field strength [5], but relies on multiple preparation pulses which might be less effective at 7T due to the inherent B_1 inhomogeneities. In contrast to QISS, the implemented version of the UGRE uses just inherent saturation effects of the GRE readout and no preparation RF pulses to generate the basic MRA contrast. This might provide sufficient contrast even in areas were desired flip angles cannot be met. Additionally, UGRE is more time-efficient because no time interval QI is necessary. By that, higher flexibility in dealing with different heart rates should be possible.

Materials and Methods

Ethics Statement

The study was conducted in conformance with the Declaration of Helsinki and approved by the Ethics Commission of the Medical Faculty of the University Duisburg-Essen (study number 11-4898-BO). Written informed consent was obtained from each volunteer before the examination.

Measurement configuration

Examinations were performed on a 7T whole-body system (Magnetom 7T, Siemens, Erlangen, Germany) with a 16-channel transmit/receive coil based on [23]. Five stripline meander elements were placed dorsally on the patient table and eleven meander elements were placed on a rigid, semicircular former above the table. A RF shimming system with 8 channels similar to [24] was used to drive the coil with an 8-channel variable power combiner (VPC) interfaced to a 16-channel Butler matrix. Eight of the 16 inputs of the 16-channel Butler matrix corresponding to the highest transmit signal in the corresponding transmit modes were connected to the VPC [23,25]. In this way the 8-channel transmit system could be used to drive a 16-channel coil. The same configuration as in [17] was used.

Image acquisition was performed with a AngioSURF table [26,27] with 2 m length by positioning the volunteers feet-first supine and manually moving the AngioSURF table to all required body positions through the RF coil, which remained stationary at the isocenter connected to the original patient table. To reduce total acquisition time (TA), a general B_0 shim that was determined at the uppermost station was used for all stations [17].

For compliance with the International Electrotechnical Commission (IEC) guidelines, SAR calculations (CST Microwave Studio, Darmstadt, Germany) were performed in human adult male and female body models of the Virtual Family and the Visible Human [28,29]. Full-wave simulations were applied with exact dimensions and characteristics of the 16-channel RF coil, and maximum permitted input power levels for each station were calculated from the simulations of the corresponding body models. Based on these simulations, a standardized SAR file was integrated into the SAR monitoring system [24].

Periodic vessel signal fall-offs over short segments, particularly observable in coronal MIP images, were reported in [17]. To counter this issue, triggering with a phonocardiogram [19–21] was used for UGRE and QISS imaging. As both sequences acquire individual slices in single-shot acquisition started by the cardiac trigger event, the center of k-space can be acquired in approximately the same time point of the cardiac cycle. To compare the impact on the artifact, GRE is acquired without cardiac triggering.

Consistent signal loss in the middle third of the thigh were observed in [17], which is suspected to be caused by RF wave interferences within the FOV due to the variable anatomy of pelvis and legs along the longitudinal axis. In those volunteers where the aforementioned problem was encountered, dedicated TIAMO shims [16] were calculated based on acquired B_1^+ maps in the same imaging position. The two shims were calculated to adjust the phases of the 8 transmit channels in such a way that in one shim the B_1^+ was maximized in a circular region of interest around the right superficial femoral artery, while in the other shim the B_1^+ in a circular region of interest around the left superficial femoral artery was maximized. The remaining stations were acquired by combining the CP^+ and CP^{2+} modes, the first- and second-order circularly-polarized modes.

Sequence modifications

TIAMO imaging was implemented in the UGRE sequence code by enabling trigger pulses that cause the RF shimming system to switch between the different modulator states. As the UGRE protocol is intended to acquire one slice in a single shot between two heartbeats, the TIAMO trigger was set after each acquired imaging slice. In this way, the same slice is acquired with the two imaging modes sequentially before the next slice is excited and acquired with both modes sequentially.

Additionally, the UGRE sequence had to be further modified. RF pulses for the suppression of the venous system were implemented into the sequence. To minimize the duration of the protocol and to be able to adjust the required TR to the heartbeat rate of the volunteers, saturation pulses could be applied sparsely (i.e. only every n-th line of k-space, where n can be flexibly chosen in the protocol). The normally used saturation pulse was exchanged with another sinc pulse with lower time-bandwidth product (TBWP) (3.6 instead of 7.8). Thus, a shorter pulse was achieved without increasing its SAR contribution at the cost of the exactness of the excitation profile, which is not relevant as long as the suppression ability is not affected. A flexible RF saturation

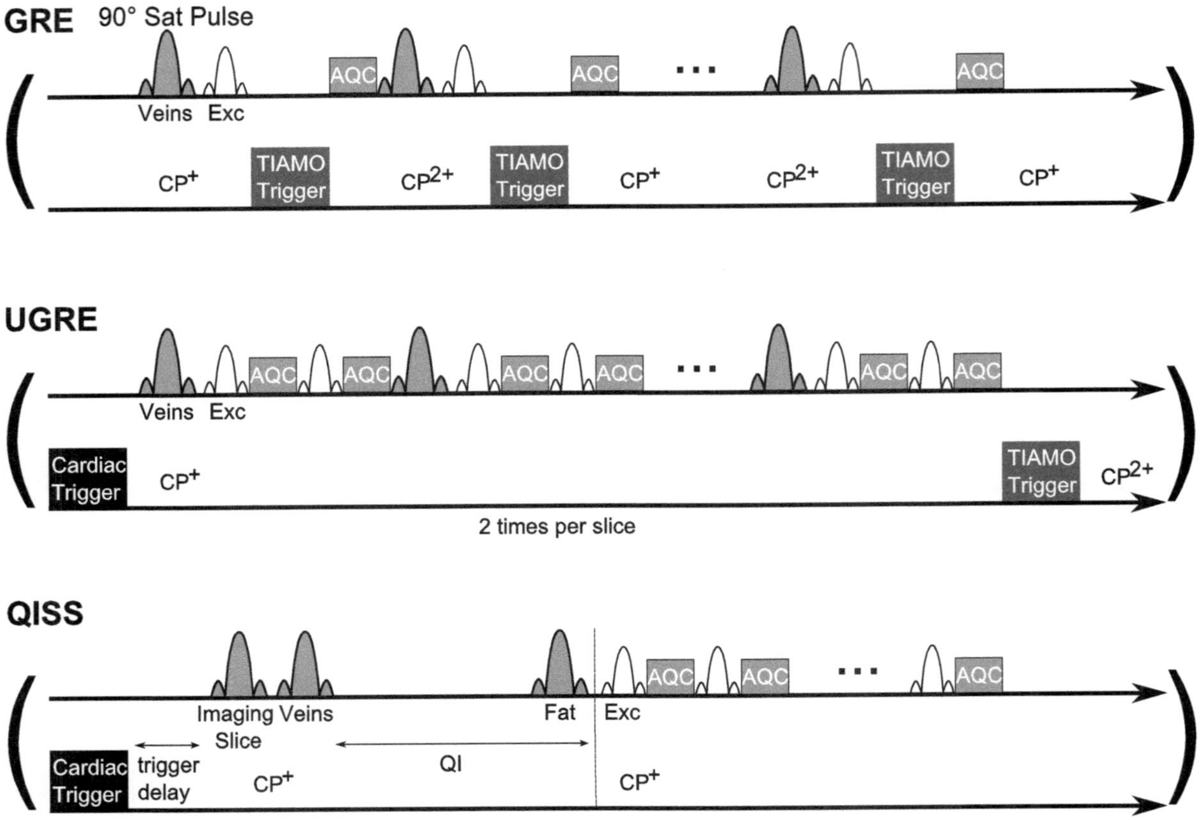

Figure 1. Sequence diagrams of GRE, UGRE and QISS. In GRE, no cardiac triggering is used. Here, the TIAMO trigger changes the excitation mode directly after every excitation pulse, which means that both modes needed for a complete slice are acquired in an interleaved fashion. Saturation pulses are applied every TR. In UGRE, the cardiac trigger event starts the acquisition of a complete slice in a single shot. Due to TIAMO, this acquisition has to be repeated to acquire the same slice with the second mode. Venous saturation RF pulses are applied only sparsely. QISS uses three different saturation pulses to prepare the image contrast: In the imaging slice to suppress background tissue, a travelling venous saturation pulse below the imaging slice and a fat saturation pulse in the imaging slice. After the venous saturation, a time interval QI allows unsaturated arterial blood spins to enter the imaging slice. No saturation pulses are applied during the single-shot slice acquisition. The duration of the trigger events is shorter than pictured in these diagrams.

pulse duration was implemented between 800 μs and 5000 μs with a default value of 3840 μs. For further reduction of the TR, the duration of the spoiling gradients following the saturation RF was made flexible (500 μs to 2000 μs).

As the QISS sequence is a vendor-provided work-in-progress at 7 T, no source code was available and no modifications could be implemented. Hence, TIAMO imaging could not be realized, and the protocol was run with the CP^+ mode of the 16-channel coil and 1 average instead of the two or more that are necessary for TIAMO. The original QISS sequence proposed by Hodnett et al. [5] used a steady-state free precession (SSFP) readout. In this study, a GRE readout was used to avoid known artifacts and SAR limitations of SSFP at 7T [30].

Imaging protocols

All protocols used a nominal flip angle of 80° and a FOV of 384 mm by 288 mm to acquire 60 transversal slices with 2 mm thickness using a matrix of 384 by 288 pixels and thus an in-plane resolution of 1 mm^2. Parallel image acceleration with a GRAPPA factor of 4 utilizing 32 integrated auto-calibration lines was used. To account for inaccuracies in the manual positioning of the AngioSURF table, the different stations were scanned with an overlap that for an exact shift would lead to the lowermost 10 slices being overlapped with the uppermost 10 slices of the subsequent station. Slice overlap, which is routinely applied e.g. in time-of-flight MRA or QISS, was not used; slices within a station were acquired with no overlap (distance factor = 0) to allow for a faster coverage. Separate from the parameters that were kept the same for all three techniques, the protocols were adapted individually to the shortest TE/TR possible without affecting image quality/ contrast.

Currently we are limited to 8 kW power which is not enough to perform abdominal imaging with arbitrary flip angles. Here, we used 80% of the maximum available power or 100% of the available peak power (which in this case corresponds to a nominal flip angle of 80° in the protocol). We concluded from preceding volunteer measurements that this power level gives us satisfying MRA contrast.

GRE. TR was set to 14 ms, TE to 5.26 ms, and the bandwidth to 1300 Hz/px. Image slices were acquired sequentially and in ascending order (feet to head) additionally using flow compensation. An RF pulse of nominal 90° for the suppression of the veins was applied every TR with a thickness of 116 mm and positioned at a distance of 10 mm below the imaging slice, travelling with the current slice position. TIAMO imaging [15,16] used CP^+ and CP^{2+} except for the stations of the upper thigh in volunteers where dedicated TIAMO shims had to be calculated. Hence, every slice was acquired twice. The TIAMO trigger changes excitation mode after every excitation RF pulse. The total acquisition time per station (12 cm coverage) amounted to 2 min 41 s.

UGRE. A TR of 700 ms per slice, a TE of 3.45 ms, and a bandwidth of 930 Hz/px were chosen. Image slices were acquired sequentially and in ascending order using flow compensation. Due to shorter flow compensation gradients, a shorter TE than in GRE could be reached; UGRE also used shorter spoiling gradients for remaining transversal magnetization than GRE. No inversion RF pulses for contrast preparation were used. The same RF pulse settings for venous suppression as in the GRE protocol were used except that the duration was only 2000 μs instead of 3840 μs and a pulse was applied only every 2nd excitation and using a shortened spoiler gradient of 1 ms length with a gradient moment of about 18 ms mT/m compared to 135 ms mT/m and ~6 ms duration in the original implementation and 15 ms mT/m in ~0.5 ms in GRE. TIAMO imaging [15,16] again used the CP^+ and CP^{2+} modes except for the stations of the upper thigh in volunteers where dedicated TIAMO shims had to be calculated. The sequence was gated by using the acoustic cardiac triggering device in such a way that one complete slice was acquired after the trigger signal. Due to TIAMO, each slice has to be acquired twice to combine both modes. In this protocol the two modes are acquired consecutively. After a single trigger signal, one complete slice is acquired in the first mode before the same slice excited by the second mode follows after the next trigger event. Total acquisition time for each station was on average ~3 minutes, depending on the heart rate of the volunteer. Without cardiac triggering, 1 min 24 s would be achievable.

QISS. A TR of 800 ms per slice, a TE of 2.74 ms, and a bandwidth of 183 Hz/px was applied. Image slices were acquired sequentially with GRE readout using a partial Fourier factor of 5/8. After the saturation RF pulses, a subsequent time interval (QI, here, 350 ms) is applied to wait for non-saturated blood spins to enter the imaging region. The sequence was gated using the acoustic cardiac triggering device. A time delay of 100 ms followed the trigger event. As in UGRE, a single slice is completely acquired beginning with the trigger event. Total acquisition time for each station was on average ~2 minutes depending on the heart rate of the volunteer. Without cardiac triggering, 48 s would be achievable. The protocol was run with only the CP^+ mode applied to the 16-ch coil and only 1 average (instead of the 2 that were necessary for TIAMO in the other protocols). An overview of the relevant sequence parameters of GRE, UGRE and QISS can be found in Table 1.

To compare the three sequences, 10 volunteers (4 female and 6 male, average age: 26.7 years, range: 20 to 38 years; average weight: 70.7 kg, range: 53 to 90 kg; average height: 1.75 m, range: 1.65 to 1.87 m) were examined by acquiring all three sequences consecutively at the same station before moving the AngioSURF table to the next station beginning at the hip and proceeding toward the feet.

For quantitative comparison of the three sequences, ROIs were placed in a single artery and in the tissue directly next to that artery for each station in both legs individually. The same artery and tissue positions were chosen for every sequence. Using the two ROIs, a vessel-to-background ratio ($VBR = Signal_{Vessel}/Signal_{Tissue}$ [31]) could be calculated, where values >1 are desirable to distinguish vessels, especially when looking at MIPs. The higher the VBR, the better the visibility of the vessel. For each station, the VBR was determined at 3 positions within the imaged region: In the central slice as well as in the slices located 5 slices toward the borders of the imaged region to avoid effects caused by gradient nonlinearity or B_1 inhomogeneities which are expected to be especially apparent in the outermost slices. As in the QISS sequence TIAMO could not be used, to minimize the influence of B_1 inhomogeneity in the evalutation of the QISS sequence, arteries were chosen that were not impaired by B_1 inhomogeneities.

To check for statistical significant differences between the three sequences, a t-test was performed [32].

Results

In seven volunteers 10 stations were acquired, in two volunteers 11 stations, and in one volunteer 12 stations. On average 124 ROIs were placed per volunteer and sequence. In total, 1242 ROIs per sequence were evaluated. Figure 2 presents maximum intensity projections (MIPs) of all acquired stations for one volunteer. For the UGRE sequence, the sparse application of the venous saturation pulses combined with the shorter spoiler gradient and saturation RF pulse permitted acquisition of one complete slice across two heartbeats. Owing to TIAMO, two averages needed to be acquired to utilize both excitation modes. Due to the consecutive acquisition of both modes, excitation and saturation pulses are always run in the same mode. Nevertheless, sufficient suppression of the venous system could be realized in the final image. The inherent saturation effects of the GRE readout in the UGRE permitted suppression of the static background tissue including fat, even though no fat suppression RF pulses were applied.

The individual heart rate dictates the total acquisition time for triggered sequences, but on average, UGRE imaging took 2 min 54 s per station while QISS took only 2 min 9 s. Without triggering 36 s would be the difference between the two sequences (although UGRE acquires two acquisitions), amounting to 45 s on average when using cardiac triggering. This means, QISS was prolonged by a factor of 2.7 on average while UGRE is prolonged by a factor of 2.1 compared to imaging without any triggering.

As observed in [17], the use of a general B_0 shim for all stations as determined at the uppermost station did not lead to perceivable image distortions.

For all volunteers, VBR was averaged over all stations and both legs using the standard deviation of the signal intensities inside the measured ROIs as error. For every volunteer UGRE performed better than GRE, while QISS achieved the lowest values in all volunteers (Table 2). In GRE and UGRE, fluctuation of VBR between different slices within a station as well as in between different stations is much higher than in QISS imaging. This is reflected in the overall higher errors for the calculated VBR in Table 2. Highest vessel signal could be observed in the QISS sequence, but also the highest tissue signal, which taken together led to the lowest VBR. Between different stations no relevant deviation and no tendency within a station (e.g. high VBR in uppermost slice and then decrease in signal) could be observed, except that vessels were harder to identify in the lowest stations at the level of the feet. In four volunteers for all sequences, delineation of arteries was not possible in the complete lowermost station, and in three volunteers delineation was not possible in the lowermost slices. In QISS images identification of the arteries in the lowermost station was not possible in four volunteers (in one of them also not possible for GRE). Averaged over all volunteers (and stations), GRE reached a VBR of 4.18±0.05, UGRE 5.20±0.06, and QISS 2.72±0.03 (Table 2).

To test for statistically significant differences between the three techniques, a t-test was performed. The resulting P values provided an estimation for the significance of differences, and P values less than 0.05 can be considered as statistically significant. The results of the t-test showed that the differences between all

Table 1. Sequence parameters.

	GRE	UGRE	QISS
TR [ms]	14	700 per slice	800 per slice
TE [ms]	5.26	3.84	2.74
Bandwidth [Hz/px]	1300	930	183
Slice orientation	Transversal	Transversal	Transversal
Slices	60	60	60
Slice acquisition	Sequential/ascending	Sequential/ascending/single shot	Sequential/ascending/single shot
FOV [mm²]	390×293	390×293	390×293
Voxel volume [mm³]	1.0×1.0×2.0	1.0×1.0×2.0	1.0×1.0×2.0
Acquisition matrix	384×288	384×288	384×288
Parallel imaging with GRAPPA: acceleration factor/reference lines	4/32	4/32	4/32
Partial Fourier factor	-	-	5/8
Fat suppression	-	-	Yes
Venous saturation	Prior to every excitation	Prior to every 2nd excitation	Prior to single-shot slice acquisition
Cardiac triggering	-	Phonocardiogram	Phonocardiogram
TIAMO	Yes: CP^+/CP^{2+} (dedicated shims in the upper thigh if necessary)	Yes: CP^+/CP^{2+} (dedicated shims in the upper thigh if necessary)	No: CP^+ (dedicated shim in the upper thigh if necessary)
Averages (TIAMO)	2	2	1
TA per station [min:s]	2:41	1:24≤TA≤~4:00 2:54 on average	0:48≤TA≤~3:30 2:09 on average

Overview of relevant protocol parameters for GRE, UGRE and QISS sequence. The total acquisition time TA of GRE and QISS depended on the individual's general heart rate and amounted to max about 4 min/3 min 30 s; without cardiac triggering 1 min 24 s/48 s would be necessary.

techniques are statistically significant. Paired comparisons led to P = 0.02/0.03 for GRE compared to UGRE/QISS and P<0.001 for UGRE compared to QISS.

Flow artifacts were very severe in GRE images (Fig. 3, 4), while in UGRE and QISS only a slight broadening in the phase-encode direction could be observed in some slices (Fig. 3). In UGRE images weak aliasing artifacts could be observed (Fig. 4). Since no TIAMO could be used for QISS imaging, clearly visible B_1 inhomogeneities are present which are considerably less pronounced or not visible in GRE and UGRE (Fig. 3, 4). Additionally, vessel contours appeared slightly blurred in QISS imaging (Fig. 4). Also, veins are often visible whereas they are nearly completely suppressed in GRE and UGRE (Fig. 2). Due to the blurring and the lower VBR in QISS, vessels were more poorly delineated or weren't even visible (Fig. 3, 4).

In six volunteers (3 female, 3 male), dedicated TIAMO shims for the upper thighs were calculated based on individual B_1 maps to improve the visibility of the arteries (Fig. 5). After detection of the impaired vessel visibility, the scan was interrupted and restarted with the new shims after B_1 maps were acquired and the dedicated RF shims were calculated. The acquisition of the B_1 maps and the calculation took less than 2 minutes. The remaining stations were examined with the CP^+ and CP^{2+} modes. The use of TIAMO imaging in conjunction with dedicated shims in the upper thighs of certain volunteers led to nearly homogenous images over all stations.

Discussion

The use of cardiac triggering in conjunction with both the UGRE and QISS sequences suppressed intravascular signal variations [17] at the cost of measurement time. The triggering itself (due to time intervals between two triggers) and variations in current heart rate prolong the measurement time depending on the individual's general heart rate. If the succeeding trigger event occurs too early and k-space data sets are not acquired completely, a time delay until the next trigger event must be introduced. The acquisition time per station ranged from approximately 1 min 30 s to 3 min. In the QISS sequence, the gating and the thereby induced time delay is reflected in signal variations of the background tissue (cf. Fig. 2). A very fast heart rate could also potentially lead to a relevant amount of interrupted data acquisition due to the gating. This would require triggering on only every 2nd heartbeat, prolonging the measurement time even more. Especially for fast heart rates, the possibility to use the saturation pulses sparsely as well as the shorter spoiler gradient and the shorter saturation RF pulse were essential. For the given UGRE protocol, the fastest possible heart rate is 85 bpm, limited by the inverse of the TR of 700 ms. The TR also determines the acquirable image resolution and correspondingly holds for the QISS sequence which is reflected in the factor the total acquisition time per station was prolonged (2.1 for a TR of 700 ms in the UGRE and 2.7 for a TR of 800 ms in the QISS). To speed up the UGRE sequence further, a lower resolution or a more sparsely applied saturation sequence segment would be possible. However, the latter would sooner or later lead to more pronounced vein visibility. Further investigation of the relationship between heart rate and the necessary minimum number of applied saturation pulses could be pursued, but a relevant benefit is not expected. The pragmatic way to acquire data from volunteers with higher heart rates would be to trigger only every 2nd heartbeat, concomitantly enabling a resolution increase at the cost of a longer acquisition time. A general increase of the image resolution would require sparser triggering, depending on the heart rate.

The use of a general B_0 shim that was determined at the uppermost station was robust enough to be used for all following

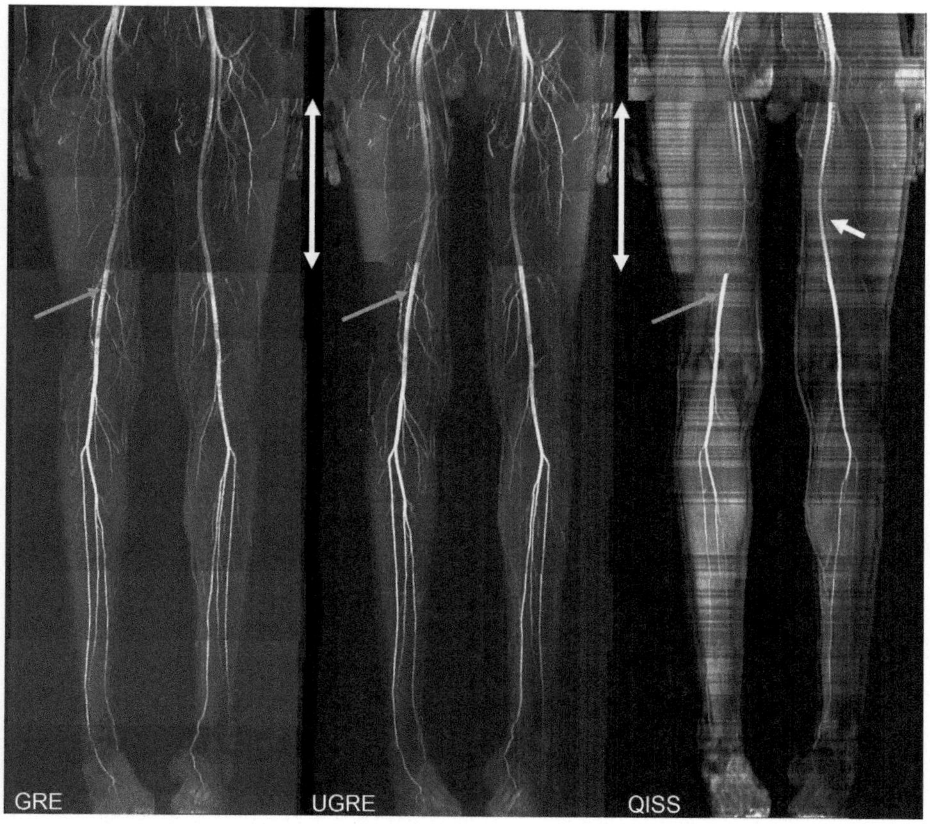

Figure 2. Complete MIPs of GRE, UGRE and QISS of one volunteer. MIPs of all acquired stations merged together manually in one volunteer for GRE, UGRE, and QISS. In this volunteer, the two stations covering the upper part of the thighs (marked by white double-headed arrows) used individual RF shims to prevent complete artery signal dropout. Vessel signal fluctuation in GRE could be mostly avoided in UGRE and QISS due to cardiac triggering (grey arrows). Tissue signal intensity fluctuation in QISS is most probably due to time delay induced by heartbeat triggering giving the surrounding tissue time to relax. White arrow in QISS shows vein visible in QISS sequence, as only one of the TIAMO RF shim modes could be used, preventing complete venous suppression.

stations without perceivable image distortions, thus helping to moderate total acquisition time as the B_0 shim procedure did not need to be repeated.

The comparison of the measured VBR shows that the UGRE sequence performed best, as it showed only moderate artifacts and led overall to the highest VBR of all sequences. It provided the best artery visibility of all sequences, as the GRE was impaired by flow artifacts combined with signal dropouts due to the lack of triggering. In one of the 10 volunteers GRE performed equally to UGRE in terms of VBR (V9 in Table 2), but UGRE was still preferable as GRE was strongly impaired by flow artifacts. The QISS protocol showed a comparatively smaller number of vessels with blurred contour. UGRE performed statistically significant better than GRE and QISS, while VBR for UGRE and GRE were quite comparable and clearly higher than for QISS. The fact that the vessel signals acquired with QISS were the highest of all sequences shows the potential of this sequence. Unfortunately, the preparation RF pulses do not seem to work as effective as for lower field strength in suppressing the background tissue. As the QISS protocol is a vendor-provided work-in-progress at 7T, the actual VBR can only be treated as preliminary result and could improve with further optimizations at this field strength; in particular, implementation of the TIAMO technique would be expected to significantly reduce B_1 artifacts.

In the lowermost station at the level of the feet, depiction of the arterial vessels was not possible in all slices (in seven cases for all

Table 2. Averaged VBR of all volunteers.

	V1	V2	V3	V4	V5	V6	V7	V8	V9	V10	Average
GRE	4.53±0.17	4.22±0.17	4.85±0.26	3.69±0.12	3.08±0.16	4.47±0.17	4.17±0.17	3.46±0.14	5.42±0.17	3.85±0.13	**4.18±0.05**
UGRE	4.90±0.19	6.08±0.23	5.56±0.30	4.90±0.16	3.46±0.13	5.44±0.21	5.88±0.21	4.82±0.19	5.58±0.19	5.37±0.17	**5.20±0.06**
QISS	2.47±0.08	3.29±0.16	2.24±0.10	3.11±0.08	1.85±0.06	2.96±0.14	3.23±0.11	3.51±0.11	2.29±0.05	2.26±0.05	**2.72±0.03**

Averaged VBR over all stations and both legs for the ten volunteers. In the far right column, the average over all volunteers is given. Standard deviation of the signal intensities inside the measured ROIs were used as error. Error values in this table were calculated via rules for propagation of uncertainty. The QISS sequence led to the lowest VBR in all cases, whereas UGRE performed best. Overall, UGRE reached relevantly higher values than GRE.

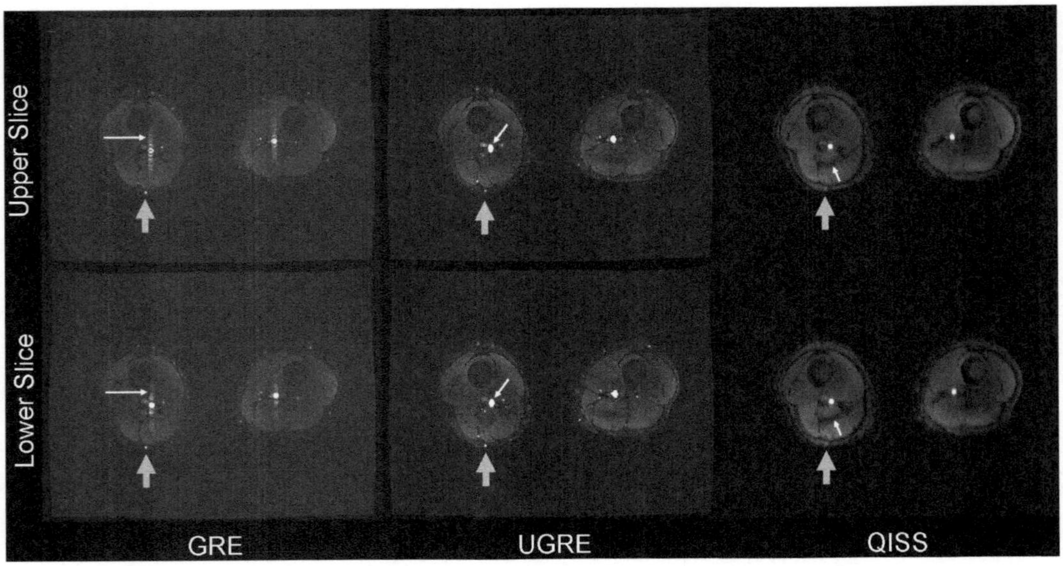

Figure 3. Signal variation flow artifact. Signal variation flow artifact (white arrow in GRE) shown for consecutive axial slices at position of the grey arrow in Fig. 1 compared to the corresponding images in UGRE and QISS. In UGRE large arteries seem to be slightly broadened (white arrow). In the QISS images, B_1 inhomogeneities are considerably more pronounced as TIAMO could not be used (white arrows). For GRE and UGRE, especially the smaller vessels can be more easily delineated than for QISS (grey arrows). The upper row shows the slice position superior to the images of the lower row.

sequences). Here, a higher imaging resolution, at the cost of prolonged total acquisition time, might help to identify more vessels. Apart from the narrow vessel diameters near the feet, a technical reason for this problem could be a relevant difference in loading of the RF coil with the feet compared to the region of the pelvis.

The absence of heartbeat triggering in the GRE sequence led to the same flow artifacts as reported in [17], which are most probably induced by an interference between individual heart rate and image acquisition frequency. GRE images are acquired covering the whole cardiac cycle and therefore a strong variation in flow velocity is present which leads to differences in flow compensation efficiency. This issue can be avoided mostly in UGRE and QISS via cardiac triggering. The weak aliasing artifacts that were visible in the UGRE sequence did not disturb the image quality, especially when looking at MIPs. The reason for the aliasing artifact is that the saturation RF pulse is applied only every second TR which leads to two different effective TRs. This

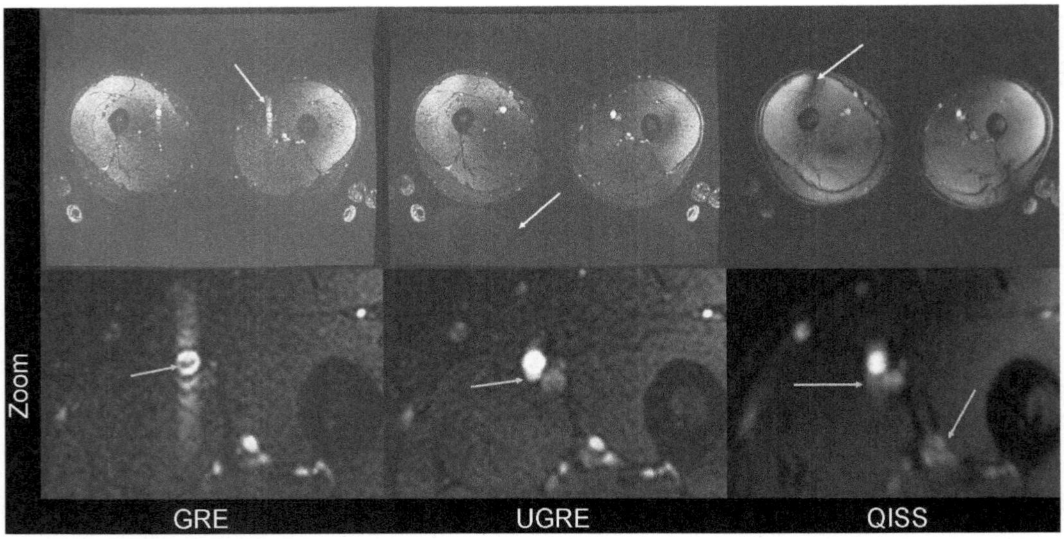

Figure 4. Artifacts in GRE, UGRE and QISS. The upper row visualizes the flow artifact in GRE images, aliasing in UGRE, and B_1 inhomogeneity in QISS, in each case marked by a white arrow. Due to use of TIAMO, the B_1 inhomogeneity could be ameliorated in GRE and UGRE. Zoomed images of the left thigh in the lower row show GRE, where the flow artifact in the phase-encode direction and a small signal dropout inside the vessel lumen are clearly visible (grey arrow), UGRE and QISS. For UGRE, slight broadening of the arteries can be observed (grey arrow). In the QISS image, blurring of the vessel walls is clearly observed (grey arrows). Artery circumference can be delineated best in UGRE.

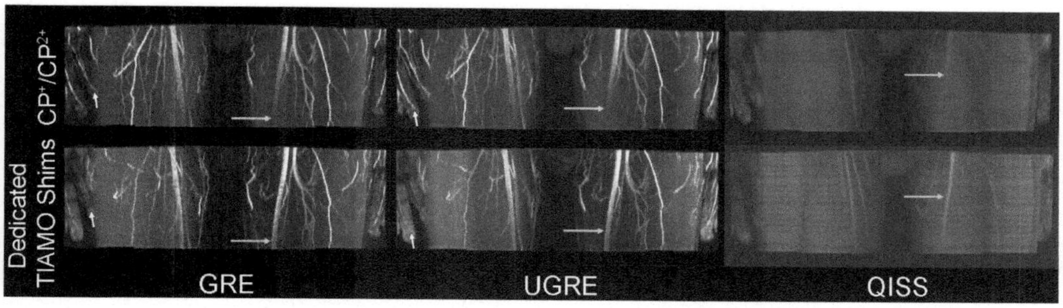

Figure 5. Dedicated TIAMO shims. MIPs showing the first station of the thigh. The upper row shows images acquired using TIAMO with the CP^+ and CP^{2+} modes. In the case of QISS, only CP^+ was used. In the lower row, dedicated TIAMO shims were calculated after the acquisition of B_1 maps. In the case of QISS, only one of the two modes could be used. One can clearly see that the left superficial femoral artery can be delineated throughout the entire station with the dedicated B_1 shims (grey arrows), whereas the finger arteries lost signal (short white arrow in GRE and UGRE).

leads to a periodic signal variation: Every second line in k-space is acquired with slightly lower signal which results in an artifact in axial slices which appears similar to aliasing. A possibility to prevent that would be to excite with two different flip angles and/or using a different k-space ordering. But as the artifact is only slightly visible in the axial images and not visible in the MIPs, this was not implemented yet and might be topic of future study. The slight vessel broadening visible in the phase-encode direction in UGRE was not visible in the coronal MIPs. The reason for the latter artifact is most probably that, despite cardiac triggering, the blood flow velocities are not constant during acquisition of the whole slice and thus the pronounced flow artifact observed in GRE remains in small parts visible in UGRE. In general, as two consecutively excited modes contribute to one individual slice the UGRE sequence is more prone to volunteer movements than GRE. On the other side, the consecutive acquisition ensures application of excitation and saturation pulses in the same mode, simplifying sparse application of the saturation pulses and leading to sufficient venous suppression in the final image. In the QISS images blurring of the vessels was observed which led to poorer vessel delineation, and especially smaller vessels could not be delineated at all. Regarding artifacts, UGRE would be the most preferable sequence.

Six of the examined volunteers required calculation of individual TIAMO RF shim settings for the station at the level of the thighs to improve the visibility of the superficial femoral artery in both legs; this extra step required the acquisition of B_1 maps. Another possible solution for this issue may be the use of high-permittivity pads to increase the transmit field homogeneity [33]. The remaining stations could be examined with the CP^+ and CP^{2+} modes, indicating that the combination of the CP^+ and CP^{2+} mode is relatively robust for TIAMO imaging. The most probable reason for the need of individual RF shimming is the variable anatomy at the transition from pelvis to the legs along the longitudinal axis. Also, this might depend on the leg circumference and/or the ratio between fat and muscle.

In conclusion, the UGRE sequence variant performed best for non-enhanced MRA of the lower extremity vessels, as the observed artifacts were only moderate and the highest average VBR was reached with a statistically significant difference to the compared sequences. The QISS sequence performed worst regarding VBR, while GRE showed the most severe flow artifacts despite reaching satisfactory VBR values. This study also revealed that the calculation of individual RF shim settings in a large proportion of volunteers as well as cardiac triggering, both of which prolong measurement time, are essential for the continuous depiction of the lower extremity arteries with non-enhanced MRA at 7T.

Acknowledgments

We would like to thank the Ultra-High Field team of Siemens, especially Thomas Benner, for their technical support and Michael Schwarz of the Department of General Psychology: Cognition, University of Duisburg-Essen, Duisburg, Germany, for the support on the statistical analysis.

Author Contributions

Conceived and designed the experiments: SJ SM AF SO LS LU TL KN ML. Performed the experiments: SJ SM SO AF LS. Analyzed the data: SJ AF SM LS. Contributed reagents/materials/analysis tools: SJ AF SM SO LS LU TL KN. Wrote the paper: SJ SM SO ML.

References

1. Gutzeit A, Sutter R, Froehlich JM, Roos JE, Sautter T, et al. (2011) ECG-triggered non-contrast-enhanced MR angiography (TRANCE) versus digital subtraction angiography (DSA) in patients with peripheral arterial occlusive disease of the lower extremities. Eur Radiol 21: 1979–1987.
2. Thomsen HS (2006) Nephrogenic systemic fibrosis: A serious late adverse reaction to gadodiamide. Eur Radiol 16: 2619–2621.
3. Prince MR, Zhang HL, Roditi GH, Leiner T, Kucharczyk W (2009) Risk factors for NSF: a literature review. J Magn Reson Imaging 30: 1298–1308.
4. Lanzman RS, Blondin D, Schmitt P, Orzechowski D, Godehardt E, et al. (2010) Non-Enhanced 3D MR Angiography of the Lower Extremity using ECG-Gated TSE Imaging with Non-Selective Refocusing Pulses - Initial Experience. Rofo 182: 861–867.
5. Hodnett PA, Koktzoglou I, Davarpanah AH, Scanlon TG, Collins JD, et al. (2011) Evaluation of Peripheral Arterial Disease with Nonenhanced Quiescent-Interval Single-Shot MR Angiography. Radiology 260: 282–293.
6. Fan ZY, Sheehan J, Bi XM, Liu X, Carr J, et al. (2009) 3D Noncontrast MR Angiography of the Distal Lower Extremities Using Flow-Sensitive Dephasing (FSD)-Prepared Balanced SSFP. Magn Reson Med 62: 1523–1532.
7. Nakamura K, Miyazaki M, Kuroki K, Yamamoto A, Hiramine A, et al. (2011) Noncontrast-enhanced Peripheral MRA: Technical Optimization of Flow-Spoiled Fresh Blood Imaging for Screening Peripheral Arterial Diseases. Magn Reson Med 65: 595–602.
8. Cukur T, Lee JH, Bangerter NK, Hargreaves BA, Nishimura DG (2009) Non-contrast-Enhanced Flow-Independent Peripheral MR Angiography with Balanced SSFP. Magn Reson Med 61: 1533–1539.
9. Maderwald S, Ladd SC, Gizewski ER, Kraff O, Theysohn JM, et al. (2008) To TOF or not to TOF: strategies for non-contrast-enhanced intracranial MRA at 7 T. MAGMA 21: 159–167.
10. Nowinski WL, Puspitasaari F, Volkau I, Marchenko Y, Knopp MV (2013) Comparison of Magnetic Resonance Angiography Scans on 1.5, 3, and 7 Tesla Units: A Quantitative Study of 3-Dimensional Cerebrovasculature. Journal of Neuroimaging 23: 86–95.

11. Hoult DI, Phil D (2000) Sensitivity and power deposition in a high-field imaging experiment. J Magn Reson Imaging 12: 46–67.
12. Van De Moortele PF, Akgun C, Adriany G, Moeller S, Ritter J, et al. (2005) B-1 destructive interferences and spatial phase patterns at 7 T with a head transceiver array coil. Magn Reson Med 54: 1503–1518.
13. Vaughan TT, Snyder CJ, DelaBarre LJ, Bolan PJ, Tian J, et al. (2009) Whole-Body Imaging at 7T: Preliminary Results. Magn Reson Med 61: 244–248.
14. Umutlu L, Maderwald S, Kinner S, Kraff O, Bitz AK, et al. (2013) First-pass contrast-enhanced renal MRA at 7 Tesla: initial results. Eur Radiol 23: 1059–1066.
15. Orzada S, Maderwald S, Poser BA, Bitz AK, Quick HH, et al. (2010) RF excitation using time interleaved acquisition of modes (TIAMO) to address B1 inhomogeneity in high-field MRI. Magn Reson Med 64: 327–333.
16. Orzada S, Maderwald S, Poser BA, Johst S, Kannengiesser S, et al. (2012) Time-interleaved acquisition of modes: an analysis of SAR and image contrast implications. Magn Reson Med 67: 1033–1041.
17. Fischer A, Maderwald S, Orzada S, Johst S, Schafer LC, et al. (2013) Nonenhanced magnetic resonance angiography of the lower extremity vessels at 7 tesla: initial experience. Invest Radiol 48: 525–534.
18. Frauenrath T, Hezel F, Renz W, d'Orth TD, Dieringer M, et al. (2010) Acoustic cardiac triggering: a practical solution for synchronization and gating of cardiovascular magnetic resonance at 7 Tesla. Journal of Cardiovascular Magnetic Resonance 12(1):67.
19. Maderwald S, Orzada S, Lin Z, Schäfer L, Bitz A, et al. 7 Tesla Cardiac Imaging with a Phonocardiogram Trigger Device. ISMRM 19th Annual Meeting; 2011; Montreal, Canada. pp. 1322.
20. Nassenstein K, Orzada S, Haering L, Czylwik A, Zenge M, et al. (2012) Cardiac MRI: evaluation of phonocardiogram-gated cine imaging for the assessment of global und regional left ventricular function in clinical routine. European Radiology 22: 559–568.
21. Nassenstein K, Orzada S, Haering L, Czylwik A, Jensen C, et al. (2012) Cardiac magnetic resonance: is phonocardiogram gating reliable in velocity-encoded phase contrast imaging? European Radiology 22: 2679–2687.
22. Edelman RR, Sheehan JJ, Dunkle E, Schindler N, Carr J, et al. (2010) Quiescent-interval single-shot unenhanced magnetic resonance angiography of peripheral vascular disease: Technical considerations and clinical feasibility. Magn Reson Med 63: 951–958.
23. Orzada S, Maderwald S, Kraff O, Brote I, Ladd ME, et al. 16-Channel Tx/Rx Body Coil for RF Shimming with Selected Cp Modes at 7T. ISMRM 18th Annual Meeting; 2010; Stockholm, Sweden. pp. 50.
24. Bitz AK, Brote I, Orzada S, Kraff O, Maderwald S, et al. An 8-channel add-on RF shimming system for whole-body 7 tesla MRI including real-time SAR monitoring. ISMRM 17th Annual Meeting; 2009; Hawai, USA. pp. 4767.
25. Yazdanbakhsh P, Fester M, Oppelt R, Bitz AK, Kraff O, et al. Variable Power Combiner for a 7T Butler Matrix Coil Array; 2009; Honolulu, Hawaii. pp. 397.
26. Herborn CU, Goyen M, Quick HH, Bosk S, Massing S, et al. (2004) Whole-body 3D MR angiography of patients with peripheral arterial occlusive disease. AJR Am J Roentgenol 182: 1427–1434.
27. Quick HH, Vogt FM, Maderwald S, Herborn CU, Bosk S, et al. (2004) High spatial resolution whole-body MR angiography featuring parallel imaging: initial experience. Rofo 176: 163–169.
28. Ackerman MJ, Spitzer VM, Scherzinger AL, Whitlock DG (1995) The Visible Human data set: an image resource for anatomical visualization. Medinfo 8 Pt 2: 1195–1198.
29. Christ A, Kainz W, Hahn EG, Honegger K, Zefferer M, et al. (2010) The Virtual Family–development of surface-based anatomical models of two adults and two children for dosimetric simulations. Physics in medicine and biology 55: N23–38.
30. Snyder CJ, DelaBarre L, Metzger GJ, van de Moortele PF, Akgun C, et al. (2009) Initial Results of Cardiac Imaging at 7 Tesla. Magn Reson Med 61: 517–524.
31. Johst S, Wrede KH, Ladd ME, Maderwald S (2012) Time-of-flight magnetic resonance angiography at 7 T using venous saturation pulses with reduced flip angles. Invest Radiol 47: 445–450.
32. Rasch D, Guiard V (2004) The robustness of parametric statistical methods. Psychology Science 46: 175–208.
33. Teeuwisse WM, Brink WM, Webb AG (2012) Quantitative assessment of the effects of high-permittivity pads in 7 Tesla MRI of the brain. Magn Reson Med 67: 1285–1293.

Coronary Plaque Burden, as Determined by Cardiac Computed Tomography, in Patients with Myocardial Infarction and Angiographically Normal Coronary Arteries Compared to Healthy Volunteers: A Prospective Multicenter Observational Study

Elin B. Brolin[1]*, Tomas Jernberg[2], Torkel B. Brismar[1], Maria Daniel[3], Loghman Henareh[2], Jonaz Ripsweden[1], Per Tornvall[4], Kerstin Cederlund[1]

1 Department of Radiology, Karolinska University Hospital Huddinge and Department of Clinical Science, Intervention and Technology, Division of Medical Imaging and Technology at Karolinska Institutet, Stockholm, Sweden, **2** Department of Medicine, Section of Cardiology, Karolinska University Hospital Huddinge and Karolinska Institutet, Stockholm, Sweden, **3** Cardiology Unit, Department of Medicine, Karolinska University Hospital Solna and Karolinska Institutet, Stockholm, Sweden, **4** Institution for Clinical Science and Education at Södersjukhuset, Karolinska Institutet, Stockholm, Sweden

Abstract

Objectives: Patients presenting with acute myocardial infarction and angiographically normal coronary arteries (MINCA) represent a diagnostic and a therapeutic challenge. Cardiac computed tomography (CT) allows detection of coronary artery disease (CAD) even in the absence of significant stenosis. We aimed to investigate whether patients suffering from MINCA had a greater coronary plaque burden, as determined by cardiac CT, than a matched group of healthy volunteers.

Methods: Consecutive patients, aged 45 to 70, with MINCA were enrolled in the Stockholm metropolitan area. Patients with myocarditis were excluded using cardiovascular magnetic resonance imaging. Remaining patients underwent cardiac CT, as did a reference group of healthy volunteers matched by age and gender, with no known cardiovascular disease. Plaque burden was evaluated semi-quantitatively on a per patient and a per segment level.

Results: Despite a higher prevalence of smoking and hypertension, patients with MINCA did not have more CAD than healthy volunteers. Among 57 MINCA patients and 58 volunteers no signs of CAD were found in 24 (42%) and 25 (43%) respectively. On a *per segment* level, MINCA patients had less segments with stenosis ≥20% (2% vs. 5%, $p<0.01$), as well as a smaller proportion of large (2% vs. 4%, $p<0.05$) and mixed type plaques (1% vs. 4%, $p<0.01$). The median coronary calcium score did not differ between MINCA patients and healthy volunteers (6 vs. 8, *ns*).

Conclusions: MINCA patients with no or minimal angiographic stenosis do not have more coronary atherosclerosis than healthy volunteers, and a large proportion of these patients do not have any signs of CAD, as determined by cardiac CT. The MINCA patient group is probably heterogeneous, with a variety of different underlying mechanisms. Non-obstructive CAD is most likely not the most prevalent cause of myocardial infarction in this patient group.

Editor: Rozemarijn Vliegenthart, University of Groningen, Netherlands

Funding: This work was supported by the Swedish Heart-Lung Foundation (www.hjart-lungfonden.se) and by the regional agreement on medical training and clinical research (ALF) between Stockholm County Council and Karolinska Institutet. The funders had no role in study design, data collection and analysis, decision to publish, or preparation of the manuscript.

Competing Interests: The authors have declared that no competing interests exist.

* E-mail: elin.bacsovics.brolin@ki.se

Introduction

In a considerable number of patients presenting with acute myocardial infarction who undergo conventional coronary angiography, no significant coronary artery stenoses are found. This condition is called MINCA (myocardial infarction and angiographically normal coronary arteries) or MINOCA (myocardial infarction and non-obstructed coronary arteries). Depending on the definition, the reported prevalence of MINCA ranges between 3% and 18% of all acute myocardial infarctions. [1–5] In women, however, the prevalence has been reported to be as high as 33%. [4,5] A number of underlying mechanisms have been proposed, including vasospasm, embolism, disturbed endothelial function and coronary artery disease (CAD) with occult rupture of non-stenotic plaque. [6–8] In a clinical setting, Takotsubo cardiomyopathy can be considered a subtype of MINCA. For this condition, often provoked by stress, additional underlying mechanisms have been suggested, such as exaggerated sympathetic stimulation and catecholamine toxicity. [9,10] Although awareness of MINCA has increased, there is still a lack of data clarifying its different aetiologies and mechanisms.

The development of diagnostic imaging methods has provided new means for understanding MINCA and its underlying causes. The use of cardiovascular magnetic resonance imaging (CMR) for instance, enables differentiation between myocarditis and myocardial infarction, as well as diagnosis of Takotsubo cardiomyopathy. [1,11] Cardiac computed tomography (CT) has evolved substantially during the last few years, and has now achieved very good accuracy when it comes to diagnosing stenoses of the coronary arteries, as compared to coronary angiography. [12] Cardiac CT has also proven highly sensitive in detecting atherosclerotic plaques in the proximal segments of the coronary arteries, when compared to intravascular ultrasound. [13] An important difference between conventional coronary angiography and cardiac CT is the fact that the former only shows the lumen of the artery, whilst the latter permits visualization of the vascular wall as well as the lumen. Cardiac CT allows detection and characterization of coronary atherosclerotic plaques even when they do not give rise to stenoses and whether they are calcified or not. Accordingly, cardiac CT makes it possible to assess atherosclerotic plaques undetected by conventional coronary angiography.

Previous studies, using intravascular ultrasound or cardiac CT, have suggested that CAD is an important underlying cause of MINCA. [7,14–16] However, none of these studies included a control group. Since other cardiac CT studies including asymtomatic subjects have demonstrated a non negligible prevalence of CAD, the question remains whether the CAD shown in MINCA patients was necessarily the cause of the myocardial infarction. [17–19].

The present study is a substudy of the SMINC (Stockholm Myocardial Infarction with Normal Coronaries) study and aims to examine whether patients suffering from MINCA have more coronary atherosclerosis, as assessed by cardiac CT, than a reference group of healthy volunteers [22].

Materials and Methods

Ethics Statement

The study conforms to the principles of the Declaration of Helsinki and was approved by the Regional Ethical Review Board in Stockholm (www.epn.se) and by the Radiation Protection Committee of the Karolinska University Hospital. Written informed consent was obtained from all patients and healthy volunteers.

Study Group

Between June 2007 and May 2011, patients with MINCA were screened for the SMINC study at five different coronary care units in the Stockholm metropolitan area, as described by Collste *et al.* [22] Patients were eligible to take part in the study if they were between 35 and 70 years of age, fulfilled the criteria for acute myocardial infarction according to the universal definition of myocardial infarction, [20] and underwent a coronary angiography showing no or minimal signs of atherosclerosis (defined as the presence of plaque discernible on coronary angiography, but no stenosis exceeding 30% by visual estimation). Coronary angiography was performed at the time of initial hospital admission, according to clinical routines, and evaluated using the modified American Heart Association 17 segment classification. [21] Exclusion criteria were a patient history of structural or coronary heart disease, chronic obstructive lung disease, renal disease, the use of a pacemaker and an electrocardiogram (ECG) on admission showing non sinus rhythm or a clinical diagnosis of pulmonary embolism. CMR was performed on all patients in order to exclude those with myocarditis. [22] After patient inclusion, the coronary angiogram as well as the clinical diagnosis of acute myocardial infarction were re-evaluated by an additional investigator. A reference group of healthy volunteers, matched by age and gender, with no known cardiovascular disease, was recruited using a registry comprising all Stockholm residents. Persons of the same age and gender as MINCA patients were contacted by mail. If they were willing to participate and had no history of cardiovascular disease they underwent an exercise stress test, and if the test was normal they were invited to take part in the study.

Out of 152 patients screened for the SMINC study, 100 MINCA patients were after exclusions described above considered for the present cardiac CT substudy, as well as 100 healthy volunteers. Accordingly, the MINCA patients of the present study form a subgroup of the patients studied by Collste *et al.* [22] Additional exclusion criteria for the CT study were age under 45 (due to considerations of radiation dose; 5 MINCA patients and 5 control persons), previous adverse reaction to iodinated contrast media (1 MINCA patient) and an irregular heart rate (jeopardizing the diagnostic quality of the CT scan; 1 control person). Out of 100 MINCA patients and 100 healthy volunteers, 61 and 58 respectively agreed to take part in the present study. The CT examinations of the MINCA patients were performed between 3 and 6 months after the acute event.

Cardiac CT Data Acquisition

Examinations were performed on a 64-slice CT scanner (LightSpeed VCT XT; GE Healthcare, Milwaukee, WI, USA). A prospectively ECG-triggered scan protocol was used: detector configuration 64×0.625 mm, rotation time 350 ms, tube potential 120 kV, tube current 450–650 mA (according to patient size). The scans were performed in diastole, in general at 70–75% of the RR interval, with a padding of 100–200 ms, depending on heart rate and variability. The contrast agent used was iodixanol 320 mg I/ml (Visipaque, GE Healthcare, Stockholm, Sweden), which was administered using a dual-head injector (Medrad, Stellant Dual Head Injector, Pittsburgh, PA, USA) and a triple-phase protocol. The contrast agent was individually dosed, based on body weight (400 mg I/kg, 75–100 ml iodixanol), with a fixed injection time (15 s), resulting in an injection rate of 5–7 ml/s. This was followed by a 50 ml mixture of 40% iodixanol and 60% saline and finally by a 50 ml saline chaser. In the absence of contraindications and depending on the initial heart rate, patients received metoprolol (25–100 mg) per os prior to the examination. Patients also received sublingual nitroglycerine (0.4 mg) 4 minutes before the scan.

To assess the coronary calcium score, a non-enhanced scan was performed, using a prospectively ECG-triggered scan protocol: tube potential 120 kV, tube current 200 mA.

Cardiac CT Data Analysis

The Cardiac CT exam was analysed independently by three readers (two experienced readers with level 2 and one reader with level 1 according to ACCF/AHA levels of competence), [23] who were blinded to all clinical information. A subsequent joint reading was performed and a consensus reached.

Cardiac CT data analysis was performed using the CardIQ Xpress software on the Advantage Workstation 4.4 (GE Healthcare, Milwaukee, WI, USA). Axial source images, multiplanar and curved multiplanar reformats as well as thin-slab maximum intensity projections were used. The optimal image display setting for lumen and plaque assessment was chosen on an individual basis, but in general at a window width of 800–1000 HU and a level of 100–200 HU. Coronary arteries were subdivided into 17 segments, according to the modified American Heart Association classification. [21] Initially, each segment was assessed regarding image quality and evaluability. Segments were considered non-evaluable if artifacts prevented reliable assessment of the lumen or the vessel wall (e. g. due to motion, image noise or heavy calcification). Secondly, each segment was visually evaluated with regard to the presence of stenosis (A), plaque size (B) and composition (C). A plaque was defined as any structure, discernible in at least two planes, within or adjacent to the vessel lumen, which could be clearly separated from the vessel lumen and from adjacent soft tissue.

A. Lesions were quantified for stenosis by visual estimation, comparing the minimal lumen of the stenotic area with the lumen of the adjacent proximal unaffected segment, and expressed in terms of diameter stenosis: <20%, 20–50% or ≥ 50%.
B. The size of the atherosclerotic plaque was determined by measuring the length of the plaque on longitudinal sections and arbitrarily classified as: small (<4 mm), medium (4–8 mm) or large (≥8 mm).
C. Plaque composition was visually assessed based on the presence or absence of calcified elements: non-calcified coronary artery plaque, mixed coronary artery plaque or calcified coronary artery plaque, the latter with ≥50% calcified tissue. [24].

In the case of more than one atherosclerotic plaque in a single segment, only the greatest degree of stenosis, the largest plaque size and the most pronounced calcification was considered.

Coronary Calcium Score

The coronary calcium score was calculated using semi-automatic software (SmartScore 4.0, GE Healthcare, Milwaukee, WI, USA) on the Advantage Workstation 4.4 (GE Healthcare, Milwaukee, WI, USA). The total calcium burden of the coronary arteries was reported in terms of AJ-130 score, based on the scoring algorithm of Agatston et al. [25].

Statistical Analysis

In order to evaluate hypotheses of variables in contingency tables, the chi-square test was used or, in the case of small expected frequencies, Fisher's exact two-sided test. Statistical comparisons for testing differences between two independent groups were made using the Student's t-test for uncorrelated means, after validation of normal distribution by use of the Shapiro Wilk test. In the case of non-normal distribution the Mann-Whitney test was used. In addition, descriptive statistics was used to characterize the data. All analyses were carried out using the SAS system and the 5% levels of significance were considered. In the case of a statistically significant result the probability value (p-value) has been given. Due to the nature of the study, an initial exploratory study, the sample size was not determined based on power or clinical difference. The number of patients participating in the study was chosen for practical reasons, not statistical. However, in order to estimate statistical power, one could consider the per segment analysis (n = 765+781) and a binomial endpoint (segment with or without CAD) and a 5% level of significance. Anticipating a prevalence of CAD of 10% in the control group and 15% in the MINCA group would yield a power of 85%.

Results

Of the 119 (61 MINCA+58 volunteers) cardiac CT exams performed, 4 exams of MINCA patients had to be excluded, 3 due to motion artifacts resulting in <7 evaluable segments and 1 due to the heart not being completely covered by the scan. Thus, cardiac CT exams of 57 MINCA patients and 58 healthy volunteers were further analyzed. From these exams 15 (1.9%) individual segments in the MINCA group and 11 (1.4%) in the reference group were non-evaluable and excluded from analyses. Figure 1 shows an example of a coronary artery in a MINCA patient, as visualized by cardiac CT and by conventional coronary angiography. Figure 2 shows examples of different plaque types as seen by cardiac CT.

Baseline characteristics of patients with MINCA and healthy volunteers are compared in Table 1. Current smoking and treated hypertension were more common in the MINCA group. Regarding all other variables the two groups were comparable. Out of 57 MINCA patients, 56 presented with no signs of heart failure (Killip class 1) and only one with heart failure, consistent with Killip class 2. Signs of acute ischemia (ST-T changes or left bundle branch block) on admission ECG were present in 31 (54%) MINCA patients, of whom 10 had ST elevations. The median (IQR) maximum troponin level was 18 (7–43) times greater than the upper limit of normal. Myocardial infarction was detectable with CMR in 11 (19%) patients. The criteria for Takotsubo cardiomyopathy was fulfilled in 15 (26%).

The cardiac CT plaque burden analyses are presented in Tables 2 and 3, on per patient (Table 2) and per segment (Table 3) basis, comparing the MINCA group with the reference group. On a *per patient* level there were no statistically significant differences in severity or extent of CAD. Twentyfour (42%) MINCA patients and 25 (43%) healthy subjects had no signs of CAD. When analyzing the data on a *per segment* level, however, there were statistically significant differences regarding degree of stenosis, plaque size and plaque composition. MINCA patients had less segments with stenosis ≥20% compared to healthy volunteers (2% vs 5%, $p<0.01$) They also exhibited a smaller proportion of large plaques (2% vs 4%, $p<0.05$) and mixed type coronary artery plaques (1% vs 4%, $p<0.01$). The calcium scores within each group were diverse, but no significant differences were found between the groups. No differences were found regarding CT plaque burden when MINCA patients with and without MI detected by CMR were compared or when MINCA patients with and without ST elevations were compared (Table S1). Nor were there any differences in plaque burden between MINCA patients with and without a diagnosis of Takotsubo cardiomyopathy (Table S1). No statistically significant difference was demonstrated regarding peak troponin levels between MINCA patients with and without CAD. There were no differences in terms of baseline characteristics when MINCA patients without CAD were compared to those with CAD demonstrated by cardiac CT (Table S2).

Discussion

This study is the first to analyze coronary plaque burden in patients with MINCA by means of cardiac CT, with a matched reference group for comparison. The most important finding was the fact that patients with MINCA did not have more coronary atherosclerosis than healthy volunteers, despite a higher frequency of smoking and hypertension in the MINCA group. In addition, a high proportion of MINCA patients (42%) did not exhibit any signs of CAD, as demonstrated by cardiac CT, which strongly suggests that there are underlying causes other than CAD in a significant number of MINCA patients. A finding that further strengthens this hypothesis was the fact that MINCA patients had

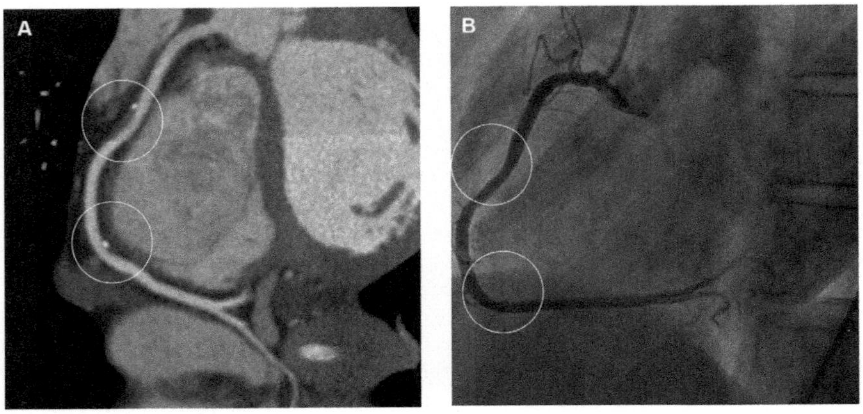

Figure 1. The right coronary artery in a patient presenting with acute myocardial infarction. Cardiac computed tomography (A) shows a large atherosclerotic plaque and more distally a small plaque, both with <20% stenosis. Coronary angiography (B) shows only minimal signs of atherosclerosis.

a lower rate of large size atherosclerotic plaques and mixed type coronary artery plaques compared to healthy volunteers. Such plaque characteristics have been shown to imply a more vulnerable plaque, more prone to rupture [26–28].

In the literature there are several definitions and terms used to designate myocardial infarction in the absence of significant CAD. The term MINOCA (myocardial infarction and non-obstructed coronary arteries) is often used, since many studies have included patients with <50% angiographic stenosis. However, the term MINCA has been chosen for this study, in order to stress the fact that only patients with no or minimal signs of atherosclerosis on coronary angiography were included.

The findings of the current study partly contradict findings of a recent study by Aldrovandi *et al.*, where only 16% of MINCA patients had no signs of CAD when examined with cardiac CT. [16] However, this difference can probably be explained by different inclusion criteria. In the previous study patients with < 50% angiographic diameter stenosis were included, whereas in the current study a more rigorous definition was used, including only patients with no or minimal signs of atherosclerosis. The mean degree of stenosis, as determined by cardiac CT, was >30% in the previous study, whereas the median degree of stenosis in the present study was <20%. Hence, applying a more rigorous definition of "normal coronary angiogram" seems useful in order to identify a patient group that is far less likely to have CAD. In addition, only patients with evidence of myocardial infarction on CMR were included in the study by Aldrovandi *et al.*, whereas the present study also included patients with smaller myocardial infarctions, proven by biochemical markers but not detectable by CMR.

A study by Reynolds *et al.* supports that CAD is a major cause of myocardial infarction in patients with higher degrees of non-obstructive stenosis (<50%) at coronary angiography, but not necessarily in patients with no or minimal signs of atherosclerosis. [7] In their study women with myocardial infarction without angiographically obstructive CAD underwent intravascular ultrasound, which revealed plaque ruptures and ulcerations in 38% of patients. A higher degree of stenosis was found in patients with plaque disruption (median degree of stenosis 40%) compared to patients without plaque disruption. One third of patients had no signs of atherosclerosis on coronary angiography and, interestingly, none of these patients had plaque disruption. Consequently, it seems likely that the frequency of plaque disruption would be smaller in the present study group, with less severe CAD.

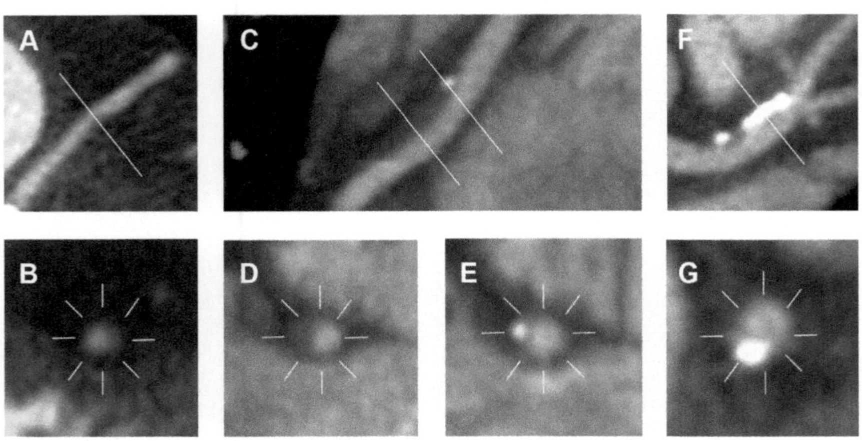

Figure 2. Different plaque types, as seen by cardiac computed tomography. A non-calcified plaque is shown in longitudinal and cross section (A and B). The degree of stenosis was 20–50%. A large mixed plaque is shown in longitudinal section (C) and in cross section at the level of non calcified (D) and calcified (E) components. A large calcified plaque is shown to the right. (F and G). The mixed and calcified plaques (C to G) were both eccentric in location and the degree of stenosis was <20%.

Table 1. Baseline characteristics.

	MINCA, n = 57	Healthy subjects, n = 58
Age (years)	60±5	61±6
Female	42 (74%)	39 (67%)
Present smoking	10 (18%)	2 (3%)*
Prior smoking	17 (30%)	23 (40%)
Family history of CAD	16 (28%)	14 (24%)
Diabetes mellitus	1 (2%)	0 (0%)
Treated hypertension	19 (33%)	6 (10%)†
Treated hyperlipidemia	8 (14%)	3 (5%)
BMI (kg/m^2)	25.8±3	25.8±3

Abbreviations: MINCA, myocardial infarction with angiographically normal coronary arteries; CAD, coronary artery disease; BMI, body mass index; SD, standard deviation. Data are presented as mean ± SD or absolute value (percentage).
*$P<0.05$,
†$P<0.01$, using Fisher's exact test.

This study cannot explain the underlying cause of MINCA. One explanation could be that an important proportion of MINCA cases are in fact Takotsubo cardiomyopathy, which was found in 26% of the study group. For the MINCA patients who had CAD, this may at least for some patients have been the cause of the myocardial infarction. Plaque disruption with transient thrombus formation might be one plausible mechanism and vasospasm another. [7] There was a higher frequency of smoking in the MINCA group, which may in turn increase the risk of thrombosis, as well as vasoconstriction. An increased resistance to activated protein C has been reported in MINCA patients, which supports the theory that thrombosis is involved in the aetiology of MINCA [4].

The present study has limitations. Although being the largest study of its kind, the sample size was limited. Thus, lack of significant differences may still be caused by lack of power to detect such differences. However, the data show a tendency towards more severe CAD in the reference group compared to the MINCA-group, rather than the other way round.

The fact that MINCA patients, on a per segment level, showed a lower frequency of stenoses ≥20% than healthy subjects can probably be explained by the selection process, where MINCA patients per definition had no or minimal stenosis as determined

Table 2. Cardiac CT plaque burden per patient.

		MINCA patients, n = 57	Healthy volunteers, n = 58	*P*
Severity of CAD*	No CAD	24 (42%)	25 (43%)	*ns*
	Stenosis <20%	22 (39%)	23 (40%)	
	Stenosis 20–50%	11 (19%)	9 (16%)	
	Stenosis ≥50%	0 (0%)	1 (2%)	
All CAD†	0 segments	24 (42%)	25 (43%)	*ns*
	1 segments	14 (25%)	10 (17%)	
	2 segments	8 (14%)	12 (21%)	
	3 segments	4 (7%)	6 (10%)	
	4 segments	2 (4%)	0 (0%)	
	5 segments	3 (5%)	1 (2%)	
	6 segments	0 (0%)	0 (0%)	
	7 segments	0 (0%)	0 (0%)	
	8 segments	2 (4%)	1 (2%)	
	9 segments	0 (0%)	1 (2%)	
	10 segments	0 (0%)	2 (3%)	
Calcium score (AJ-130)		6 (0–778)	8 (0–1882)	*ns*

Abbreviations: Cardiac CT, cardiac computed tomography; MINCA, myocardial infarction with angiographically normal coronary arteries; CAD, coronary artery disease; *ns*, non significant. Values are presented as absolute value (percentage) or median (range).
*refers to the maximum diameter stenosis;
†refers to obstructive and non-obstructive CAD.

Table 3. Cardiac CT plaque burden per segment.

		MINCA patients, 765 segments	Healthy volunteers, 781 segments	*P*
Severity of CAD	No CAD	684 (89%)	687 (88%)	<0.01*
	Stenosis <20%	68 (9%)	58 (7%)	
	Stenosis 20–50%	13 (2%)	35 (4%)	
	Stenosis ≥50%	0 (0%)	1 (0.1%)	
Plaque size	No CAD	684 (89%)	687 (88%)	0.04*
	Small	41 (5%)	31 (4%)	
	Medium	24 (3%)	29 (4%)	
	Large	16 (2%)	34 (4%)	
Plaque composition	No CAD	684 (89%)	687 (88%)	0.04*
	Non-calcified plaque	10 (1%)	10 (1%)	
	Mixed plaque	10 (1%)	28 (4%)	
	Calcified plaque	61 (8%)	56 (7%)	

Abbreviations: Cardiac CT, cardiac computed tomography; MINCA, myocardial infarction with angiographically normal coronary arteries; CAD, coronary artery disease; Values are presented as absolute value (percentage).
*P-values apply to the comparison of the four categories in the two columns to the left of the value, using the chi-square test.

by conventional coronary angiography. One could argue that the reference group should have been selected by excluding individuals with angiographic coronary stenoses. This was however not achievable, since it is not ethically possible to perform invasive coronary angiography on healthy volunteers. Still, on a per patient level there were roughly equal numbers of MINCA patients (19%) and healthy controls (18%) with stenosis ≥20%. Only 57 of the initial 100 MINCA patients were included in the cardiac CT analyses. There were however no differences in baseline characteristics when these patients were compared with the 43 MINCA patients who did not participate in the cardiac CT study (Table S3). The study population mainly reflects a northern European ethnic group, the majority being women, which might affect generalizability. However, the female predominance is not surprising, since it reflects the higher prevalence of MINCA in women compared to men. Although 64 detector cardiac CT has proven highly sensitive in detecting atherosclerotic plaques, its spatial resolution is limited, which makes it hazardous to assess very small structures. A study comparing cardiac CT plaque detection and quantification with IVUS measures showed a very good diagnostic accuracy for cardiac CT to detect atherosclerotic plaques on a segmental level. However, the sensitivity decreased for smaller plaques and for plaques located more distally in the coronary arteries. [29] Hence, early coronary atherosclerosis, with very subtle changes of the vessel wall, as well as distal lesions might remain undetected by cardiac CT. For the MINCA patients there was a time span of 3 to 6 months between the acute event and the CT examination, which might have had minor influence on the results. A semi-quantitative method was used to estimate plaque burden. It could be debated whether an automated, non-user dependent method should have been used. However, such automated approaches have not been thoroughly validated, whilst semi-quantitative methods relying on visual assessment for plaque detection and characterization have been described in several studies and have been found to entail good intra- and interobserver variability [30].

The current findings together with findings of previous studies suggest that patients with MINCA compose a heterogeneous group, with a variety of underlying causes of the myocardial infarction. It seems that in patients with moderate angiographic coronary stenosis, CAD with plaque disruption might be an important cause of the myocardial infarction, whilst in patients with no or minimal angiographic stenosis the myocardial infarction is more likely to have other causes than established CAD. It is now well recognized that atherosclerosis is a heterogeneous process, including for instance inflammation and endothelial dysfunction, and additional research is warranted in order to investigate the role of these processes in the MINCA patient group.

Since the prognosis for patients suffering from MINCA is not benign, [31,32] it is of great importance to further clarify the underlying mechanisms, in order to offer patients appropriate treatment and care.

Supporting Information

Table S1 Cardiac CT plaque burden, comparing subgroups of MINCA patients.

Table S2 Baseline characteristics for MINCA patients with and without CAD.

Table S3 Baseline characteristics for MINCA patients that participated and did not participate in the CT substudy.

Author Contributions

Conceived and designed the experiments: EBB TJ TBB MD LH JR PT KC. Performed the experiments: EBB JR KC. Analyzed the data: EBB TJ TBB PT KC. Contributed reagents/materials/analysis tools: EBB MD LH JR PT KC. Wrote the paper: EBB TJ TBB PT KC.

References

1. Stensaeth KH, Fossum E, Hoffmann P, Mangschau A, Klow NE (2011) Clinical characteristics and role of early cardiac magnetic resonance imaging in patients with suspected ST-elevation myocardial infarction and normal coronary arteries. Int J Cardiovasc Imaging 27: 355–365.
2. Gehrie ER, Reynolds HR, Chen AY, Neelon BH, Roe MT, et al. (2009) Characterization and outcomes of women and men with non-ST-segment elevation myocardial infarction and nonobstructive coronary artery disease: Results from the can rapid risk stratification of unstable angina patients suppress adverse outcomes with early implementation of the ACC/AHA guidelines (CRUSADE) quality improvement initiative. Am Heart J 158: 688–694.
3. Larsen AI, Galbraith PD, Ghali WA, Norris CM, Graham MM, et al. (2005) Characteristics and outcomes of patients with acute myocardial infarction and angiographically normal coronary arteries. Am J Cardiol 95: 261–263.
4. Agewall S, Daniel M, Eurenius L, Ekenback C, Skeppholm M, et al. (2012) Risk factors for myocardial infarction with normal coronary arteries and myocarditis compared with myocardial infarction with coronary artery stenosis. Angiology 63: 500–503.
5. Chokshi NP, Iqbal SN, Berger RL, Hochman JS, Feit F, et al. (2010) Sex and race are associated with the absence of epicardial coronary artery obstructive disease at angiography in patients with acute coronary syndromes. Clin Cardiol 33: 495–501.
6. Ong P, Athanasiadis A, Hill S, Vogelsberg H, Voehringer M, et al. (2008) Coronary artery spasm as a frequent cause of acute coronary syndrome: The CASPAR (coronary artery spasm in patients with acute coronary syndrome) study. J Am Coll Cardiol 52: 523–527.
7. Reynolds HR, Srichai MB, Iqbal SN, Slater JN, Mancini GBJ, et al. (2011) Mechanisms of myocardial infarction in women without angiographically obstructive coronary artery disease. Circulation 124: 1414–1425.
8. Kardasz I, De Caterina R (2007) Myocardial infarction with normal coronary arteries: A conundrum with multiple aetiologies and variable prognosis: An update. J Intern Med 261: 330–348.
9. Wittstein IS, Thiemann DR, Lima JA, Baughman KL, Schulman SP, et al. (2005) Neurohumoral features of myocardial stunning due to sudden emotional stress. N Engl J Med 352: 539–548.
10. Prasad A, Lerman A, Rihal CS (2008) Apical ballooning syndrome (tako-tsubo or stress cardiomyopathy): A mimic of acute myocardial infarction. Am Heart J 155: 408–417.
11. Laissy JP, Hyafil F, Feldman LJ, Juliard JM, Schouman-Claeys E, et al. (2005) Differentiating acute myocardial infarction from myocarditis: Diagnostic value of early- and delayed-perfusion cardiac MR imaging. Radiology 237: 75–82.
12. Mowatt G, Cook JA, Hillis GS, Walker S, Fraser C, et al. (2008) 64-slice computed tomography angiography in the diagnosis and assessment of coronary artery disease: Systematic review and meta-analysis. Heart 94: 1386–1393.
13. Voros S, Rinehart S, Qian Z, Joshi P, Vazquez G, et al. (2011) Coronary atherosclerosis imaging by coronary CT angiography: Current status, correlation with intravascular interrogation and meta-analysis. JACC Cardiovasc Imaging 4: 537–548.
14. Caussin C, Ohanessian A, Lancelin B, Rahal S, Hennequin R, et al. (2003) Coronary plaque burden detected by multislice computed tomography after acute myocardial infarction with near-normal coronary arteries by angiography. Am J Cardiol 92: 849–852.
15. Aldrovandi A, Cademartiri F, Menozzi A, Ugo F, Lina D, et al. (2008) Evaluation of coronary atherosclerosis by multislice computed tomography in patients with acute myocardial infarction and without significant coronary artery stenosis a comparative study with quantitative coronary angiography. Circ Cardiovasc Imaging 1: 205–211.
16. Aldrovandi A, Cademartiri F, Arduini D, Lina D, Ugo F, et al. (2012) Computed tomography coronary angiography in patients with acute myocardial infarction without significant coronary stenosis. Circulation 126: 3000–3007.
17. Hwang Y, Kim Y, Chung IM, Ryu J, Park H (2010) Coronary heart disease risk assessment and characterization of coronary artery disease using coronary CT angiography: Comparison of asymptomatic and symptomatic groups. Clin Radiol 65: 601–608.
18. Hadamitzky M, Meyer T, Hein F, Bischoff B, Martinoff S, et al. (2010) Prognostic value of coronary computed tomographic angiography in asymptomatic patients. Am J Cardiol 105: 1746–1751.
19. Neefjes LA, Ten Kate GJ, Rossi A, Galema-Boers AJ, Langendonk JG, et al. (2011) CT coronary plaque burden in asymptomatic patients with familial hypercholesterolaemia. Heart 97: 1151–1157.
20. Thygesen K, Alpert JS, White HD, Jaffe AS, Apple FS, et al. (2007) Universal definition of myocardial infarction. Circulation 116: 2634–2653.
21. Austen WG, Edwards JE, Frye RL, Gensini GG, Gott VL, et al. (1975) A reporting system on patients evaluated for coronary artery disease. Report of the ad hoc committee for grading of coronary artery disease, council on cardiovascular surgery, american heart association. Circulation 51: 5–40.
22. Collste O, Sorensson P, Frick M, Agewall S, Daniel M, et al. (2013) Myocardial infarction with normal coronary arteries is common and associated with normal findings on cardiovascular magnetic resonance imaging: Results from the stockholm myocardial infarction with normal coronaries study. J Intern Med 273: 189–196.
23. Budoff MJ, Cohen MC, Garcia MJ, Hodgson JM, Hundley WG, et al. (2005) ACCF/AHA clinical competence statement on cardiac imaging with computed tomography and magnetic resonance. Circulation 112: 598–617.
24. Leber AW, Knez A, Becker A, Becker C, von Ziegler F, et al. (2004) Accuracy of multidetector spiral computed tomography in identifying and differentiating the composition of coronary atherosclerotic plaques: A comparative study with intracoronary ultrasound. J Am Coll Cardiol 43: 1241–1247.
25. Agatston AS, Janowitz WR, Hildner FJ, Zusmer NR, Viamonte M Jr, et al. (1990) Quantification of coronary artery calcium using ultrafast computed tomography. J Am Coll Cardiol 15: 827–832.
26. Pundziute G, Schuijf JD, Jukema JW, Decramer I, Sarno G, et al. (2008) Evaluation of plaque characteristics in acute coronary syndromes: Non-invasive assessment with multi-slice computed tomography and invasive evaluation with intravascular ultrasound radiofrequency data analysis. Eur Heart J 29: 2373–2381.
27. Pflederer T, Marwan M, Schepis T, Ropers D, Seltmann M, et al. (2010) Characterization of culprit lesions in acute coronary syndromes using coronary dual-source CT angiography. Atherosclerosis 211: 437–444.
28. Virmani R, Burke AP, Farb A, Kolodgie FD (2006) Pathology of the vulnerable plaque. J Am Coll Cardiol 47: C13–18.
29. Papadopoulou SL, Neefjes LA, Schaap M, Li HL, Capuano E, et al. (2011) Detection and quantification of coronary atherosclerotic plaque by 64-slice multidetector CT: A systematic head-to-head comparison with intravascular ultrasound. Atherosclerosis 219: 163–170.
30. Maurovich-Horvat P, Ferencik M, Bamberg F, Hoffmann U (2009) Methods of plaque quantification and characterization by cardiac computed tomography. J Cardiovasc Comput Tomogr 3 Suppl 2: S91–98.
31. Bugiardini R, Manfrini O, De Ferrari GM (2006) Unanswered questions for management of acute coronary syndrome: Risk stratification of patients with minimal disease or normal findings on coronary angiography. Arch Intern Med 166: 1391–1395.
32. Larsen AI, Nilsen DW, Yu J, Mehran R, Nikolsky E, et al. (2013) Long-term prognosis of patients presenting with ST-segment elevation myocardial infarction with no significant coronary artery disease (from the HORIZONS-AMI trial). Am J Cardiol 111: 643–648.

Cardiovascular Magnetic Resonance Imaging of Scar Development Following Pulmonary Vein Isolation

Jeff Hsing[1]¶, Dana C. Peters[1,3]*¶, Benjamin R. Knowles[1], Warren J. Manning[1,2], Mark E. Josephson[1]

1 Department of Medicine, Cardiovascular Division, Beth Israel Deaconess Medical Center, Harvard Medical School, Boston, Massachusetts, United States of America, **2** Department of Radiology, Beth Israel Deaconess Medical Center, Harvard Medical School, Boston, Massachusetts, United States of America, **3** Department of Radiology, Yale Medical School, New Haven, Connecticut, United States of America

Abstract

Aims: Cardiovascular magnetic resonance (MR) provides non-invasive assessment of early (24-hour) edema and injury following pulmonary vein isolation (by ablation) and subsequent scar formation. We hypothesize that 24-hours after ablation, cardiovascular MR would demonstrate a pattern of edema and injury due to ablation and the severity would correlate with subsequent scar.

Methods: Fifteen atrial fibrillation patients underwent cardiovascular MR prior to pulmonary vein isolation, 24-hours post ($N=11$) and 30-days post ($N=7$) ablation, with T2-weighted (T2W) and late gadolinium enhancement (LGE) imaging. Left atrial wall thickness, edema enhancement ratio and LGE enhancement were assessed at each time point. Volumes of LGE and edema enhancement were measured, and the circumferential presence of injury was assessed at 24-hours, including comparison with LGE enhancement at 30 days.

Results: Left atrial wall thickness was increased 24-hours post-ablation (10.7 ± 4.1 mm vs. 7.0 ± 1.8 mm pre-PVI, $p<0.05$). T2W enhancement at 24-hours showed increased edema enhancement ratio (1.5 ± 0.4 for post-ablation, vs. 0.9 ± 0.2 pre-ablation, $p<0.001$). Edema and LGE volumes at 24-hours were correlated with 30-day LGE volume ($R=0.76$, $p=0.04$, and $R=0.74$, $p=0.09$, respectively). Using a 16 segment model for assessment, 24-hour T2W had sensitivity, specificity, and accuracy of 82%, 63%, and 79% respectively, for predicting 30-day LGE. 24-hour LGE had sensitivity, specificity, and accuracy of 91%, 47%, and 84%.

Conclusions: Increased left atrial wall thickening and edema were characterized on cardiovascular MR early post-ablation, and found to correlate with 30-day LGE scar.

Editor: Rory Edward Morty, University of Giessen Lung Center, Germany

Funding: This work was supported by in part by grants from the NIH (NHLBI R21 HL 098573 & R21 HL103463). The funders had no role in study design, data collection and analysis, decision to publish, or preparation of the manuscript.

Competing Interests: The authors have declared that no competing interests exist.

* Email: dana.peters@yale.edu

¶ These authors contributed equally to this work.

Introduction

Atrial fibrillation (AF) is the most common sustained arrhythmia, with substantial associated morbidity and mortality [1]. Pulmonary vein isolation (PVI) has been advocated as a therapy for AF, with freedom from AF reported in 60% to 85% of patients with paroxysmal AF [2]. Recurrence also depends on follow-up duration [3].

A suspected cause of AF recurrence is incomplete circumferential PVI ablation with associated electrical reconnection of the PVs to the left atrium (LA) [4–6]. One hypothesis to explain early (<30 days) (but not late) isolation after PVI is that the PVI procedure causes early focal *reversible* edema without permanent injury, resulting in only temporary electrical isolation. After the edema resolves, the PVs are electrically reconnected. During the PVI procedure, the extent of injury that is created during PVI is unknown, as neither fluoroscopy nor electroanatomical mapping allows for discrimination of the ablation lesions.

Cardiovascular magnetic resonance (CMR) is a non-invasive imaging modality that allows for identification of myocardial scar [7,8], and edema [9] using late gadolinium enhancement (LGE) and T2-weighted (T2w) imaging, respectively. Animal studies have shown a close correspondence between CMR and injury after RF ablation [10,11].

LGE CMR is also able to identify LA and PV scar late (≥30 days) after ablation, showing a trend of more extensive scarring in subjects who later recur [12–14]. Further, in patients undergoing redo procedures, isolated PVs had greater amount of ostial scar by LGE (43%) vs. those which were reconnected (21%) [15]. Therefore, it may be valuable to acutely identify PVs which will exhibit insufficient chronic scarring. Recent CMR studies have examined and characterized the development of LGE after ablation, comparing early and later imaging findings [11–13,16,17]. A critical issue for the important goal of CMR-guided ablation—whether as adjunct to catheterization or ablation within the CMR suite [18–22] — is to identify early imaging findings that are predictive of late LA wall scar after PVI.

Acute ablation lesions may consist of inflammation, coagulation necrosis and hemorrhage. Acute post-PVI imaging findings include an increase in LA wall thickness, likely due to edema [23,24]. Other findings include LGE enhancement or dark no-reflow regions (where contrast agent is completely excluded, also called microvascular obstruction (MVO) [25]) and enhancement on T2W imaging. Knowles et al. visualized acute LA wall edema after PVI in humans [16], and found that T2W evidence of edema was more wide spread than acute LGE enhancement. Acute LGE patterns have been compared to subsequent/late LGE patterns [17], showing a more widespread and less intense enhancement on early LGE, and the transition of MVO acutely to enhancement on subsequent LGE [26]. This has also been reported in animal studies of acute ablation, where MVO persists for more than 45 minutes [10], with acutely injured necrotic tissue very slowly enhancing.

Little is known regarding the relationship of early injury (i.e. edema/necrosis) with late LGE scarring (i.e. fibrosis). Late LGE imaging (1 to 3 months) after PVI demonstrates a pattern of scarring in the LA [12], which correlates with clinical outcomes and to ablation locations [27–29]. Evidence shows that at 1 month post-PVI, edema has resolved [23]. LGE patterns do not change from 3 to 6–9 months [17].

We hypothesized that early (24 hours) after PVI, the PVs and LA would demonstrate transient injury, characterized by CMR enhancement on T2W and LGE images and that some of these changes would correlate with 30-day LGE scar. We sought to replicate prior studies of the correlation between acute LGE and acute T2W imaging [16], and between acute and late LGE imaging [30]. Further we sought to add to the existing knowledge of the relationship of acute T2w to 30-day LGE.

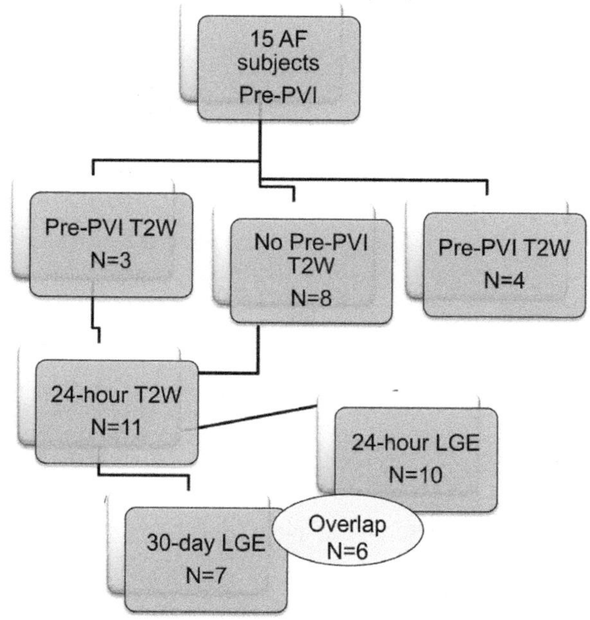

Figure 1. Flow chart describing the number of patients with T2W and LGE images at each time-point for the entire cohort. T2W = T2-weighted imaging. LGE = Late gadolinium enhancement. PVI = pulmonary vein isolation. Data from all available studies were used in all analyses.

Methods

Patients

Fifteen AF patients referred for their first PVI were prospectively studied, although not all images were acquired at each time-point (see Figure 1). Written informed consent for CMR was provided by all subjects and the study was approved by the Beth Israel Deaconess Medical Center Committee on Clinical Investigations. The study complies with the Declaration of Helsinki.

Pulmonary Vein Isolation (PVI) Procedure

In brief, as described elsewhere [31], a 3.5 mm Biosense Thermocool (Biosense, Webster, Diamond Bar, CA, USA) irrigated catheter was advanced witin a long sheath into the LA, using intracardiac echocardiography guidance. A lasso catheter was advanced through a second long sheath and placed at each PV ostium for guiding the ablations and to confirming PV entrance and exit block. Radiofrequency (RF) ablation lesions were made 5–10 mm outside of each PV ostium in a circumferential fashion. Each PV was isolated. Maximal power was set at 30 W and 40°C and ablation lesions were generated using a maximum of 15–30 seconds at each site based on changes in the local electrogram. Electroanatomic mapping was performed using CARTO XP (Biosense Webster, Diamond Bar, California). The ablation duration was reduced to 10–15 seconds during ablation of the posterior LA wall and near the esophagus as identified by intracardiac echocardiography. The ablation goal was the loss of all PV potentials and failure to capture the atrium during pacing all bipolar poles of the lasso with a pulse width of 5 ms at 10 mA. Additional lines were only made if left sided atrial flutter could be induced. Posterior wall debulking and targeting of complex fractionated atrial electrograms were not performed. Intracardiac echocardiography was performed prior to and after PVI to confirm the absence of pericardial effusions. All PVI procedures were performed by a single operator (MEJ).

CMR Imaging Protocol

CMR was performed on a Philips 1.5T CMR scanner (Achieva, Phillips Healthcare, Best, The Netherlands). Prior to contrast injection, ECG-triggered navigator-gated, fat-saturated, T2W 2D black blood fast spin echo imaging was performed in a stack of axial images covering the LA. Image parameters included: 300 mm FOV, 192×192 matrix (1.5×1.5 mm^2 zero-filled to 0.6×0.6 in-plane resolution), 5 mm slice thickness, 33 echo train length, echo spacing 5.4 ms, 90° flip, TE = 60 ms, 1 average, 15 slices with no gaps, imaging in diastole. Coil-sensitivity correction was used on the T2W images. LGE imaging was performed ~20 minutes after the injection of 0.2 mmol/kg Gd-DTPA (N = 6; Magnevist, Bayer Healthcare, Leverkusen, Germany; or 0.2 mmol/kg Gd-BOPTA (N = 1; MultiHance; Bracco, Princeton, NJ). The LGE sequence was an ECG-triggered navigator-gated 3D inversion recovery gradient echo sequence with fat saturation. Imaging parameters included: 320 mm FOV, 224×224 matrix, 4 mm slice thickness (spatial resolution 1.4×1.4×4 mm zero-filled to 0.6×0.6×2 mm^3), TR/TE/θ = 5.3 ms/2.1 ms/25°, centric acquisition, with 100–150 ms acquisition window in diastole.

The inversion time was set to null LV myocardium, using a Look-Locker sequence [32].

Image Analyses

Image analyses were performed using ImageJ (NIH Image, Bethesda, MD) and 3D Slicer (v3.6, NA-MIC, Boston, MA).

LA Wall Thickness

LA wall thickness was measured at one location pre- and post-PVI, in an unmatched cohort (see Figure 1). Posterior LA wall thickness measurements at the level of the right superior PV (RSPV) were made on T2W images by a blinded observer. The RSPV location (Figure 2A,B) was chosen to correspond to the location described by Okada et al. [23]. Thickness was measured by an experienced reader, on twice-zoomed images, with the line tool. Thickness measurement reproducibility was tested by repeating measurements (but not imaging) on a different day.

Edema Enhancement Ratio (EER): $T2_W$ Image Analysis Pre- vs. Post-PVI

To investigate the development of edema post-PVI, the signal in a small region-of-interest (ROI) of about 60 pixels containing the brightest region of each PV ostial wall was measured on T2W images by a blinded observer on pre- and 24-hour post-PVI images. The edema enhancement ratio (EER; Equation 1), the ratio of LA wall (Figure 2C, D) to LV myocardial signal (Figure 2E) was calculated, as previously described [33].

$$\text{EER} = \text{LA wall Signal} \div \text{LVmyocardium signal} \qquad (\text{Eq.1})$$

The EER threshold for edema was chosen as 1.4, based on pre-PVI EER measurements (mean +3SDS, see Results).

CNR Comparison of 24-Hour vs. 30-Day LGE

In a similar fashion, the contrast-to-noise (CNR; scar to blood, Figure 2F) was measured, using a small region-of-interest (ROI) for scar, containing the most enhanced region of each PV ostial wall on LGE images. The measurement was performed by a blinded observer on 24-hour and 30-day post-PVI images (excluding data from the single patient who received Gd-BOPTA). Mean blood pool signal was measured, and the standard deviation of signal in air-space was used to estimate noise.

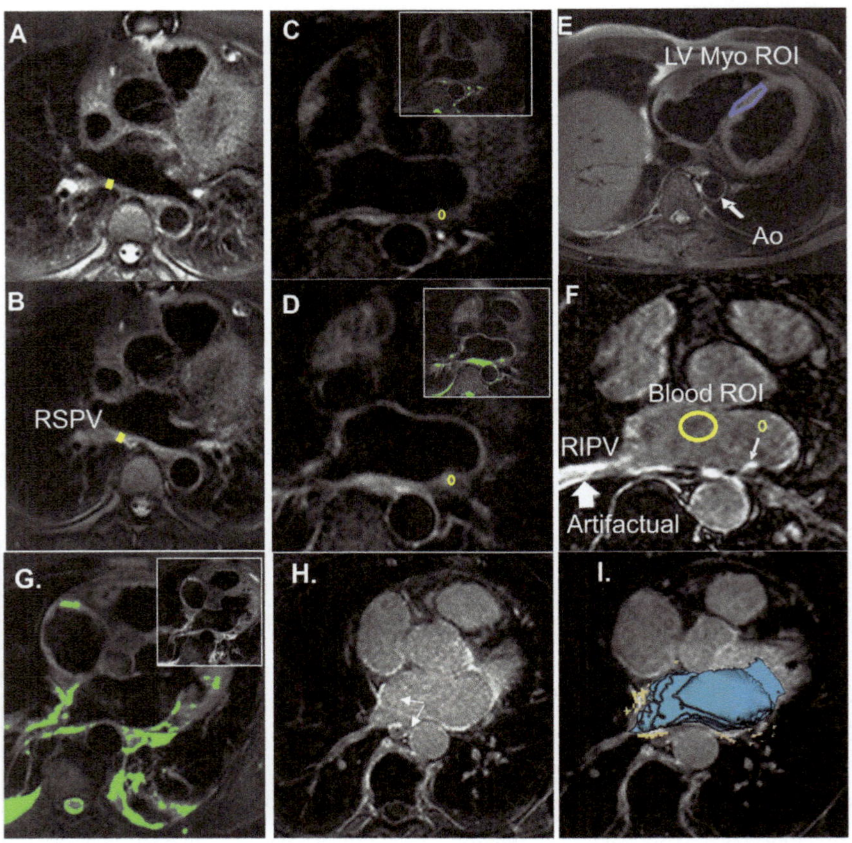

Figure 2. Methods of data analysis. A-B) T2W images from a subject imaged pre pulmonary vein isolation (PVI) (A) and 24-hour post PVI (B), used for measuring right superior PV wall thickness, as shown; note the prominent LA wall thickening. C-F) Another subject imaged pre-pulmonary vein isolation (PVI), 24-hour post-PVI, and 30-day post-PVI. C) Pre-PVI T2W image. D) 24-hours post -PVI T2W image shows enhancement where none is observed pre-PVI. Colored insets highlight regions where signal exceeds the edema threshold in C and D. ROIs were placed on the T2W images, as shown in (C, D). E) Axial T2-weighted (T2W) image at the level of the mid left ventricle (LV) with the region of interest (ROI) used for calculating the edema threshold (defined as 1.4 times the mean LV myocardium signal). F) Late gadolinium enhancement (LGE) 30-days post-PVI demonstrating scar. A left lower PV wall ROI, and blood pool ROI are shown. G) Color) Early post-PVI, the T2W image shows enhancement. Regions above the EER threshold (1.4) are highlighted in green. H) 30-day LGE appears to correlate 24-hour T2W. I) By registration of 24-hour T2W and 30-day LGE, the correlation between acute edema and later scar is more easily quantified, using matched ROIs. The blue shell represents the LA cavity segmented from the 30-day LGE images. The segmented edema (orange) is overlaid on the 30-day LGE image.

Correlation between 24-Hour T2W and LGE Findings and 30-day LGE in the LA

CNR and EER comparison at matched locations. To compare signal on the 24-hour and 30-day post-PVI images, the 30-day post-PVI LGE images were registered to the 24-hour LGE images using 3D Slicer (v3.6, NA-MIC), with a 3D rigid registration based on mutual information; the resulting transformation also registered the 30-day LGE to 24-hour T2W images. After registration, signal intensity in a small ROI was measured in two locations each with and without LGE enhancement/scar on 30-day LGE. The small ROI containing PV ostia wall (see Figure 2F,D) was placed on all images, at well-matched locations. For the T2W images, the EER was calculated. For LGE images, the wall-blood CNR was calculated.

In order to assess the adequacy of contrast in the LGE images, and compare 30 day and 24 hour LGE contrast, valvular CNR was measured using an ROI in a visible mitral valve segment, vs. the blood signal.

Qualitative agreement of injury on 24-hour and 30-day images, in a 16 segment model. The presence of injury was assessed in a 16 segment model (Figure 3): 4 quadrants (anterior, posterior, inferior and superior) around each of 4 PVs. Blinded assessment was performed in all patients (4*4*7 = 112 total), on 24-hour T2W and LGE images, and 30-day LGE. These segments included PV wall territory within a radius ±1 cm from the ostia.

The presence of injury was assessed on T2W images, by using an EER>1.4. LGE was assessed visually, by noting enhancement having a CNR>~3.5. A global threshold of CNR>3.5 SDs above the mean blood pool signal was used for LGE, based on a single mid-volume measurement (Figure 2F). This threshold choice has been demonstrated to optimally correlate with low voltage on post-ablation electroanatomic mapping [35]. When right PV ostial enhancement was apparent but adjacent to artifacts, the region was included as "injury" [34]. Since MVO has been shown to develop into scar [26], the presence of MVO was noted, and included as "injury". For both T2w and LGE, any sizable enhanced territory (>3 mm diameter—excluding small islands) was classified as "injury" in that segment. The power of 24-hour T2W and LGE to predict late scar was studied using the 30-day LGE as the reference. Intra-observer variability was measured by repeating the qualitative analysis on a different day.

Quantitative volumetric comparison of 24-hour and 30-day injury. On all post-PVI T2W and LGE images, the entire LA cavity was traced, extending inferior to the most inferior PV, and superior to the LSPV, excluding the LA appendage, with care taken to exclude areas of artifactual enhancement (i.e. where enhanced wall is proximal to artifactually enhanced blood pool, Figure 2F). Using this tracing and a threshold of CNR>3.5, the volume of LGE enhancement was measured at 24-hours and 30-days. This semi-automated LGE segmentation method has been described in detail [36] and shown to outperform competing methods. For T2W images, a similar tracing was used, and an EER>1.4 was used to indicate enhancement. Enhancement volumes, normalized as a percent of the total LA blood pool cavity volume, were calculated and compared.

Statistical Analyses

Data analyses were performed using Excel (Microsoft 2010, Redmond, WA) or Stata/IC 10.0 (Stata Corporation, College Station, TX). Continuous variables are presented as mean ± one standard deviation. The relationship between in LGE and T2W enhancement was compared between time-points on a segment basis using Pearson's chi-squared test. LA wall thickness comparisons were made using a two-tailed Student's t-test. Linear regression was used to compare volumes of enhancement. Cohen's kappa and intra-class correlation coefficient were used to characterize the reproducibility of categorical and ordinal measurements, respectively. A p value ≤0.05 was considered statistically significant, without Bonferroni correction.

Results

Table 1 describes the 11/15 subjects who underwent post-PVI imaging. All available studies as described in Figure 1 were analyzed. Table 2 summarizes some of the results. The raw data supporting all results, and sample images, are provided as (Figures S1-S3, and Table S1).

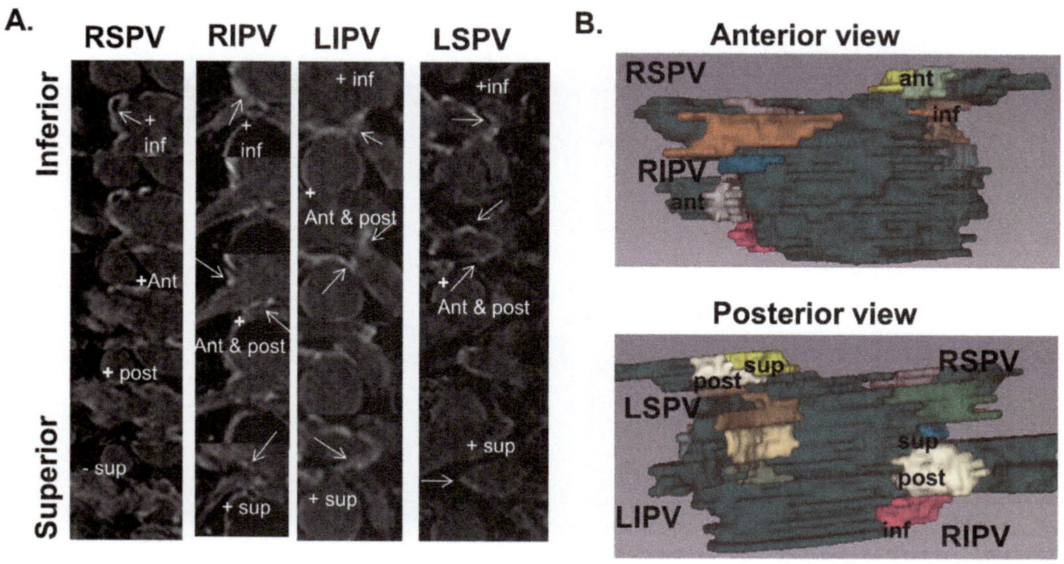

Figure 3. 16 segment model showing the 4 regions evaluated around each pulmonary vein. A) Zoomed and cropped slices labeled by region. B) 3D color-coded display, showing 4 regions about each PV, with explicit labeling for the right inferior and left superior PV.

Figure 4 shows matched slices at 3 time-points in a single subject. At 24-hours post PVI, T2W and LGE imaging display multiple areas of enhancement in the PV ostia and posterior LA wall indicating edema and injury. There was also visual correspondence between 30-day and 24-hour LGE, with a less intense pattern of enhancement on 24-hour LGE.

Figure 2G-I shows how matched locations were obtained in another subject, through registration. The registration achieved between 30-day LGE (blue shell) and 24-hour T2W (orange segmented pixels) was good. The correlation between the 24-hour T2W enhancement and 30-day LGE enhancement is demonstrated.

LA Wall Thickness

The LA wall thickness, measured at the posterior wall of the RPSV, was increased by about 4 mm 24-hours after PVI (Table 2). Wall thickness measurement intraobserver variability was good: $R = 0.88$, and bias ± 2SDs of -0.4 ± 2.2 mm, and intra-class correlation coefficient of 0.69 (strong agreement).

Edema Enhancement Ratio: Pre- vs. 24-Hour Post-PVI

For pre-PVI AF patients, the average T2W EER of the LA wall to the LV myocardium was significantly lower than for 24-hour post-PVI patients (Table 2). The pre-PVI EER measurements were used to choose EER = 1.4 as the threshold for edema, using the mean +3SDs (0.87+3*0.18 = 1.41).

CNR Comparison: 24-Hour vs. 30-Day LGE

The PV ostial CNR (LA wall to blood) of enhanced regions for 30-day LGE was greater than for 24-hour LGE (Table 2). Figure 2 and 4 demonstrate that some regions enhanced on 30-day LGE but not on 24-hour LGE (yellow arrows, Figure 4C,D), and that enhancement at 30 days had higher CNR, and better conspicuity. The CNR of the mitral valve was measured to be similar on 24 hour vs. 30 day LGE (Table 2).

Correlation between 24-Hour T2W and LGE Findings and 30-day LA Wall LGE Enhancement at Matched Locations

The EER was higher in locations in which 30-day LGE enhancement developed compared to locations without later scar, as was the 24-hour LGE CNR (Table 2).

Qualitative Assessment in 16 Segment Model

Pre-PVI, T2W imaging demonstrated 8% of PV quadrants were enhanced (>1.4 ER), with one-third of these regions located on the posterior wall of the right inferior PV (Figure 2C). At 24-hours post-PVI, 75% of quadrants had T2W enhancement and 84% of regions had findings on LGE. Agreement between 24-hour T2W enhancement and 24-hour LGE enhancement or MVO was found in 79% of quadrants, with a Kappa value of 0.37 (fair).

Ninety six quadrants (86%) were scarred by 30-day LGE. Using 30-day LGE as reference standard, the 24-hour T2W images had 82% sensitivity, 63% specificity, and an accuracy of 79% to predict 30-day LGE enhancement, on a per quadrant basis. The 24-hour LGE images had 91% sensitivity, 47% specificity and 84% accuracy. Agreement of 30 day LGE with acute LGE and T2W was significantly correlated by chi-squared test ($p = 0.005$ and $p = 0.002$, respectively). Table 2 summarizes these regional results.

Intraobserver agreement for qualitative assessments was 88% for T2W, 93% for 24-hour LGE, and 94% for 30-day LGE, with kappa values of 0.66, 0.68, and 0.71 for the three datasets, respectively (all substantial agreement).

Volumetric Comparison of Enhancement on LGE and T2W

30-day LGE enhancement volume significantly correlated with 24-hour edema ($R = 0.76$, $p = 0.047$), but did not correlate significantly for 24-hour LGE ($R = 0.74$, $p = 0.092$) (Figure 5).

Table 1. Patient characteristics and MRI findings for patients with post-PVI imaging.

Patient Characteristic	N = 11
Age (years)	52±11
Male gender, N (%)	9 (82%)
LV EF (%)*	56.0±9.3
LA dimension)	43±9
Ablation time (secs)	2900±1100
Paroxysmal AF, N (%)	8 (73%)
Anti-arrhythmic Medications, N (%)	10 (91%)
Hypertension, N (%)	5 (45%)
LGE and T2W measurements	All available
# segments enhanced (16 segment model)	
30-day LGE	13.7±1.8
24-hour LGE	13.6±1.1
24-hour T2W	12.1±3.2
Volume of enhancement (% of LA volume)	
30-day LGE	6.6±5.4
24-hour LGE	5.7±3.7
24-hour T2W	7.8±4.1

AF = atrial fibrillation, LA = left atrium, LV EF = left ventricular ejection fraction.

Table 2. Summary of Results.

	Pre-PVI	Post-PVI	P-value
LA wall thickness (mm)	7.0±1.8	10.7±4.1	0.038
Average EER	0.87±0.18	1.52±0.38	<0.001
% with 24-hour LGE	—	84%	
% with 24-hour T2W	8%	75%	
% with 30-day LGE	—	86%	
	24-hour	**30-day**	**p-value**
PV ostial LGE CNR	8.2±3.6	11.4±4.1	0.01
Valve LGE CNR	3.3±1.0	3.7±1.1	0.46
	30-day LGE +	**30-day LGE -**	**p-value**
24-hour EER	1.5±0.3	1.2±0.3	0.004
24-hour LGE CNR	7.3±3.3	3.0±5.8	0.037
	Sensitivity*	**Specificity***	**Accuracy***
24-hour EER>1.4	82% (75%–89% CI)	63% (54%–71% CI)	79%
24-hour LGE CNR>3.5	91% (86%–97% CI)	47% (40%–60% CI)	84%

* vs. 30-day LGE.

Discussion

In this prospective study of AF patients referred for their first PVI, we demonstrate the ability of CMR to visualize early edema and injury using T2W and LGE of the pulmonary veins and LA wall, confirming prior studies [16,17]. Further, we demonstrate a correlation between patterns of injury on 24-hour imaging and 30-day LGE, a finding that has not been previously reported. The purpose of this study is to evaluate the feasibility of using acute CMR to predict chronic ablation patterns. The goal of PVI is to electrically isolate the PV by creating permanent scar around the pulmonary veins. Our study highlights that there is a relationship between early and later findings of post PVI injury, which is evident in the linear correlation between volume of scar on 30-day LGE, to volume of 24-hour edema, and the ability of LGE and T2W at 24-hours to predict later scarring. Whether the relationship is strong enough to provide peri-procedural guidance to improve ablation patterns is uncertain, since potentially even small gaps might result in PV reconnection [37], and since the accuracy of 24-hour imaging appears limited.

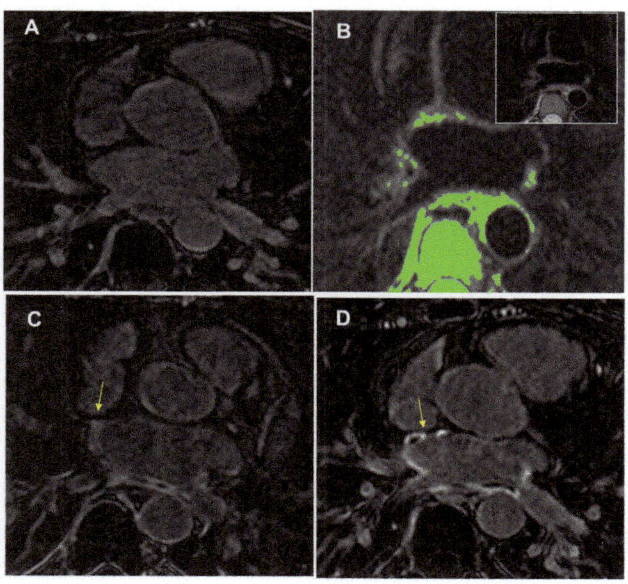

Figure 4. Axial CMR images demonstrating the progression of scar development of a single patient after PVI. A) Pre-PVI LGE scan shows no baseline scar. B) 24-hour post PVI T2W image showing areas of edema, highlighted in green, which had an EER>1.4. Inset shows original image. C) 24-hour LGE. D) 30-day post PVI LGE showing enhancement in the pulmonary veins which corresponded to 24-hour edema location. Note the less intense enhancement pattern of 24-hour LGE compared to 30-day LGE, with some enhancement not visible at 24-hours and dark "no-reflow "regions both early and late after PVI (yellow arrows).

Correlation of 24-Hour Enhancement with 30-Day in the LA and PVs

We found high sensitivity (91% and 82%) but lower specificity (47% and 63%) for both 24-hour LGE and 24-hour T2W imaging, respectively, for predicting LGE at 30 days. The low specificity suggests that some acute injury resolves. 24-hour T2W had greater specificity (fewer false positives) than LGE, which is perhaps most critical.

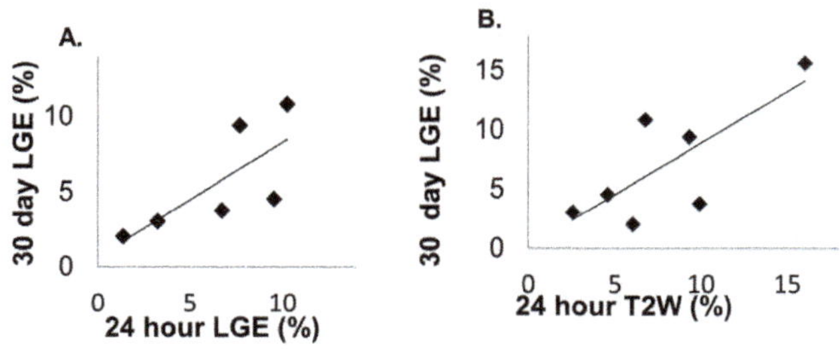

Figure 5. Linear correlations between volumes of LGE enhancement at 30 days, and volumes measured at 24-hours. A) 24-hour LGE vs. 30-day LGE (R = 0.76, p = 0.09). B) 24-hour T2W vs. 30-day LGE volume (R = 0.74, p = 0.04). All volumes of edema/injury were normalized by the patient's LA volume.

Relationship to Prior Reports

This study found acute wall-thickening after PVI. Using electron beam computed tomography (CT), Okada et al. [23] reported the increased thickness of the right posterior wall after circumferential ablation was 5 mm, similar to our finding in the same location. Yokokawa et al. found an increase in LA roof thickness of 1–2 mm [24]. While our baseline measured wall thickness of 7 mm is greater than that reported by CT imaging (1–4 mm) [38,39]. This is likely due to 5 mm slice thickness which could cause partial-voluming of the LA wall with other tissues, or increased apparent thickness due to the LA wall curvature. However, the relative change in thickness after PVI is similar to previous CT reports [23].

Badger et al. compared early LGE and very late LGE (3 months) and found no correlation, while early LGE appeared as a diffuse (i.e. wide-spread, low CNR) signal [17]. In agreement, we found that the CNR of the injured regions was higher on the 30-day vs. 24-hour LGE, despite that the valvular CNRs were not different. This is likely due to the very slow enhancement of acutely ablated tissue [10], requiring ~45 minute to full enhancement, which is longer than the delay of 20–25 minutes used for LGE imaging [10]. Our study, in agreement with [26], found that 24-hour MVO regions developed into 30-day LGE enhancement (Figure 3); however, even at 30 days, MVO regions remained present and common (Figures 2–3). Finally, our study examined 24-hour T2W and correlated this with 30-day LGE, finding a significant relationship.

Regions with LGE and T2W edema spatially overlap in imaging ablation sites [10,11]—this is known. An unanswered question is whether acute LGE or T2W is more predictive of later ablation patterns, and later outcome. Another question is whether some edema resolves without fibrosis development. Arujuna et al. [40] found evidence that acute edema without acute LGE indicates reversible injury, potentially predicting later recurrence. They found that patients with greater T2W edema ostial encirclement at an acute stage experienced AF recurrence, while those with more extensive LGE at the acute stage were free from AF at follow-up. They found widespread edema compared to LGE, acutely. Our studied differed from this prior study, in that we did not find that edema was more widespread than LGE, acutely. This difference could be explained by the use of TE = 60 ms and an EER threshold of 1.4 in our study, compared to use of a TE = 120 ms, and a edema threshold of 3 SDs above mean myocardial signal. Our threshold for edema was set more stringently, based on data from controls, and our TE was lower. We found that edematous regions with a greater EER were more likely to develop into LGE than regions with lower EER, i.e. evidence that minimal edema does not result in later fibrosis, agreeing with the prior work. Therefore, apparent differences—i.e. a good correlation of acute edema with later LGE in the present study—might be related to a higher threshold for edema in our study.

Limitations

Our study population was small, mainly because recruitment of patients immediately after the PVI procedure is highly challenging. However, this study is unique in that both T2W and LGE images were available acutely, for comparison with 30-day LGE. T2W images were not routinely obtained prior to PVI for comparison with the 24-hour images, and therefore we could not perform a paired analysis of T2W findings pre and post-PVI. However, this cannot be expected to affect our findings that EER increases acutely after PVI, and that the LA wall thickens.

Our rigid registration of T2W and LGE images at 24-hours and 30-days may result in imperfectly matched locations for measuring and comparing signal intensity. Furthermore, the thicker slices used in T2W imaging is also a source of location mismatch. However, in spite of the possible mismatch, we found higher 24-hour T2W EER and LGE CNR in regions which exhibited 30-day LGE enhancement. Finally, it is possible that some enhancement on T2W is related to pericardial fluid-filled recesses [41], or diffuse inflammatory response associated with AF.

In conclusion, increased LA wall thickening and edema and injury are characterized on CMR early post-PVI with correlation to 30-day LGE scar.

Supporting Information

Figure S1 24-hour LGE patient image.

Figure S2 30-day LGE patient image.

Figure S3 24-hour T2W patient image.

Table S1 Raw measurements. A) Data of Figure 4. B) Data on regional assessment of injury using 16 segment model. C) CNR and EER measurements.

Acknowledgments

The authors gratefully acknowledge Beth Goddu, R.T. and Kraig V. Kissinger, RT, and Lois Goepfert, R.N. for their assistance with CMR scanning; the authors thank Jaime S. Shaw, B.S. for her help with patient studies.

Author Contributions

Conceived and designed the experiments: DCP WJM MEJ JH BRK. Performed the experiments: JH DCP. Analyzed the data: JH DCP BRK. Contributed reagents/materials/analysis tools: MEJ WJM DCP BRK JH. Wrote the paper: MEJ WJM DCP BRK JH.

References

1. Peters NS, Schilling RJ, Kanagaratnam P, Markides V (2002) Atrial fibrillation: strategies to control, combat, and cure. Lancet 359: 593–603.
2. Verma A, Marrouche NF, Natale A (2004) Pulmonary vein antrum isolation: intracardiac echocardiography-guided technique. Journal of cardiovascular electrophysiology 15: 1335–1340.
3. Sorgente A, Tung P, Wylie J, Josephson ME (2012) Six year follow-up after catheter ablation of atrial fibrillation: a palliation more than a true cure. The American journal of cardiology 109: 1179–1186.
4. Ouyang F, Antz M, Ernst S, Hachiya H, Mavrakis H, et al. (2005) Recovered pulmonary vein conduction as a dominant factor for recurrent atrial tachyarrhythmias after complete circular isolation of the pulmonary veins: lessons from double Lasso technique. Circulation 111: 127–135.
5. Nanthakumar K, Plumb VJ, Epstein AE, Veenhuyzen GD, Link D, et al. (2004) Resumption of electrical conduction in previously isolated pulmonary veins: rationale for a different strategy? Circulation 109: 1226–1229.
6. Verma A, Kilicaslan F, Pisano E, Marrouche NF, Fanelli R, et al. (2005) Response of atrial fibrillation to pulmonary vein antrum isolation is directly related to resumption and delay of pulmonary vein conduction. Circulation 112: 627–635.
7. Simonetti OP, Kim RJ, Fieno DS, Hillenbrand HB, Wu E, et al. (2001) An improved MR imaging technique for the visualization of myocardial infarction. Radiology 218: 215–223.

8. Kim RJ, Fieno DS, Parrish TB, Harris K, Chen EL, et al. (1999) Relationship of MRI delayed contrast enhancement to irreversible injury, infarct age, and contractile function. Circulation 100: 1992–2002.
9. Abdel-Aty H, Zagrosek A, Schulz-Menger J, Taylor AJ, Messroghli D, et al. (2004) Delayed enhancement and T2-weighted cardiovascular magnetic resonance imaging differentiate acute from chronic myocardial infarction. Circulation 109: 2411–2416.
10. Dickfeld T, Kato R, Zviman M, Lai S, Meininger G, et al. (2006) Characterization of radiofrequency ablation lesions with gadolinium-enhanced cardiovascular magnetic resonance imaging. J Am Coll Cardiol 47: 370–378.
11. Dickfeld T, Kato R, Zviman M, Nazarian S, Dong J, et al. (2007) Characterization of acute and subacute radiofrequency ablation lesions with nonenhanced magnetic resonance imaging. Heart Rhythm 4: 208–214.
12. Peters DC, Wylie JV, Hauser TH, Kissinger KV, Botnar RM, et al. (2007) Detection of pulmonary vein and left atrial scar after catheter ablation with three-dimensional navigator-gated delayed enhancement MR imaging: initial experience. Radiology 243: 690–695.
13. McGann CJ, Kholmovski EG, Oakes RS, Blauer JJ, Daccarett M, et al. (2008) New magnetic resonance imaging-based method for defining the extent of left atrial wall injury after the ablation of atrial fibrillation. J Am Coll Cardiol 52: 1263–1271.
14. Hunter RJ, Jones DA, Boubertakh R, Malcolme-Lawes LC, Kanagaratnam P, et al. (2013) Diagnostic accuracy of cardiac magnetic resonance imaging in the detection and characterization of left atrial catheter ablation lesions: a multicenter experience. Journal of cardiovascular electrophysiology 24: 396–403.
15. Malcolme-Lawes LC, Juli C, Karim R, Bai W, Quest R, et al. (2013) Automated analysis of atrial late gadolinium enhancement imaging that correlates with endocardial voltage and clinical outcomes: A 2-center study. Heart Rhythm.
16. Knowles BR, Caulfield D, Cooklin M, Rinaldi CA, Gill J, et al. (2010) 3-D visualization of acute RF ablation lesions using MRI for the simultaneous determination of the patterns of necrosis and edema. IEEE transactions on bio-medical engineering 57: 1467–1475.
17. Badger TJ, Oakes RS, Daccarett M, Burgon NS, Akoum N, et al. (2009) Temporal left atrial lesion formation after ablation of atrial fibrillation. Heart Rhythm 6: 161–168.
18. Vergara GR, Vijayakumar S, Kholmovski EG, Blauer JJ, Guttman MA, et al. (2011) Real-time magnetic resonance imaging-guided radiofrequency atrial ablation and visualization of lesion formation at 3 Tesla. Heart Rhythm 8: 295–303.
19. Kolandaivelu A, Lardo AC, Halperin HR (2009) Cardiovascular magnetic resonance guided electrophysiology studies. J Cardiovasc Magn Reson 11: 21.
20. Schmidt EJ, Mallozzi RP, Thiagalingam A, Holmvang G, d'Avila A, et al. (2009) Electroanatomic mapping and radiofrequency ablation of porcine left atria and atrioventricular nodes using magnetic resonance catheter tracking. Circulation Arrhythmia and electrophysiology 2: 695–704.
21. Nordbeck P, Quick HH, Ladd ME, Ritter O (2013) Real-time magnetic resonance guidance of interventional electrophysiology procedures with passive catheter visualization and tracking. Heart Rhythm 10: 938–939.
22. Schmidt EJ, Fung MM, Ciris PA, Song T, Shankaranarayanan A, et al. (2013) Navigated DENSE strain imaging for post-radiofrequency ablation lesion assessment in the swine left atria. Europace.
23. Okada T, Yamada T, Murakami Y, Yoshida N, Ninomiya Y, et al. (2007) Prevalence and severity of left atrial edema detected by electron beam tomography early after pulmonary vein ablation. J Am Coll Cardiol 49: 1436–1442.
24. Yokokawa M, Tada H, Koyama K, Ino T, Naito S, et al. Thickening of the left atrial wall shortly after radiofrequency ablation predicts early recurrence of atrial fibrillation. Circ J 74: 1538–1546.
25. Wu KC, Zerhouni EA, Judd RM, Lugo-Olivieri CH, Barouch LA, et al. (1998) Prognostic significance of microvascular obstruction by magnetic resonance imaging in patients with acute myocardial infarction. Circulation 97: 765–772.
26. McGann C, Kholmovski E, Blauer J, Vijayakumar S, Haslam T, et al. Dark regions of no-reflow on late gadolinium enhancement magnetic resonance imaging result in scar formation after atrial fibrillation ablation. J Am Coll Cardiol 58: 177–185.
27. Badger TJ, Daccarett M, Akoum NW, Adjei-Poku YA, Burgon NS, et al. Evaluation of left atrial lesions after initial and repeat atrial fibrillation ablation: lessons learned from delayed-enhancement MRI in repeat ablation procedures. Circulation Arrhythmia and electrophysiology 3: 249–259.
28. Peters DC, Wylie JV, Hauser TH, Nezafat R, Han Y, et al. (2009) Recurrence of atrial fibrillation correlates with the extent of post-procedural late gadolinium enhancement: a pilot study. Jacc 2: 308–316.
29. Taclas JE, Nezafat R, Wylie JV, Josephson ME, Hsing J, et al. (2010) Relationship between intended sites of RF ablation and post-procedural scar in AF patients, using late gadolinium enhancement cardiovascular magnetic resonance. Heart Rhythm 7: 489–496.
30. Badger TJ, Adjei-Poku YA, Burgon NS, Kalvaitis S, Shaaban A, et al. (2009) Initial experience of assessing esophageal tissue injury and recovery using delayed-enhancement MRI after atrial fibrillation ablation. Circulation Arrhythmia and electrophysiology 2: 620–625.
31. Essebag V, Wylie JV Jr, Reynolds MR, Baldessin F, McClennen S, et al. (2006) Bi-directional electrical pulmonary vein isolation as an endpoint for ablation of paroxysmal atrial fibrillation. J Interv Card Electrophysiol 17: 111–117.
32. Look D, Locker D (1970) Time savings in measure of NMR and EPR relaxation times. Rev Sci Instrum 41: 250–251.
33. Gutberlet M, Spors B, Thoma T, Bertram H, Denecke T, et al. (2008) Suspected chronic myocarditis at cardiac MR: diagnostic accuracy and association with immunohistologically detected inflammation and viral persistence. Radiology 246: 401–409.
34. Peters DC, Shaw JL, Knowles BR, Moghari MH, Manning WJ (2012) Respiratory bellows-gated late gadolinium enhancement of the left atrium. J Magn Reson Imaging doi:10.1002/jmri.23954
35. Malcolme-Lawes LC, Lim PB, Wright I, Kojodjojo P, Koa-Wing M, et al. (2013) Characterization of the left atrial neural network and its impact on autonomic modification procedures. Circulation Arrhythmia and electrophysiology 6: 632–640.
36. Karim R, Housden RJ, Balasubramaniam M, Chen Z, Perry D, et al. (2013) Evaluation of current algorithms for segmentation of scar tissue from late Gadolinium enhancement cardiovascular magnetic resonance of the left atrium: an open-access grand challenge. J Cardiovasc Magn Reson 15: 105.
37. Ranjan R, Kato R, Zviman MM, Dickfeld TM, Roguin A, et al. (2011) Gaps in the ablation line as a potential cause of recovery from electrical isolation and their visualization using MRI. Circulation Arrhythmia and electrophysiology 4: 279–286.
38. Beinart R, Abbara S, Blum A, Ferencik M, Heist K, et al. (2011) Left atrial wall thickness variability measured by CT scans in patients undergoing pulmonary vein isolation. Journal of cardiovascular electrophysiology 22: 1232–1236.
39. Suenari K, Nakano Y, Hirai Y, Ogi H, Oda N, et al. (2013) Left atrial thickness under the catheter ablation lines in patients with paroxysmal atrial fibrillation: insights from 64-slice multidetector computed tomography. Heart and vessels 28: 360–368.
40. Arujuna A, Karim R, Caulfield D, Knowles B, Rhode K, et al. (2012) Acute pulmonary vein isolation is achieved by a combination of reversible and irreversible atrial injury after catheter ablation: evidence from magnetic resonance imaging. Circulation Arrhythmia and electrophysiology 5: 691–700.
41. Truong MT, Erasmus JJ, Gladish GW, Sabloff BS, Marom EM, et al. (2003) Anatomy of pericardial recesses on multidetector CT: implications for oncologic imaging. Ajr 181: 1109–1113.

Heterogeneity of Tumor Vasculature and Antiangiogenic Intervention: Insights from MR Angiography and DCE-MRI

Wenlian Zhu[1], Yoshinori Kato[1,2], Dmitri Artemov[1,2]*

1 Division of Cancer Imaging Research, The Russell H. Morgan Department of Radiology and Radiological Science, The Johns Hopkins University School of Medicine, Baltimore, Maryland, United States of America, 2 Department of Oncology, The Sidney Kimmel Comprehensive Cancer Center, The Johns Hopkins University School of Medicine, Baltimore, Maryland, United States of America

Abstract

Purpose: Solid tumor vasculature is highly heterogeneous, which presents challenges to antiangiogenic intervention as well as the evaluation of its therapeutic efficacy. The aim of this study is to evaluate the spatial tumor vascular changes due to bevacizumab/paclitaxel therapy using a combination approach of MR angiography and DCE-MRI method.

Experimental Design: Tumor vasculature of MCF-7 breast tumor mouse xenografts was studied by a combination of MR angiography and DCE-MRI with albumin-Gd-DTPA. Tumor macroscopic vasculature was extracted from the early enhanced images. Tumor microvascular parameters were obtained from the pharmacokinetic modeling of the DCE-MRI data. A spatial analysis of the microvascular parameters based on the macroscopic vasculature was used to evaluate the changes of the heterogeneous vasculature induced by a 12 day bevacizumab/paclitaxel treatment in mice bearing MCF-7 breast tumor.

Results: Macroscopic vessels that feed the tumors were not affected by the bevacizumab/paclitaxel combination therapy. A higher portion of the tumors was within close proximity of these macroscopic vessels after the treatment, concomitant with tumor growth retardation. There was a significant decrease in microvascular permeability and vascular volume in the tumor regions near these vessels.

Conclusion: Bevacizumab/paclitaxel combination therapy did not block the blood supply to the MCF-7 breast tumor. Such finding is consistent with the modest survival benefits of adding bevacizumab to current treatment regimens for some types of cancers.

Editor: Francesco Bertolini, European Institute of Oncology, Italy

Funding: This study was supported by NIH RO1 CA154738 (PI Dmitri Artemov) and NIH 2P50CA103175 (PI Zaver Bhujwalla). The funders had no role in study design, data collection and analysis, decision to publish, or preparation of the manuscript.

Competing Interests: The authors have declared that no competing interests exist.

* E-mail: dmitri@mri.jhu.edu

Introduction

Intratumoral vascular heterogeneity is an important feature of the solid tumors [1,2] and needs to be considered when the therapeutic response to a targeted antiangiogenic regimen is evaluated. Contrast-enhanced MR angiography (MRA) is an ideal tool with which to investigate the heterogeneity of the tumor vasculature due to its ability to visualize the static macroscopic vessels of the tumor with high spatial resolution and strong contrast [3]. Combining MRA with a dynamic contrast-enhanced MRI (DCE-MRI) study of the microvasculature, it is possible to obtain a more comprehensive picture of the tumor vascular function [4]. Nevertheless, the current common practice is to use DCE-MRI results only to evaluate the treatment response to single or combination antiangiogenic treatment. Although the American College of Radiology Breast Imaging Reporting and Data System Atlas (BI-RADS® Atlas) lexicon did utilize the internal enhancement pattern as well as the dynamic curve characteristics in the diagnosis of malignancy [5], therapeutic efficacy of targeted antiangiogenic treatments is conventionally measured by changes in statistical values representing microvascular permeability, averaged over the entire tumor or large tumor regions like hot spots only [6]. Such a global analysis typically results in poor correlation with clinical outcomes [6]. One of the reasons could be that any significant local and regional vascular changes due to the therapy may be masked and lost in the averaging process. Indeed, it is time to rethink the approach of using a single number to quantitatively measure the efficacy of a targeted antiangiogenic regimen without considering intratumoral heterogeneity.

Another obstacle in using averaged values, such as mean or median in therapeutic assessment, is that tumor microvascular parameters often have an abnormal skewed distribution over the entire tumor due to the spatial heterogeneity [7]. Direct comparison of the longitudinal mean or median of the same tumor, or of different tumors, is not meaningful, as these values cannot represent the complexity of non-normal distribution. There have been some exploratory efforts to quantify tumor vascular heterogeneity in order to characterize the tumor vascular network more accurately and to detect the differential regional microenvironment changes in the tumor in response to treatments [7,8,9]. Initial vascular heterogeneity quantification attempts were either region-based, in which the tumor was divided into multiple concentric bands of less spatial variability [10] or histogram-based [11]. Other approaches, such as principle component analysis, texture analysis, and Rényi fractal dimension and geometrical property analysis, were proposed as well [12]. The region-based method is mostly useful in animal models of solid tumors where a "rim enhancement pattern" is commonly observed, so that the tumor can be segmented into a poorly enhancing core and a strongly enhancing periphery or rim in an "onion-peeling" manner [8]. While histograms constructed from the voxel-by-voxel DCE-MRI parametric maps adequately depict the heterogeneity within the tumor, quantitative analysis of such histograms in response to treatment remains arbitrary and challenging [13]. As such, neither region- nor histogram-based methods have addressed the intrinsic spatial complexity of the intratumoral heterogeneity and thus, have not produced reliable quantitative biomarkers of prognostic value.

The mismatch between tumor growth and vascular supply leads to hypoxia and the up-regulation of multiple cytokines, such as vascular endothelial growth factor A (VEGF-A), which increases microvascular permeability and plays a dominant role in angiogenesis [14]. Significant hypoxia tends to occur in low-perfusion areas [15]. One study showed that mean interstitial pH and mean oxygen pressure decreased at an increased distance from a blood vessel [16]. The largest proportion of hypoxia was found at distances beyond 100 μm from perfused vessels in a human glioma mouse model [17]. To address the unique connection between vascular perfusion and microvascular permeability within the tumor, we proposed using a spatial analysis of the tumor microvascular parameters based on the macroscopic vascular architecture detected by contrast-enhanced MRI with a macromolecular contrast agent (MMCA), albumin-Gd-DTPA. Tumor *macrovasculature* composed of these macroscopic vessels was extracted using early time-point DCE-MRI images and tumor microvascular parameters were analyzed voxel-by-voxel based on the distance from the voxel to the nearest macroscopic blood vessels. Vascular changes were evaluated in a human breast tumor MCF-7 mouse model treated with bevacizumab/paclitaxel combination therapy. Although a similar approach had been adapted in the immunohistochemical analysis of the spatial relationship between hypoxia and the perfused vascular network [17], to our best knowledge this is the first application of this method to the analysis of the *in vivo* functional microvascular parameters. The present study provided clear imaging evidence that the tumor blood supply was not blocked by the bevacizumab/paclitaxel combination treatment in the MCF-7 breast tumor mouse model, and corroborated the modest survival benefits of adding bevacizumab to current treatment regimens for some types of cancers.

Materials and Methods

Human Breast Cancer Xenografts in Mice

The human breast MCF-7 mouse xenografts were established as described previously [18]. Briefly, 3×10^6 MCF-7 cells (in 0.05 ml of Hanks' balanced salt solution) were inoculated into the thoracic mammary fat pad of the SCID mice 48 hours after the implantation of one-half of a 17β-estradiol pellet in the back of the mouse.

Ethics Statement

All animal experiments in this study were approved and performed in accordance with the Guidelines for Animal Experimentation of the Johns Hopkins University School of Medicine and every effort was made to minimize suffering.

Treatment and Scanning Schedule

Combination therapy with bevacizumab and paclitaxel was initiated after tumors reached approximately 150 mm^3 in volume. MCF-7 breast tumor xenograft-bearing mice were treated with three doses of bevacizumab and paclitaxel by intraperitoneal injection, each at a dose of 10 mg/kg every four days ($n = 7$). DCE-MRI scanning was performed prior to the treatment and on day 12 after the initiation of the treatment. Mice in the control group were treated with equal volumes of saline and were subjected to the same scanning protocol ($n = 6$) [18]. Tumor volumes were determined from the length of the longest axis and the width of the vertical axis, measured with a slide caliper, as described previously [19]. Overall, 14 mice were scanned prior to the treatment, 7 and 6 mice were scanned at day 12 for the combination treatment and the control group, respectively [18].

MRI Data Acquisition and Analysis

MRI data acquisition and analysis were performed as described earlier [18]. Briefly, 3D DCE-MRI images were acquired using a highly T1-weighted, saturation recovery, short delay gradient echo sequence. The total acquisition time for a 3D image set was about six minutes, with a field of view of $12\times12\times10$ mm, a matrix size of $128\times64\times48$, and six averages. A baseline image was acquired before the intravenous administration of albumin-Gd-DTPA at 0.16 mmol (Gd)/kg, and dynamic contrast-enhanced images were acquired for 30 min after the injection. Raw data were processed with an in-house IDL program (Exelis) to a final image size of $128\times128\times128$. The contrast concentration in voxels was calculated directly from the equilibrium magnetization M_0 map, pre and post-contrast signal amplitudes, and the blood relaxation rate as described [18]. Images were visualized using the ImageJ (National Institutes of Health) and Amira (Visage Imaging) packages.

Modeling CA Pharmacokinetics from DCE-MRI Data

Under the above experimental conditions, the tumor vascular volume (*VV*) and vascular permeability-surface area product (*PS*) for each voxel can be derived directly from the intersect and slope of the linear regression of the enhanced intensity versus elapsed time after administration of albumin-Gd-DTPA, respectively, as described previously [20,21]. Only positive intercepts and slopes were retained as physically relevant *VV* and *PS* values [18].

Segmentation of Tumor Macrovasculature and Heterogeneity Analysis

A binary map of the macroscopic tumor blood vasculature was generated semi-automatically from the initial enhanced images acquired immediately after the administration of albumin-Gd-DTPA based on a combination of threshold, cluster size, and boundary identification process. The segmented continuous voxels above a set threshold formed the binary macrovasculature map. A 3D voxel-by-voxel distance map was subsequently created by calculating the distance from each voxel to the nearest macroscopic blood vessel. The tumor microvascular parameters, *VV* and *PS*, were then analyzed based on the distance from the nearest blood vessel. Statistical analysis was performed using the non-parametric Wilcoxon signed-rank test. The tumor macrovascular vessel volume ratio was calculated, using the total voxel counts of segmented vessels and total tumor volumes determined slice-by-slice from the T1-weighted images.

Results

Segmentation of the Tumor Macrovasculature

The vasculature of MCF-7 tumors was, indeed, quite heterogeneous. Tumor angiograms were obtained from the early dynamic enhanced images, acquired within six minutes after the administration of albumin-Gd-DTPA, when the leakage of the MMCA to the tumor interstitium was minimal. The macroscopic vessel/background contrast threshold ratio varied slightly between the mice in our investigation, possibly due to the individual fluctuations in the albumin-Gd-DTPA injection dose, and mouse cardiac and kidney functions. Nevertheless, the strong contrast between the macroscopic vessels and the remainder of the tumor allowed the unambiguous segmentation of the tumor macrovasculature using a semi-automatic IDL program, adapting a threshold in the range of the upper 15–20 percentiles of the enhancement. An example of a 3D rendering of the aforementioned enhanced image is shown in Fig. 1, on the left, while the corresponding binarized segmented macrovasculature map is shown on the right. Noticeably, strongly enhanced macroscopic feeding vessels were detected extending from the body flank into the tumor periphery in all mice in both the bevacizumab and paclitaxel combination treatment and saline control groups in various time points. The images in Fig. 1 were acquired prior to the treatments.

Distance to the Nearest Macroscopic Vessel

A central slice from the 3D distance map that depicts the distance from each pixel to the nearest macroscopic vessel within the tumor, is shown in Fig. 2, as well as the corresponding early enhanced image. Fig. 2 shows that a sizable portion of the tumor peripheral area is in close vicinity to the macroscopic vessels, while the tumor core area is generally poorly enhanced and farther away from these vessels. Similar distance maps were observed in the pre- and post-treatment mice that received either saline or the bevacizumab and paclitaxel combination treatment. The images in Fig. 2 were acquired prior to the treatments.

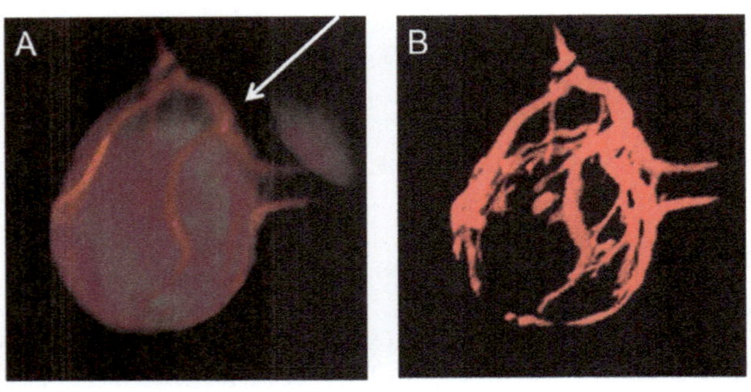

Figure 1. Segmentation of the tumor macrovasculature. A: A representative 3D rendering of the images of MCF-7 tumor orthotopically grown in a female SCID mouse acquired immediately after the injection of albumin-Gd-DTPA. B: corresponding segmented binary macrovasculature map. The arrow indicates where the tumor was attached to the mouse body.

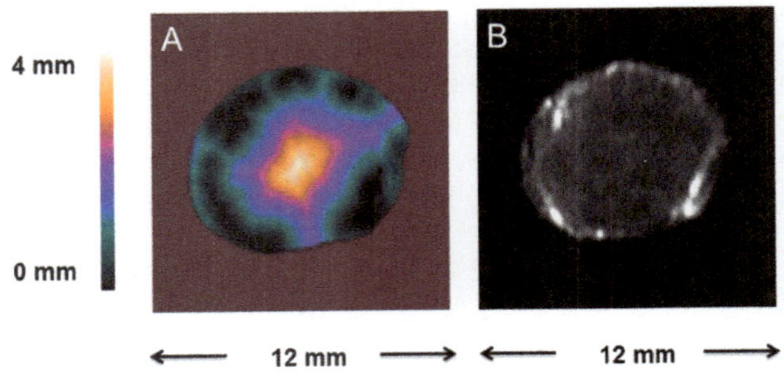

Figure 2. Generation of the distance map. A: A representative central slice from a 3D tumor distance map that depicts the distance of each pixel to the nearest segmented macroscopic vessel. B: the corresponding early enhanced image.

Distribution of the Tumor Microvascular Parameters

Charts that plot representative average regional tumor *VV* and *PS*, as well as the corresponding voxel counts, stratified by the distance to the nearest enhanced vessel are shown in Fig. 3. Not surprisingly, areas in the vicinity of the tumor macroscopic vessels displayed the highest average vascular volume. Tumor areas close to these vessels also generally showed higher average *PS* values. Average *VV* decreased rapidly with increasing distance to the vessels and leveled off at around 250 μm. Treatment with bevacizumab/paclitaxel combination therapy did not have a significant impact on the overall distribution pattern of the tumor microvascular parameters, Fig. 3.

Vascular Changes Induced by the Bevacizumab/Paclitaxel Combination Therapy

Bevacizumab/paclitaxel combination therapy appeared to have induced barely any changes in the tumor macrovascular network, as evidenced by the tumor angiograms from different treatment groups shown in Fig. 4. The average macrovascular volume fraction was 4.4% (±1%) of the total tumor volume prior to the start of the treatment, and was 4.2% (±1%) and 4.8% (±1%) at the end of the treatment for the saline control and the bevacizumab/paclitaxel group, respectively. Overall, 18% (±5%) of the entire tumor volume was within 250 μm of an enhancing vessel at the initiation of the treatment, with an average tumor volume of 170 mm^3. Twelve days later, at the end of the treatment, 23% (±3%) of the total tumor volume remained within 250 μm of the nearest enhancing vessel in mice that received bevacizumab/paclitaxel, with an average tumor size of 160 mm^3. In control mice that received saline, the average tumor volume was 300 mm^3 and the fraction of tumor within a 250 μm range of an enhancing vessel was 17% (±5%).

A trend of decreasing permeability *PS*, averaged over the entire tumor, was observed in the mice received the bevacizumab/paclitaxel combination treatment, in comparison to the *PS* in the pre-treated or the saline controlled mice [18]. However, a consistent decrease in both *VV* and *PS* in the treated mice was apparent when the stratified average values were compared base on the distance to the nearest vessel, as shown in Fig. 5. The overall albumin-Gd-DTPA enhancement in the tumor core was very low [18]. As such, the determination of *VV* and *PS* in these regions, with the distance to the nearest vessel above approximately 1 mm, was mainly dominant by the signal intensity fluctuation due to the noise. When these core regions were excluded from the analysis, the decreases in *VV* and *PS* in the group of treated *vs.* controlled mice were significant in the tumor

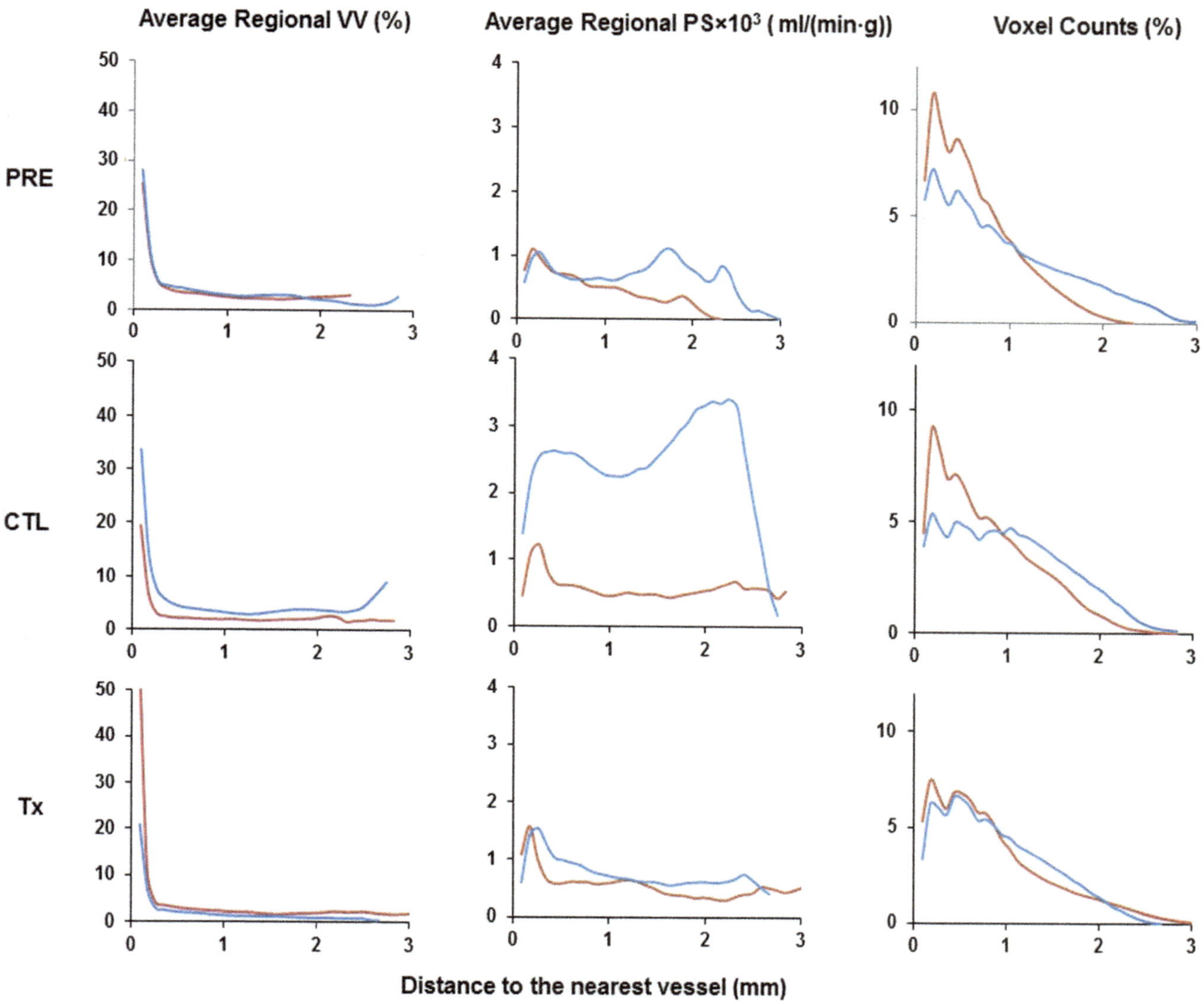

Figure 3. Representative distribution of average tumor VV and PS as a function of the distance to the nearest segmented vessel. Results for two mice, shown in red and blue lines, from the pre-treatment (PRE), day 12 of saline control (CTL), and day 12 of bevacizumab/paclitaxel combination (Tx) groups are shown.

area within 1 mm to the nearest enhancing vessel with p values less than $2 \cdot 10^{-5}$, respectively.

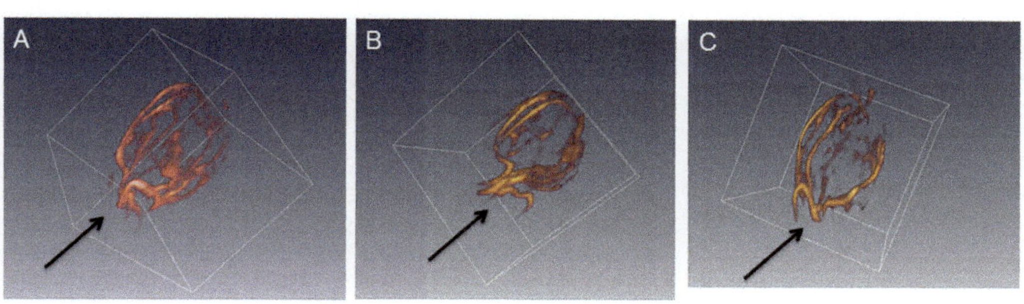

Figure 4. Tumor macrovasculature extracted from the 3D T1-weighted images acquired immediately after the administration of albumin-Gd-DTPA. A: pre-treatment, B: day 12 of saline control, C: day 12 of bevacizumab/paclitaxel combination treatment. The arrows indicate where the tumor was attached to the mouse body.

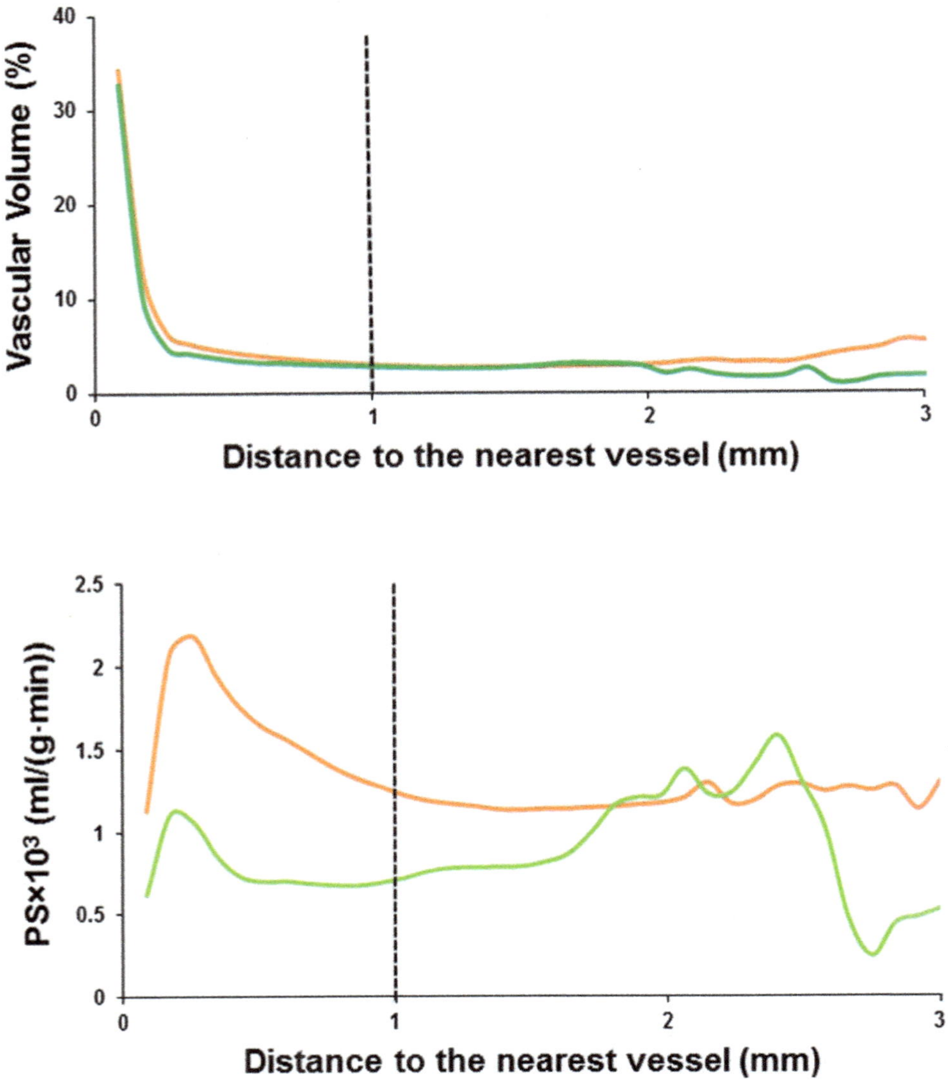

Figure 5. Distribution of group average VV and PS values of the control (orange) and the treated mice (green) relative to the distance to the segmented nearest vessel. The control group was the combination of the pre-treatment and day 12 of saline treated mice.

Discussion

DCE-MRI with an MMCA, albumin-Gd-DTPA, enabled the noninvasive acquisition of high-resolution 3D tumor angiograms (macrovasculature) as well as determination of the functional microvascular tumor parameters. Although it has been suggested that tumor blood supply and therapeutic intervention that targets the tumor vasculature may be more accurately assessed with a combination of DCE-MRI and MR angiography [4], past studies focused primarily on the microvascular changes only [6]. Our study is one of the few attempts to provide a more complete *in vivo* mapping of the tumor vasculature that includes larger vessels and small leaky capillaries, each an indispensable part of a functional vascular network. While MR angiography can detect only the macroscopic enhancing blood vessels that are close to or larger than the spatial MRI resolution, on the order of 100 μm in our study, DCE-MRI can reveal the presence and the permeability of micro-capillaries that are well below the imaging resolution by the kinetic analysis of the contrast concentration [22].

In this study, we detected a general trend of decreased *VV* and *PS* with increasing distance from large enhancing blood vessels. It has been reported that the diffusion limit for oxygen and nutrients is around 100 to 200 μm from the blood vessels [23,24], and tumors could not grow to more than 1–2 mm^3 without neovascularization [2,25,26]. Consistent with this diffusion limit, our results showed that *VV*, a measurement of the total macro- and microvascular volume, drastically decreased at increasing distance from the vessels and leveled off around 250 μm.

Inadequate vascular supply and the subsequently induced hypoxia are the driving force of angiogenesis and increased vascular permeability [2]. While the general trend of decreased *PS* observed in the current study appears in contradiction with the possible severe hypoxia at increasing distance from macrovasculature [15,16,17], the product of vascular permeability and vascular surface area, *PS*, is also related to the vascular volume. Low *PS* values observed might be partially due to the low vascular surface area in the poorly perfused regions with low vascular volume and might not have reflected the possible high vascular permeability in these regions.

A significant decrease in average *VV* and *PS* values were detected in the vicinity of the macroscopic vessels within the tumor after the bevacizumab/paclitaxel combination treatment. However, as demonstrated by Fig. 4, the tumor macrovasculature is largely unresponsive to the bevacizumab/paclitaxel combination treatment. This is not surprising, as the feeder vessels and draining veins are considered to have originated from remodeling and enlargement of the preexisting arteries and veins [27]. Such blood vessels are mature and are less angiogenically active [27]. These vessels can survive antiangiogenic therapy, replenish the blood and nutrient supply to the remaining tumor cells, and maintain an avenue for tumor growth and expansion. An increased portion of the MCF-7 tumor was within the close distance of a macroscopic blood vessel after the bevacizumab/paclitaxel combination treatment, possibly due the tumor growth retardation. Previous study also shows that treatment with antiangiogenic agent SU5416 results in larger vessel perimeter and vessel area in a rat mammary cancer model [28]. The persistence of such macroscopic vessels in the established tumors diminishes the significance of any microvascular changes by a targeted antiangiogenic regimen. Indeed, bevacizumab treatment was initiated within 24 hours of the tumor cell inoculation in one of the first reports that demonstrated the potent efficacy of this VEGF antibody in a mouse model of human cancer, prior to the establishment of any tumor vasculature [29]. Clinical trials showed that the addition of bevacizumab to neoadjuvant chemotherapy for the early stage breast cancer patients resulted in a modest but significant increase in the rate of pathological complete response [30,31]. However, bevacizumab is currently indicated for the first- or second-line treatment of patients with advanced stage metastatic carcinoma [32]. It is possible that the indifference of the mature macroscopic vessels in the well-established tumors towards bevacizumab contributes to the marginal improvement in overall survival rates when it is added to a treatment regimen for late stage metastatic breast cancer patients [33,34,35,36]. The inhibition of angiogenesis may only improve progression-free survival rates temporarily in such situation [33,34,35,36].

The tumor angiogram observed here showed that MCF-7 tumors are supplied by large vessels on the MRI resolution scale, which closely paralleled the normal organs such as muscles, kidney and brain. Areas outside the major vessels remained less enhanced, yet these organs can carry out their normal functions while any vascular occlusion can have serious consequences. Similarly, permanent occlusion of feeding arteries and draining veins in solid mouse tumors by vascular targeted photodynamic therapy leads to tumor necrosis and eradication within 24–48 hours [37]. Our combined angiogram and DCE-MRI results reaffirm the need to identify new tumor blood vessel type-specific targets for a more comprehensive therapeutic intervention at different stages of tumor developments [27,38]. Our approach also stresses the importance of developing robust prognostic imaging biomarkers to design and evaluate treatment options based on tumor characteristics.

Acknowledgments

We would like to thank Mr. Meiyappan Solaiyappan, Dr. Jiangyang Zhang, Dr. Arvind P. Pathak, and Dr. Zaver M. Bhujwalla for helpful discussions. We are also grateful to Mr. Gary Cromwell for mouse tumor inoculation, Dr. Noriko Mori for the preparation of the albumin-Gd-DTPA used in this study, and Ms. Mary McAllister for editing the manuscript.

Author Contributions

Conceived and designed the experiments: WZ YK DA. Performed the experiments: WZ YK. Analyzed the data: WZ YK DA. Contributed reagents/materials/analysis tools: WZ YK DA. Wrote the paper: WZ YK DA.

References

1. Marusyk A, Almendro V, Polyak K (2012) Intra-tumour heterogeneity: a looking glass for cancer? Nat Rev Cancer 12: 323–334.
2. Goel S, Duda DG, Xu L, Munn LL, Boucher Y, et al. (2011) Normalization of the vasculature for treatment of cancer and other diseases. Physiol Rev 91: 1071–1121.
3. Brubaker LM, Bullitt E, Yin C, Van Dyke T, Lin W (2005) Magnetic resonance angiography visualization of abnormal tumor vasculature in genetically engineered mice. Cancer Res 65: 8218–8223.
4. van Vliet M, van Dijke CF, Wielopolski PA, ten Hagen TL, Veenland JF, et al. (2005) MR angiography of tumor-related vasculature: from the clinic to the micro-environment. Radiographics 25 Suppl 1: S85–97; discussion S97–88.
5. Erguvan-Dogan B, Whitman GJ, Kushwaha AC, Phelps MJ, Dempsey PJ (2006) BI-RADS-MRI: a primer. AJR Am J Roentgenol 187: W152–160.
6. O'Connor JP, Jackson A, Parker GJ, Jayson GC (2007) DCE-MRI biomarkers in the clinical evaluation of antiangiogenic and vascular disrupting agents. Br J Cancer 96: 189–195.
7. Jackson A, O'Connor JP, Parker GJ, Jayson GC (2007) Imaging tumor vascular heterogeneity and angiogenesis using dynamic contrast-enhanced magnetic resonance imaging. Clin Cancer Res 13: 3449–3459.
8. Yang X, Knopp MV (2011) Quantifying tumor vascular heterogeneity with dynamic contrast-enhanced magnetic resonance imaging: a review. J Biomed Biotechnol 2011: 732848.
9. Leach MO, Brindle KM, Evelhoch JL, Griffiths JR, Horsman MR, et al. (2005) The assessment of antiangiogenic and antivascular therapies in early-stage clinical trials using magnetic resonance imaging: issues and recommendations. Br J Cancer 92: 1599–1610.
10. Benjaminsen IC, Graff BA, Brurberg KG, Rofstad EK (2004) Assessment of tumor blood perfusion by high-resolution dynamic contrast-enhanced MRI: a preclinical study of human melanoma xenografts. Magn Reson Med 52: 269–276.
11. Chang YC, Huang CS, Liu YJ, Chen JH, Lu YS, et al. (2004) Angiogenic response of locally advanced breast cancer to neoadjuvant chemotherapy evaluated with parametric histogram from dynamic contrast-enhanced MRI. Phys Med Biol 49: 3593–3602.
12. Rose CJ, Mills SJ, O'Connor JP, Buonaccorsi GA, Roberts C, et al. (2009) Quantifying spatial heterogeneity in dynamic contrast-enhanced MRI parameter maps. Magn Reson Med 62: 488–499.
13. Li KL, Wilmes LJ, Henry RG, Pallavicini MG, Park JW, et al. (2005) Heterogeneity in the angiogenic response of a BT474 human breast cancer to a novel vascular endothelial growth factor-receptor tyrosine kinase inhibitor: assessment by voxel analysis of dynamic contrast-enhanced MRI. J Magn Reson Imaging 22: 511–519.
14. Dvorak HF (2002) Vascular permeability factor/vascular endothelial growth factor: a critical cytokine in tumor angiogenesis and a potential target for diagnosis and therapy. J Clin Oncol 20: 4368–4380.
15. Gillies RJ, Schornack PA, Secomb TW, Raghunand N (1999) Causes and effects of heterogeneous perfusion in tumors. Neoplasia 1: 197–207.
16. Helmlinger G, Yuan F, Dellian M, Jain RK (1997) Interstitial pH and pO2 gradients in solid tumors in vivo: high-resolution measurements reveal a lack of correlation. Nat Med 3: 177–182.
17. Rijken PF, Bernsen HJ, Peters JP, Hodgkiss RJ, Raleigh JA, et al. (2000) Spatial relationship between hypoxia and the (perfused) vascular network in a human glioma xenograft: a quantitative multi-parameter analysis. Int J Radiat Oncol Biol Phys 48: 571–582.
18. Zhu W, Kato Y, Artemov D (2013) Water exchange-minimizing DCE-MRI protocol to detect changes in tumor vascular parameters: effect of bevacizumab/paclitaxel combination therapy. Magn Reson Mater Phy.
19. Oku N, Doi K, Namba Y, Okada S (1994) Therapeutic effect of adriamycin encapsulated in long-circulating liposomes on Meth-A-sarcoma-bearing mice. Int J Cancer 58: 415–419.
20. Bhujwalla ZM, Artemov D, Natarajan K, Solaiyappan M, Kollars P, et al. (2003) Reduction of vascular and permeable regions in solid tumors detected by macromolecular contrast magnetic resonance imaging after treatment with antiangiogenic agent TNP-470. Clin Cancer Res 9: 355–362.
21. Pathak AP, Penet MF, Bhujwalla ZM (2010) MR molecular imaging of tumor vasculature and vascular targets. Adv Genet 69: 1–30.
22. Tofts PS (1997) Modeling tracer kinetics in dynamic Gd-DTPA MR imaging. J Magn Reson Imaging 7: 91–101.
23. Carmeliet P, Jain RK (2000) Angiogenesis in cancer and other diseases. Nature 407: 249–257.

24. Tannock IF (1972) Oxygen diffusion and the distribution of cellular radiosensitivity in tumours. Br J Radiol 45: 515–524.
25. Folkman J, Long DM, Jr., Becker FF (1963) Growth and metastasis of tumor in organ culture. Cancer 16: 453–467.
26. Folkman J (1990) What is the evidence that tumors are angiogenesis dependent? J Natl Cancer Inst 82: 4–6.
27. Nagy JA, Dvorak HF (2012) Heterogeneity of the tumor vasculature: the need for new tumor blood vessel type-specific targets. Clin Exp Metastasis.
28. Kan Z, Phongkitkarun S, Kobayashi S, Tang Y, Ellis LM, et al. (2005) Functional CT for quantifying tumor perfusion in antiangiogenic therapy in a rat model. Radiology 237: 151–158.
29. Presta LG, Chen H, O'Connor SJ, Chisholm V, Meng YG, et al. (1997) Humanization of an anti-vascular endothelial growth factor monoclonal antibody for the therapy of solid tumors and other disorders. Cancer Res 57: 4593–4599.
30. von Minckwitz G, Eidtmann H, Rezai M, Fasching PA, Tesch H, et al. (2012) Neoadjuvant chemotherapy and bevacizumab for HER2-negative breast cancer. N Engl J Med 366: 299–309.
31. Bear HD, Tang G, Rastogi P, Geyer CE, Jr., Robidoux A, et al. (2012) Bevacizumab added to neoadjuvant chemotherapy for breast cancer. N Engl J Med 366: 310–320.
32. Shih T, Lindley C (2006) Bevacizumab: an angiogenesis inhibitor for the treatment of solid malignancies. Clin Ther 28: 1779–1802.
33. Miles DW, Chan A, Dirix LY, Cortes J, Pivot X, et al. (2010) Phase III study of bevacizumab plus docetaxel compared with placebo plus docetaxel for the first-line treatment of human epidermal growth factor receptor 2-negative metastatic breast cancer. J Clin Oncol 28: 3239–3247.
34. Robert NJ, Dieras V, Glaspy J, Brufsky AM, Bondarenko I, et al. (2011) RIBBON-1: randomized, double-blind, placebo-controlled, phase III trial of chemotherapy with or without bevacizumab for first-line treatment of human epidermal growth factor receptor 2-negative, locally recurrent or metastatic breast cancer. J Clin Oncol 29: 1252–1260.
35. Brufsky AM, Hurvitz S, Perez E, Swamy R, Valero V, et al. (2011) RIBBON-2: a randomized, double-blind, placebo-controlled, phase III trial evaluating the efficacy and safety of bevacizumab in combination with chemotherapy for second-line treatment of human epidermal growth factor receptor 2-negative metastatic breast cancer. J Clin Oncol 29: 4286–4293.
36. Burstein HJ (2011) Bevacizumab for Advanced Breast Cancer: All Tied Up With a RIBBON? Journal of Clinical Oncology 29: 1232–1235.
37. Madar-Balakirski N, Tempel-Brami C, Kalchenko V, Brenner O, Varon D, et al. (2010) Permanent occlusion of feeding arteries and draining veins in solid mouse tumors by vascular targeted photodynamic therapy (VTP) with Tookad. PLoS One 5: e10282.
38. Sitohy B, Nagy JA, Dvorak HF (2012) Anti-VEGF/VEGFR therapy for cancer: reassessing the target. Cancer Res 72: 1909–1914.

14

A Prospective Study of Treatment Patterns and 1-Year Outcome of Asian Age-Related Macular Degeneration and Polypoidal Choroidal Vasculopathy

Chui Ming Gemmy Cheung[1,2,3,4*], Xiang Li[2,5], Ranjana Mathur[1], Shu Yen Lee[1], Choi Mun Chan[1], Ian Yeo[1], Boon Kwang Loh[1], Rachel Williams[6], Edmund Yick-Mun Wong[1], Doric Wong[1], Tien Yin Wong[1,2,3,4]

1 Vitreoretinal Service, Singapore National Eye Centre, Singapore, Singapore, **2** Singapore Eye Research Institute, Singapore, Singapore, **3** Department of Ophthalmology, Yong Loo Lin School of Medicine, National University of Singapore, Singapore, Singapore, **4** Ophthalmology Academic Clinical Program, Duke-NUS Graduate Medical School, Singapore, Singapore, **5** Department of Statistics and Applied Probability, National University of Singapore, Singapore, Singapore, **6** Worldwide Epidemiology, R&D Projects, Clinical Platforms & Sciences, GlaxoSmithKline, Pennsylvania, United States of America

Abstract

Objective: To study the treatment patterns and visual outcome over one year in Asian patients with choroidal neovascular membrane secondary to age-related macular degeneration (AMD-CNV) and polypoidal choroidal vasculopathy (PCV).

Design: Prospective cohort, non-interventional study.

Methods: 132 treatment-naïve patients who received treatment for AMD-CNV and PCV were included. All patients underwent standardized examination procedures including retinal imaging at baseline and follow-up. AMD-CNV and PCV were defined on fundus fluorescein angiography and indocyanine green angiography at baseline. Patients were treated according to standard of care.We report the visual acuity (VA) and optical coherence tomography (OCT) measurements at baseline, month 3 and month 12 The factors influencing month 12 outcomes were analyzed.

Main Outcome Measure: Type of treatment, number of Anti-vascular endothelial growth factor (VEGF) treatments, visual outcome over one year.

Results: Anti-VEGF monotherapy was the initial treatment in 89.1% of AMD-CNV, but only 15.1% of PCV. The mean number of anti-VEGF injections up to month 12 was 3.97 (4.51 AMD-CNV, 3.43 PCV, $p = 0.021$). Baseline OCT, month 3 OCT and month 3 VA were significant in determining continuation of treatment after month 3. At month12, mean VA improved from 0.82 (~20/132) at baseline to 0.68 (~20/96) at month 12 (mean gain 6.5 ETDRS letters, $p = 0.002$). 34.2% of eyes (38/113 eyes) gained ≥15 ETDRS letters and 14.4% (16/113 eyes) lost ≥15 ETDRS letters. There were no significant differences in visual outcome between AMD-CNV and PCV ($p = 0.51$). Factors predictive of month 12 visual outcome were baseline VA, baseline OCT central macular thickness, month 3 VA and age.

Conclusions: There is significant variation in treatment patterns in Asian eyes with exudative maculopathy. There is significant visual improvement in all treatment groups at one year. These data highlight the need for high quality clinical trial data to provide evidence-based management of Asian AMD.

Editor: Pedro Gonzalez, Duke University, United States of America

Funding: This study was supported by National Medical Research Council grant: NMRC/NIG/1003/2009; GlaxoSimthKline Research and Development Protocol WEUSKOP5855. The funders had no role in study design, data collection and analysis, decision to publish, or preparation of the manuscript.

Competing Interests: REW is employed by and holds stock in GlaxoSmithKline. The remaining authors have no competing interest.

* Email: gemmy.cheung.c.m@snec.com.sg

Introduction

Age-related macular degeneration (AMD) is one of the major causes of blindness worldwide [1–4]. The efficacy of ranibizumab, bevacizumab and aflibercept, have been confirmed by landmark clinical trials and these agents are now the mainstay of treatment for exudative AMD [5–11]. However, frequent follow-up and retreatment remain challenging in clinical setting. Data from the US Medicare and several European registries have highlighted these in the form of high treatment discontinuation rate within the first year and low mean number of injections [11–18].

There are few studies which have examined treatment pattern and outcomes of exudative maculopathy specifically in Asians, although it is often assumed that similar results with anti-VEGF therapy can be expected for eyes with choroidal neovascularization secondary to typical AMD (AMD-CNV) while different treatment appears to be required for the polypoidal choroidal vasculopathy (PCV) subtype [19–20]. In addition, lack of government funded reimbursement in many Asian countries, potential differences in patient understanding and expectation, and uncertainties of the role of anti-VEGF mono-therapy in PCV, may all affect the pattern of therapy in an Asian setting [20–24]. Furthermore, because photodynamic therapy (PDT) has been suggested to have superior angiographic, and possibly visual outcome in the PCV subtype [25–28], PDT is recommended as preferred treatment in PCV [29], in contrast to declining usage in Western populations. Therefore, significant heterogeneity remains in the management of Asian eyes with exudative maculopathy, in terms of diagnosis, optimal treatment and outcome.

There are few prospective studies which have examined treatment patterns and outcomes in a "real life" setting in Asians. To address this gap, we performed a prospective observational clinical study to document the current treatment pattern and outcomes of Asian exudative maculopathy, comparing in particular AMD-CNV and PCV.

Methods

Study Design and Population

The Asian AMD Phenotyping Study is a prospectively planned, cohort study approved by the SingHealth Centralized Institutional Review Board (protocol number R697/47/2009). All patients provided written informed consent to participate in this research. Specifically, the Asian AMD Phenotyping Study aimed to investigate prospectively a consecutive series of treatment-naïve Asian patients with exudative maculopathy secondary to AMD-CNV or PCV [30]. Consecutive patients were recruited from the retinal clinic of the Singapore National Eye Centre. Recruitment started on March 01 2010 and is still ongoing.

Clinical Examination and Investigations

Participants received treatment according to standard of care by individual physicians, and treatment was not altered by entering into the study. Patients were followed up prospectively according to clinical need, but minimum reviews at month 1, month 3 and month 12 were mandated by the protocol to ensure minimal data collection. Additional visits were allowed if indicated by clinical needs. All patients underwent a complete standardized ophthalmic examination at baseline and follow-up. This included visual acuity, dilated fundus examination, color fundus photography and optical coherence tomography (OCT), fundus fluorescein angiography (FFA), and indocyanine angiography (ICGA), according to a standardized protocol at baseline.

Fundus photography was performed using a digital mydriatic retinal camera (TRC-50X/IMAGEnet 2000, Topcon, Tokyo, Japan). Spectral domain optical Coherence Tomography (OCT) was performed with the Cirrus OCT (Carl Zeiss Meditec, Dublin, CA) using the 512×128-volume cube setting. Central macular thickness (CMT) was recorded. Fundus angiography with fluorescein and indocyanine green is performed using a fundus camera (TRC-50X/IMAGEnet 2000, Topcon, Tokyo, Japan) or confocal SLO (Heidelberg Retina Angiograph Spectralis; Heidelberg Engineering, Heidelberg, Germany).

Best corrected visual acuity (BCVA) was tested with Snellen chart and converted to LogMAR. Repeat fundus photography and OCT were performed at each follow-up visit and repeat fluorescein and ICGA was performed as deemed appropriate by the treating retinal specialist.

Angiographic Grading

AMD-CNV and PCV were diagnosed clinically and by FFA and ICGA. Both the primary diagnosis and treatment decision were made by the treating clinician, all of whom are fellowship-trained retinal specialist. Presence or absence of CNV was graded using criteria from the Macular Photocoagulation Study [31]. The diagnosis of definitive PCV lesions was based on the angiographic criteria from the Japanese Study Group guidelines, which defined PCV as characteristic polypoidal lesions on ICGA [32] To reflect the 'real-world' scenario, no secondary level grading was used in this analysis.

Treatment Strategies

Treatment was recommended by one of the retinal specialists in the department, all of whom were fellowship-trained. However, patients decided their final treatment after considering their visual need and financial situation. Typically, anti-VEGF therapy was recommended in the presence of subretinal or intraretinal fluid or hemorrhage associated with active AMD-CNV. In cases of PCV, anti-VEGF was recommended where there was significant fluid or hemorrhage subfoveally. In addition, focal laser was recommended if polyps were localized extrafoveally. Where PCV lesions were extensive and not amenable to focal laser, PDT was recommended. Anti-VEGF monotherapy was used in patients who could not afford PDT for subfoveal or juxtafoveal PCV. In selected cases, individual retinal specialist might recommend anti-VEGF monotherapy if polyps were small and vision was good.

Patients were followed-up at intervals determined by their treating physician. A variety of regimens were used, including monthly with prn retreatment, treat-and –extend, and sometimes less frequent follow-up. Retreatment was based on visual acuity, clinical examination and OCT morphology, usually if there is persistent subretinal or intraretinal fluid or hemorrhage. Loading with 3 initial monthly injections was not compulsory.

Anti-VEGF treatment was given intravitreally either as ranibizumab (Lucentis, Novartis) 0.5 mg/0.05 ml or bevacizumab (Avastin, Roche) 1.25 mg/0.05 ml in pre-aliquoted syringes using local compounding pharmacy.

All focal laser treatment was performed by retinal specialists. Generally, treatment was performed with a green laser with a focal contact lens, using the following parameters: 100 to 200 µm spot size, 0.15 to 0.3 millisecond duration to achieve a greyish-white burn to the active polypoidal lesions identified on ICGA. Laser may be repeated at more than one session if closure is felt to be incomplete at follow-up. Laser was not performed on the associated branching network.

PDT was performed with verteporfin (Visudyne, Novartis, Basel, Switzerland) according to the protocol of the TAP study [33]. The greatest linear dimension (GLD) was measured based on FA for CNV lesions, according to TAP protocol. For eyes with PCV, the GLD included the entire area of abnormal choroidal vasculature on the ICGA. The diameter of the laser spot size selected to be 1000 µm more than the GLD. Patients were followed-up 3-monthly after the initial PDT.

Statistical analysis

Statistical analysis was performed using standard statistical software (Statistical Package for Social Science, SPSS version 16, Illinois, Chicago) and R version 2.15.2 (R Development Core Team, Vienna, Austria, 2012). Characteristics of the study population were examined using proportions or means and standard deviation (SD). Wilcoxon rank sum test (Kruskal-Wallis rank sum test if number of groups is more than 2) or Chi-square test (Fisher's exact test if there is any entry with expected number less than 5) was performed to test the difference between diagnosis results (AMD-CNV vs. PCV) or between different treatment patterns. Factors influencing continuation of treatment after month 3 were analyzed by applying recursive partitioning tree model using R package "rpart" (Recursive Partitioning), to the factors of age, gender, initial treatment, OCT CMT (baseline, month 3 and change at month 3) and VA (baseline, month 3 and change at month 3). Decision tree was pruned after built to avoid overfitting.

Linear mixed-effect model was used to analyze longitudinal data of visual acuity over the first year to account for the repeated measurements made on the same eye. Both random and fixed effects of number of injections were added to control the heterogeneous effect among eyes. Stepwise model selection (forward and backward selection) was performed to investigate the effect on visual acuity at month 12, from a set of variables, including age, gender, VA at baseline, VA at month 3, change of VA at month 3, OCT CMT at baseline, OCT CMT at month 3, change of OCT CMT at month 3. Akaike information criterion (AIC) and recursive partitioning and regression tree model were used to select the important predictors for visual acuity at month 12.

Results

From March 1st 2010 to July 31st 2011, a total of 167 study eyes from 167 patients were included (participation rate of 77.7%). The mean age of the subjects was 69.5 years, with a slight male dominance (58.1%). The presenting visual acuity was 0.85 (~20/132). The proportion presenting with 0.3 (~6/12) or better was 13.2%, and the proportion presenting with vision 1.0 (~6/60) or worse was 35.3%. Sixty five eyes (38.9%) had typical AMD-CNV and 102 eyes (61.1%) had PCV. Baseline characteristics are summarized in **Table 1**.

Initial Treatment Pattern for All Eyes

Treatment was initiated between baseline visit and 3-month visit in one hundred and thirty-two eyes (79%). At least 1 anti-VEGF injection was received by 97 of these 132 eyes (73.5%) during the first 3 months (**Table 2**). Of these 97 eyes treated with anti-VEGF, 54 eyes were as monotherapy, and the remainder was in combination with laser (12 eyes) or PDT (29 eyes) or both PDT and laser (2 eyes). After the initial 3 months, only 46.2% (61 eyes) received further treatment, most with continuation of anti-VEGF monotherapy (70.5%, 43 eyes). Data at 1 year was available from 87/97 eyes that were commenced on anti-VEGF therapy. The mean number of injections was 2.46 (3 months), 3.15 (6 months) and 3.97 (12 months) (**Table 3**). The mean cumulative numbers of out-patient visits were 3.08, and 8.03 at month 3 and month 12 (**Table 3**). Among eyes treated with any anti-VEGF, 83.2% received bevacizumab, and the remaining received ranibizumab. Thirty-four out of 41 patients initially treated with PDT remained on follow-up at one year. The mean cumulative number of PDT sessions was 1.29 (range 1–3) during the first year of treatment. Of the 35 eyes that initially did not receive treatment before their month-3 visit, 10 were eventually treated due to increase in activity or patient's change of mind, 8 patients defaulted and the remaining patients continued to be observed.

One-Year Treatment Outcomes for All Eyes

VA at month 12 was available in 113 (of 132) treated patients. The mean VA improved from 0.82 (~20/132) at baseline to 0.68 (~20/96) at month 12 (mean gain 6.5 ETDRS letters, p = 0.002, **Table 4, Fig 1**). 34.2% gained ≥15 ETDRS letters and 14.4% lost ≥15 ETDRS letters. VA at month 3 was available in 75 eyes (**Table 4**) and generally are similar to VA at month 12. At month 12, 48% of 98 eyes (including 58.5% of AMd-CNV eyes and 41.3% of PCV eyes) had activity when graded into categories of active and inactive. Central macular thickness measured using

Table 1. Baseline Characteristics, comparing eyes with Age-related Macular Degeneration (AMD-CNV) and Polypoidal Choroidal Vasculopathy (PCV).

	All (N = 167)	AMD-CNV (N = 65)	PCV (N = 102)	P
Age	69.5 (9.94)	70.47 (12.05)	68.88 (8.34)	0.08
Gender				
Men	97 (58.1%)	37 (56.9%)	60 (58.8%)	0.81
Ethnicity				
Chinese	145 (86.8%)	55 (84.6%)	90 (88.2%)	0.32
Indian	2 (1.2%)	1 (1.5%)	1 (1%)	
Malay	17 (10.2%)	9 (13.8%)	8 (7.8%)	
Others	3 (1.8%)	0 (0%)	3 (2.9%)	
Prior involvement of Fellow eye *	13 (7.8%)	8 (12.3%)	5 (4.9%)	0.08
Pseudophakia in affected eye	40 (24.1%) n = 166	20 (30.8%)	20 (19.8%) n = 101	0.11
Visual Acuity (affected eye)	0.85 (0.56),	**0.95 (0.55)**	**0.78 (0.57)**	**0.018**
% Visual Acuity 6/12 (0.3 LogMAR) or better	22 (13.2%)	6 (9.2%)	16 (15.7%)	0.23
% Visual Acuity 6/60 (1.0 LogMAR) or worse	59 (35.3%)	**29 (44.6%)**	**30 (29.4%)**	**0.045**
Visual acuity (fellow eye)	0.52 (0.64), n = 165	0.59 (0.7)	0.47 (0.59), n = 100	0.38
OCT CMT (affected eye)†	310.61 (98.51), n = 132	331.02 (106.33), n = 51	297.75 (91.61), n = 81	0.08
OCT CMT (fellow eye)	260.53 (80.05), n = 127	247.4 (65.14), n = 50	269.05 (87.75), n = 77	0.27

*Indicating whether a scar was present in the fellow eye.
†Exclude statistically outlier values of 18, 23, 785.
AMD-age-related macular degeneration, PCV- polypoidal choroidal vasculopathy, OCT- optical coherence tomography; CMT - central macular thickness.

Table 2. Initial Treatment Pattern from Baseline to Month 3, comparing eyes with Age-related Macular Degeneration (AMD-CNV) and Polypoidal Choroidal Vasculopathy (PCV).

	All (N = 167)	AMD-CNV (N = 65)	PCV (N = 102)	P value[†]
Initial treatment*				0.036
No	35 (21%)	19 (29.2%)	16 (15.7%)	
Yes	132 (79%)	46 (70.8%)	86 (84.3%)	
Eyes with initial treatment	n = 132	n = 46	n = 86	<0.001
Any anti-VEGF	97 (73.5%)	44 (95.7%)	51 (59.3%)	
Anti-VEGF monotherapy	54 (40.9%)	41 (89.1%)	13 (15.1%)	
PDT monotherapy	9 (6.8%)	2 (4.3%)	7 (8.1%)	
Laser monotherapy	25 (18.9%)	0 (0%)	25 (29.1%)	
Anti-VEGF & PDT	29 (22.0%)	0 (0%)	29 (33.7%)	
Anti-VEGF & laser	12 (9.1%)	3 (6.5%)	9 (10.5%)	
PDT & laser	1 (0.8%)	0 (0%)	1 (1.2%)	
Anti-VEGF & PDT & laser	2 (1.5%)	0 (0%)	2 (2.3%)	

* Treatment given before month 3 (inclusive).
[†]P value to test the distribution of initial treatment between AMD and PCV, Fisher's exact test.
AMD-age-related macular degeneration, PCV- polypoidal choroidal vasculopathy, anti-VEGF- anti-vascular endothelial growth factor, PDT-photodynamic therapy.

Cirrus OCT (available in 74 eyes) was significantly reduced from baseline to month 12 (300.86 µm vs 264.68 µm, $p<0.001$). The proportion of eyes with vision 0.3 (~6/12) or better increased from 15.3% to 31.5%, and the proportion of eyes with vision 1.0 (~6/60) or worse decreased from 33.3% at baseline to 22.5%. In the subgroup of 85 eyes treated with anti-VEGF, visual outcome was similar compared to the whole group, with mean gain of 7.0 letters at month 12. 32.9% (28/85) gained ≥15 letters and 12.9% (11/85) lost ≥15 letters.

Comparison of Treatment Patterns for AMD-CNV and PCV

Presenting vision was significantly worse in AMD-CNV than PCV (0.95 vs 0.78, $p = 0.018$) (**Table 1**) and more eyes with AMD-CNV had vision worse than 6/60 (44.6%) than PCV (29.4%, $p = 0.045$). However, within the group of treated eyes with at least one year follow-up (n = 113), the baseline vision was similar. There was no significant difference in age, gender, OCT thickness, proportion of previous involvement in fellow eyes and lens status. However after excluding 35 patients who did not receive treatment (29 AMD-CNV, 16 PCV), the presenting vision was similar in the remaining eyes (0.79 AMD-CNV, 0.83 PCV, $p = 0.89$) (**Table 4**).

Initial treatment choice was markedly different between AMD-CNV and PCV groups (**Table 2**, **Figure 2**). Anti-VEGF monotherapy was used in the majority of AMD-CNV (89.1%, 41/46 eyes), but only 15.1% (13/86) of PCV. Within the PCV group, the single most commonly used treatment was anti-VEGF and PDT combination (33.7%, 29/86), followed by laser monotherapy (29.1%, 25/86). Overall, 59.3% of eyes with PCV received anti-VEGF therapy alone or in combination. The mean cumulative number of anti-VEGF injections was significantly lower in PCV group (4.51 for AMD-CNV, 3.43 for PCV, $p = 0.021$).

Mean vision at month 12 was similar between AMD-CNV and PCV group (0.70 AMD-CNV, 0.67 PCV, $p = 0.94$) (**Table 3**). The mean change in vision and proportion gaining and losing ≥ 15 ETDRS letters were also similar. (**Table 3**)

Factors Influencing Treatment Patterns

Factors that influenced the choice of initial therapy were diagnosis (see above, AMD-CNV compared to PCV) and OCT CMT at baseline. Eyes treated with anti-VEGF monotherapy had thicker OCT CMT at baseline compared to eyes treated with combination. (367.62 µm vs 291.68 µm, $p = 0.001$). These two factors remained significant (diagnosis, $p<0.001$; OCT CMT $p = 0.004$) after adjusting for age, gender, baseline OCT and diagnosis Baseline VA and previous fellow eye involvement were not significantly related to treatment choice.

Factors that influenced the cumulative number of injections included diagnosis, choice of initial treatment and OCT CMT measurement at month 3. PCV eyes had significantly less injections than AMD eyes (3.43 vs 4.51 at 1 year, $p = 0.021$) This difference remained after controlling age, gender and the OCT CMT at month 3. Eyes treated with anti-VEGF combinations had significantly lower number of injections than eyes treated with anti-VEGF monotherapy only in the PCV group (3.03 vs 4.70 at 1 year, $p = 0.008$). Each 100 µm increase in OCT CMT at month 3 was associated with additional 0.925 injections after month 3 ($p = 0.029$).This remains significant after controlling for diagnosis and the baseline OCT CMT ($p = 0.025$).

Factors Influencing One-Year Visual Outcome

Using recursive partitioning and regression tree method, baseline VA, baseline OCT thickness and month 3 VA were significant predictors of VA at month 12. Eyes with baseline VA of ≥1.0 had worse vision at month 12 compared to eyes with better baseline VA (1.13 vs 0.46, $p<0.001$). However they experienced larger improvement in VA (18.5 letters vs 1 letter, $p = 0.002$) and had a larger proportion experiencing at least 15 letters gain (54.1% vs 24.3%, $p = 0.002$).

In addition, we performed a longitudinal analysis, utilizing all available data at different time points over the first year. Visual

Table 3. Cumulative number of Anti-vascular endothelial growth factor (anti-VEGF) injections and follow-up visits to month 12, comparing eyes with Age-related Macular Degeneration (AMD-CNV) and Polypoidal Choroidal Vasculopathy (PCV).

	Month 3	Month 6	Month 12
All Anti-VEGF (N = 87)			
Number of injections	2.46 (1.13)	3.15 (1.47)	3.97 (2.07)
Number of visits	3.08 (1.31)	4.11 (2.00)	8.03 (1.90)
Stratified by Diagnosis & Treatment mode			
AMD-CNV (N = 43)			
Number of injections	2.70 (1.19)	3.63 (1.63)	4.51 (2.25)
Number of visits	2.794 (1.41)	3.86 (2.17)	5.51 (2.76)
AMD-CNV treated with Anti-VEGF monotherapy (n = 33)			
Number of injections	2.73 (1.13)	3.55 (1.6)	4.45 (2.31)
Number of visits	2.52 (1.42)	3.33 (2.16)	4.91 (2.82)
AMD-CNV treated with combination therapy (n = 10)			
Number of injections	2.6 (1.43)	3.9 (1.79)	4.7 (2.21)
Number of visits	3.7 (0.95)	5.6 (0.97)	7.5 (1.27)
P value* for number of injections comparing monotherapy vs combination in AMD-CNV			
	1.000	0.536	0.511
PCV (N = 44)			
Number of injections	2.23 (1.03)	2.68 (1.14)	3.43 (1.73)
Number of visits	3.36 (1.16)	4.36 (1.81)	6.20 (2.36)
PCV treated with Anti-VEGF monotherapy (n = 10)			
Number of injections	3.1 (0.57)	3.8 (1.03)	4.8 (1.99)
Number of visits	3.7 (0.95)	5.2 (1.81)	7.3 (2.67)
PCV treated with combination therapy (n = 34)			
Number of injections	1.97 (1)	2.35 (0.95)	3.03 (1.45)
Number of visits	3.26 (1.21)	4.12 (1.75)	5.88 (2.2)
P value* for number of injections comparing monotherapy vs combination in PCV			
	0.002	0.001	0.008
P value* for number of injections between AMD-CNV and PCV			
	0.003	**0.002**	**0.017**

*P value based on Wilcoxon rank sum test.
AMD-age-related macular degeneration, PCV- polypoidal choroidal vasculopathy, anti-VEGF- anti-vascular endothelial growth factor, PDT-photodynamic therapy.

acuity was weakly correlated with number of injections and age. For each additional injection received, there was on average an additional 1.7 letters improvement in VA at month 12 ($p = 0.05$). Every year increase in age was associated with a 0.6 letter worsening of VA ($p = 0.05$). OCT CMT measurement was significantly correlated with visual acuity ($p < 0.001$). Each 100 µm increase in OCT CMT was correlated to a drop of 3.62 ETDRS letters in visual acuity. There was no significant difference in Month 12 VA or change in VA whether anti-VEGF therapy was alone or in combination.

Discussion

This prospective study reports the current treatment pattern and outcome for exudative maculopathy in an Asian population over a one year period. While it has been documented that anti-VEGF monotherapy is now the most common treatment for exudative AMD in the USA and Europe [11], similar data from an Asian population are limited. In addition, it is unclear how anti-VEGF usage may be affected by issues including the high prevalence of PCV in Asian populations, the apparent superior efficacy of PDT in causing polyp regression, and the uncertainty of the role of anti-VEGF monotherapy [20–29]. Recently, health authorities from some Asian countries have excluded PCV from the treatment label of anti-VEGF agents. Therefore, a clearer understanding of the management patterns and outcome of Asian eyes with exudative maculopathy is important in accurately planning eye care provision, research strategies, labelling of medications and re-imbursement of therapies.

Our study population can be compared to similar registry and insurance-based data, mostly from Western countries with largely white populations (**Table 5**). Our study population was generally younger (mean age 69.6 years), had higher male subjects (58.1%) and had lower presenting vision (44.0 ETDRS letters). Overall, 72.0% of treated eyes received at least one anti-VEGF treatment. While the widespread use of anti-VEGF is comparable to data from US [11], only 40.9% of cases received anti-VEGF as monotherapy. This pattern is remarkably different compared to reports in white people [11]. However, when stratified by diagnosis, the vast majority of AMD-CNV cases were treated with anti-VEGF monotherapy (89.1%). Therefore the lower monotherapy rate can be attributed largely to the higher

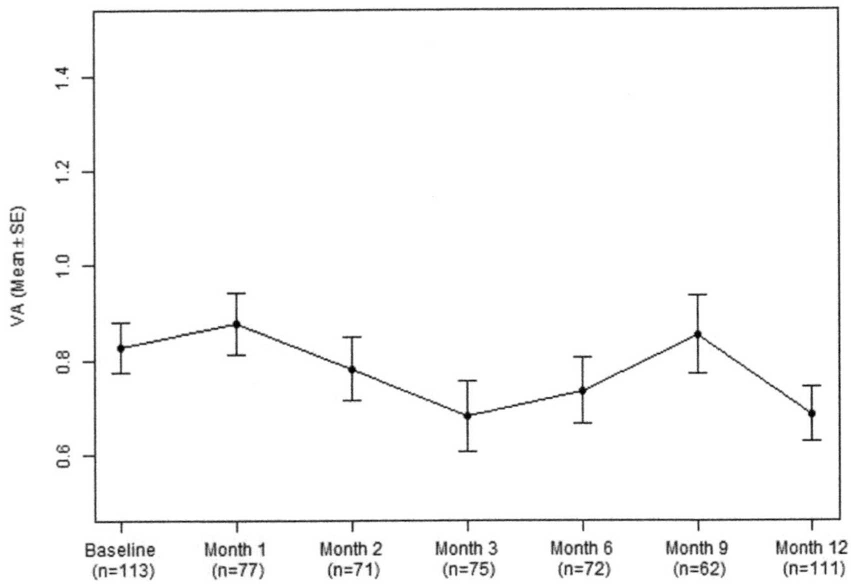

Figure 1. Mean visual acuity of all treated eyes from baseline to month 12. The number of eyes with OCT available at each timepoint is indicated by n.VA Visual acuity; SE standard error.

Table 4. Visual Acuity and Optical Coherence Tomography Central Macular Thickness at Month 3 and Month 12, stratified by Diagnosis.

	All	AMD-CNV	PCV	P
Visual acuity	N = 113	N = 43	N = 70	
Baseline	0.82 (0.57)	0.79 (0.53)	0.83 (0.59)	0.89
Month 3	0.68 (0.65) (n = 75)	0.76 (0.79) (n = 25)	0.64 (0.57) (n = 50)	0.94
Month 12	0.68 (0.6)	0.7 (0.64)	0.67 (0.57)	0.94
Change at month 3	−0.16 (0.47)	0.03 (0.52)	−0.26 (0.42)	0.15
Change at month 12	−0.13 (0.51)	−0.09 (0.52)	−0.16 (0.51)	0.51
Gain ≥15 letters at Month 3	25 (33.3%)	9(36.0%)	16 (32.0%)	0.73
Gain ≥15 letters at Month 12	38 (34.2%)	14 (34.1%)	24 (34.3%)	0.99
Loss ≥15 letters at month 3	7 (9.3%)	6 (24.0%)	1 (2.0%)	0.005
Loss ≥15 letters at Month 12	16 (14.4%)	6 (14.6%)	10 (14.3%)	0.96
Proportion with VA 0.3 or better				
Baseline	17 (15.3%)	7 (17.1%)	10 (14.3%)	0.69
Month 3	29 (38.7%	11 (44.0%)	18 (36.0%)	0.50
Month 12	35 (31.5%)	14 (34.1%)	21 (30%)	0.65
Proportion with VA 1.0 or worse				
Baseline	37 (33.3%)	13 (31.7%)	24 (34.3%)	0.781
Month 3	17 (22.7%)	6 (24.0%)	11 (22.0%)	0.85
Month 12	25 (22.5%)	11 (26.8%)	14 (20%)	0.406
OCT CMT	N = 76	N = 26	N = 50	
Baseline	300.86 (98.29)	317.62 (94.79)	292.14 (99.88)	0.26
Month 12	264.68 (89.82)	272.81 (71.18)	260.46 (98.54)	0.16
Change at month 12	−36.17 (93.99)	−44.81 (79.52)	−31.68 (101.17)	0.68

P value based Wilcoxon rank sum test or Chi-square test.
AMD-age-related macular degeneration, PCV- polypoidal choroidal vasculopathy, OCT- optical coherence tomography, CMT - central macular thickness.

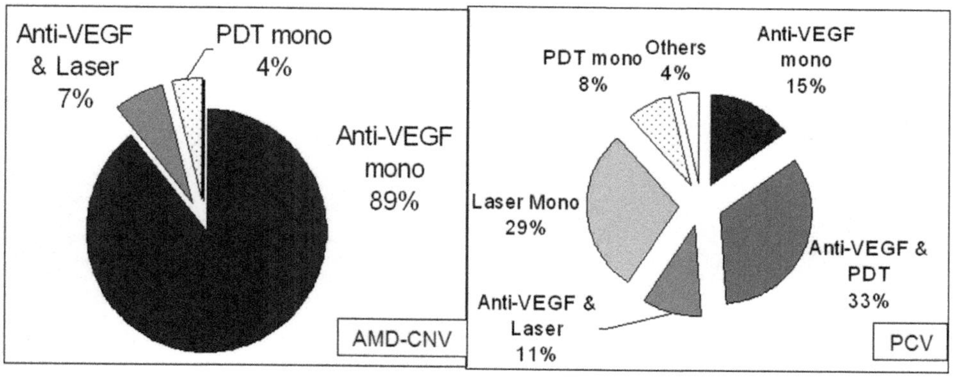

Figure 2. Distribution of Initial Treatment Modalities by diagnosis of Age-related Macular Degeneration (AMD-CNV) (left) and Polypoidal Choroidal Vasculopathy (PCV) (right).

proportion of patients needing specific PCV treatment, of which only 15.1% received anti-VEGF monotherapy. Despite the lower proportion of anti-VEGF monotherapy, a further 44.2% of PCV eyes received anti-VEGF in combination with PDT (33.7%) or laser (10.5%). Thus, an key observation of this study is that anti-VEGF therapy constitutes a significant part of treatment for PCV eyes (59.3%), although more commonly in combination with other treatments.

The overall number of injections was low at 3.97 (range 1–9) over 12 months. Even after separating PCV eyes from AMD-CNV eyes, the mean number of injections was only 4.51 injections over 12 months in AMD-CNV eyes. However, these figures are not far off published data from USA and European registries (**Table 5**) [11–18]. These data highlight the challenges in translating clinical trial results into "real life" clinical practice. As in most countries, the utilization of anti-VEGF is affected by reimbursement structure and retreatment criteria. In addition to low retreatment number, the number of follow-up visits during the first year was also low (mean 8 visits). Although only three mandatory visits were included in the study protocol (at months 1, 3 and 12), most patients attended much more frequently due to clinical need (mean 8.03 visits). However,it is likely this lack of follow-up and under-treatment contributed significantly towards the low injection numbers, as 48% of eyes still had activity on OCT at month 12, However, similar low follow-up visits (8.06 visits) had been reported from France [17], highlighting the adherence to follow-up is also a challenge in the delivery of AMD care.

We report the mean VA improved significantly by 6.5 letters, with 34.2% gaining 15 ETDRS letters and 14.4% losing ≥15 ETDRS letters. When outcome was analyzed by diagnosis of AMD-CNV versus PCV, there was no significant difference in mean VA change, or of the proportion gaining and losing 15 letters. Visual outcome from several European registries have been summarized in **Table 5** for comparison. In addition to mean change in VA, it is also important to note that patients from the current study had generally worse presenting visual acuity than those from European registries [12–18]. Despite significant mean visual gain, the vision at 1 year remained significantly lower than those from European registries [12–18]. Lower public awareness of AMD and generally later presentation in Asian setting is likely to be a significant explanation for these findings. It is also interesting to note that 35 patients did not receive treatment initially (before their month-3 visit). The most common reasons were poor prognosis (10/19 eyes in the AMD-CNV group and 6/15 eyes in the PCV group), and limited activity at presentation (3/19 in the AMD-CNV group and 8/15 in the PCV group) reason in the PCV group (8/15 eyes). The remaining patients defaulted their follow up. Of these 35 eyes, 10 eyes eventually received treatment from month 4 onwards.

In terms of predictive factors for visual outcome, we identified OCT measurement at baseline and VA at month 3 as significant predictors for both the need to continue treatment beyond month 3 and also vision at month 12. Each 100 μm increase in OCT CMT was correlated to a drop of 3.6 ETDRS letters in visual acuity ($p<0.001$). OCT CMT measurement at month 3 was also predictive of whether treatment was continued after 3 months. Each 100 μm increase in OCT CMT at month 3 was associated with 0.925 additional injections after month 3 ($p=0.025$). The number of injection was only weakly correlated with visual outcome at month 12. Each additional injection was associated with a further 1.7 letters gain in vision at month 12.

In our study, 61.1% of eyes had PCV. Apart from features on ICGA and worse baseline VA in AMD-CNV (0.95 in AMD-CNV vs 0.78 in PCV, $p=0.018$), there were no significant differences in baseline characteristics in terms of age, gender, fellow eye involvement or lens status between AMD-CNV and PCV eyes. These results highlight the importance to screen for PCV with ICGA in an Asian population. Our results showed several major findings regarding PCV treatment in our centre. First, a variety of treatment modalities are currently employed in treating PCV. Second, anti-VEGF use was common, but appears to require less injection number when used as combination therapy. Third, the visual outcome was similar in PCV and AMD-CNV eyes in the anti-VEGF era. Therefore, the role of anti-VEGF therapy in PCV, as monotherapy or as adjunct to occlusive therapies, should be further studied.

There are limitations to this study. The observational design aims to capture the current treatment pattern of exudative AMD in an Asian setting in Singapore. Variations in treatment preference between individual clinicians, between countries and regions are to be expected. Variations in reimbursement systems between countries will also influence the treatment pattern. Practice pattern, such as injection number, is likely to evolve with time and injection numbers may increase with increasing acceptance of the need for long-term therapy. We did not perform secondary grading of PCV but decided to follow the initial clinical diagnosis by the treating clinician. Therefore PCV diagnosis may be less stringent, and some of the PCV cases in this series may represent possible/probable PCV (mixed cases) in addition to definite PCV cases. Due to logistic constraints, OCT examination was performed using SD-OCT other than the Cirrus OCT in some cases. Therefore the OCT thickness measurements in these

Table 5. Comparison of Patient Characteristics and Anti-VEGF Utilization during the First Year of Treatment.

Study origin	USA (2008) [11]	Germany (2008) [12,13]	UK (2007) [14]	UK (2007) [14]	Sweden (2007) [12,15]	Belgium (2008) [12,16]	Netherlands (2008) [12,16]	France (2007) [17]	Beirut (2005) [18]	Korea (2007) [19]	Singapore, Current study (2010)	Singapore, Current study (2010)
Sample size	91,628	3,470	897 (pretreated n = 125)	897 (no pretreatment n = 772)	471	253	243	122	60	41	132 (AMD-CNV, n = 43)	132 (PCV, n = 87)
Mean age, years (SD)	81.1 (7.0)	77.6 (7.8)	75.0 (8.4)		78.1 (8.0)	78.7 (6.8)	77.9 (8.0)	78.3 (7.0)	72.2	70.3 (7.9)	69.6 (10.5)	
Female, %	63.8%	64.6%	-		66.0%	62.1%	59.3%	70.0%	43.1%	51.2%	41.9%	
Mean baseline VA ETDRS letters (SD)	NA	48.8 (18.7)	50.4	54.1	58.3 (12.2)	56.3 (14.2)	45.1 (21.5)	56.2 (14.0)	45.7	42.1	45.5	43.5
Mean VA at 1 year ETDRS letters (SD)	NA	48.0 (11.7)	53.1	57.9	59.3 (16.2)	58.8 (17.9)	50.7 (24.0)	56.9 (17.0)	53.1	46.0	50.0	51.5
Mean number of injections at 1 year (SD)			6.2 (2.6)	5.2 (2.7)							4.51 (2.25)	3.43 (1.73)

Formula of conversion from LogMAR to ETDRS letters: 85-50LogMAR.
AMD - age-related macular degeneration; PCV- polypoidal choroidal vasculopathy; SD standard deviation.

eyes were not incorporated into the current analysis. Post treatment ICGA would have been informative in all cases. However ICGA was only repeated post treatment if there is clinical suspicion (based on fundoscopy, visual acuity and OCT findings) of residual activity.

In conclusion, our prospective study showed significant variation in treatment patterns in Asian eyes with exudative maculopathy. AMD-CNV was treated predominantly with anti-VEGF monotherapy, whereas a variety of treatment modalities were used to treat PCV. Low overall injection numbers over 1 year suggest that many patients may be under-treated in the "real life" setting, a situation not dissimilar to US and European countries. Despite these variations, relatively good visual outcomes at 1 year were achieved in both AMD-CNV and PCV. Nevertheless, these data highlight the need for high quality clinical trial data to provide evidence-based guidelines to optimize the management of Asian AMD.

Acknowledgments

The authors would like to acknowledge Mr. Joseph Ho, principal ophthalmic imaging specialist, Singapore National Eye Centre, for performing the angiography for the Singapore patients.

Author Contributions

Conceived and designed the experiments: CMGC TYW. Performed the experiments: CMGC RM SYL CMC IY BKL EW DW TYW. Analyzed the data: CMGC XL RW TYW. Contributed reagents/materials/analysis tools: CMGC RM SYL CMC IY BKL RW EW DW TYW. Wrote the paper: CMGC.

References

1. Lim LS, Mitchell P, Seddon JM, Holz FG, Wong TY (2012) Age-related macular degeneration. Lancet379: 1728–38
2. Klein R, Klein BE, Knudtson MD, Wong TY, Cotch MF, et al. (2006)Prevalence of age related macular degeneration in 4 racial/ethnic groups in the Multi-ethnic Study of Atherosclerosis. Ophthalmology 113: 373–80.
3. Mitchell P, Smith W, Attebo K, Wang JJ (1995) Prevalence of age-related maculopathy in Australia. The Blue Mountains Eye Study. Ophthalmology 102: 1450–60.
4. Kawasaki R, Yasuda M, Song SJ, Cheng SJ, Jonas JB, et al (2010) The Prevalence of Age-Related Macular Degeneration in Asians. Ophthalmology 117: 921–927.
5. Rosenfeld PJ, Brown DM, Heier JS, Boyer DS, Kaiser PK, et al (2006) Ranibizumab for neovascular age-related macular degeneration. N Eng J Med 355: 1419–31.
6. Brown DM, Kaiser PK, Michels M, Soubrane G, Heier JS, et al (2006) Ranibizumab versus verteportin for neovascular age-related macular degeneration. N Eng J Med 355: 1432–44.
7. The CATT Research Group (2011) Ranibizumab and bevacizumab for neovascular age-related macular degeneration. N Eng J Med 364: 1897–908.
8. The CATT Research Group (2012) Ranibizumab and bevacizumab for neovascular age-related macular degeneration: Two-year results. Ophthalmology 119: 1388–98.
9. Chakravarthy U, Harding SP, Rogers CA, Downes SM, Lotery AJ, et al (2013) Alternative treatments to inhibit VEGF in age-related choroidal neovascularisation: tow-year findings of the IVAN randomised controlled trial. The Lancet. 382: 1258–67.
10. Heier JS, Brown DM, Chong V, Korobelnik JF, Kaiser PK, et al (2012) Intravitreal aflibercept (VEGF trap-eye) in wet age-related macular degeneration. Ophthalmology 119: 2537–48.
11. Curtis LH, Hammill BG, Qualls LG, DiMartino LD, Wang F, et al (2012) Treatment patterns for neovascular age-related macular degeneration: Analysis of 284380 Medicare Beneficiaries. Am J Ophthalmol 153: 1116–1124.
12. Holz FG, Bandello F, Gillies M, Mitchell P, Osborne A, et al (2013) Safety of ranibizumab in routine clinical practice: 1-year retrospective pooled analysis of four European neovascular AMD registries within the LUMINOUS programme. Br J Ophthalmol 97: 1161–7.
13. Finger RP, Wiedemann P, Blumhage F, Pohl K, Holz FG (2013) Treatment patterns, visual acuity and quality-of-life outcomes of the WAVE study- a noninterventional study of ranibizumab treatment for neovascular age-related macular degeneration in Germany. Acta Ophthalmologica 91: 540–6.
14. Pushpoth S, Sykakis E, Merchant K, Browning AC, Gupta R, et al (2012) Measuring the benefit of 4 years of Intravitreal Ranibizumab treatment for neovascular age-related macular degeneration. Br J Ophthalmol 96: 1469–73.
15. Hjelmqvist L, Lindberg C, Kanulf P, Dahlgren H, Johansson I, et al (2011) One-year outcomes using ranibizumab for neovascular age-related macular degeneration. J Ophthalmol 2011: 405724.
16. Rakic JM, Leys A, Brie H, Denhaerynck K, Pacheco C, et al (2013). Real-world variability in ranibizumab treatment and associated clinica, quality of life, and safety outcomes over 24 months in patients with neovascular age-related macular degeneration: the HELIOS study. Clin Ophthalmol 7: 1849–58.
17. Cohen SY, Dubois L, Tadayoni R, Fajnkuchen F, Nghiem-Buffet S, et al (2009) Results of one-year's treatment with ranibizumab for exudative age-related macular degeneration in a clinical setting. Am J Ophthalmol 148: 409–413.
18. Bashshur ZF, Haddad ZA, Schakal A, Jaafar RF, Saab M, et al (2008) Intravitreal bevacizumab for treatment of neovascular age-related macular degeneration: A one-year prospective study. Am J Ophthalmol 145: 249–256.
19. Kang S, Roh YJ (2011) Ranibizumab treatment administered as needed for occult and minimally classic neovascular membranes in age-related macular degeneration. Jpn J Ophthalmol 55: 123–7.
20. Cheung CM, Wong TY (2011) Anti-VEGF Debate: Limitation in Asia New Eng J Med 365: 2237.
21. Lamoureux EL, Mitchell P, Rees G, Cheung G, Yeo I, et al (2011) Impact of early and late age-related macular degeneration on vision-specific function. Br J Ophthalmol 95: 666–70.
22. Laude A, Cackett PD, Vithana EN, Yeo IY, Wong D, et al (2010) Polypoidal choroidal vasculopathy and neovascular age-related macular degeneration: Same or deifferent disease? Prof Ret Eye Res 29: 19–29.
23. Gomi F, Sawa M, Sakaguchi H, Tsujikawa M, Oshima Y, et al (2008) Efficacy of intravitreal bevacizumab for polypoidal choroidal vasculopathy. Br J Ophthalmol 92: 70–73.
24. Lai TY, Chan WM, Liu DT, Luk FO, Lam DS (2008) Intravitreal bevacizumab (Avastin) with or without photodynamic therapy for the treatment of polypoidal choroidal vasclopathy. Br J Ophthalmol 92: 661–666.
25. Koh A, Lee WK, Chen LJ, Chen SJ, Hashad Y, et al (2012) EVEREST STUDY: Efficacy and Safety of Verteporfin Photodynamic Therapy in Combination with Ranibizumab or Alone Versus Ranibizumab Monotherapy in Patients with Symptomatic Macular Polypoidal Choroidal Vasculopathy. Retina. 32: 1453–64
26. Chan WM, Lam DS, Lai TY, Liu DT, Li KK, et al (2004) Photodynamic therapy with verteporfin for symptomatic polypoidal choroidal vasculopathy one-year results of a prospective case series. Ophthalmology 111: 1576–1584.
27. Gomi F, Ohji M, Sayanagi K, Sawa M, Sakaguchi H, et al (2008) One-year outcomes of photodynamic therapy in age-related macular degeneration and polypoidal choroidal vasculopathy in Japanese patients. Ophthalmology 115: 141–146.
28. Kurashige Y, Otani A, Sasahara M, Yodoi Y, Tamura H, et al (2008) Two-year results of photodynamic therapy for polypoidal choroidal vasculopathy. Am J Ophthalmol 146: 513–519.
29. Koh AH, Chen LJ, Chen SJ, Chen Y, Giridhar A, et al (2013) Polypoidal choroidal vasculopathy: Evidence-based guidelines for clinical diagnosis and treatment. Retina 33: 686–716.
30. Cheung CM, Bhargava M, Li X, Mathur R, Mun CC, et al (2013) Six Month Visual Prognosis in Eyes with Submacular Hemorrhage secondary to Age-Related Macular Degeneration or Polypoidal Choroidal Vasculopathy. Graefes Arch Clin Exp Ophthalmol 251: 19–25.
31. Macular Photocoagulation Study Group (1991) Laser photocoagulation of subfoveal neovascular lesions in age-related macular degeneration: Results of a randomized clinical trial. Arch Ophthalmol 109: 1219–1230.
32. Japanese Study Group of Polypoidal Choroidal Vasculopathy (2005) Criteria for diagnosis of polypoidal choroidal vasculopathy. Nippon Ganka Gakkai Zasshi [Japanese] 109: 417–427.
33. Treatment of Age-Related Macular Degeneration with Photodynamic Therapy (TAP) Study Group (1999) Photodynamic therapy of subfoveal choroidal neovascularization in age-related macular degeneration with verteporfin. One-year results of 2 randomized clinical trials- TAP report 1. Arch Ophthalmol 117: 1329–45.

15

Motion of the Esophagus Due to Cardiac Motion

Jacob Palmer, Jinzhong Yang, Tinsu Pan, Laurence E. Court*

Department of Radiation Physics, Unit 94, The University of Texas MD Anderson Cancer Center, Houston, Texas, United States of America

Abstract

When imaging studies (e.g. CT) are used to quantify morphological changes in an anatomical structure, it is necessary to understand the extent and source of motion which can give imaging artifacts (e.g. blurring or local distortion). The objective of this study was to assess the magnitude of esophageal motion due to cardiac motion. We used retrospective electrocardiogram-gated contrast-enhanced computed tomography angiography images for this study. The anatomic region from the carina to the bottom of the heart was taken at deep-inspiration breath hold with the patients' arms raised above their shoulders, in a position similar to that used for radiation therapy. The esophagus was delineated on the diastolic phase of cardiac motion, and deformable registration was used to sequentially deform the images in nearest-neighbor phases among the 10 cardiac phases, starting from the diastolic phase. Using the 10 deformation fields generated from the deformable registration, the magnitude of the extreme displacements was then calculated for each voxel, and the mean and maximum displacement was calculated for each computed tomography slice for each patient. The average maximum esophageal displacement due to cardiac motion for all patients was 5.8 mm (standard deviation: 1.6 mm, maximum: 10.0 mm) in the transverse direction. For 21 of 26 patients, the largest esophageal motion was found in the inferior region of the heart; for the other patients, esophageal motion was approximately independent of superior-inferior position. The esophagus motion was larger at cardiac phases where the electrocardiogram R-wave occurs. In conclusion, the magnitude of esophageal motion near the heart due to cardiac motion is similar to that due to other sources of motion, including respiratory motion and intra-fraction motion. A larger cardiac motion will result into larger esophagus motion in a cardiac cycle.

Editor: Zhuoli Zhang, Northwestern University Feinberg School of Medicine, United States of America

Funding: The authors have no support or funding to report.

Competing Interests: The authors have declared that no competing interests exist.

* E-mail: lecourt@mdanderson.org

Introduction

Many groups have investigated the respiratory motion of radiation targets (i.e., tumors) and normal tissues in the thoracic cavity and the impact of this motion in diagnostic imaging and radiation therapy [1,2,3,4,5,6]. Only a few studies have assessed the effect of cardiac motion in radiation therapy [1,3,7], and, to our knowledge, none have assessed the impact of cardiac motion on esophageal motion. The effects from cardiac and respiratory motions may not generally be separable as most therapy sessions are performed with free-breathing. Also, although respiratory motion can be minimized by either breathhold techniques or abdominal compression, any motion due to cardiac pulsing will remain. This may give a blurring of the dose in radiation therapy (where treatments are several minutes long); the effect in imaging studies will depend on the temporal resolution of the imaging study, but could include blurring or local geometric distortion. This may be particularly important for longitudinal studies that attempt to examine local morphological changes at the voxel level.

There are several reasons why it may be important to accurately image the esophagus – some examples in radiation therapy are given here. The esophagus can be an important dose-limiting structure in radiation therapy treatment planning, but its dose-response characteristics have not been well characterized. That is, although it is known that volumes of the esophagus receiving more than 40–50 Gy correlate significantly with acute esophagitis [8], the impact of the spatial distribution is not yet understood. Some studies have shown that circumferential metrics (i.e., the esophageal length receiving a certain full-circumference dose) are statistically significant [9,10], but they have not been shown to be superior to dose-volume metrics. One likely reason for this is that the spatial extent (location) and severity of esophagitis is currently unknown, so easily determining the exact impact of the spatial dose distribution on the local tissue is not possible. Several imaging techniques could be used to do this on a voxel-by-voxel basis, thus allowing the calculation of a true voxel-by-voxel dose-response curve. One such technique uses computed tomography (CT) images to measure the esophageal swelling that occurs as a result of radiation damage [11]. Another possible technique is the use of positron emission tomography (PET) images. Although this second technique has yet to be used to assess esophageal toxicity, it has been successfully used to show a relationship between dose and standardized uptake values (SUV) for radiation-induced lung toxicity [12]. The effects of motion (attributed to respiration or some other source) on these techniques is complex, and will depend on details of the imaging technique used, but could include blurring (depending on temporal resolution) or local geometric distortions in the esophageal shape. These effects could be particularly relevant when trying to assess changes in the esophagus (CT or PET, etc.) on a voxel-by-voxel level). Thus, it is important to understand the effects of motion prior to using imaging (CT or PET) to understand the dose-response of the esophagus. Therefore, we initiated this study to assess the impact of cardiac motion on the esophagus as an important step toward understanding the different causes of motion uncertainty.

Materials and Methods

Patient data

A total of 26 patients who had received contrast-enhanced CT-based coronary angiography with retrospective electrocardiographic gating had been randomly selected in a previous study [7]. The use of these data for the current study was approved by the Institutional Review Board at The University of Texas MD Anderson Cancer Center (PA12-0340), including a specific waiver to obtain written consent from the patient for this retrospective data review study. The images were taken using a GE LightSpeed VCT 64-slice CT scanner (GE Healthcare, Waukesha, WI) and deep-inspiration breath hold with patients' arms raised above their shoulders, in a position similar to that used for radiation therapy. For each patient, 10 CT data sets were reconstructed over a cardiac cycle from the carina to the bottom of the heart. These images had 1.25-mm slice thickness and 0.35×0.35 mm^2 pixel size. The images corresponding to the diastolic phases of cardiac motion were imported into a Pinnacle[3] treatment planning system (Philips Medical Systems, Fitchburg, WI), and the esophagus was delineated on a single, consistent phase using standard delineation tools.

Motion analysis

For each patient the image sets comprised 10 CT data sets ($T_0, T_{10}, \ldots, T_{90}$) over a cardiac cycle. (The images are reconstructed from multiple cardiac cycles. The phases of the images are over a cardiac cycle from 0% to 90% like the ones in 4D-CT.) We used an in-house deformable image registration tool to perform the motion analysis based on the 10 phases of CT images. An accelerated Demons algorithm [13] was applied to sequentially register the 10 CT images and generate 10 displacement fields ($T_0 \rightarrow T_{10}$, $T_{10} \rightarrow T_{20}$, ... $T_{90} \rightarrow T_0$). We validated the deformation visually by comparing the deformed images with the original image. The 10 displacement fields were concatenated to form the motion trajectory for each voxel in a cardiac cycle. The voxel-level motion trajectory is illustrated in Figure 1. The motion magnitudes in three directions—left-right (LR), anterior-posterior (AP), and superior-inferior (SI)—were computed for each voxel by measuring the maximum range of the trajectory in all three directions. The total motion magnitude for each voxel was computed as

$$M_T = \sqrt{M_{LR}^2 + M_{AP}^2 + M_{SI}^2},$$

where M_{LR}, M_{AP}, and M_{SI}, are the motion magnitudes in the LR, AP, and SI directions, respectively. The motion trajectory for voxels inside the esophagus contour constitutes the esophageal motion. For each patient, and for each CT slice, the mean and maximum motions at each direction (LR, AP, and SI) and the total motion magnitudes were calculated. Then, for each patient, the maximum values of these mean and maximum motions over all slices were calculated. Finally, the mean, standard deviation, and maximum range of these values were calculated for the overall patient population. Note, when calculating the motion in a slice, we noticed that the motion in SI direction was not reliable and difficult to validate its accuracy. Therefore, we reported the motion in the transverse direction without taking into account the SI motion. In addition, the esophagus motion of each cardiac phase was analyzed, which might be beneficial for determining the optimal imaging temporal resolution or acquisition phase in a future study. For each patient, the maximum motion of esophagus was determined from the 10 displacement fields for each phase, and the averaged maximum motion was calculated from the overall patient population for comparison among different phases.

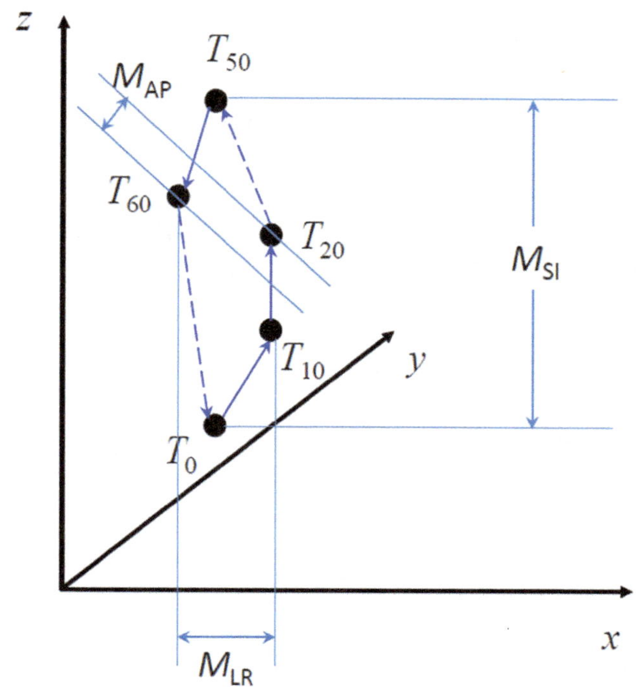

Figure 1. Illustration of voxel-level motion trajectory. The displacement vectors from $T_0 \rightarrow T_{10}$, $T_{10} \rightarrow T_{20}$, ... $T_{90} \rightarrow T_0$ are concatenated together to form this motion trajectory. The motion magnitudes in three directions, M_{LR}, M_{AP}, and M_{SI}, were computed by measuring the maximum range of the trajectory in all three directions: left-right (LR), anterior-posterior (AP), and superior-inferior (SI).

Results

The maximum esophageal displacement due to cardiac motion varied between patients, up to 10 mm in the transverse direction. The average maximum esophageal displacement due to cardiac motion for all patients was 5.8 mm (standard deviation: 1.6 mm) in the transverse direction. The extent of motion is patient specific. Table 1 shows the analyzed results for all 26 patients. The mean and maximum peak-to-peak motion of the esophagus was a function of the superior-inferior position, as shown in the example of Figure 2. For 21 of the 26 patients, the largest esophageal motion was found in the inferior region. For the remaining 5 patients, the esophageal peak-to-peak motion was constant (within ~1 mm) throughout the imaged region. When viewing individual axial slices, the largest esophageal motion was in the esophageal wall closest to the heart or the aorta. Figure 3 showed the averaged maximum esophagus motion versus cardiac phase over 26 patients, including total motion magnitude and motions in LR, AP, and SI directions. The motion was found maximum at T80 with 3.6 mm and minimum at T60 with 2.2 mm. Overall, the motion was larger at phases T0, T10, T80, and T90, where the electrocardiogram R-wave occurs. Figure 3 also showed that SI direction had slightly larger motion than LR and AP directions, but this might not be true because images used for analysis had

Table 1. The analyzed results for 26 patients.

No.	Mean motion (mm)					Maximum motion (mm)				
	LR	AP	SI	Axial	Total	LR	AP	SI	Axial	Total
1	1.8	2.9	5.0	3.4	6.1	5.3	5.3	12.7	6.0	12.9
2	2.0	1.6	2.0	2.5	3.3	6.3	3.4	6.4	6.7	8.4
3	1.6	2.7	2.9	3.2	3.8	4.0	6.5	8.7	7.0	9.8
4	1.4	1.3	2.1	1.9	2.8	3.1	2.6	5.8	3.8	6.0
5	1.5	1.2	2.1	1.9	2.7	4.6	3.8	4.5	5.9	7.1
6	1.1	1.1	2.5	1.6	2.9	3.0	3.1	7.4	3.7	7.5
7	2.1	2.2	2.5	3.0	3.5	4.8	4.0	6.1	5.8	8.3
8	2.0	1.7	2.4	2.5	3.4	5.8	4.5	4.9	6.3	7.7
9	1.6	1.9	4.0	2.5	4.7	6.2	5.5	8.6	8.2	10.2
10	2.1	1.9	3.5	2.8	4.5	6.5	4.9	10.4	7.4	11.6
11	1.4	1.3	2.1	1.8	2.7	4.6	2.9	6.4	5.3	6.9
12	1.7	1.6	3.4	2.2	4.0	4.1	3.8	8.4	5.0	8.4
13	1.0	1.3	1.8	1.6	2.4	3.2	3.6	5.0	4.8	6.2
14	3.1	2.5	4.9	4.0	6.3	8.8	5.6	9.8	10.0	13.7
15	1.3	1.5	1.9	2.0	2.8	3.8	4.5	5.0	4.8	5.7
16	3.3	5.3	4.3	6.2	7.6	6.0	7.4	7.1	8.7	11.0
17	1.5	1.3	2.4	2.0	3.1	4.3	3.6	8.2	5.1	9.4
18	2.5	2.1	3.9	3.3	5.2	6.6	4.5	11.3	6.9	12.8
19	1.8	1.6	2.1	2.2	3.1	3.3	3.8	4.0	4.0	5.5
20	1.4	1.6	1.8	1.9	2.5	4.7	3.4	3.7	5.5	6.0
21	1.6	1.5	3.7	2.2	4.3	5.1	3.7	7.8	5.4	9.4
22	1.2	1.5	1.9	1.8	2.6	2.6	2.8	4.0	3.3	4.9
23	1.7	1.3	2.4	2.2	3.3	6.4	3.8	4.9	6.6	8.0
24	1.6	1.9	3.1	2.5	4.0	3.6	4.5	9.4	5.5	9.9
25	1.1	1.1	1.6	1.5	2.2	3.0	3.0	4.9	4.0	5.2
26	1.3	1.4	2.9	1.7	3.4	3.3	2.8	6.1	3.8	6.6
Mean	1.7	1.8	2.8	2.5	3.7	4.7	4.1	7.0	5.8	8.4
SD	0.6	0.9	1.0	1.0	1.3	1.5	1.2	2.4	1.6	2.5

For each patient, and for each CT slice, the mean and maximum motions at each direction—left-right (LR), anterior-posterior (AP), and superior-inferior (SI)—and the total motion magnitudes were calculated. Then, for each patient, the maximum values of these mean and maximum motions over all slices were calculated and presented in this table. The mean and standard deviation (SD) were calculated for all 26 patients as well. Because the motion in SI direction was not reliable and difficult to validate, we also reported the motion in the transverse (Axial) direction without taking into account the SI motion.

1.25 mm resolution in SI dimension but 0.35 mm in LR and AP dimensions, thus resulting the motion calculation in SI direction was less accurate than LR and AP directions.

Discussion

The results of this study showed that parts of the esophagus move more than the rest of the esophagus due to cardiac motion. To our knowledge, this is the first study to assess the impact of cardiac motion on the position of the esophagus. In fact, only a few studies have assessed the impact of cardiac motion on radiation therapy at any site. Steppenwolde et al. reported that the cardiac beat can cause a displacement of 1–4 mm in the position of markers in the lung, depending on their location, which ranged from 15 mm to 65 mm from the cardiac or aortic wall [1].

The esophagus is subject to other sources of motion, including respiratory motion and intrafraction motion (e.g., relative shifts in position over an interval of several minutes). Pan et al. reported that the esophagus clearly moves during breathing, and the magnitude depends largely on the individual and on the level of the esophagus, ranging from 5 mm in the AP and LR directions at the thoracic inlet to larger than 10 mm at the gastroesophageal junction in these two directions [14]. Several authors have evaluated the respiratory motion of esophageal cancers (rather than healthy esophagus studied here). Yaremko et al. [15] used deformable registration to map the respiratory motion of the gross tumor volume for distal esophageal cancer and found that the mean tumor motion was 9 mm (95th percentile: 20 mm) for a total motion magnitude. Patel et al. conducted a similar study that included several tumors in the proximal two-thirds of the esophagus (corresponding closer to the anatomic region we assessed in our study), and the total displacements due to respiratory motion were less than 4 mm in the transverse direction [16]. Cohen et al. evaluated the intrafraction motion of the esophagus [4]. They compared CT images taken using a CT-on-rails system before and after radiotherapy and found that intrafraction motion of the esophagus in LR and AP directions was greater than 5 mm for 13% of cases and greater than 10 mm

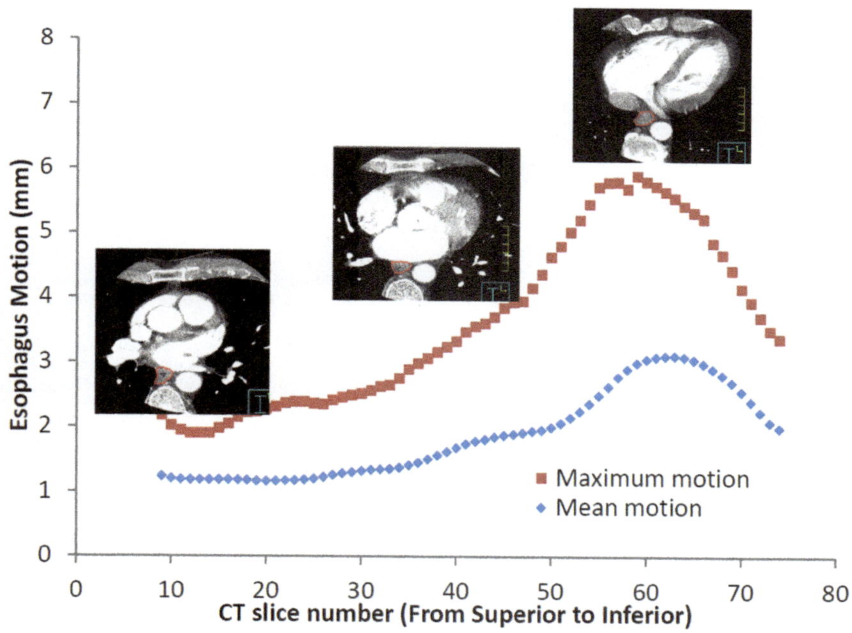

Figure 2. Variation of mean and maximum esophageal motion as a function of CT slice number.

for 4% of cases. Thus, for some parts of the esophagus that are in the vicinity of the heart, the impact of cardiac motion (from our study) appears to be comparable to that of respiratory motion (compared with the data of Pan et al). Away from the heart, in the distal region, respiratory motion likely dominates, although our study did not include images away from the heart.

Conclusion

In conclusion, cardiac motion results in displacements of 5–10 mm for some parts of the esophagus, depending on patient and location. This magnitude is similar to that of other sources of motion, including respiratory motion and intrafraction motion. A

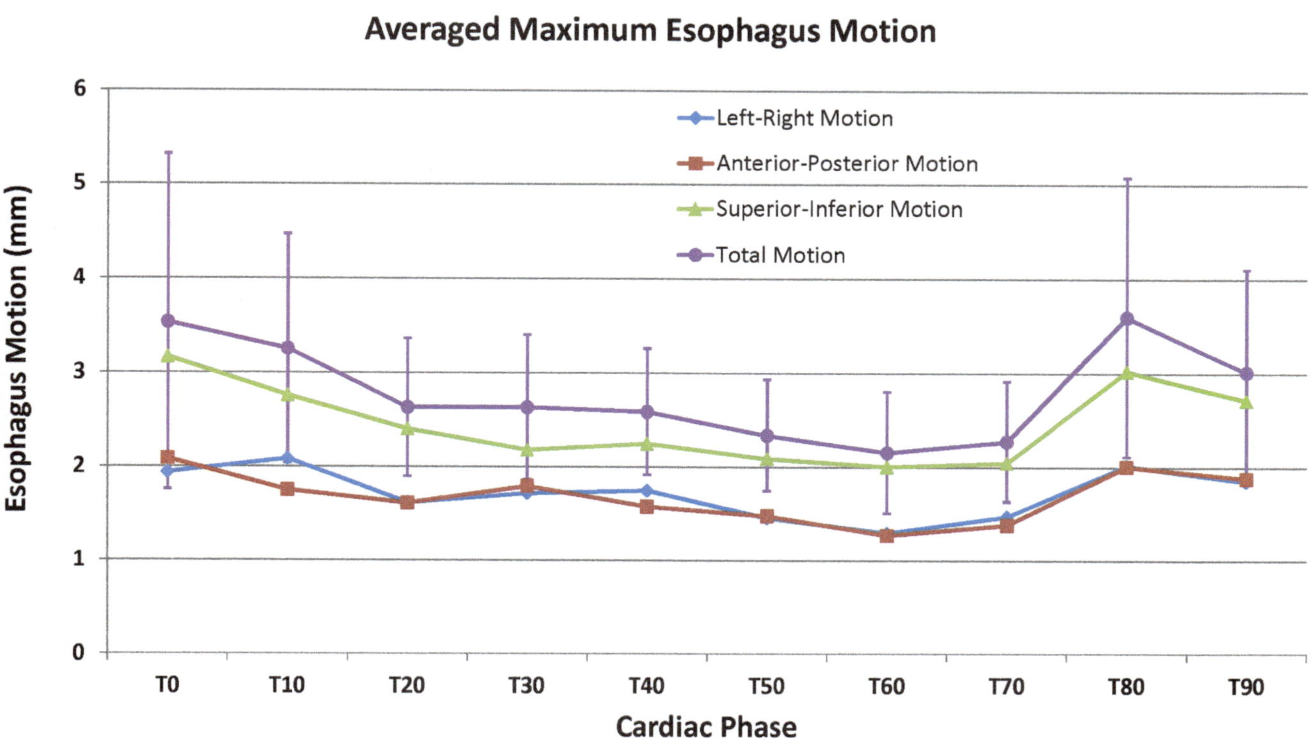

Figure 3. Averaged maximum esophagus motion versus cardiac phase over 26 patients. Error bars for total motion indicate the standard deviation over 26 patients.

larger cardiac motion will result into larger esophagus motion in a cardiac cycle.

Author Contributions

Conceived and designed the experiments: LEC JP JY TP. Performed the experiments: JP JY. Analyzed the data: JP JY LEC. Contributed reagents/materials/analysis tools: JY. Wrote the paper: LEC JY JP TP.

References

1. Seppenwoolde Y, Shirato H, Kitamura K, Shimizu S, van Herk M, et al. (2002) Precise and real-time measurement of 3D tumor motion in lung due to breathing and heartbeat, measured during radiotherapy. International Journal of Radiation Oncology Biology Physics 53: 822–834.
2. Langen KM, Jones DTL (2001) Organ motion and its management. International Journal of Radiation Oncology*Biology*Physics 50: 265–278.
3. Korreman SS (2012) Motion in radiotherapy: photon therapy. Physics in Medicine and Biology 57: R161–R191.
4. Cohen RJ, Paskalev K, Litwin S, Price RA Jr, Feigenberg SJ, et al. (2010) Original article: Esophageal motion during radiotherapy: quantification and margin implications. Diseases of the Esophagus 23: 473–479.
5. Callahan J, Kron T, Schneider-Kolsky M, Hicks RJ (2011) The clinical significance and management of lesion motion due to respiration during PET/CT scanning. Cancer Imaging 11: 224–236.
6. Bettinardi V, Picchio M, Di Muzio N, Gianolli L, Gilardi MC, et al. (2010) Detection and compensation of organ/lesion motion using 4D-PET/CT respiratory gated acquisition techniques. Radiotherapy and Oncology 96: 311–316.
7. Wang XC, Pan TS, Pinnix C, Zhang SX, Salehpour M, et al. (2012) Cardiac Motion during Deep-Inspiration Breath-Hold: Implications for Breast Cancer Radiotherapy. International Journal of Radiation Oncology Biology Physics 82: 708–714.
8. Werner-Wasik M, Yorke E, Deasy J, Nam J, Marks LB (2010) Radiation Dose-Volume Effects in the Esophagus. International Journal of Radiation Oncology*Biology*Physics 76: S86–S93.
9. Ahn S-J, Kahn D, Zhou S, Yu X, Hollis D, et al. (2005) Dosimetric and clinical predictors for radiation-induced esophageal injury. International Journal of Radiation Oncology*Biology*Physics 61: 335–347.
10. Belderbos J, Heemsbergen W, Hoogeman M, Pengel K, Rossi M, et al. (2005) Acute esophageal toxicity in non-small cell lung cancer patients after high dose conformal radiotherapy. Radiotherapy and Oncology 75: 157–164.
11. Court LE, Tucker SL, Gomez D, Liao ZX, Zhang J, et al. (2013) A technique to use CT images for in vivo detection and quantification of the spatial distribution of radiation-induced esophagitis. Journal of Applied Clinical Medical Physics 14: 91–98.
12. Guerrero T, Johnson V, Hart J, Pan T, Khan M, et al. (2007) Radiation pneumonitis: Local dose versus [F-18]-fluorodeoxyglucose uptake response in irradiated lung. International Journal of Radiation Oncology Biology Physics 68: 1030–1035.
13. Wang H, Dong L, Lii MF, Lee AL, de Crevoisier R, et al. (2005) Implementation and validation of a three-dimensional deformable registration algorithm for targeted prostate cancer radiotherapy. International Journal of Radiation Oncology*Biology*Physics 61: 725–735.
14. Pan CC, Kashani R, Hayman JA, Kessler ML, Balter JM (2004) Intra- and inter-fraction esophagus motion in 3D-conformal radiotherapy: Implications for ICRU 62 definitions of internal target volume and planning organ at risk volume. International Journal of Radiation Oncology*Biology*Physics 60: S580–S581.
15. Yaremko BP, Guerrero TM, McAleer MF, Bucci MK, Noyola-Martinez J, et al. (2008) Determination of Respiratory Motion for Distal Esophagus Cancer Using Four-Dimensional Computed Tomography. International Journal of Radiation Oncology*Biology*Physics 70: 145–153.
16. Patel AA, Wolfgang JA, Niemierko A, Hong TS, Yock T, et al. (2009) Implications of Respiratory Motion as Measured by Four-Dimensional Computed Tomography for Radiation Treatment Planning of Esophageal Cancer. International Journal of Radiation Oncology*Biology*Physics 74: 290–296.

The Diagnostic Performance of Coronary Artery Angiography with 64-MSCT and Post 64-MSCT

Min Li[1]*[⁹], Xiang-min Du[2⁹], Zhi-tao Jin[3], Zhao-hui Peng[1], Juan Ding[1], Li Li[1]

1 Department of Medical Imaging, Jinan Military General Hospital, Jinan, Shandong Province, China, **2** Department of Medical Engineering, Jinan Military General Hospital, Jinan, Shandong Province, China, **3** Department of Cardiology, General Hospital of the Second Artillery, Beijing, China

Abstract

Purpose: To comprehensively investigate the diagnostic performance of coronary artery angiography with 64-MDCT and post 64-MDCT.

Materials and Methods: PubMed was searched for all published studies that evaluated coronary arteries with 64-MDCT and post 64-MDCT. The clinical diagnostic role was evaluated by applying the likelihood ratios (LRs) to calculate the post-test probability based on Bayes' theorem.

Results: 91 studies that met our inclusion criteria were ultimately included in the analysis. The pooled positive and negative LRs at patient level were 8.91 (95% CI, 7.53, 10.54) and 0.02 (CI, 0.01, 0.03), respectively. For studies that did not claim that non-evaluable segments were included, the pooled positive and negative LRs were 11.16 (CI, 8.90, 14.00) and 0.01 (CI, 0.01, 0.03), respectively. For studies including uninterruptable results, the diagnostic performance decreased, with the pooled positive LR 7.40 (CI, 6.00, 9.13) and negative LR 0.02 (CI, 0.01, 0.03). The areas under the summary ROC curve were 0.98 (CI, 0.97 to 0.99) for 64-MDCT and 0.96 (CI, 0.94 to 0.98) for post 64-MDCT, respectively. For references explicitly stating that the non-assessable segments were included during analysis, a post-test probability of negative results >95% and a positive post-test probability <95% could be obtained for patients with a pre-test probability of <73% for coronary artery disease (CAD). On the other hand, when the pre-test probability of CAD was >73%, the diagnostic role was reversed, with a positive post-test probability of CAD >95% and a negative post-test probability of CAD <95%.

Conclusion: The diagnostic performance of post 64-MDCT does not increase as compared with 64-MDCT. CTA, overall, is a test of exclusion for patients with a pre-test probability of CAD<73%, while for patients with a pre-test probability of CAD> 73%, CTA is a test used to confirm the presence of CAD.

Editor: Rozemarijn Vliegenthart, University of Groningen, Netherlands

Funding: These authors have no support or funding to report.

Competing Interests: The authors have declared that no competing interests exist.

* E-mail: liminyingxiang@163.com

⁹ These authors contributed equally to this work.

Introduction

Coronary artery disease (CAD) is the leading illness threating human health in developed countries and it is increasingly becoming a significant public health problem in developing countries [1]. With the development of the 16-multi-detector CT (MDCT), a non-invasive approach of coronary CT angiography (CTA), it has been applied widely to avoid the complications of invasive coronary angiography (ICA), which is generally believed to be the gold standard in evaluating CAD [2].

Several meta-analysis studies have proven that single source 64-MDCT with improved parameters has a better ability to predict the stenosis of coronary artery lumen than that of 16-MDCT [3–5]. With the emergence and wider application of dual source 64-, 128-, 256-, and 320-MDCT it is hoped that the improvement will lead to a greater diagnostic accuracy than 64-MDCT. To our knowledge, no study has statistically proven that this claim is correct.

In particular, the CAD diagnosis is not only dependent upon the accuracy of CTA, but also upon pre-test probability, which is estimated according to the symptoms and examinations [3,6–8]. The pre-test probability categorization is important because of its significant impact on the post-test probability of disease and the selection of a diagnostic test [8]. Appropriate application of CTA may improve patients' clinical outcomes, while the inappropriate utilization of CTA may generate extra radiation exposure to patients and unwarranted costs. Since there are already a number of risk algorithms available to evaluate the detailed pre-test probability [9–12], we evaluated the diagnostic role of CTA based on the diagnostic performance of CTA and the precise pre-test probability to provide a more practical patient-relevant utility of CTA.

Materials and Methods

Generally, we followed a standard protocol based on the Preferred Reporting Items for Systematic Reviews and Meta-analyses (PRISMA) statement [13].

Selection of Studies

PubMed was searched for all published studies that examined patients with 64-MDCT and post-64-MDCT. The language was limited to English and the search terms were, "computed tomography," "multi-slice computed tomography," "multi-section computed tomography," "multi-detector computed tomography," and "coronary angiography."

The literature search ranged from 2004 to 2013, as 64-MDCT was first introduced into clinical practice in 2004. The references of published systematic reviews and meta-analyses were also screened. Two readers examined the studies to exclude potential duplicate or overlapping data.

Study Eligibility

The title and abstract were reviewed first. If considered suitable or in doubt, the full text was screened. The inclusion criterion were listed as follows: 64-MDCT or post-64-MDCT was applied as a test to diagnose stenostic CAD (stenosis >50%); the absolute numbers of true-positive, false-positive, true-negative, and false-negative results were presented or can be calculated from the detailed data; and ICA served as the reference standard. Studies were excluded for the following reasons: they included patients who had undergone bypass graft surgery (CABG), percutaneous coronary intervention (PCI), or prior heart transplantation; they were retrospective studies.

Data Extraction

Two investigators extracted the data independently. The following information was extracted from each study: first author, year of publication, country, number of patients, sex, age, heart rate, calcium scoring, the type and brand of machine used, temporal resolution, electrocardiographic (ECG) triggered scanning protocols, prevalence of CAD as well as non-diagnostic segments, and numbers of true-positive, true-negative, false-positive, and false-negative values. While most studies applied a 15-segment scheme of the coronary artery tree, several articles used other alternative protocols, such as 13-, 14-, 16-, and 17-segment models. The scheme of the coronary arterial tree for stenostic analysis was also extracted. Two readers assessed methodological quality independently and according to the QUADAS items [14].

Data Synthesis and Statistical Analysis

Cohen κ test was conducted to evaluate the inter-observer agreement. The publication bias was assessed by the method developed by Deeks, et al. [15]. The heterogeneity across studies was evaluated by I^2 test [16] and the impact of potential covariates was examined using meta-regression. Possible sources of heterogeneity were predefined based on QUADAS items, average age, gender, vendor, temporal resolution, number of slices, the scheme used to evaluate the coronary arterial tree, non-assessable segments, calcium score, protocol of ECG-triggered scanning, prevalence of CAD, and study quality score. A hierarchical summary receiver operating characteristic curves (sROC) was conducted based on the parameters estimated by the bivariate model. The area under the sROC (AUROC) serves as a global measure of CTA performance [17].

The available data was synthesized by an exact binomial rendition of the bivariate mixed-effects regression model [18-20]. We mainly calculated the positive and negative likelihood ratios (LRs) and 95% confidence intervals (CIs) to eliminate the influence of the prevalence of CAD [21] and to compute post-test probability. The LRs indicate by how much a given test would raise or lower the probability of having the disease.

Furthermore, the clinical, or patient-relevant, utility of the diagnostic test was evaluated by using the LRs and the pre-test probability of CAD to calculate the post-test probability based on Bayes' theorem [22]. The log-odds of the posterior probability, which show the chance to diagnose the disease after the test, is a linear function of the log-odds of prior probability and the log likelihood ratio of the target test, which is depicted visually with Fagan's nomogram [23]. The Fagan's nomogram plots an axis on the left with the prior log-odds, an axis in the middle representing the log likelihood ratio of the test, and an axis on the right representing the posterior log-odds. A straight line is drawn from the prior probability on the left axis through the likelihood ratios in the middle and extended to the posterior probability on the right. Thus, the posterior probability is estimated from the prior probability and the likelihood ratio of the test. The pre-test and post-test probabilities are both subjective estimates of the presence of a disease before and after a diagnostic test. The detailed pre-test probability of CAD could be calculated from clinical data and one or more proceeding tests [9,10]. The post-test probability, in turn, can be calculated, depending on whether CTA falls out as a positive test or a negative test. If the positive or negative post-test probability is larger than 95%, the test is treated as an effective tool to confirm or exclude CAD. The overall diagnostic role of CTA at artery and segment levels was represented graphically by an LR scattergram introduced by Stengel et al. [24].

The data was analyzed using STATA (version 12), MetaDiSc (version 1.4), as well as SPSS (version 16.0).

Results

The Characteristics of CT Studies

91 studies that met our inclusion criteria were finally included in the analysis (Figure 1 shows the literature search and selection algorithm). 48 studies performed CTA with single source, 64-MDCT; 26 studies with dual source, 64-MDCT; 6 with dual source, 128-MDCT; 9 with single source, 320-MDCT; 1 with single and dual source, 64-MDCT; and 1 with single source, 64-MDCT and 320-MDCT. 55 studies scanned the coronary artery with retrospective ECG gating, 21 studies with prospective protocol, 4 studies with retrospective and prospective ECG gating, and 11 studies did not report the detailed information. 36 studies reported a calcium score ranging from 47.7 to 821. The radiation dose ranged from 0.76 mSv to 21.4 mSv. Further information on the characteristics of each study is illustrated in Table 1.

Methodological Quality

The inter-observer agreement for assessing quality items was good ($\kappa = 0.83$). According to the QUADAS tool, 62 studies had a quality score of $\geqq 10$ and 29 studies had a quality score of <10. Table S1 demonstrates the QUADAS quality of the included studies.

Data Synthesis and Statistical Analysis

A total of 126,615 segments, 21,834 vessels, and 9,696 patients were analyzed. The publication bias was significant at the patient, artery and segment levels ($P = 0.004$, 0.001 and 0.005 respectively). The pooled positive and negative LRs at patient level were

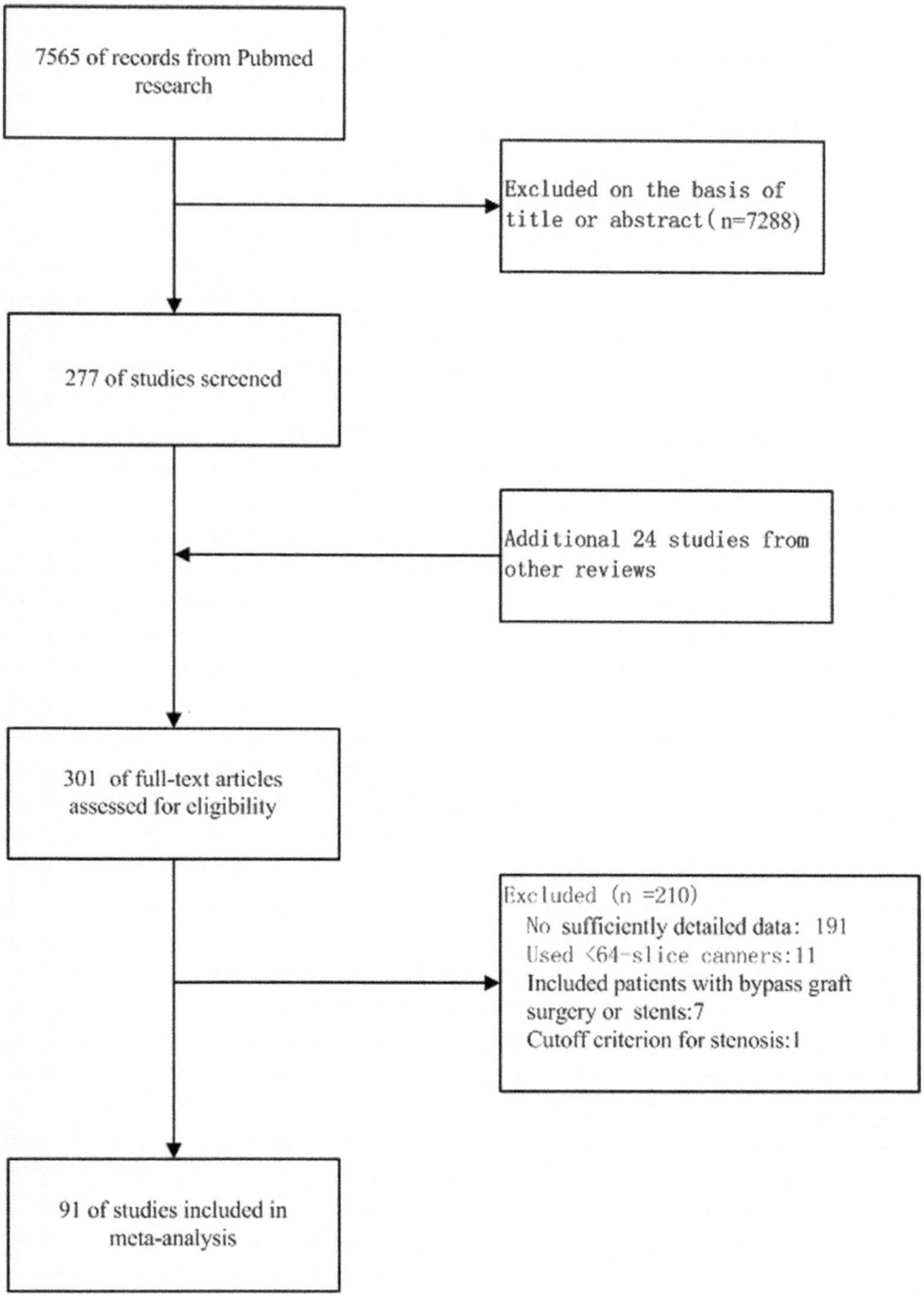

Figure 1. The flow chart for references searching and selection. After careful searching and selection, 91 studies were finally included in the analysis.

8.91 (95% CI, 7.53, 10.54) and 0.02 (CI, 0.01, 0.03), respectively. At the patient level, significant heterogeneity was detected for positive and negative LRs (Q = 976.63; $P<0.001$; $I^2 = 88.58\%$ [CI, 88.58%, 91.55%]; Q = 476.01; $P<0.001$; $I^2 = 79.62\%$ [CI, 75.88%, 83.37%], respectively).

As methodological quality may significantly influence diagnostic accuracy, we investigated the impact of QUADAS items on the heterogeneity. We found that item 13 was the only key factor for heterogeneity (P = 0.02). In the present study, item 13 was defined as, "How authors handled uninterpretable results." For studies that did not claim that non-evaluable segments were included, the pooled positive and negative LRs at patient level were 11.16 (CI, 8.90, 14.00) and 0.01 (CI, 0.01, 0.03), respectively. Slight heterogeneity was detected for positive and negative LRs (Q = 67.06; $P<0.001$; $I^2 = 89.78\%$ [CI, 89.78%, 92.36%]; Q = 78.23; $P<0.001$; $I^2 = 38.64\%$ [CI, 17.37%, 59.91%], respectively).

Table 1. Characteristics of Included Studies.

Authors	Year	Country	Male/ female	Mean age(y)	Scanner	Temporal resolusion(ms)	ECG triggered protocol	NO. of slice	HR(bpm)	Calcium score	Undiagnosis segments	Scheme to evaluate coronary tree	Radiation dose(mSv)
Leber[41]	2005	Germany	...	64	Siemens	165	R	64	62	...	0	15	10–14
Leschka[42]	2005	Switzerland	2.84	60	Siemens	165	R	64	66	...	0	15	...
Mollet[43]	2005	Netherlands	1.89	58	Siemens	165	R	64	58	231	0	16	15.2–21.4
Pugliese[44]	2005	Netherlands	1.5	61	Siemens	165	R	64	58		0.03	17	15–20
Raff[45]	2005	United States	3.12	59	Siemens	165	R	64	65	326	0.12	15	13–18
Ehara[46]	2006	Japan	3.06	67	Siemens	165	R	64	72	...	0.05	14	...
Ghostine[47]	2006	France	1.54	69	Siemens	165	R	64	67	...	0.06	15	7
Meijboom[48]	2006	Netherlands	2.33	63	Siemens	165	R	64	60	214	...	17	15.2 –21.4
Nikolaou[49]	2006	Germany	4.54	63	Siemens	165	R	64	61	...	0.1	15	8.8–13.6
Plass[50]	2006	Switzerland	3.54	66	Siemens	165	R	64	65	...	0.03	11	...
Ropers[51]	2006	Germany	1.63	58	Siemens	83	R	64	59	...	0.04	17	7.45–10.24
Scheffel[52]	2006	Switzerland	4	63.1	Siemens	83	R	64	70.3	821	0.014	...	...
Schuijf[53]	2006	Netherlands	3.29	60	Toshiba	200	R	64	60	423	0.014	...	...
Cademartiri[54]	2007	Italy	1.12	53.9	Siemens	165	R	64	60.6	47.7	0.004	17	15.2–21.4
Herzog[55]	2007	Germany	1.12	67	Siemens	165	R	64	64	...	0.076	15	...
Herzog[56]	2007	Germany	1.22	61	Siemens	165	R	64	72	...	...	15	...
Heuschmid[57]	2007	Germany	2.64	64	Siemens	83	R	64	65	779	0.046	13	...
Johnson[58]	2007	Germany	2.18	60	Siemens	83	R	64	68	...	0.02	15	4.6–7.8
Leber[59]	2007	Germany	1.73	58	Siemens	83	R	64		...	...	13	9.6
Meijboom[60]	2007	Netherlands	2.06	56.2	Siemens	165	R	64	59	...	...	17	13.4–17
Meijboom[61]	2007	Netherlands	2.59	58	Siemens	165	R	64	58	450	...	17	15.2–21.4
Oncel1[62]	2007	Turkey	3.21	56	Siemens	165	R	64	58	...	0	15	...
Ropers[63]	2007	Italy	1.70	61	Siemens	83	R	64	64	...	...	...	15.3
Scheffel[64]	2007	Switzerland	3.17	54	Siemens	165	...	64	65.5	136	0.018	15	8.8–13.6
Schlosser[65]	2007	Germany	1.86	62.4	Siemens	165	...	64	57	...	0.01	15	...
Weustink[66]	2007	Netherlands	3.76	61	Siemens	83	R	64	68	...	0.06	17	11.1–14.4
Achenbach[67]	2008	Germany	0.8	65	Siemens	165	R	64	64.5	...	0.12	17	12.6
Achenbach[67]	2008	Germany	1.78	61	Siemens	83	R	64	64.3	...	0.04	17	14.7
Alkadhi[68]	2008	Switzerland	2.19	62.9	Siemens	83	R	64	68.5	309	0.019	16	7–9
Brodoefel[69]	2008	Germany	4	62	Siemens	83	R	64	64.9	786.5	0.098	15	...
Han[70]	2008	Taiwan	...	59.64	GE	175	R	64	...	...	...	15	...
Herzog[71]	2008	Switzerland	1.73	58.8	GE	175	P	64	55.7	...	0.04	16	2.1
Leschka[72]	2008	Switzerland	0.54	64.1	Siemens	165	R	64	63.9	...	0.014	15	...
Leschka[73]	2008	Switzerland	2.077	61.9	Siemens	83	R	64	67.7	720	0.021	15	7–9

Table 1. Cont.

Authors	Year	Country	Male/ female	Mean age(y)	Scanner	Temporal resolusion(ms)	ECG triggered protocol	NO. of slice	HR(bpm)	Calcium score	Undiagnosis segments	Scheme to evaluate coronary tree	Radiation dose(mSv)
Maruyama[74]	2008	Japan	2.73	69.1	GE	175	R	64	56.1	...	0.045	15	21.1
Maruyama[74]	2008	Japan	1.62	69.9	GE	175	P	64	54.6	...	0.034	15	4.3
Miller[75]	2008	Multi-countries	2.83	59	Toshiba	200	R	64	60	80	...	19	13.8–15.2
Pugliese[76]	2008	Netherlands	3.25	59	Siemens	165	R	64	58	440	0.026	17	15–20
Pundziute[77]	2008	Netherlands	0.98	60	Toshiba	200	R	64	...	216	...	17	...
Ravipati[78]	2008	United States	1.94	66	Siemens	83	...	64	...	...	...	...	...
Scheffel[79]	2008	Switzerland	1.44	68	Siemens	83	P	64	59	238	0.017	...	1.6
Stolzmann[80]	2008	Switzerland	0.72	65.8	Siemens	83	P	64	60.7	316	0.04	16	2.6
Dewey[81]	2009	Germany	2.63	61	Toshiba	175	P	320	59.9	384	0	16	4.2
Gaudio[82]	2009	Italy	1.68	65	Siemens	165	R	64	...	...	...	...	10.6
Herzog[83]	2009	Switzerland	2.23	62	GE	165	P	64	55.4	...	0.0282	16	2.1
Leschka[84]	2009	United States	4	62	Siemens	75	P	128	58	...	0.01	16	0.9
Meng[85]	2009	China	1.66	63	Siemens	83	...	64	71.8	821	0.02	15	...
Pontone[86]	2009	Italy	7	64.8	GE	175	P	64	54.7	375	0.04	15	5.7
Pontone[86]	2009	Italy	4.33	64.3	GE	175	R	64	57.4	334	0.03	...	20.5
Reimann[87]	2009	Germany	2.75	62	Siemens	83	R	64	62.7	707	0	13	...
Rixe[88]	2009	Germany	1.62	65	Siemens	83	R	64	68	337	0.007	16	13.8–14.3
Sheikh[89]	2009	Kuwait	4.62	60	GE	165	R	64	...	...	...	13	...
Weustink[29]	2009	Switzerland	2.24	61.5	Siemens	165	R	64	69.8	...	...	17	14.2
Weustink[29]	2009	Switzerland	2.21	61.9	Siemens	165	P	64	68.8	...	...	17	10.7
Alkadhi[33]	2010	Switzerland	3.17	62	Siemens	75	P	128	58	...	0.014	16	1.4
Alkadhi[33]	2010	Switzerland	2.57	63	Siemens	75	P	128	56	...	0.011	16	0.9
Andreini[90]	2010	Italy	7.08	65.4	GE	165	R	64	61.2	479	...	15	14.3
Andreini[90]	2010	Italy	7.08	63.3	GE	165	R	64	58	356	...	15	...
Cademartiri[91]	2010	Italy	1.13	53.6	Siemens	165	R	64	58	151	...	15	15–21
Cademartiri[92]	2010	Italy	0.52	48	Siemens	165	R	64	59.4	...	...	17	15–22
Carrascosa[93]	2010	United States	1.94	62.4	Philips	200	P	64	54.9	...	0.021	17	3.4
Chen[94]	2010	China	1.62	60.7	Siemens	83	...	64	86.4	...	0.014	15	...
de Graaf[95]	2010	Netherlands	1.13	61	Toshiba	175	P	320	60	184	0.01	17	3.9–6
Donati[96]	2010	Switzerland	4.22	64	Siemens	83	R	64		...	0.005	16	2.5
Fang[97]	2010	China	1.78	59.6	Siemens	83	R	64	88	...	0.012	15	...
Husmann[98]	2010	Switzerland	1.54	61	GE	175	P	64	56	481	...	16	2.1
Kajander[99]	2010	Finland	1.49	63.5	GE	175	R	64	...	...	...	17	7.6
Nasis[100]	2010	Australia	1.52	63.2	Toshiba	175	P	320	65	...	0.02	17	5.4

Table 1. Cont.

Authors	Year	Country	Male/ female	Mean age(y)	Scanner	Temporal resolusion(ms)	ECG triggered protocol	NO. of slice	HR(bpm)	Calcium score	Undiagnosis segments	Scheme to evaluate coronary tree	Radiation dose(mSv)
Nazeri[101]	2010	Iran	1.68	58	Siemens	165	R	64	62	…	0	15	…
Ovrehus[102]	2010	Denmark	1.28	61	Siemens	83	…	64	61	…	0.025	16	8.4
Sato[103]	2010	Japan.	2.33	67	Toshiba	200	R	64	…	…	…	…	…
Scheffel[104]	2010	Switzerland	2.45	56	Siemens	83	…	64	67.3	126	0.009	16	…
Scheffel[105]	2010	Switzerland	3.78	64	Siemens	83	P	64	61	…	0.014	16	…
Xu[106]	2010	China	2.23	64.6	Siemens	83	R	64	71.4	…	…	15	16.1
Yang[107]	2010	China	3.6	62	Siemens	83	…	64	59	…	…	15	…
Zhang[108]	2010	China	2.65	64	Siemens	165	R	64	76	136.7	0.038	15	16.51
Achenbach[109]	2011	Germany	2.13	59	Siemens	75	P	128	71	…	0	…	0.76
Bamberg[110]	2011	Multi-countries	…	68.1	Siemens	75	P	128	72.2		0.04	17	3.1
Gang[111]	2011	China	1.73	68	Toshiba	175	R	320	73.7	653	0.021	15	12.5
Kerl[112]	2011	United States	1.31	65	Siemens	165	R	64	66	…	0.028	15	…
Moon[113]	2011	Korea	1.85	60.5	Siemens	83	R	64	58.9	…	0.02	15	5.8
Stolzmann[114]	2011	Switzerland	1.38	68	Siemens	83	P	64	58	…	0.016	16	2.2
van Velzen[115]	2011	Netherlands	1.78	57	Toshiba	175	P	320/64	…	…	0.04	17	3.2–7.1
van Velzen[116]	2011	Netherlands	2.03	57	Toshiba	175	P	320	58	139	0.036	17	6–12
Vavere[117]	2011	Multi-countries	3.03	61	Toshiba	175	R	64	61	…	0.096	19	…
Xu[118]	2011	China	0.76	60.4	Toshiba	175	P	320	60.4	…	0.03	15	13
Zhang[119]	2011	China	…	…	Toshiba	200	R	64	60.5	…	…	15	19.88
Zhang[119]	2011	China	…	…	Toshiba	175	P	320	60.9	…	…	15	4.27
Dharampal[120]	2012	Netherlands.	1.18	58	Siemens	165	…	128	66	252	…	17	12
Kadokami[121]	2012	Japan.	2.5	70	Toshiba	200	…	640	70	…	…	15	16.
Kerl[122]	2012	Germany	1.08	67	Siemens	165	R	64	64	…	…	15	…
Maffei[123]	2012	Italy	1.13	61.2	Siemens	75	R	128	64.3	178	…	17	8.9
Maffei[124]	2012	Italy	1.8	59.3	Siemens	75	…	64	58	444	…	17	…
Sohns[125]	2012	Germany.	2.18	57	Siemens	…	R	64	84		…	15	…
Uehara[126]	2012	…	2.12	64.4	Toshiba	175	…	320	65.2	180	…	15	…
van Velzen[127]	2012	Netherlands.	2.03	57	Toshiba	175	P	64	58	…	0.04	17	12.0
Gueret[128]	2013	France	2.44	61	GE/Philips	…	…	64	63	396	…	…	17.2
Pelliccia[129]	2013	Italy	1.95	61	Toshiba	175	P	64	…	…	…	16	…

Note. —ECG = electrocardiographic, R = retrospective, P = prospective, HR = heart rate.

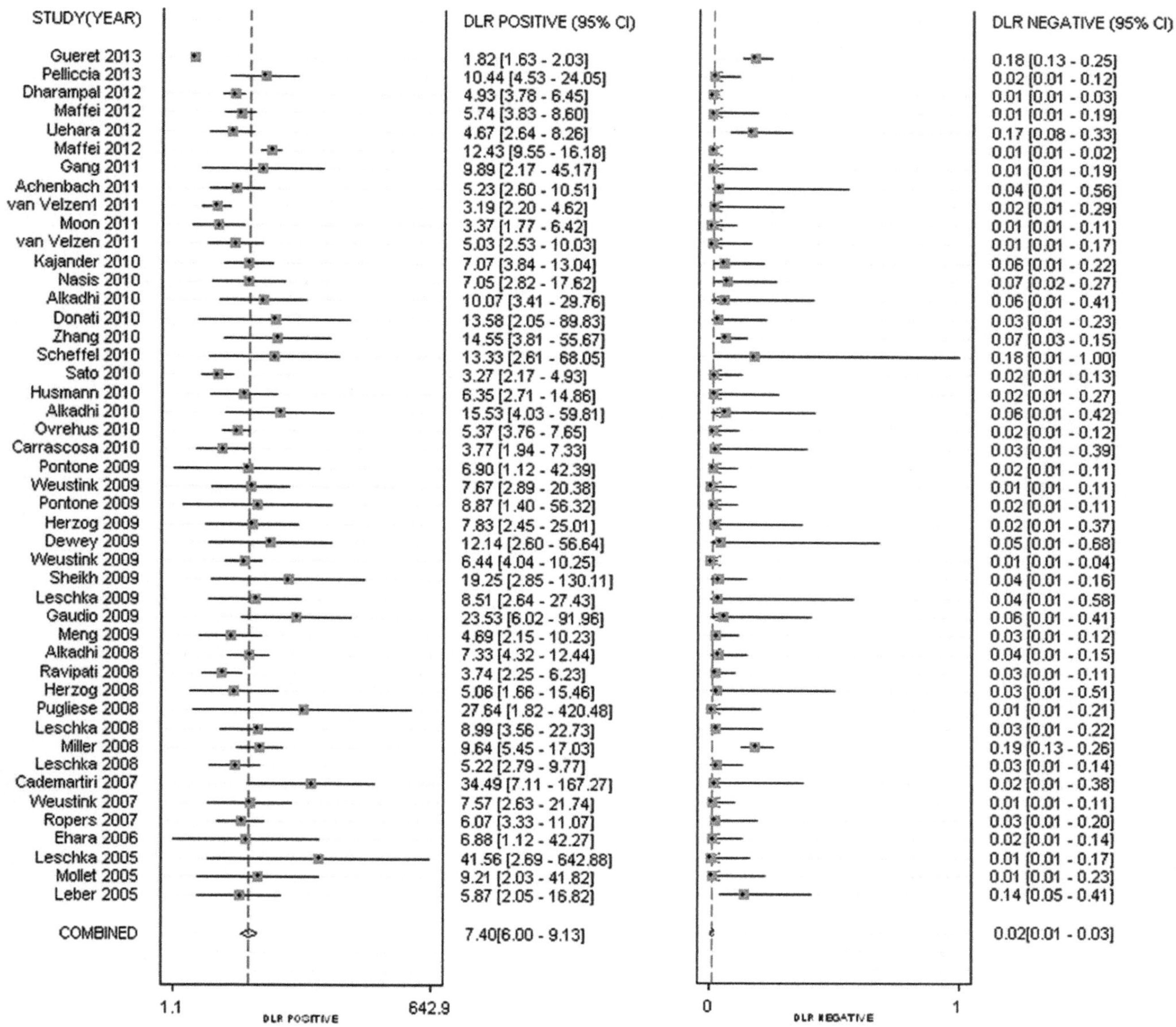

Figure 2. Forest plots showing positive and negative LRs at the patient level. For studies including uninterpretable results, the pooled positive LR was 7.40 (CI, 6.00, 9.13) and negative LR was 0.02 (CI, 0.01, 0.03), respectively.

For studies including uninterpretable results, the diagnostic performance decreased, with the pooled positive LR 7.40 (CI, 6.00, 9.13) and negative LR 0.02 (CI, 0.01, 0.03). Moderate heterogeneity was found for positive LR (Q = 705.71; $P<0.001$; $I^2 = 91.75\%$ [CI, 91.75%, 94.37%]) and significant heterogeneity for negative LR (Q = 346.89; $P<0.001$; $I^2 = 85.87\%$ [CI, 82.59%,

Table 2. Overall Diagnostic Performance of CT Angiography.

	All references		**References excluding non-diagnostic image**		**References including non-diagnostic image**	
	Positive LR (95% CI)	**Negative LR (95% CI)**	**Positive LR (95% CI)**	**Negative LR (95% CI)**	**Positive LR (95% CI)**	**Negative LR (95% CI)**
Patient level	8.91(7.53, 10.54)	0.02 (0.01, 0.03)	11.16(8.90, 14.00)	0.01(0.01, 0.03)	7.40(6.00, 9.13)	0.02(0.01, 0.03)
Artery level	15.22(12.44, 18.64)	0.05(0.04, 0.07)	16.27(12.37, 21.42)	0.05(0.03, 0.08)	14.45(10.83, 19.27)	0.05(0.04, 0.08)
Segment level	31.57(26.92, 37.02)	0.08(0.07, 0.10)	39.76(31.84, 49.63)	0.08(0.06, 0.11)	23.91(19.62, 29.14)	0.08(0.07, 0.11)

Note. —LR = likelihood ratio.

Table 3. Pooled Summary Results by Subgroups.

	Patient level (95% CI)		Artery level (95% CI)		Segment level (95% CI)	
	Positive LR	Negative LR	Positive LR	Negative LR	Positive LR	Negative LR
Temporal resolution						
<100ms	7.23(5.74, 9.09)	0.02(0.01, 0.03)	14.21(9.86, 20.48)	0.05(0.03, 0.07)	25.55(19.49, 33.50)	0.08(0.06, 0.10)
>100ms	7.83(6.03, 10.16)	0.02(0.01, 0.03)	15.61(10.29, 23.66)	0.05(0.03, 0.10)	23.01(17.60, 30.09)	0.08(0.06, 0.12)
ECG-triggered protocol						
Retrospective	8.41(5.83, 12.13)	0.02(0.01, 0.04)	17.10(10.71, 27.30)	0.06(0.03, 0.12)	23.74(18.79, 30.00)	0.08(0.05, 0.12)
Prospective	5.95(4.52, 7.84)	0.03(0.02, 0.06)	12.41(8.22, 18.72)	0.05(0.03, 0.08)	25.64(17.895, 36.77)	0.107(0.07, 0.13)
Gender						
Male/female<3	7.01(5.59, 8.80)	0.02(0.01, 0.03)	16.52(12.43, 21.95)	0.05(0.03, 0.08)	25.148(19.58, 32.30)	0.08(0.06, 0.12)
Male/female>3	11.02(6.56, 18.52)	0.02(0.01, 0.04)	9.43(4.49, 19.82)	0.05(0.03, 0.09)	19.87(14.20, 27.81)	0.08(0.05, 0.12)
Scheme of coronary tree						
≦16-segments	7.82(6.17, 9.93)	0.02(0.01, 0.04)	16.75(11.07, 25.34)	0.06(0.04, 0.08)	24.89(18.81, 32.93)	0.09(0.07, 0.12)
>16-segments	7.33(5.53, 9.72)	0.01(0.00, 0.03)	12.28(8.65, 17.44)	0.05(0.02, 0.12)	22.50(16.57, 30.54)	0.06(0.05, 0.08)
Heart rate						
<65bpm	7.55(5.52, 10.34)	0.02(0.01, 0.04)	13.09(9.32, 18.40)	0.06(0.04, 0.11)	21.79(17.46, 27.19)	0.10(0.07, 0.14)
>65bpm	6.89(5.28, 8.98)	0.02(0.01, 0.04)	18.07(9.48, 34.47)	0.03(0.02, 0.07)	26.11(18.36, 37.14)	0.06(0.05, 0.09)
Calcium score						
<400	7.23(5.86, 8.92)	0.02(0.01, 0.03)	13.97(8.22, 23.72)	0.06(0.03, 0.15)	22.36(15.31, 32.65)	0.08(0.04, 0.15)
>400	11.51(9.13, 14.53)	0.01(0.01, 0.02)	16.37(7.00, 38.30)	0.04(0.02, 0.09)	19.43(12.28, 30.72)	0.06(0.03, 0.12)
Prevalence of CAD						
<0.5	7.50 (5.32, 10.58)	0.05(0.02, 0.08)	18.27(13.11, 25.48)	0.06(0.03, 0.11)	28.35(21.32, 37.71)	0.09(0.06, 0.15)
>0.5	7.18(5.62, 9.17)	0.01(0.01, 0.02)	11.48(7.473, 17.64)	0.05(0.03, 0.07)	20.06(15.36, 26.21)	0.08(0.06, 0.11)
Prevalence of non-assessable segments						
<0.02	9.12(6.41, 12.96)	0.03(0.01, 0.05)	18.73(13.76, 25.50)	0.05(0.03, 0.08)	33.303(25.574, 43.369)	0.08(0.05, 0.11)
>0.02	6.36(4.32, 9.36)	0.01(0.01, 0.04)	12.21(7.19, 20.74)	0.04(0.02, 0.07)	17.62(14.14, 21.94)	0.09(0.06, 0.12)

Note. —TP = true-positive, FP = false-positive, TN = true-negative, FN = false-negative, LR = likelihood ratio, ECG = electrocardiographic, bpm = beat per minute, BMI = body mass index, CAD = coronary artery disease.

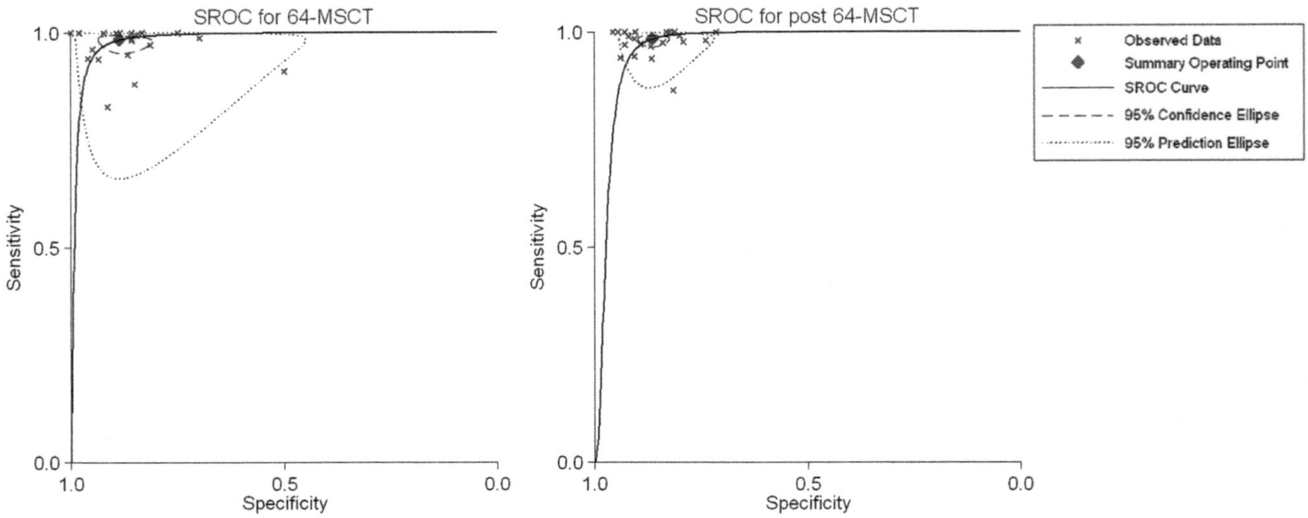

Figure 3. sROC for 64-MDCT and post 64-MDCT. sROC demonstrated the diagnostic performance of 64-MDCT and post 64-MDCT at the patient level (sROC = summary receiver operating characteristic).

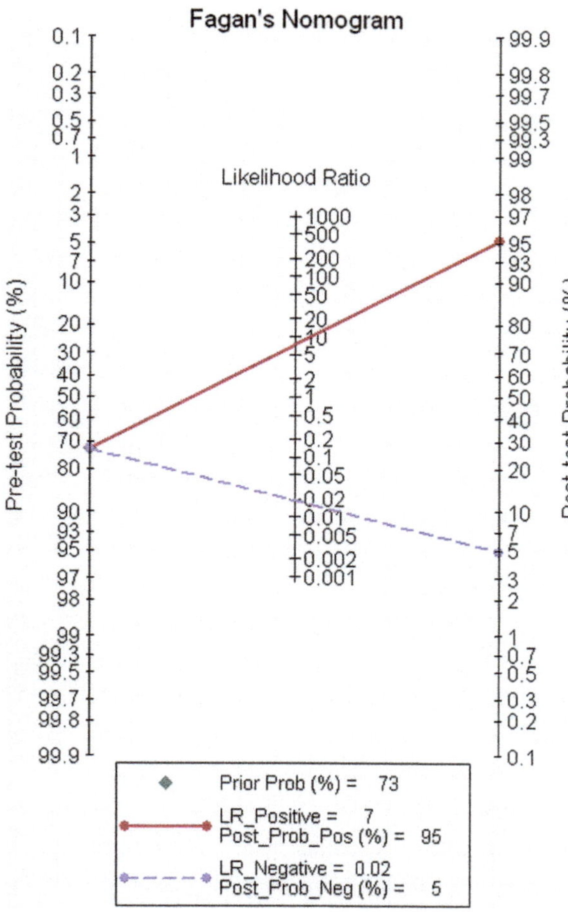

Figure 4. Fagan's nomogram for CTA. For patients with a pre-test probability of CAD<73%, the post-test probability of negative results was larger than 95%. However, when the pre-test probability was larger than 73%, the diagnostic role was reversed, with a positive post-test probability of larger than 95% and a negative post-test probability of less than 95%.

89.16%]) (Figure 2). The detailed diagnostic accuracy at patient, artery and segment levels is presented in Table 2 as well as in Table S2.

Using the pre-specified potential sources of heterogeneity as covariates in the random effects models, we found that gender, heart rate, scheme of the coronary arterial tree for stenostic analysis, temporal resolution, calcium score, the proportion of non-assessable segments, and the protocol of ECG-triggered scanning were significant predictors, while age did not impact diagnostic accuracy (Table S3). The results for the subgroups in patient-based analyses are shown in Table 3.

We added the generation of CT scanners as a covariate to the bivariate model to compare the performance of 64-MDCT and post 64-MDCT. The result showed that, with new techniques used in the newer generations of CT scanners, the overall accuracy of post 64-MDCT at the patient level decreased ($P<0.001$, the area under the summary ROC curve were 0.98 [CI, 0.97 to 0.99] for 64-MDCT and 0.96 [CI, 0.94 to 0.98] for post 64-MDCT, respectively) (Figure 3). Further analysis indicated that the decreased index was positive LRs (8.71 [5.76, 13.12] versus 7.24 [5.92, 8.85]), while the negative LRs were similar (0.02 [0.01, 0.04] versus 0.02 [0.01, 0.03]). Importantly, the heterogeneity of 64-MDCT was larger than that of post 64-MDCT ($I^2 = 96.26\%$ versus 30.2%; 91.89% versus 56.79% for positive and negative LRs, respectively).

We evaluated the post-test probability for studies that explicitly stated that the non-assessable segments were included during analysis, as it is common practice to classify a segment as diseased if there is any doubt. The relationship between pre-test probability and post-test probability was depicted by visual Fagan's nomogram [23]. As we can see from Figure 4, for patients with a pre-test probability of CAD<73%, the post-test probability of negative results was larger than 95%, while the post-test probability of positive results was less than 95%, which indicated that the CT angiography was only an effective tool to exclude patients with CAD. On the other hand, when the pre-test probability was larger than 73%, the diagnostic role was reversed, with a positive post-test probability of larger than 95% and a negative post-test probability of less than 95%, which implied that when there was a pre-test probability of CAD >73%, the role of CTA changed from a test of exclusion to a confirmatory tool.

The likelihood ratio scattergram showed that at the artery and segment levels, the likelihood ratio profile of CTA was both a test of exclusion and a confirmatory test tool to diagnose stenosis > 50% (positive likelihood ratio >10; negative likelihood ratio <0.1), while CTA was generally a test of exclusion to rule out significant stenosis at the patient level (positive likelihood ratio <10; negative likelihood ratio <0.1) (Figure 5) [24].

The sensitivity analysis was conducted at the patient level to investigate the influence of each individual study on the overall meta-analysis summary estimate. No study influenced the pooled sensitivity and specificity larger than 0.02 (Figure S1).

Discussion

The present study analyzed studies of 64-MDCT and post 64-MDCT to shed new light on the following critical questions: (1) What is the role of CTA in patients with different pre-test probabilities? (2) Can post 64-MDCT lead to a better diagnostic accuracy than 64-MDCT?

The hypothesis, which states that CTA can exclude individuals with suspected CAD for patients with low to intermediate pre-test likelihood, has been argued widely in previous studies [3,20]. The present study showed that not all patients with an intermediate pre-test likelihood of CAD could be excluded by CTA. After assessing the precise analysis based on Bayes' theorem, the results show that the pre-test probability of 73% is the cut off value for the diagnostic role of CTA. When pre-test probability is <73%, CTA is an effective tool to exclude CAD. Of note, the positive LR is comparatively low and CTA may be still applied to determine the presence of obstructive CAD in patients with a pre-test probability of CAD>73%. The confirmatory application of CTA also plays an important role for clinical diagnosis, especially for patients with stable angina when revascularization is not preferred at the present time [25]. CTA, therefore, may provide more evidence to confirm the presence of CAD and avoid the major complications associated with ICA [2,25]. As there are several studies providing detailed algorithms to quantify pre-test risk [9–12], a precise evaluation of the diagnostic role of CTA according to pre-test probability will improve the cost-effectiveness of CTA. Moreover, the present analysis demonstrates that CTA is both a test of exclusion and confirmatory test on both artery and segment levels, which provides detailed information for prognostic evaluation [26,27] or for the selection of a revascularization strategy [28].

The results indicate that the exclusive performance of post 64-MDCT does not increase. Rather, the confirmatory accuracy of post 64-MDCT decreases. The main reason may be that the

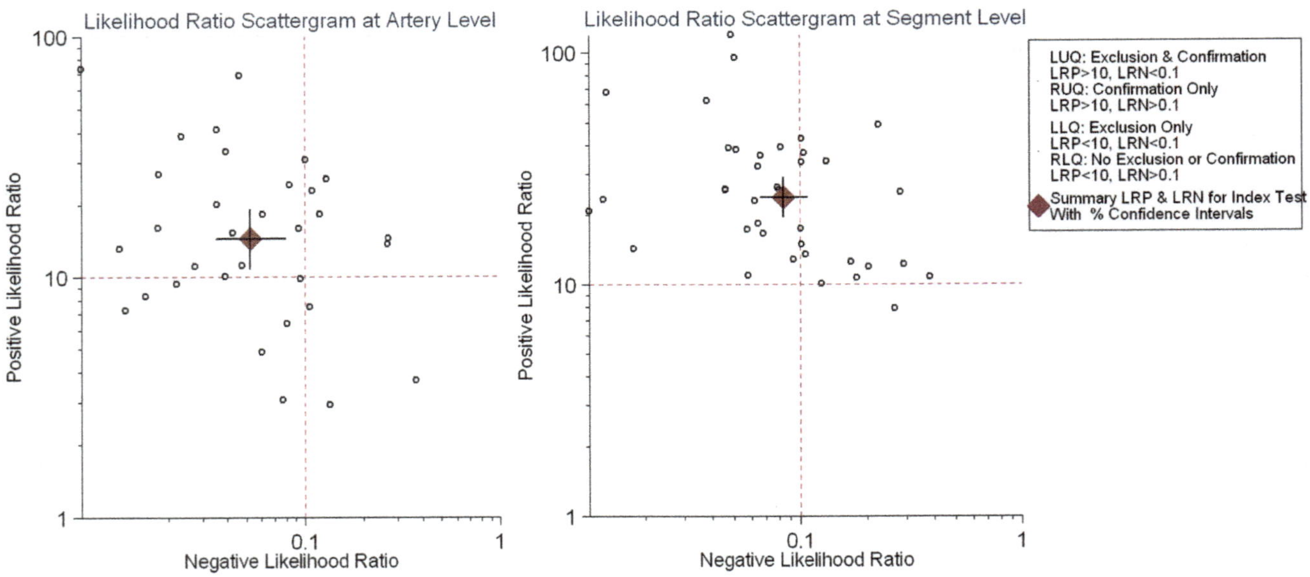

Figure 5. Illustration chart indicating the diagnostic role for accuracy of CTA at the artery and segment levels. At the artery and segment levels, the likelihood ratio profile of CT was both an exclusion and s confirmation test to diagnose stenosis >50% (positive likelihood ratio > 10; negative likelihood ratio <0.1), while CTA was generally a test of exclusion to rule out significant stenosis at the patient level (LRP = positive likelihood ratio, LRN = negative likelihood ratio, LLQ = left lower quadrant, LUQ = left upper quadrant, RLQ = right lower quadrant, RUQ = right upper quadrant).

improved techniques mainly focuses on the motion artifacts. For example, DSCT, with two detectors arranged at angles of 90°, effectively doubles the temporal resolution [29]. Additionally, 320-MDCT, with 16-cm wide volume coverage, enabled whole coronary arteries covered with one heartbeat, which eliminated the motion artifact effectively [30]. The spatial resolution, however, is not improved and the beam hardening artifacts still present a primary shortcoming of CTA. As is apparent from the results, the heterogeneity of post 64-MDCT was significantly larger than that of 64-MDCT. The decreased positive LR of post 64-MDCT may be caused by a different prevalence of calcified plaques, which are not, however, provided by most studies. Further analysis with information regarding the individual may illustrate the question more clearly. Another potential reason for the decreased pooled positive LR may be that with an improved technique of post 64-MDCT, the inclusion criteria of patients was broader than that of 64-MDCT. With dual-source, 64-slice CT, it could be theoretically possible to scan without lowering the heart rate [31]. Nevertheless, in reality, the heart rate still needs to remain low for good image quality since the temporal resolution of this scanner is still too low. In addition, a low heart rate is also suggested for 128-MDCT or 320-MDCT due to the technical specifications of the scanners. Nevertheless, with wider detection, prospective ECG gating is more feasible. Combined with iterative construction, the radiation dose of post 64-MDCT was significantly lower than that of 64-MDCT [32,33].

Schueler et al. reported that item referring to how authors handled "Uninterpretable Results" (QUADAS item 13) had a significant influence on diagnostic accuracy values and that exclusion of uninterpretable results may overestimate the diagnostic abilities of the method being investigated[34], which has also been proven by our analysis. Salavati et al., on the other hand, did not detect a difference between studies including and excluding uninterpretable segments[35]. The potential reason might be the lower proportion of uninterpretable segments achieved by DSCT[35]. The present study, with 64- and post 64-MDCT included, evaluates the diagnostic performance mainly through studies that clearly claim that coronary arterial segments with non-diagnostic image quality were treated as positive for disease, as it is a common practice to classify a segment as diseased if it is non-diagnostic, which guarantees the validity of the conclusion reached.

Our meta-analysis has limitations. First, we did not analyze the diagnostic accuracy of CTA for stable angina and ACS respectively, as most studies include all symptomatic patients without further classification of clinical features. In addition, though the clinical diagnoses were different, the morphologic images of angiography were both indicative of stenosis of the coronary lumen. Second, although the present study is aimed at illustrating the diagnostic role of CTA by pre-test probability, information on symptoms, however, are not provided by most references. However, the main conclusion was not impacted as we mainly used Bayes' theorem and the positive and negative LRs, instead of the sensitivity and specificity, to evaluate the diagnostic role of CT angiography. Such LRs have advantages for the following reasons: they are less likely to change with the prevalence of CAD and they can be calculated for several levels of the symptom/sign. Third, the conclusion was conducted by using ICA as standard references. Recent studies indicate that fractional flow reserve (FFR)-guided treatment may lead to a better prognosis than that of an ICA-guided strategy [36,37]. Several studies, however, demonstrate that the accuracy to diagnose ischemic stenosis, with FFR as a reference, was poor [38-40]. Further meta-analysis is therefore required to explore the different capacities of CTA for detecting morphological and functional stenosis.

In conclusion, the diagnostic performance of post 64-MDCT does not increase as compared with 64-MDCT. CTA, overall, is a test of exclusion for patients with a pre-test probability of CAD< 73%, while for patients with a pre-test probability of CAD>73%, CTA is a test used to confirm the presence of CAD.

Supporting Information

Figure S1 The Serrbar Illustrating a Sensitivity Analysis in which the Meta-Analysis was Re-estimated by Omitting Each Study in Turn. The sensitivity analysis indicates that no study influenced the pooled sensitivity and specificity larger than 0.02.

Table S1 Quality Assessment of Studies Enrolled to Diagnostic Accuracy.

Table S2 Detailed Diagnostic Information for Each Study.

Table S3 Results of the Multivariate Meta-Regression Analysis for Identifying Covariates to Explain Heterogeneity at Patient Level.

Checklist S1 PRISMA Checklist.

Author Contributions

Conceived and designed the experiments: ML XD. Analyzed the data: ML XD ZJ. Contributed reagents/materials/analysis tools: ZJ JD. Wrote the paper: ML XD ZJ JD ZP LL.

References

1. Naghavi M, Libby P, Falk E, Casscells SW, Litovsky S, et al. (2003) From vulnerable plaque to vulnerable patient: a call for new definitions and risk assessment strategies: Part I. Circulation 108: 1664–1672.
2. Mowatt G, Cummins E, Waugh N, Walker S, Cook J, et al. (2008) Systematic review of the clinical effectiveness and cost-effectiveness of 64-slice or higher computed tomography angiography as an alternative to invasive coronary angiography in the investigation of coronary artery disease. Health Technol Assess 12: iii-iv, ix-143.
3. Schuetz GM, Zacharopoulou NM, Schlattmann P, Dewey M (2010) Meta-analysis: noninvasive coronary angiography using computed tomography versus magnetic resonance imaging. Annals of internal medicine 152: 167–177.
4. Hamon M, Morello R, Riddell JW (2007) Coronary arteries: diagnostic performance of 16- versus 64-section spiral CT compared with invasive coronary angiography–meta-analysis. Radiology 245: 720–731.
5. Vanhoenacker PK, Heijenbrok-Kal MH, Van Heste R, Decramer I, Van Hoe LR, et al. (2007) Diagnostic performance of multidetector CT angiography for assessment of coronary artery disease: meta-analysis. Radiology 244: 419–428.
6. Schlattmann P, Schuetz GM, Dewey M (2011) Influence of coronary artery disease prevalence on predictive values of coronary CT angiography: a meta-regression analysis. Eur Radiol 21: 1904–1913.
7. von Ballmoos MW, Haring B, Juillerat P, Alkadhi H (2011) Meta-analysis: diagnostic performance of low-radiation-dose coronary computed tomography angiography. Annals of internal medicine 154: 413–420.
8. Weustink AC, de Feyter PJ (2011) The role of multi-slice computed tomography in stable angina management: a current perspective. Neth Heart J 19: 336–343.
9. Budaj A, Dean V, Deckers J, Dickstein K (2006) Guidelines on the management of stable angina pectoris. European Heart Journal: 1–63.
10. Cheng VY, Berman DS, Rozanski A, Dunning AM, Achenbach S, et al. (2011) Performance of the traditional age, sex, and angina typicality-based approach for estimating pretest probability of angiographically significant coronary artery disease in patients undergoing coronary computed tomographic angiography: results from the multinational coronary CT angiography evaluation for clinical outcomes: an international multicenter registry (CONFIRM). Circulation 124: 2423–2432, 2421–2428.
11. Pryor DB, Shaw L, McCants CB, Lee KL, Mark DB, et al. (1993) Value of the history and physical in identifying patients at increased risk for coronary artery disease. Annals of internal medicine 118: 81–81.
12. Diamond GA, Forrester JS (1979) Analysis of probability as an aid in the clinical diagnosis of coronary-artery disease. N Engl J Med 300: 1350–1358.
13. Moher D, Liberati A, Tetzlaff J, Altman DG (2009) Preferred reporting items for systematic reviews and meta-analyses: the PRISMA statement. Ann Intern Med 151: 264–269, W264.
14. Whiting P, Rutjes A, Reitsma J, Bossuyt P, Kleijnen J (2003) The development of QUADAS: a tool for the quality assessment of studies of diagnostic accuracy included in systematic reviews. BMC medical research methodology 3: 1–13.
15. Deeks JJ, Macaskill P, Irwig L (2005) The performance of tests of publication bias and other sample size effects in systematic reviews of diagnostic test accuracy was assessed. Journal of clinical epidemiology 58: 882–893.
16. Higgins J, Thompson SG, Deeks JJ, Altman DG (2003) Measuring inconsistency in meta-analyses. Bmj 327: 557.
17. Swets JA (1988) Measuring the accuracy of diagnostic systems. Science 240: 1285–1293.
18. Chu H, Cole SR, Reitsma J, Zwinderman A (2006) Bivariate meta-analysis of sensitivity and specificity with sparse data: a generalized linear mixed model approach. Authors' reply. Journal of clinical epidemiology 59: 1331–1333.
19. Reitsma JB, Glas AS, Rutjes AWS, Scholten RJPM, Bossuyt PM, et al. (2005) Bivariate analysis of sensitivity and specificity produces informative summary measures in diagnostic reviews. Journal of clinical epidemiology 58: 982–990.
20. von Ballmoos MW, Haring B, Juillerat P, Alkadhi H (2011) Meta-analysis: diagnostic performance of low-radiation-dose coronary computed tomography angiography. Ann Intern Med 154: 413–420.
21. Skupski DW, Rosenberg CR, Eglinton GS (2002) Intrapartum Fetal Stimulation Tests: A Meta-Analysis. Obstetrics & Gynecology 99: 129–134.
22. Jaeschke R, Guyatt GH, Sackett DL, Guyatt G, Bass E, et al. (1994) Users' guides to the medical literature. JAMA: the journal of the American Medical Association 271: 703–707.
23. Fagan TJ (1975) Letter: Nomogram for Bayes theorem. The New England journal of medicine 293: 257.
24. Stengel D, Bauwens K, Sehouli J, Ekkernkamp A, Porzsolt F (2003) A likelihood ratio approach to meta-analysis of diagnostic studies. J Med Screen 10: 47–51.
25. Moscariello A, Vliegenthart R, Schoepf UJ, Nance JW, Jr., Zwerner PL, et al. (2012) Coronary CT angiography versus conventional cardiac angiography for therapeutic decision making in patients with high likelihood of coronary artery disease. Radiology 265: 385–392.
26. Andreini D, Pontone G, Mushtaq S, Bartorelli AL, Bertella E, et al. (2012) A long-term prognostic value of coronary CT angiography in suspected coronary artery disease. JACC: Cardiovascular Imaging 5: 690–701.
27. Nance JW, Jr., Schlett CL, Schoepf UJ, Oberoi S, Leisy HB, et al. (2012) Incremental prognostic value of different components of coronary atherosclerotic plaque at cardiac CT angiography beyond coronary calcification in patients with acute chest pain. Radiology.
28. Moscariello A, Vliegenthart R, Schoepf UJ, Nance JW, Jr., Zwerner PL, et al. (2012) Coronary CT angiography versus conventional cardiac angiography for therapeutic decision making in patients with high likelihood of coronary artery disease. Radiology.
29. Weustink AC, Mollet NR, Neefjes LA, van Straten M, Neoh E, et al. (2009) Preserved diagnostic performance of dual-source CT coronary angiography with reduced radiation exposure and cancer risk. Radiology 252: 53–60.
30. Chen MY, Shanbhag SM, Arai AE (2013) Submillisievert median radiation dose for coronary angiography with a second-generation 320-detector row CT scanner in 107 consecutive patients. Radiology 267: 76–85.
31. Hsiao EM, Rybicki FJ, Steigner M (2010) CT coronary angiography: 256-slice and 320-detector row scanners. Curr Cardiol Rep 12: 68–75.
32. Yoneyama K, Vavere AL, Cerci R, Ahmed R, Arai AE, et al. (2012) Influence of image acquisition settings on radiation dose and image quality in coronary angiography by 320-detector volume computed tomography: the CORE320 pilot experience. Heart Int 7: e11.
33. Alkadhi H, Stolzmann P, Desbiolles L, Baumueller S, Goetti R, et al. (2010) Low-dose, 128-slice, dual-source CT coronary angiography: accuracy and radiation dose of the high-pitch and the step-and-shoot mode. Heart 96: 933–938.
34. Schueler S, Walther S, Schuetz GM, Schlattmann P, Dewey M (2013) Methodological quality of diagnostic accuracy studies on non-invasive coronary CT angiography: influence of QUADAS (Quality Assessment of Diagnostic Accuracy Studies included in systematic reviews) items on sensitivity and specificity. Eur Radiol 23: 1603–1622.
35. Salavati A, Radmanesh F, Heidari K, Dwamena BA, Kelly AM, et al. (2011) Dual-source computed tomography angiography for diagnosis and assessment of coronary artery disease: Systematic review and meta-analysis. J Cardiovasc Comput Tomogr.
36. Tonino PA, De Bruyne B, Pijls NH, Siebert U, Ikeno F, et al. (2009) Fractional flow reserve versus angiography for guiding percutaneous coronary intervention. N Engl J Med 360: 213–224.
37. Pijls NH, Fearon WF, Tonino PA, Siebert U, Ikeno F, et al. (2010) Fractional flow reserve versus angiography for guiding percutaneous coronary intervention in patients with multivessel coronary artery disease: 2-year follow-up of the FAME (Fractional Flow Reserve Versus Angiography for Multivessel Evaluation) study. J Am Coll Cardiol 56: 177–184.
38. Meijboom WB, Van Mieghem CA, van Pelt N, Weustink A, Pugliese F, et al. (2008) Comprehensive assessment of coronary artery stenoses: computed tomography coronary angiography versus conventional coronary angiography and correlation with fractional flow reserve in patients with stable angina. J Am Coll Cardiol 52: 636–643.

39. Ko BS, Cameron JD, Meredith IT, Leung M, Antonis PR, et al. (2012) Computed tomography stress myocardial perfusion imaging in patients considered for revascularization: a comparison with fractional flow reserve. Eur Heart J 33: 67–77.
40. Min JK, Leipsic J, Pencina MJ, Berman DS, Koo BK, et al. (2012) Diagnostic accuracy of fractional flow reserve from anatomic CT angiography. JAMA 308: 1237–1245.
41. Leber AW, Knez A, von Ziegler F, Becker A, Nikolaou K, et al. (2005) Quantification of Obstructive and Nonobstructive Coronary Lesions by 64-Slice Computed Tomography: A Comparative Study With Quantitative Coronary Angiography and Intravascular Ultrasound. Journal of the American College of Cardiology 46: 147–154.
42. Leschka S, Alkadhi H, Plass A, Desbiolles L, Grunenfelder J, et al. (2005) Accuracy of MSCT coronary angiography with 64-slice technology: first experience. Eur Heart J 26: 1482–1487.
43. Mollet NR, Cademartiri F, van Mieghem CAG, Runza G, McFadden EP, et al. (2005) High-resolution spiral computed tomography coronary angiography in patients referred for diagnostic conventional coronary angiography. Circulation 112: 2318–2323.
44. Pugliese F, Mollet NRA, Runza G, Mieghem C, Meijboom WB, et al. (2005) Diagnostic accuracy of non-invasive 64-slice CT coronary angiography in patients with stable angina pectoris. European radiology 16: 575–582.
45. Raff GL, Gallagher MJ, O'Neill WW, Goldstein JA (2005) Diagnostic accuracy of noninvasive coronary angiography using 64-slice spiral computed tomography. Journal of the American College of Cardiology 46: 552–557.
46. Ehara M, Surmely JF, Kawai M, Katoh O, Matsubara T, et al. (2006) Diagnostic accuracy of 64-slice computed tomography for detecting angiographically significant coronary artery stenosis in an unselected consecutive patient population: comparison with conventional invasive angiography. Circulation journal: official journal of the Japanese Circulation Society 70: 564–571.
47. Ghostine S, Caussin C, Daoud B, Habis M, Perrier E, et al. (2006) Non-invasive detection of coronary artery disease in patients with left bundle branch block using 64-slice computed tomography. J Am Coll Cardiol 48: 1929–1934.
48. Meijboom WB, Mollet NR, Van Mieghem CA, Kluin J, Weustink AC, et al. (2006) Pre-operative computed tomography coronary angiography to detect significant coronary artery disease in patients referred for cardiac valve surgery. J Am Coll Cardiol 48: 1658–1665.
49. Nikolaou K, Knez A, Rist C, Wintersperger BJ, Leber A, et al. (2006) Accuracy of 64-MDCT in the diagnosis of ischemic heart disease. American Journal of Roentgenology 187: 111–117.
50. Plass A, Grunenfelder J, Leschka S, Alkadhi H, Eberli F, et al. (2006) Coronary artery imaging with 64-slice computed tomography from cardiac surgical perspective. European Journal of Cardio-Thoracic Surgery 30: 109–116.
51. Ropers D, Rixe J, Anders K, Küttner A, Baum U, et al. (2006) Usefulness of multidetector row spiral computed tomography with 64-×0.6-mm collimation and 330-ms rotation for the noninvasive detection of significant coronary artery stenoses. The American journal of cardiology 97: 343–348.
52. Scheffel H, Alkadhi H, Plass A, Vachenauer R, Desbiolles L, et al. (2006) Accuracy of dual-source CT coronary angiography: First experience in a high pre-test probability population without heart rate control. Eur Radiol 16: 2739–2747.
53. Schuijf JD, Pundziute G, Jukema JW, Lamb HJ, van der Hoeven BL, et al. (2006) Diagnostic accuracy of 64-slice multislice computed tomography in the noninvasive evaluation of significant coronary artery disease. Am J Cardiol 98: 145–148.
54. Cademartiri F, Maffei E, Palumbo A, Malagò R, Alberghina F, et al. (2007) Diagnostic accuracy of 64-slice computed tomography coronary angiography in patients with low-to-intermediate risk. La Radiologia Medica 112: 969–981.
55. Herzog C, Zwerner PL, Doll JR, Nielsen CD, Nguyen SA, et al. (2007) Significant Coronary Artery Stenosis: Comparison on Per-Patient and Per-Vessel or Per-Segment Basis at 64-Section CT Angiography. Radiology 244: 112–120.
56. Herzog C, Nguyen SA, Savino G, Zwerner PL, Doll J, et al. (2007) Does Two-Segment Image Reconstruction at 64-Section CT Coronary Angiography Improve Image Quality and Diagnostic Accuracy? Radiology 244: 121–129.
57. Heuschmid M, Burgstahler C, Reimann A, Brodoefel H, Mysal I, et al. (2007) Usefulness of noninvasive cardiac imaging using dual-source computed tomography in an unselected population with high prevalence of coronary artery disease. Am J Cardiol 100: 587–592.
58. Johnson TR, Nikolaou K, Busch S, Leber AW, Becker A, et al. (2007) Diagnostic accuracy of dual-source computed tomography in the diagnosis of coronary artery disease. Invest Radiol 42: 684–691.
59. Leber AW, Johnson T, Becker A, von Ziegler F, Tittus J, et al. (2007) Diagnostic accuracy of dual-source multi-slice CT-coronary angiography in patients with an intermediate pretest likelihood for coronary artery disease. Eur Heart J 28: 2354–2360.
60. Meijboom WB, van Mieghem CA, Mollet NR, Pugliese F, Weustink AC, et al. (2007) 64-slice computed tomography coronary angiography in patients with high, intermediate, or low pretest probability of significant coronary artery disease. J Am Coll Cardiol 50: 1469–1475.
61. Meijboom WB, Mollet NR, Van Mieghem CA, Weustink AC, Pugliese F, et al. (2007) 64-Slice CT coronary angiography in patients with non-ST elevation acute coronary syndrome. Heart 93: 1386–1392.
62. Oncel D, Oncel G, Tastan A, Tamci B (2007) Detection of significant coronary artery stenosis with 64-section MDCT angiography. European journal of radiology 62: 394–405.
63. Ropers U, Ropers D, Pflederer T, Anders K, Kuettner A, et al. (2007) Influence of heart rate on the diagnostic accuracy of dual-source computed tomography coronary angiography. J Am Coll Cardiol 50: 2393–2398.
64. Scheffel H, Leschka S, Plass A, Vachenauer R, Gaemperli O, et al. (2007) Accuracy of 64-slice computed tomography for the preoperative detection of coronary artery disease in patients with chronic aortic regurgitation. Am J Cardiol 100: 701–706.
65. Schlosser T, Mohrs OK, Magedanz A, Nowak B, Voigtlander T, et al. (2007) Noninvasive coronary angiography using 64-detector-row computed tomography in patients with a low to moderate pretest probability of significant coronary artery disease. Acta Radiol 48: 300–307.
66. Weustink AC, Meijboom WB, Mollet NR, Otsuka M, Pugliese F, et al. (2007) Reliable high-speed coronary computed tomography in symptomatic patients. Journal of the American College of Cardiology 50: 786–794.
67. Achenbach S, Ropers U, Kuettner A, Anders K, Pflederer T, et al. (2008) Randomized comparison of 64-slice single- and dual-source computed tomography coronary angiography for the detection of coronary artery disease. JACC Cardiovasc Imaging 1: 177–186.
68. Alkadhi H, Scheffel H, Desbiolles L, Gaemperli O, Stolzmann P, et al. (2008) Dual-source computed tomography coronary angiography: influence of obesity, calcium load, and heart rate on diagnostic accuracy. European Heart Journal 29: 766–776.
69. Brodoefel H, Burgstahler C, Tsiflikas I, Reimann A, Schroeder S, et al. (2008) Dual-source CT: effect of heart rate, heart rate variability, and calcification on image quality and diagnostic accuracy. Radiology 247: 346–355.
70. Han SC, Fang CC, Chen Y, Chen CL, Wang SP (2008) Coronary computed tomography angiography–a promising imaging modality in diagnosing coronary artery disease. J Chin Med Assoc 71: 241–246.
71. Herzog BA, Husmann L, Burkhard N, Gaemperli O, Valenta I, et al. (2008) Accuracy of low-dose computed tomography coronary angiography using prospective electrocardiogram-triggering: first clinical experience. European Heart Journal 29: 3037–3042.
72. Leschka S, Scheffel H, Husmann L, Gämperli O, Marincek B, et al. (2008) Effect of decrease in heart rate variability on the diagnostic accuracy of 64-MDCT coronary angiography. American Journal of Roentgenology 190: 1583–1590.
73. Leschka S, Scheffel H, Desbiolles L, Plass A, Gaemperli O, et al. (2008) Combining dual-source computed tomography coronary angiography and calcium scoring: added value for the assessment of coronary artery disease. Heart 94: 1154–1161.
74. Maruyama T, Takada M, Hasuike T, Yoshikawa A, Namimatsu E, et al. (2008) Radiation dose reduction and coronary assessability of prospective electrocardiogram-gated computed tomography coronary angiography: comparison with retrospective electrocardiogram-gated helical scan. Journal of the American College of Cardiology 52: 1450–1455.
75. Miller JM, Rochitte CE, Dewey M, Arbab-Zadeh A, Niinuma H, et al. (2008) Diagnostic performance of coronary angiography by 64-row CT. N Engl J Med 359: 2324–2336.
76. Pugliese F, Mollet NR, Hunink M, Cademartiri F, Nieman K, et al. (2008) Diagnostic Performance of Coronary CT Angiography by Using Different Generations of Multisection Scanners: Single-Center Experience. Radiology 246: 384–393.
77. Pundziute G, Schuijf JD, Jukema JW, van Werkhoven JM, Boersma E, et al. (2008) Gender influence on the diagnostic accuracy of 64-slice multislice computed tomography coronary angiography for detection of obstructive coronary artery disease. Heart 94: 48–52.
78. Ravipati G, Aronow WS, Lai H, Shao J, DeLuca AJ, et al. (2008) Comparison of sensitivity, specificity, positive predictive value, and negative predictive value of stress testing versus 64-multislice coronary computed tomography angiography in predicting obstructive coronary artery disease diagnosed by coronary angiography. Am J Cardiol 101: 774–775.
79. Scheffel H, Alkadhi H, Leschka S, Plass A, Desbiolles L, et al. (2008) Low-dose CT coronary angiography in the step-and-shoot mode: diagnostic performance. Heart 94: 1132–1137.
80. Stolzmann P, Scheffel H, Leschka S, Plass A, Baumuller S, et al. (2008) Influence of calcifications on diagnostic accuracy of coronary CT angiography using prospective ECG triggering. AJR Am J Roentgenol 191: 1684–1689.
81. Dewey M, Zimmermann E, Deissenrieder F, Laule M, Dubel HP, et al. (2009) Noninvasive coronary angiography by 320-row computed tomography with lower radiation exposure and maintained diagnostic accuracy: comparison of results with cardiac catheterization in a head-to-head pilot investigation. Circulation 120: 867–875.
82. Gaudio C, Mirabelli F, Pelliccia F, Francone M, Tanzilli G, et al. (2009) Early detection of coronary artery disease by 64-slice multidetector computed tomography in asymptomatic hypertensive high-risk patients. Int J Cardiol 135: 280–286.
83. Herzog BA, Wyss CA, Husmann L, Gaemperli O, Valenta I, et al. (2009) First head-to-head comparison of effective radiation dose from low-dose 64-slice CT with prospective ECG-triggering versus invasive coronary angiography. Heart 95: 1656–1661.

84. Leschka S, Stolzmann P, Desbiolles L, Baumueller S, Goetti R, et al. (2009) Diagnostic accuracy of high-pitch dual-source CT for the assessment of coronary stenoses: first experience. Eur Radiol 19: 2896–2903.
85. Meng L, Cui L, Cheng Y, Wu X, Tang Y, et al. (2009) Effect of heart rate and coronary calcification on the diagnostic accuracy of the dual-source CT coronary angiography in patients with suspected coronary artery disease. Korean J Radiol 10: 347–354.
86. Pontone G, Andreini D, Bartorelli AL, Cortinovis S, Mushtaq S, et al. (2009) Diagnostic accuracy of coronary computed tomography angiography: a comparison between prospective and retrospective electrocardiogram triggering. Journal of the American College of Cardiology 54: 346–355.
87. Reimann AJ, Tsiflikas I, Brodoefel H, Scheuering M, Rinck D, et al. (2009) Efficacy of computer aided analysis in detection of significant coronary artery stenosis in cardiac using dual source computed tomography. Int J Cardiovasc Imaging 25: 195–203.
88. Rixe J, Rolf A, Conradi G, Moellmann H, Nef H, et al. (2009) Detection of relevant coronary artery disease using dual-source computed tomography in a high probability patient series: comparison with invasive angiography. Circ J 73: 316–322.
89. Sheikh M, Ben-Nakhi A, Shukkur AM, Sinan T, Al-Rashdan I (2009) Accuracy of 64-multidetector-row computed tomography in the diagnosis of coronary artery disease. Med Princ Pract 18: 323–328.
90. Andreini D, Pontone G, Bartorelli AL, Agostoni P, Mushtaq S, et al. (2010) Comparison of the diagnostic performance of 64-slice computed tomography coronary angiography in diabetic and non-diabetic patients with suspected coronary artery disease. Cardiovasc Diabetol 9: 80.
91. Cademartiri F, Maffei E, Palumbo A, Seitun S, Martini C, et al. (2010) Coronary calcium score and computed tomography coronary angiography in high-risk asymptomatic subjects: assessment of diagnostic accuracy and prevalence of non-obstructive coronary artery disease. Eur Radiol 20: 846–854.
92. Cademartiri F, Maffei E, Palumbo A, Martini C, Seitun S, et al. (2010) Diagnostic accuracy of computed tomography coronary angiography in patients with a zero calcium score. European radiology 20: 81–87.
93. Carrascosa P, Capuñay C, Deviggiano A, Goldsmit A, Tajer C, et al. (2010) Accuracy of low-dose prospectively gated axial coronary CT angiography for the assessment of coronary artery stenosis in patients with stable heart rate. Journal of Cardiovascular Computed Tomography 4: 197–205.
94. Chen HW, Fang XM, Hu XY, Bao J, Hu CH, et al. (2010) Efficacy of dual-source CT coronary angiography in evaluating coronary stenosis: initial experience. Clin Imaging 34: 165–171.
95. de Graaf FR, Schuijf JD, van Velzen JE, Kroft LJ, de Roos A, et al. (2010) Diagnostic accuracy of 320-row multidetector computed tomography coronary angiography in the non-invasive evaluation of significant coronary artery disease. Eur Heart J 31: 1908–1915.
96. Donati OF, Scheffel H, Stolzmann P, Baumuller S, Plass A, et al. (2010) Combined cardiac CT and MRI for the comprehensive workup of hemodynamically relevant coronary stenoses. AJR Am J Roentgenol 194: 920–926.
97. Fang XM, Chen HW, Hu XY, Bao J, Chen Y, et al. (2010) Dual-source CT coronary angiography without heart rate or rhythm control in comparison with conventional coronary angiography. Int J Cardiovasc Imaging 26: 323–331.
98. Husmann L, Herzog BA, Burger IA, Buechel RR, Pazhenkottil AP, et al. (2010) Usefulness of additional coronary calcium scoring in low-dose CT coronary angiography with prospective ECG-triggering: impact on total effective radiation dose and diagnostic accuracy. Academic radiology 17: 201–206.
99. Kajander S, Joutsiniemi E, Saraste M, Pietila M, Ukkonen H, et al. (2010) Cardiac positron emission tomography/computed tomography imaging accurately detects anatomically and functionally significant coronary artery disease. Circulation 122: 603–613.
100. Nasis A, Leung MC, Antonis PR, Cameron JD, Lehman SJ, et al. (2010) Diagnostic accuracy of noninvasive coronary angiography with 320-detector row computed tomography. Am J Cardiol 106: 1429–1435.
101. Nazeri I, Shahabi P, Tehrai M, Sharif-Kashani B, Nazeri A (2010) Impact of calcification on diagnostic accuracy of 64-slice spiral computed tomography for detecting coronary artery disease: a single center experience. Arch Iran Med 13: 373–383.
102. Ovrehus KA, Munkholm H, Bottcher M, Botker HE, Norgaard BL (2010) Coronary computed tomographic angiography in patients suspected of coronary artery disease: impact of observer experience on diagnostic performance and interobserver reproducibility. J Cardiovasc Comput Tomogr 4: 186–194.
103. Sato A, Nozato T, Hikita H, Miyazaki S, Takahashi Y, et al. (2010) Incremental value of combining 64-slice computed tomography angiography with stress nuclear myocardial perfusion imaging to improve noninvasive detection of coronary artery disease. J Nucl Cardiol 17: 19–26.
104. Scheffel H, Stolzmann P, Plass A, Leschka S, Grunenfelder J, et al. (2010) Coronary artery disease in patients with cardiac tumors: preoperative assessment by computed tomography coronary angiography. Interact Cardiovasc Thorac Surg 10: 513–518.
105. Scheffel H, Stolzmann P, Alkadhi H, Azemaj N, Plass A, et al. (2010) Low-dose CT and cardiac MR for the diagnosis of coronary artery disease: accuracy of single and combined approaches. Int J Cardiovasc Imaging 26: 579–590.
106. Xu Y, Tang L, Zhu X, Xu H, Tang J, et al. (2010) Comparison of dual-source CT coronary angiography and conventional coronary angiography for detecting coronary artery disease. Int J Cardiovasc Imaging 26 Suppl 1: 75–81.
107. Yang X, Gai LY, Li P, Chen YD, Li T, et al. (2010) Diagnostic accuracy of dual-source CT angiography and coronary risk stratification. Vasc Health Risk Manag 6: 935–941.
108. Zhang LJ, Wu SY, Wang J, Lu Y, Zhang ZL, et al. (2010) Diagnostic accuracy of dual-source CT coronary angiography: The effect of average heart rate, heart rate variability, and calcium score in a clinical perspective. Acta Radiol 51: 727–740.
109. Achenbach S, Goroll T, Seltmann M, Pflederer T, Anders K, et al. (2011) Detection of coronary artery stenoses by low-dose, prospectively ECG-triggered, high-pitch spiral coronary CT angiography. JACC Cardiovasc Imaging 4: 328–337.
110. Bamberg F, Becker A, Schwarz F, Marcus RP, Greif M, et al. (2011) Detection of Hemodynamically Significant Coronary Artery Stenosis: Incremental Diagnostic Value of Dynamic CT-based Myocardial Perfusion Imaging. Radiology 260: 689–698.
111. Gang S, Min L, Li L, Guo-Ying L, Lin X, et al. (2011) Evaluation of CT coronary artery angiography with 320-row detector CT in a high-risk population. Br J Radiol.
112. Kerl JM, Schoepf UJ, Zwerner PL, Bauer RW, Abro JA, et al. (2011) Accuracy of coronary artery stenosis detection with CT versus conventional coronary angiography compared with composite findings from both tests as an enhanced reference standard. European radiology 21: 1895–1903.
113. Moon JH, Park E-A, Lee W, Yin YH, Chung JW, et al. (2011) The Diagnostic Accuracy, Image Quality and Radiation Dose of 64-Slice Dual-Source CT in Daily Practice: a Single Institution's Experience. Korean Journal of Radiology 12: 308–318.
114. Stolzmann P, Goetti R, Baumueller S, Plass A, Falk V, et al. (2011) Prospective and retrospective ECG-gating for CT coronary angiography perform similarly accurate at low heart rates. Eur J Radiol 79: 85–91.
115. van Velzen JE, Schuijf JD, de Graaf FR, Boersma E, Pundziute G, et al. (2011) Diagnostic performance of non-invasive multidetector computed tomography coronary angiography to detect coronary artery disease using different endpoints: detection of significant stenosis vs. detection of atherosclerosis. Eur Heart J 32: 637–645.
116. van Velzen J, de Graaf F, Kroft L, de Roos A, Reiber JHC, et al. (2011) Performance and efficacy of 320-row computed tomography coronary angiography in patients presenting with acute chest pain: results from a clinical registry. The International Journal of Cardiovascular Imaging (formerly Cardiac Imaging): 1–12.
117. Vavere AL, Arbab-Zadeh A, Rochitte CE, Dewey M, Niinuma H, et al. (2011) Coronary Artery Stenoses: Accuracy of 64–Detector Row CT Angiography in Segments with Mild, Moderate, or Severe Calcification—A Subanalysis of the CORE-64 Trial. Radiology 261: 100–108.
118. Xu L, Yang L, Fan Z, Yu W, Lv B, et al. (2011) Diagnostic performance of 320-detector CT coronary angiography in patients with atrial fibrillation: preliminary results. Eur Radiol 21: 936–943.
119. Zhang T, Luo Z, Wang D, Han D, Bai J, et al. (2011) Radiation dose in coronary artery angiography with 320-detector row CT and its diagnostic accuracy: comparison with 64-detector row CT. Minerva Med 102: 249–259.
120. Dharampal AS, Papadopoulou SL, Rossi A, Weustink AC, Mollet NR, et al. (2012) Computed tomography coronary angiography accuracy in women and men at low to intermediate risk of coronary artery disease. Eur Radiol 22: 2415–2423.
121. Kadokami T, Ando S, Momii H, Yoshida M, Narita S, et al. (2012) Diagnostic performance of cardiac fusion images from myocardial perfusion imaging and multislice computed tomography coronary angiography for assessment of hemodynamically significant coronary artery lesions: an observational study. Nucl Med Commun 33: 60–68.
122. Kerl JM, Schoepf UJ, Bauer RW, Tekin T, Costello P, et al. (2012) 64-slice multidetector-row computed tomography in the diagnosis of coronary artery disease: interobserver agreement among radiologists with varied levels of experience on a per-patient and per-segment basis. J Thorac Imaging 27: 29–35.
123. Maffei E, Martini C, Rossi A, Mollet N, Lario C, et al. (2012) Diagnostic accuracy of second-generation dual-source computed tomography coronary angiography with iterative reconstructions: a real-world experience. Radiol Med 117: 725–738.
124. Maffei E, Martini C, Tedeschi C, Spagnolo P, Zuccarelli A, et al. (2012) Diagnostic accuracy of 64-slice computed tomography coronary angiography in a large population of patients without revascularisation: registry data on the comparison between male and female population. Radiol Med 117: 6–18.
125. Sohns C, Kruse S, Vollmann D, Luthje L, Dorenkamp M, et al. (2012) Accuracy of 64-multidetector computed tomography coronary angiography in patients with symptomatic atrial fibrillation prior to pulmonary vein isolation. Eur Heart J Cardiovasc Imaging 13: 263–270.
126. Uehara M, Takaoka H, Kobayashi Y, Funabashi N (2012) Diagnostic accuracy of 320-slice computed-tomography for detection of significant coronary artery stenosis in patients with various heart rates and heart rhythms compared with conventional coronary-angiography. Int J Cardiol.
127. van Velzen JE, de Graaf FR, Kroft LJ, de Roos A, Reiber JH, et al. (2012) Performance and efficacy of 320-row computed tomography coronary

angiography in patients presenting with acute chest pain: results from a clinical registry. Int J Cardiovasc Imaging 28: 865–876.

128. Gueret P, Deux JF, Bonello L, Sarran A, Tron C, et al. (2013) Diagnostic performance of computed tomography coronary angiography (from the Prospective National Multicenter Multivendor EVASCAN Study). Am J Cardiol 111: 471–478.

129. Pelliccia F, Pasceri V, Evangelista A, Pergolini A, Barilla F, et al. (2013) Diagnostic accuracy of 320-row computed tomography as compared with invasive coronary angiography in unselected, consecutive patients with suspected coronary artery disease. Int J Cardiovasc Imaging 29: 443–452.

Dual-Phase CT Collateral Score: A Predictor of Clinical Outcome in Patients with Acute Ischemic Stroke

Na-Young Shin[1], Kyung-eun Kim[1], Mina Park[1], Young Dae Kim[2], Dong Joon Kim[1], Sung Jun Ahn[1], Ji Hoe Heo[2], Seung-Koo Lee[1]*

1 Department of Radiology, Severance Hospital, Yonsei University College of Medicine, Seoul, Korea, **2** Department of Neurology, Severance Hospital, Yonsei University College of Medicine, Seoul, Korea

Abstract

Background and Purpose: The presence of good collaterals on CT angiography (CTA) is a well-known predictor for favorable outcome in acute ischemic stroke. Recently, multiphase CT has been introduced as a more accurate method in assessing collaterals. The aim of this study was to assess the ability of dual-phase CT to evaluate collateral status and predict clinical outcome.

Methods: Forty-three patients who underwent both dual-phase CT and transfemoral cerebral angiography (TFCA) for occluded intracranial internal carotid artery (ICA) and/or middle cerebral artery (M1 segment) were recruited from a prospectively collected database. The collateral status on dual-phase CT was graded by using a 4-point scale: grade 0 = no collaterals; 1 = some collaterals with persistence of some defects; 2 = slow but complete collaterals; and 3 = fast and complete collaterals. Univariate and multivariate analysis were performed to define the independent predictors for favorable outcome at 3 months.

Results: Dual-phase CT collateral status ($\rho = 0.744$) showed higher correlation with TFCA collateral status than CTA collateral status ($\rho = 0.596$) and substantial interobserver agreement (weighted $\kappa = 0.776$). In the univariate analysis, age, history of hypertension, collateral scores on CTA, dual-phase CT, and TFCA, occlusion in intracranial ICA, final infarct volume, and symptomatic hemorrhage were significantly associated with outcome. Among them, only the dual-phase CT collateral score was an independent predictor for favorable outcome (OR = 26.342 (2.788–248.864); $P = 0.004$) in the multivariate analysis.

Conclusions: The collateral status on dual-phase CT can be a useful predictor for clinical outcome in acute stroke patients, especially when advanced CT techniques are not available in emergent situations.

Editor: Jean-Claude Baron, INSERM U894, Centre de Psychiatrie et Neurosciences, Hopital Sainte-Anne and Université Paris 5, France

Funding: These authors have no support or funding to report.

Competing Interests: The authors have declared that no competing interests exist.

* Email: slee@yuhs.ac

Introduction

The presence of good collateral circulation to the ischemic territory is a notable predictor for favorable long term clinical outcome as well as small infarct size and good response to treatment in patients with proximal intracranial arterial occlusion [1–6]. These beneficial roles may be attributable to preserve downstream perfusion distal to occluded vessels, to permit access of thrombolytic materials to the distal end of the clot by retrograde flow, and to augment washout of emboli in distal arteries [7–9].

Transfemoral cerebral angiography (TFCA) has been considered as a gold standard to assess collateral status owing to its temporal and spatial resolution. However, global evaluation of pial collateral flow requires catheterization of multiple vessels and, as an invasive investigation with recognized complication rate, is usually only performed when IA treatment is indicated. To aid selection of treatment strategy or to prognosticate, a method of collateral assessment for all stroke patients, not just for those undergoing intra-arterial therapy is warranted. Furthermore, accurate non-invasive assessment of collateral status prior to endovascular therapy would also be advantageous. Therefore, noninvasive assessment of collateral status before IA treatment or in patients who are not candidates for IA treatment may be helpful to select the treatment strategy and predict long term outcome.

Because of short scan times and easy accessibility, computed tomography (CT) is used as the first imaging modality in most patients with acute ischemic stroke. Diverse collateral scoring methods have been suggested in the last decades using CT angiography source images (CTA-SI) [4,5,7,10–14] and CTA maximum intensity projection (MIP) images [6,12,15,16]. Although there is no standard scoring system, CTA allows prediction of clinical outcome with moderate to excellent interobserver agreement [11–13,16,17]. To overcome limitations of CTA such

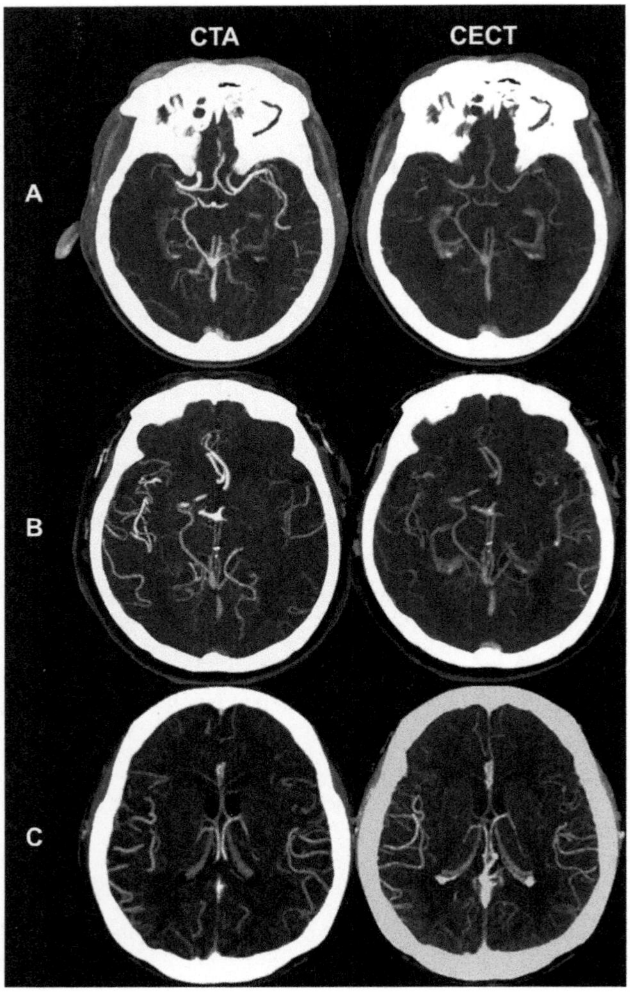

Figure 1. Representative images of collateral status on dual-phase CT. A, Some collaterals to the right MCA territory on CTA with persistence of some defects on CECT (Grade 1). B, Collaterals in part of the left MCA territory on CTA with complete filling on CECT (Grade 2). The collaterals show lower attenuation on CTA with equal to higher attenuation on CECT than unaffected vessels, suggesting slow inflow and washout of collaterals. C, Collaterals in the entire right MCA territory on both CTA and delayed CECT (Grade 3). The collateral vessels show attenuation similar to unaffected vessels on both phase images, suggesting fast velocity of collaterals.

as absence of temporal information from single phase acquisition and possible underestimation of collateral status from faster image acquisition, multi- [18,19] or tri-phase CT [20] and perfusion CT [3,21] have been proposed for assessing collateral status. At our institution, the routine CT protocol consists of noncontrast CT (NCCT), CTA, and delayed contrast enhanced CT (CECT). We empirically found that dual-phase CT composed of CTA and delayed CECT is helpful for predicting clinical outcome in patients with acute stroke. Therefore, the aim of this study was to assess the ability of dual-phase CT to evaluate collateral status and predict clinical outcome.

Materials and Methods

Patients

The patients were retrospectively selected from a prospectively collected neurointerventional database in a single institution. From February 2011 to June 2013, we recruited consecutive patients who underwent TFCA for possible thrombolysis/mechanical thrombectomy for acute ischemic stroke and met the following inclusion criteria: (1) occlusion of the intracranial ICA or M1 segment; (2) time from symptom onset to admission <6 hours; and (3) presence of a standard local CT protocol including NCCT, CTA, and delayed CECT. Exclusion criteria included bilateral anterior circulation occlusion, posterior circulation occlusion, significant stenosis in contralateral anterior circulation, and past history of stroke.

Clinical data were collected from a prospectively recorded stroke registry database. Type of stroke etiology was classified using Trial of Org 10172 in Acute Stroke Treatment (TOAST) criteria [22]. Functional outcome was assessed using the modified Rankin Scale score (mRS) at 3 months and classified as favorable (≤2) and unfavorable (>2). This study was approved by Severance hospital Institutional Review Board. The Clinical Research Ethics Committee waived the need for written informed consent from the participants because the data released from the hospital database were analyzed anonymously.

Image Acquisition

CT images were obtained on a 64 multi-detector row CT system (Sensation 64; Siemens, Erlangen, Germany). The sequential axial 3-mm NCCT was performed first with the following parameters from the skull base to the vertex: 120 kVp, 300 mAs, field of view (FOV) of 25 cm, feed/rotation 18 mm, 30×0.6 mm collimation and a H30s medium reconstruction kernel. Each of the conventional axial CT images was subsequently reconstructed into 1.2 mm slices and 1.2 mm increments. A nonionic contrast agent was administered followed by a 40 ml saline chaser at a rate of 4 ml/s by using a power injector. A bolus tracking technique was used with a marker placed at the ascending aorta, triggering at 100 Hounsfield Units (HU) above baseline with a 7 s delay prior to image acquisition. CTA from the aortic arch to the vertex was performed with the following parameters: 120 kVp, 160 mA, FOV of 18–20 cm, 0.33 s per rotation, 0.8 pitch, and a 0.6-mm section thickness. Delayed CECT was performed with the same parameters as NCCT 40 s after contrast injection. The effective dose which was calculated by the CTDI volume x the scan range x the conversion factor was 1.8 mSv for NCCT and CECT, respectively, 0.9 mSv for the cranial portion of CTA, and 3.0 mSv for the cervical portion of CTA. Therefore the total effective dose was 5.7mSv.

TFCA was performed using biplane digital subtraction angiograms (Allura Xper FD20/20; Philips Healthcare, Best, Netherlands) in all patients for the purpose of IA thrombolysis/thrombectomy via bilateral ICAs and the dominant vertebral artery.

Routine follow-up MRI was obtained 1 day after the onset of symptoms with the 3-Tesla MR system (Achieva; Philips Healthcare, Best, Netherlands). DWI was performed with single shot echo planar imaging and parameters were as follows: b-value 1000 s/mm2, TR/TE 6500–7000/65–78 ms, slice thickness 3 mm, FOV 230 mm, matrix 128×128, and NEX 1.

Image Analysis

Imaging studies at admission. *CT:* The extent of ischemic lesions on NCCT scan images at admission was rated according to the Alberta Stroke Programme Early CT Score (ASPECTS) [23].

Collaterals on dual-phase CT were graded on CTA and delayed CECT axial MIP images by using a 4-point scale [19]: Grade 0 = no collaterals to the occluded arterial territory; 1 = some collaterals to the occluded arterial territory with persistence of

Table 1. Demographic characteristics according to dual-phase collateral status.

	Collateral status on dual-phase CT				
	Incomplete (G1) (n = 10)	**Slow-complete (G2) (n = 23)**	**Rapid-complete (G3) (n = 10)**	***P* value**	**Post-hoc analysis**
Age, y, mean ± SD	75.9±6.8	70.1±10.7	61.1±11.4	0.010*	G1>G3 (*P* = 0.008)
Sex, n, M:F	4:3	13:10	6:4	0.974‡	
Risk factors					
Hypertension, n (%)	9 (90.0)	14 (60.9)	1 (10.0)	0.001‡	G1>G3 (*P* = 0.002)
Diabetes, n (%)	4 (40.0)	5 (21.7)	0 (0.0)	0.109‡	
Hypercholesterolemia, n (%)	3 (30.0)	2 (8.7)	0 (0.0)	0.147‡	
Smoking, n (%)	6 (60.0)	8 (34.8)	6 (60.0)	0.302‡	
Coronary artery disease, n (%)	3 (30.0)	10 (43.5)	3 (30.0)	0.763‡	
Clinical measures at presentation					
SBP, mmHg, median (IQR)	134.0 (111.0–161.0)	135.0 (120.0–146.5)	138.5 (112.0–149.0)	0.947†	
DBP, mmHg, mean ± SD	78.5 mmHg	76.3 mmHg	74.9 mmHg	0.680*	
Glucose, mmol/L, median (IQR)	7.25 (6.9–8.6)	6.7 (5.7–8.3)	7.1 (5.9–8.9)	0.490†	
NIHSS score, median (IQR)	16.5 (12.0–19.0)	17.0 (14.3–19.0)	14.0 (13.0–19.0)	0.210†	
TOAST classification				0.015‡	
Large artery, n (%)	1 (10.0)	2 (8.7)	6 (60.0)		
Cardioembolic, n (%)	7 (70.0)	14 (60.9)	4 (40.0)		
Undetermined, n (%)	2 (20.0)	7 (30.4)	0 (0.0)		
CT					
Time from symptom onset to CT, min, mean ± SD	170.9±106.6	209.0±91.1	170.0±87.1	0.415*	
ASPECTS, mean ± SD	6.3±1.8	7.6±1.2	8.5±1.0	0.002*	G1<G2 (*P* = 0.038), G1<G3 (*P* = 0.002)
Occluded segment					
Intracranial ICA, n (%)	5 (50.0)	4 (17.4)	0 (0.0)	0.018‡	
Proximal M1, n (%)	7 (70.0)	16 (69.6)	7 (70.0)	1.000‡	
Distal M1, n (%)	8 (80.0)	20 (87.0)	8 (80.0)	0.753‡	
Thrombus length, mm, median (IQR)	19.3 (11.9–25.5)	15.8 (8.6–18.5)	11.0 (7.3–18.8)	0.298†	
IV tPA					
IV tPA, n (%)	5 (50.0)	11 (47.8)	8 (80.0)	0.275.	
Time from symptom onset to IV tPA, min, mean ± SD	77.8±20.6	108.6±41.4	91.4±38.2	0.301*	
TFCA					
TICI ≥ 2b, n (%)	5 (50.0)	5 (21.7)	2 (20.0)	0.264	
Time from symptom onset to recanalization	385.3±198.2	375.3±106.3	304.0±103.0	0.447	
Outcome					
Final infarct volume, ml, median (IQR)	91.1 (49.1–183.2)	25.0 (10.3–76.7)	12.3 (7.5–27.8)	0.047	G1>G2 (*P* = 0.012), G1>G3 (*P* = 0.021)
Symptomatic hemorrhage	3 (30.0)	3 (13.0)	1 (10.0)	0.537	
parenchymal hematoma	5 (50.0)	4 (17.4)	2 (20.0)	0.199	
3m-mRS ≤ 2	0 (0.0)	14 (60.9)	9 (90.0)	<0.001	G1<G2 (*P* = 0.003), G1<G3 (*P*<0.001)

ASPECTS indicates Alberta Stroke Program Early CT Score; DBP, diastolic blood pressure; IQR, Interquatile range; mRS, modified Rankin Score; NIHSS, National Institutes of Health Stroke Scale; SBP indicates systolic blood pressure; TICI, thrombolysis in cerebral infarction; TOAST, Trial of Org 10172 in Acute Stroke Treatment; and tPA, tissue plasminogen activator.

* one-way ANOVA; † Kruskal Wallis test; ‡ Fisher's exact test

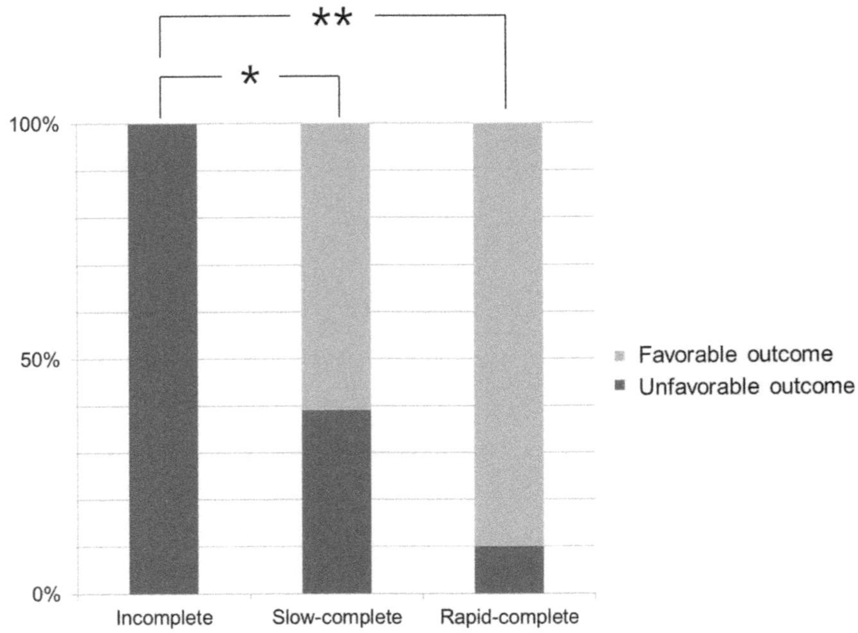

Figure 2. Clinical outcome according to collateral status. All patients with incomplete collaterals showed unfavorable outcome at 3 months. Patients with complete collaterals had favorable clinical outcome more frequently than did patients with incomplete collaterals. * $P=0.003$; ** $P<0.001$

some defects; 2 = slow but complete collaterals (detectable only on delayed CECT) without defects; and 3 = fast and complete collaterals (detectable on both CTA and delayed CECT; Figure 1). Collateral vessel scores were assessed on CTA-SI images using a scale of 0–3: 0 = absence of collateral supply to the occluded vascular territory; 1 = collateral supply filling <50% but >0% of the occluded vascular territory; 2 = collateral supply filling >50% but <100% of the occluded vascular territory; and 3 = collateral supply filling 100% of the occluded vascular territory [6]. The collateral scores on both dual-phase CT and CTA were evaluated independently by two neuroradiologist (N.Y.S. with 4 years of experience and M.P. with 1 year of experience) blinded to the clinical data. Disagreements were settled by consensus.

Occluded segments were recorded based on the location of the non-enhanced segment on delayed CECT as follows [24]: intracranial ICA; proximal M1 segment = occlusion at or proximal to the lenticulostriate arteries; and distal M1 segment = occlusion distal to the lenticulostriate arteries before MCA genu. The thrombus length was measured quantitatively on CECT curved multiplanar reformatted (MPR) images by a neuroimaging fellow (K.E.K. with 1 year of experience) blinded to the clinical data.

TFCA: The collateral flow grading system suggested by the Technology Assessment Committees of the American Society of Interventional and Therapeutic Neuroradiology and the Society of Interventional Radiology [24] was used to assess collateral vessels on TFCA: grade 0 = no collaterals to the ischemic region; 1 = slow collaterals to the periphery of the ischemic region with persistence of some defects; 2 = rapid collaterals to the periphery of the ischemic region with persistence of some defects; 3 = slow but complete collaterals to the ischemic bed by the late venous phase; and 4 = complete and rapid collaterals. The assessment of collateral flow was performed through arterial and late venous phases considering all possible collaterals from bilateral carotid and dominant vertebral angiography.

TICI score was recorded to assess recanalization using a 5-point scale [24]: 0 = no perfusion; 1 = penetration of contrast material beyond the occluded segment with minimal perfusion; 2a = partial perfusion (<2/3) of the entire vascular territory; 2b = complete but slow perfusion of the entire vascular territory; and 3 = complete perfusion and rapid clearance comparable to the uninvolved vascular territory. TICI 2b and 3 were considered recanalization.

Imaging outcome. The final infarct volume was measured on diffusion weighted images of 1-day follow-up MRI [25] using semiautomatic segmentation. The hemorrhagic transformation on follow-up CT or MRI was classified into hemorrhagic infarction or parenchymal hematoma and determined if it was symptomatic hemorrhage according to ECASS criteria [26].

Statistics

Nonparametric tests were used for non-normally distributed data. Baseline characteristics were compared according to collateral status on dual-phase CT. Continuous variables are reported as mean ± SD or as the median (interquartile range (IQR)) and were compared using one-way analysis of variance or the Kruskal-Wallis test. Categorical variables are reported as numbers (proportions, %) and were compared using the Fisher's exact test. Post hoc analysis was also performed using the Students' t-test, Mann-Whitney U test, chi-square test, or Fisher's exact test where appropriate with correction for multiple comparisons.

Spearman's rank correlation was used to assess the correlation between collateral status on dual-phase CT or CTA and collateral status on TFCA. Interobserver agreement for assessment of collateral status on CT was determined using weighted Kappa (κ) statistics [27]. The level of agreement was defined as follows: $\kappa \leq 0.2$, poor; $0.2<\kappa\leq 0.4$, fair; $0.4<\kappa\leq 0.6$, moderate; $0.6<\kappa\leq 0.8$, substantial, and $0.8<\kappa$, good.

To test the association between various clinical and imaging characteristics including collateral status on dual-phase CT and clinical outcome, univariate logistic regression was performed.

Table 2. Univariate analysis for favorable clinical outcome (mRS ≤2) at 3 months.

	Favorable (n = 23)	Unfavorable (n = 20)	Univariate analysis		
			Odds ratio	95% CI	*P* value
Age, y, mean ± SD	66.1±10.2	73.4±11.0	0.934	0.874–0.997	0.040
Male, n (%)	16 (69.6)	9 (45.0)	2.794	0.800–9.760	0.107
Risk factors					
Hypertension, n (%)	9 (39.1)	15 (75.0)	0.214	0.058–0.797	0.022
Diabetes, n (%)	4 (17.4)	5 (25.0)	0.632	0.144–2.771	0.542
Hypercholesterolemia, n (%)	1 (4.3)	4 (20.0)	0.182	0.019–1.785	0.143
Smoking, n (%)	12 (52.2)	8 (40.0)	1.636	0.487–5.500	0.426
Coronary artery disease, n (%)	11 (47.8)	5 (25.0)	2.749	0.748–10.102	0.128
Clinical measures at admission					
SBP, mmHg, median (IQR)	135.0 (114.0–144.0)	140.5 (113.5–163.5)	0.980	0.956–1.005	0.114
DBP, mmHg, mean ± SD	73.5±11.0	79.9±17.3	0.967	0.924–1.013	0.157
Glucose, mmol/L, median (IQR)	6.7 (103.0–154.3)	7.25 (121.0–152.5)	1.028	0.793–1.334	0.833
NIHSS score, median (IQR)	15.0 (13.0–16.8)	18.0 (15.5–19.0)	0.873	0.747–1.020	0.088
Delays					
Time from symptom onset to IV tPA, min, mean ± SD	96.8±39.5	96.4±36.7	1.000	0.978–1.023	0.983
Time from symptom onset to CT, min, mean ± SD	198.0±95.7	183.0±93.2	1.002	0.995–1.008	0.596
Time from symptom onset to IA treatment, min, mean ± SD	268.2±107.9	259.2±113.8	1.001	0.995–1.006	0.785
TOAST classification					
Large artery, n (%)	7 (30.4)	2 (10.0)	Reference		0.286
Cardioembolic, n (%)	12 (52.2)	13 (65.0)	0.264	0.046–1.528	0.137
Undetermined, n (%)	4 (17.4)	5 (25.0)	0.229	0.029–1.774	0.158
CT					
ASPECTS, mean ± SD	8.0±0.9	6.9±1.8	1.908	1.135–3.209	0.015
CTA Collateral score	2.0 (2.0–3.0)	1.0 (1.0–2.0)	6.077	1.926–19.167	0.002
0, n (%)	0 (0.0)	0 (0.0)			
1, n (%)	4 (17.4)	14 (70.0)			
2, n (%)	12 (52.2)	5 (25.0)			
3, n (%)	7 (30.4)	1 (5.0)			
Dual-phase CT collateral score	2.4±0.5	1.6±0.6	19.436	2.581–146.371	0.004
0, n (%)	0 (0.0)	0 (0.0)			
1, n (%)	0 (0.0)	10 (50.0)			
2, n (%)	14 (60.9)	9 (45.0)			
3, n (%)	9 (39.1)	1 (5.0)			
Occluded segment					
Intracranial ICA, n (%)	2 (8.7)	7 (35.0)	0.177	0.032–0.985	0.048
Proximal M1, n (%)	14 (60.9)	16 (80.0)	0.389	0.098–1.544	0.179
Distal M1, n (%)	20 (87.0)	16 (80.0)	1.667	0.325–8.549	0.540
Thrombus length, mm, median (IQR)	11.4 (7.4–17.6)	17.9 (10.4–22.8)	0.938	0.871–1.011	0.093
Treatment					
IV tPA only, n (%)	3 (13.0)	0 (0.0)	Reference		0.639
IA only, n (%)	8 (34.8)	11 (55.0)	0.000	0.000	0.999
IV tPA and IA, n (%)	12 (52.2)	9 (45.0)	0.000	0.000	0.999
TFCA					
TFCA collateral score	3.0 (2.3–4.0)	2.0 (1.0–2.0)	3.092	1.537–6.221	0.002
0, n (%)	0 (0.0)	0 (0.0)			
1, n (%)	2 (8.7)	8 (40.0)			

Table 2. Cont.

	Favorable (n = 23)	Unfavorable (n = 20)	Univariate analysis		
			Odds ratio	95% CI	*P* value
2, n (%)	4 (17.4)	8 (40.0)			
3, n (%)	6 (26.1)	2 (10.0)			
4, n (%)	11 (47.8)	2 (10.0)			
TICI ≥ 2b, n (%)	4 (17.4)	8 (40.0)	0.316	0.078–1.282	0.107
Time from symptom onset to recanalization, min, mean ± SD	352.0±110.6	383.0±152.3	0.998	0.993–1.003	0.998
Imaging outcome					
Final infarct volume, ml, median (IQR)	13.7 (7.2–25.0)	80.7 (34.0–144.8)	0.965	0.943–0.988	0.003
Symptomatic hemorrhage, n (%)	1 (4.3)	6 (30.0)	0.106	0.012–0.977	0.048
Parenchymal hematoma, n (%)	3 (13.0)	8 (40.0)	0.225	0.050–1.016	0.052

ASPECTS indicates Alberta Stroke Program Early CT Score; DBP, diastolic blood pressure; IQR, Interquatile range; mRS, modified Rankin Score; NIHSS, National Institutes of Health Stroke Scale; SBP indicates systolic blood pressure; TFCA, transfemoral cerebral angiography; TICI, thrombolysis in cerebral infarction; TOAST, Trial of Org 10172 in Acute Stroke Treatment; and tPA, tissue plasminogen activator.

Multivariate logistic regression with backward elimination (probability value for elimination of 0.1) was used to identify independent factors for favorable outcome. Variables significantly associated with a favorable outcome in the univariate analysis ($P<0.05$) were included in the multivariable model. To assess independent predictors before IA treatment, multivariate analysis with clinical and CT variables was also performed. Receiver operating curve (ROC) comparison was performed to compare the prediction ability of models containing either dual-phase CT collateral (model 1), CTA collateral (model 2), or TFCA collateral (model 3) scores.

All statistical analyses were performed using SAS, version 9.2 (SAS Institute, Cary, NC, USA) and SPSS, version 19 software (IBM Corp., Armonk, NY, USA). ROC curve comparison was performed by using MedCalc, Version 9.3.9.0 software (MedCalc software, Mariakerke, Belgium). *P* values less than 0.05 were considered statistically significant.

Results

Among 166 patients who underwent TFCA for possible thrombolysis/mechanical thrombectomy for acute ischemic stroke, 123 patients were excluded due to posterior circulation occlusion (n = 34), anterior cerebral arterial occlusion (n = 4), occlusion distal to the M1 segment (n = 41), proximal ICA occlusion only (n = 12), old territorial infarcts (n = 8), multiple territorial infarcts due to cardioembolism (n = 2), significant stenosis in the contralateral M1 segment (n = 1), moyamoya disease (n = 1), and only NCCT acquisition (n = 20). Therefore, a total of 43 patients were recruited for this study. The patients underwent IA treatment with stent-assisted thrombectomy (SAT; n = 29), Penumbra system (n = 1), both SAT and Penumbra system (n = 4), stent placement after mechanical thrombectomy (n = 4), Penumbra system with urokinase infusion (n = 2), and urokinase infusion only (n = 1).

Patient demographic and clinical data according to collateral status on dual-phase CT are summarized in Table 1. Ten (23.3%) patients were grouped as grade 1 (incomplete collaterals); 23 (53.5%) as grade 2 (slow-complete collaterals); and 10 (23.3%) as grade 3 (rapid-complete collaterals). No patients were classified as grade 0 (no collaterals). There was no statistical difference in the time from symptom onset to CT scan between there groups ($P = 0.415$). Patients with incomplete collaterals were older than those with rapid-complete collaterals ($P = 0.008$). Patients with less collaterals had hypertension more often, although other cardiovascular risk factors did not show differences in the prevalence across different collateral patterns. The pattern of leptomeningeal collaterals on dual-phase CT was also associated with the TOAST classification of stroke: cardioembolic infarcts were observed more often in patients with less collaterals than those with large arterial infarcts. Less collaterals were associated with lower ASPECTS on NCCT ($P = 0.002$) and the presence of intracranial ICA occlusion ($P = 0.018$). Final infarct volume was significantly larger in patients with incomplete collaterals (91.1 (IQR, 49.1–183.2) ml) than that in patients with slow-complete (25.0 (IQR, 10.3–76.7) ml) and rapid-complete (12.3 (IQR, 7.5–27.8) ml) collaterals on dual-phase CT ($P = 0.012$ and $P = 0.021$, respectively). Clinical outcome was also more favorable in patients with complete collateral patterns (Figure 2). However, there was no significant difference in recanalization rate or hemorrhagic transformation according to collateral pattern.

The dual-phase collateral scores showed higher correlation with collateral status on TFCA ($\rho = 0.744$; $P<0.001$) than that of the CTA collateral scores ($\rho = 0.596$; $P<0.001$). Interobserver agreement for the collateral scoring on dual-phase CT [weighted $\kappa = 0.776$ (0.619–0.933)] was substantial and better than that on CTA [weighted $\kappa = 0.475$ (0.285–0.665)].

Univariate analysis of patients with good and poor clinical outcome is presented in Table 2. Younger age ($P = 0.040$), absence of history of hypertension ($P = 0.022$), higher collateral scores on CTA ($P = 0.002$), dual-phase CT ($P = 0.004$), and TFCA ($P = 0.002$), absence of occlusion in intracranial ICA ($P = 0.048$), smaller final infarct volume ($P = 0.003$), and absence of symptomatic hemorrhage ($P = 0.048$) were all significantly associated with favorable clinical outcome. Multivariate analysis of all significant variables using backward elimination showed that only the collateral score on dual-phase CT [odds ratio (OR) = 26.342 (2.788–248.864); $P = 0.004$] was an independent predictor for favorable outcome with adjustment for NIHSS scores at admission [OR = 0.834 (0.679–1.025); $P = 0.085$]. Moreover, multivariate analysis with significant clinical and imaging variables before IA treatment also showed the dual-phase CT collateral score [OR = 27.117 (1.519–484.258); $P = 0.025$] as an independent

Table 3. Multivariate analysis for favorable clinical outcome (mRS ≤2) at 3 months.

	Model 1			Model 2			Model 3		
	Odds ratio	95% CI	*P* value	Odds ratio	95% CI	*P* value	Odds ratio	95% CI	*P* value
Age	0.969	0.880–1.067	0.520	0.953	0.877–1.035	0.250	0.958	0.879–1.044	0.332
Hypertension	2.682	0.294–24.508	0.382	1.435	0.187–10.993	0.728	1.164	0.171–7.939	0.877
NIHSS score at admission	0.814	0.648–1.023	0.077	0.868	0.731–1.029	0.103	0.826	0.678–1.006	0.058
ASPECTS	1.504	0.675–3.351	0.318	1.515	0.793–2.893	0.208	1.480	0.734–2.984	0.273
Occlusion of intracranial ICA	0.518	0.057–4.679	0.558	0.273	0.032–2.318	0.234	0.245	0.025–2.371	0.225
Dual-phase CT collateral score	27.117	1.519–484.258	0.025	-	-	-	-	-	-
CTA collateral score	-	-	-	4.456	0.929–21.365	0.062	-	-	-
TFCA collateral score	-	-	-	-	-	-	2.996	1.138–7.890	0.026
AUC	0.922 (0.798–0.981)			0.880 (0.745–0.959)			0.874 (0.737–0.955)		

ASPECTS indicates Alberta Stroke Program Early CT Score; AUC, area under the curve; ICA, internal carotid artery; and NIHSS, National Institutes of Health Stroke Scale.

predictor for clinical outcome even after adjustment of age, presence of hypertension, NIHSS score at admission, ASPECTS, and occlusion of intracranial ICA. Meanwhile, the CTA collateral score in model 2 was not an independent predictor ($P = 0.062$) unlike dual-phase CT collateral score in model 1. Although the TFCA collateral score was also an independent predictor [OR = 2.996 (1.138–7.890); $P = 0.026$], the area under the curve (AUC) of model 3 (0.874) was lower than that of model 1 (0.922). However, it failed to achieve a level of statistical significance ($P = 0.206$; Table 3).

Discussion

The present study suggests collateral status on dual-phase CT may be an independent predictor [OR = 26.342 (2.788–248.864); $P = 0.004$] for clinical outcome in acute ischemic stroke patients who are subjected to IA treatment. Moreover, after adjustment of clinical and CT variables measured before IA treatment, collateral status on dual-phase CT was also an independent predictor for clinical outcome [OR = 25.763 (1.342–494.601); $P = 0.031$]. On the other hand, the CTA collateral score could not independently predict clinical outcome in model 2. Also, although there was no statistical significance, the prediction model with the dual-phase CT collateral score was better than that with TFCA collateral scores.

Leptomeningeal collaterals have been considered as having a beneficial role in patients with acute stroke despite various scoring scales and different imaging modalities [17]. CT, which is noninvasive and widely available in emergency situations, has been used to evaluate collateral status. Above all, CTA-based methods are the most commonly suggested so far [4–6,10–14]. However, the prediction power of these methods can be influenced by small differences in time delay from contrast injection to image acquisition as there is no dynamic information on single phase CTA. Before the era of fast CTA acquisition, CTA images were acquired under an almost steady-state condition with maximal enhancement in arteries and tissues. Therefore, the nonenhanced area on this protocol is associated with decreased cerebral blood volume and can be a predictor for cerebral infarction [11]. After the introduction of multidetector CT that has made fast acquisition of CTA possible, slowly perfused areas via collaterals might not be enhanced on CTA images causing overestimation of infarct core [28] and thrombus length [29] as well as underestimation of collateral status [21,30]. To overcome limitations of single phase CTA, multi- [18,19] and tri-phase [20,31] CT and perfusion CT [3,21] have been suggested as a tool to assess collateral status; but the additional value of these advanced techniques over single phase CTA to predict clinical outcome lacks confirmation. Moreover, lack of ubiquitousness of these advanced sequences and post processing techniques, insufficient scan coverage, and potential radiation hazard caused by additional CT scans might be problems in daily clinical practice.

A previous study using tri-phase CT [31] graded collateral scores on each phase image and focused on identifying the best phase to predict infarct volume. A recent study with time-resolved assessment of collateral status on perfusion CT [21] also scored collateral status on early and peak phases and temporal MIP reconstruction images which were obtained by fusing contrast enhancement across the whole duration of the 4-dimensional CTA. This study classified patients into incomplete, slow-complete, and rapid-complete collateral flow groups by integrating dynamic information from various phase images. In addition, they also showed that complete collateral flow groups achieve favorable clinical outcome more often; however, the effective dose of this CT protocol was 8.5 mSv excluding NCCT. Kim et al. [19] obtained multiphase CT and evaluated collateral status on mid (23 and 32 s after contrast injection) and late (41 and 50 s after contrast injection) phase CECT images by using the same scales that were used in our study. They found high correlation between collateral status on these two phase images and TFCA. However, analysis of the effect of collateral status on multiphase CT on clinical outcome was not conducted. It is worth noting that the time delay between contrast injection and image acquisition of mid and late phases were similar to those of CTA and delayed CECT in the present study. Thus, supporting that only dual-phase CT with optimized time delay from contrast injection may have sufficient dynamic information to show collateral status.

In this study, collateral scores on dual-phase CT showed better correlation with collateral status on TFCA and higher interobserver agreement than did collateral scores on single phase CTA. Also, as mentioned above, collateral status on dual-phase CT was an independent predictor for clinical outcome; however, collateral scores on single phase CTA and even TFCA were not. On dual-phase CT, detection of collateral defects on CTA and delayed CECT was needed. On the other hand, additional detection on the degree (smaller or larger than 50% of the occluded territory) of collateral extent was required on single phase CTA. Therefore, the observers might grade collateral status more consistently on dual-phase CT. Both dual-phase CTA and TFCA provide dynamic information of collaterals; however, it is difficult to evaluate pial collaterals from whole cerebral circulation by TFCA, so the prediction power for clinical outcome might be lower than that of dual-phase CT.

Among the patients with complete collaterals on dual-phase CT, patients with rapid-complete collaterals had higher ASPECT scores at admission (7.6 vs. 8.5), smaller final infarct volume (25.0 ml vs. 12.3 ml), and more frequent favorable clinical outcome (60.9% vs. 90%) than patients with slow-complete collaterals. Although there was no significant differences between the two groups as reported in a previous study [21], the number of patients may have been too small to reach a statistically significant conclusion. Therefore, prospective studies with larger sample size and an optimized CT protocol are warranted to establish the influence of collateral velocity on clinical outcome.

There were several limitations in our study. First, this study was a retrospective study although the patients were recruited from a prospectively collected database. Also a small number of patients included in the analysis might cause a wide range of 95% CI of OR of dual-phase CT collateral status and its overestimation. Therefore, caution is needed in generalizing the results of this study. Second, more than 50% of patients were treated with IV thrombolysis. As a result of the IV treatment, potential confounding factors may have influenced the assessment of collateral status on TFCA and prediction of clinical outcome. There might be difference in thrombus extent and the collateral status between CT and TFCA. Third, there is the possibility that selection bias may exist. Patients who achieved recanalization only after IV treatment or had substantial ischemic change larger than 1/3 of the middle cerebral artery (MCA) territory were not subjected to IA treatment and excluded from this study. We also excluded considerable number of patients according to the exclusion criteria. However, our results could be applied to a relatively homogenous patient group with occlusion of distal ICA or M1 segments who are indicated for IA treatment. Fourth, we did not perform multiphase CT or perfusion CT, so direct comparison between these advanced techniques and dual-phase CT in predicting clinical outcome was not performed. Finally, our routine CT protocol was not optimized to assess collateral status in patients with acute ischemic stroke. According to a previous study using time-resolved CTA [21], alteration of time delay from contrast injection to image acquisition has the potential to impair outcome prediction. Therefore, efforts to establish an appropriate CT protocol and future studies with this optimized CT protocol in a larger scale are required.

Conclusions

In conclusion, dual-phase CT is feasible for assessing collateral status in patients with acute ischemic stroke, showing substantial interobserver agreement. Collateral status on dual-phase CT can also be a useful predictor for clinical outcome in acute stroke patients subjected to IA treatment, especially when advanced CT techniques are not available in emergency situations.

Author Contributions

Conceived and designed the experiments: NYS SKL. Performed the experiments: NYS KEK MP. Analyzed the data: NYS KEK. Contributed reagents/materials/analysis tools: YDK JHH. Contributed to the writing of the manuscript: NYS. Revising the manuscript: YDK SKL DJK SJA.

References

1. Kucinski T, Koch C, Eckert B, Becker V, Kromer H, et al. (2003) Collateral circulation is an independent radiological predictor of outcome after thrombolysis in acute ischaemic stroke. Neuroradiology 45: 11–18.
2. Bang OY, Saver JL, Kim SJ, Kim GM, Chung CS, et al. (2011) Collateral flow predicts response to endovascular therapy for acute ischemic stroke. Stroke 42: 693–699.
3. Calleja AI, Cortijo E, Garcia-Bermejo P, Gomez RD, Perez-Fernandez S, et al. (2013) Collateral circulation on perfusion-computed tomography-source images predicts the response to stroke intravenous thrombolysis. Eur J Neurol 20: 795–802.
4. Lima FO, Furie KL, Silva GS, Lev MH, Camargo EC, et al. (2010) The pattern of leptomeningeal collaterals on CT angiography is a strong predictor of long-term functional outcome in stroke patients with large vessel intracranial occlusion. Stroke 41: 2316–2322.
5. Maas MB, Lev MH, Ay H, Singhal AB, Greer DM, et al. (2009) Collateral vessels on CT angiography predict outcome in acute ischemic stroke. Stroke 40: 3001–3005.
6. Tan IY, Demchuk AM, Hopyan J, Zhang L, Gladstone D, et al. (2009) CT angiography clot burden score and collateral score: correlation with clinical and radiologic outcomes in acute middle cerebral artery infarct. AJNR Am J Neuroradiol 30: 525–531.
7. Liebeskind DS (2003) Collateral circulation. Stroke 34: 2279–2284.
8. Bang OY, Saver JL, Alger JR, Starkman S, Ovbiagele B, et al. (2008) Determinants of the distribution and severity of hypoperfusion in patients with ischemic stroke. Neurology 71: 1804–1811.
9. Caplan LR, Hennerici M (1998) Impaired clearance of emboli (washout) is an important link between hypoperfusion, embolism, and ischemic stroke. Arch Neurol 55: 1475–1482.
10. Rosenthal ES, Schwamm LH, Roccatagliata L, Coutts SB, Demchuk AM, et al. (2008) Role of recanalization in acute stroke outcome: rationale for a CT angiogram-based "benefit of recanalization" model. AJNR Am J Neuroradiol 29: 1471–1475.
11. Schramm P, Schellinger PD, Fiebach JB, Heiland S, Jansen O, et al. (2002) Comparison of CT and CT angiography source images with diffusion-weighted imaging in patients with acute stroke within 6 hours after onset. Stroke 33: 2426–2432.
12. Tan JC, Dillon WP, Liu S, Adler F, Smith WS, et al. (2007) Systematic comparison of perfusion-CT and CT-angiography in acute stroke patients. Ann Neurol 61: 533–543.
13. Wildermuth S, Knauth M, Brandt T, Winter R, Sartor K, et al. (1998) Role of CT angiography in patient selection for thrombolytic therapy in acute hemispheric stroke. Stroke 29: 935–938.
14. Knauth M, von Kummer R, Jansen O, Hahnel S, Dorfler A, et al. (1997) Potential of CT angiography in acute ischemic stroke. AJNR Am J Neuroradiol 18: 1001–1010.

15. Soares BP, Tong E, Hom J, Cheng SC, Bredno J, et al. (2010) Reperfusion is a more accurate predictor of follow-up infarct volume than recanalization: a proof of concept using CT in acute ischemic stroke patients. Stroke 41: e34–40.
16. Miteff F, Levi CR, Bateman GA, Spratt N, McElduff P, et al. (2009) The independent predictive utility of computed tomography angiographic collateral status in acute ischaemic stroke. Brain 132: 2231–2238.
17. McVerry F, Liebeskind DS, Muir KW (2012) Systematic review of methods for assessing leptomeningeal collateral flow. AJNR Am J Neuroradiol 33: 576–582.
18. Lee SJ, Lee KH, Na DG, Byun HS, Kim YB, et al. (2004) Multiphasic helical computed tomography predicts subsequent development of severe brain edema in acute ischemic stroke. Arch Neurol 61: 505–509.
19. Kim SJ, Noh HJ, Yoon CW, Kim KH, Jeon P, et al. (2012) Multiphasic perfusion computed tomography as a predictor of collateral flow in acute ischemic stroke: comparison with digital subtraction angiography. Eur Neurol 67: 252–255.
20. Lee KH, Cho SJ, Byun HS, Na DG, Choi NC, et al. (2000) Triphasic perfusion computed tomography in acute middle cerebral artery stroke: a correlation with angiographic findings. Arch Neurol 57: 990–999.
21. Frolich AM, Wolff SL, Psychogios MN, Klotz E, Schramm R, et al. (2014) Time-resolved assessment of collateral flow using 4D CT angiography in large-vessel occlusion stroke. Eur Radiol 24: 390–396.
22. Adams HP Jr, Bendixen BH, Kappelle LJ, Biller J, Love BB, et al. (1993) Classification of subtype of acute ischemic stroke. Definitions for use in a multicenter clinical trial. TOAST. Trial of Org 10172 in Acute Stroke Treatment. Stroke 24: 35–41.
23. Barber PA, Demchuk AM, Zhang J, Buchan AM (2000) Validity and reliability of a quantitative computed tomography score in predicting outcome of hyperacute stroke before thrombolytic therapy. ASPECTS Study Group. Alberta Stroke Programme Early CT Score. Lancet 355: 1670–1674.
24. Higashida RT, Furlan AJ, Roberts H, Tomsick T, Connors B, et al. (2003) Trial design and reporting standards for intra-arterial cerebral thrombolysis for acute ischemic stroke. Stroke 34: e109–137.
25. Campbell BC, Tu HT, Christensen S, Desmond PM, Levi CR, et al. (2012) Assessing response to stroke thrombolysis: validation of 24-hour multimodal magnetic resonance imaging. Arch Neurol 69: 46–50.
26. Hacke W, Kaste M, Fieschi C, von Kummer R, Davalos A, et al. (1998) Randomised double-blind placebo-controlled trial of thrombolytic therapy with intravenous alteplase in acute ischaemic stroke (ECASS II). Second European-Australasian Acute Stroke Study Investigators. Lancet 352: 1245–1251.
27. Landis JR, Koch GG (1977) The measurement of observer agreement for categorical data. Biometrics 33: 159–174.
28. Yoo AJ, Hu R, Hakimelahi R, Lev MH, Nogueira RG, et al. (2012) CT angiography source images acquired with a fast-acquisition protocol overestimate infarct core on diffusion weighted images in acute ischemic stroke. J Neuroimaging 22: 329–335.
29. Mortimer AM, Little DH, Minhas KS, Walton ER, Renowden SA, et al. (2013) Thrombus length estimation in acute ischemic stroke: a potential role for delayed contrast enhanced CT. J Neurointerv Surg.
30. Choi JY, Kim EJ, Hong JM, Lee SE, Lee JS, et al. (2011) Conventional enhancement CT: a valuable tool for evaluating pial collateral flow in acute ischemic stroke. Cerebrovasc Dis 31: 346–352.
31. Jung SL, Lee YJ, Ahn KJ, Kim YI, Lee KS, et al. (2011) Assessment of collateral flow with multi-phasic CT: correlation with diffusion weighted MRI in MCA occlusion. J Neuroimaging 21: 225–228.

Quantification of Left Ventricular Torsion and Diastolic Recoil Using Cardiovascular Magnetic Resonance Myocardial Feature Tracking

**Johannes T. Kowallick[1,8]⁹, Pablo Lamata[2,7]⁹, Shazia T. Hussain[3], Shelby Kutty[4], Michael Steinmetz[5,8], Jan M. Sohns[1,8], Martin Fasshauer[1,8], Wieland Staab[1,8], Christina Unterberg-Buchwald[6,8], Boris Bigalke[7,9], Joachim Lotz[1,8], Gerd Hasenfuß[6,8], Andreas Schuster[6,7,8]*

1 Institute for Diagnostic and Interventional Radiology, Georg-August-University Göttingen, Göttingen, Germany, **2** Department of Computer Science, University of Oxford, Oxford, United Kingdom, **3** Papworth Hospital NHS Trust, Papworth Everard, Cambridgeshire, United Kingdom, **4** Children's Hospital and Medical Center, University of Nebraska College of Medicine, Omaha, Nebraska, United States of America, **5** Department of Pediatric Cardiology and Intensive Care Medicine, Georg-August-University Göttingen, Göttingen, Germany, **6** Department of Cardiology and Pneumology, Georg-August-University Göttingen, Göttingen, Germany, **7** Division of Imaging Sciences and Biomedical Engineering, The Rayne Institute, St. Thomas' Hospital, King's College London, London, United Kingdom, **8** DZHK (German Centre for Cardiovascular Research), partner site Göttingen, Göttingen, Germany, **9** Medizinische Klinik III, Kardiologie und Kreislauferkrankungen, Eberhard-Karls-Universität Tübingen, Tübingen, Germany

Abstract

Objectives: Cardiovascular magnetic resonance feature tracking (CMR-FT) offers quantification of myocardial deformation from routine cine images. However, data using CMR-FT to quantify left ventricular (LV) torsion and diastolic recoil are not yet available. We therefore sought to evaluate the feasibility and reproducibility of CMR-FT to quantify LV torsion and peak recoil rate using an optimal anatomical approach.

Methods: Short-axis cine stacks were acquired at rest and during dobutamine stimulation (10 and 20 $\mu g \cdot kg^{-1} \cdot min^{-1}$) in 10 healthy volunteers. Rotational displacement was analysed for all slices. A complete 3D-LV rotational model was developed using linear interpolation between adjacent slices. Torsion was defined as the difference between apical and basal rotation, divided by slice distance. Depending on the distance between the most apical (defined as 0% LV distance) and basal (defined as 100% LV distance) slices, four different models for the calculation of torsion were examined: Model-1 (25–75%), Model-2 (0–100%), Model-3 (25–100%) and Model-4 (0–75%). Analysis included subendocardial, subepicardial and global torsion and recoil rate (mean of subendocardial and subepicardial values).

Results: Quantification of torsion and recoil rate was feasible in all subjects. There was no significant difference between the different models at rest. However, only Model-1 (25–75%) discriminated between rest and stress (Global Torsion: $2.7\pm1.5°cm^{-1}$, $3.6\pm2.0°cm^{-1}$, $5.1\pm2.2°cm^{-1}$, $p<0.01$; Global Recoil Rate: $-30.1\pm11.1°cm^{-1}s^{-1}$, $-46.9\pm15.0°cm^{-1}s^{-1}$, $-68.9\pm32.3°cm^{-1}s^{-1}$, $p<0.01$; for rest, 10 and 20 $\mu g \cdot kg^{-1} \cdot min^{-1}$ of dobutamine, respectively). Reproducibility was sufficient for all parameters as determined by Bland-Altman analysis, intraclass correlation coefficients and coefficient of variation.

Conclusions: CMR-FT based derivation of myocardial torsion and recoil rate is feasible and reproducible at rest and with dobutamine stress. Using an optimal anatomical approach measuring rotation at 25% and 75% apical and basal LV locations allows effective quantification of torsion and recoil dynamics. Application of these new measures of deformation by CMR-FT should next be explored in disease states.

Editor: Zhuoli Zhang, Northwestern University Feinberg School of Medicine, United States of America

Funding: AS was funded by the Research program of the Faculty of Medicine of the Georg-August-University in Göttingen. PL holds a Sir Henry Dale Fellowship jointly funded by the Wellcome Trust and the Royal Society (Grant Number 099973/Z/12/Z). The authors are grateful for the financial support provided by the DZHK (German Centre for Cardiovascular Research). The funders had no role in study design, data collection and analysis, decision to publish, or preparation of the manuscript.

Competing Interests: The authors have declared that no competing interests exist.

* Email: andreas_schuster@gmx.net

⁹ These authors contributed equally to this work.

Introduction

The prevalence of heart failure including systolic and diastolic functional impairments continues to increase representing a major health problem [1,2]. Several diagnostic techniques have been proposed to study systolic and diastolic myocardial performances [3,4,5].

Left ventricular (LV) systolic torsion and diastolic recoil describe the myocardial twisting and untwisting motion resulting from apical counter-clockwise and basal clockwise rotation during systole (when viewed from the apex and normalized for LV length). Torsion and recoil rate have shown to be sensitive markers for systolic and diastolic dysfunction [6,7,8]. The phenomenon can be captured by the simple twist angle (difference in apical and basal rotation) [9,10], the circumferential-longitudinal shear angle [11,12] or torsion (twist per cardiac length) [13,14]. Recent studies showed that torsion might represent an important compensatory mechanism to maintain an adequate systolic function in patients with chronic hypertension as examined in a large community-based population based on cardiovascular magnetic resonance (CMR) myocardial tagging [14,15]. Recoil rate seems particularly appealing to study diastolic function. Its applicability has been demonstrated in isolated diastolic dysfunction [16], in heart failure with preserved ejection fraction [17] and heart disease characterized by both systolic and diastolic dysfunction such as hypertrophic cardiomyopathy (HCM) [18]. CMR myocardial tagging is considered the reference standard for the evaluation of torsion at the current time. However, this technique has not found widespread implementation into clinical routine since practical obstacles, e.g. the need for additional sequence acquisition and time-consuming post-processing limit its clinical applicability. Recent advances in LV deformation quantification based on CMR feature tracking (CMR-FT) allow straightforward quantification of myocardial physiology from routine steady-state free precession (SSFP) images [19,20]. The technique has been used to analyse ventricular strain in health and disease [21,22]. However, the feasibility of CMR-FT for quantitative assessment of LV torsion has never previously been demonstrated.

We therefore aimed to first develop a model that allows uniform selection of apical and basal slices at standardized LV levels and to evaluate its feasibility and reproducibility to quantify LV systolic torsion and diastolic recoil at rest and during dobutamine stress using CMR-FT.

Materials and Methods

Ten healthy volunteers underwent CMR on a 1.5 Tesla scanner (Intera R 12.6.1.3, Philips Medical Systems, Best, The Netherlands). The study protocol was approved by the Institutional Review Board at the University of Nebraska Medical Center and complies with the Declaration of Helsinki. Written informed consent was obtained from all participants.

CMR Imaging

All CMR measurements were performed in the supine position using a 5-channel cardiac surface coil. LV dimensions and function were assessed with an ECG- gated SSFP cine sequence during brief periods of breath-holding in 12 to 14 equidistant short-axis planes (slice thickness 8 mm; gap 1–2 mm) completely covering the LV. The field of view was 360×480 mm and matrix size 196×172. Dobutamine stress imaging was performed as previously described [23]. Complete short-axis stacks were acquired at rest and with 10 and 20 $\mu g \cdot kg^{-1} \cdot min^{-1}$ of dobutamine.

Haemodynamic analysis

End-diastolic (EDV) and end-systolic volume (ESV), stroke volume (SV), ejection fraction and cardiac index (CI), were calculated using MassK-Mode in QMass Version 7.6 (Medis Medical Systems, Leiden, The Netherland). Ventricular volumes were adjusted to body surface area. All parameters were analysed at rest, 10 and 20 $\mu g \cdot kg^{-1} \cdot min^{-1}$ of dobutamine stress. Furthermore, heart rate and mean blood pressure were measured at rest and with both levels of dobutamine stimulation.

Cardiac magnetic resonance myocardial feature tracking

Myocardial feature tracking was performed using dedicated software (TomTec Imaging Systems, 2D CPA MR, Cardiac Performance Analysis, Version 1.1.2.36, Unterschleissheim, Germany). All short-axis slices were included in the analysis between the most apical slice showing LV cavity at end-systole and the most basal slice including a complete circumference of myocardium at end-systole. LV endocardial and epicardial borders were manually traced in all slices using a point-and-click approach with the initial contour set at end-diastole. Endocardial and epicardial border surfaces were manually delineated and the automated tracking algorithm was applied. The software automatically tracks 48 subendocardial and subepicardial tissue voxels throughout the cardiac cycle. Tracking performance was visually reviewed to ensure accurate tracking of the ventricular myocardium. In case of insufficient border tracking manual adjustments were made to the initial contour and the algorithm was reapplied. Tracking was repeated for three times in each short-axis view and results were based on the average of the three repeated measures.

Definition of torsion and recoil rate

Torsion and peak recoil rate were calculated using MATLAB software (The Math Works, MA, USA). Averaged LV rotation profiles were calculated from the angular displacement of all 48 tissue voxels in all slices. LV rotation was averaged across the three repeated measurements. The rotation of points that would typically be located in between adjacent slices was linearly interpolated resulting in a complete 3D LV model of angular displacement (**Figure 1**). When viewed from the apex, LV torsion was calculated as the difference in counter-clockwise apical rotation (ϕ_{apex}) and clockwise rotation at the base (ϕ_{base}) divided by the inter-slice distance (D) [13,14]:

$$LV\ Torsion = \frac{\phi_{apex} - \phi_{base}}{D}$$

The distance (D) was calculated as the sum of the slice thickness (8 mm) and gap (1–2 mm) of imaging planes that were located in between the basal and apical slices where rotation was measured [14] (**Figure 2 and 3**). Depending on these measurement positions of rotation obtained at different LV locations and the distance between the most apical (defined as 0% of LV distance) and the most basal slice (defined as 100% of LV distance) the following four methods to calculate torsion were examined: Model 1 (difference in rotation between 25% and 75%), model 2 (difference in rotation between 0% and 100%), model 3 (difference in rotation between 25% and 100%) and model 4 (difference in rotation between 0% to 75%) (**Figure 3**). The analysis included subepicardial and subendocardial torsion as well as LV global torsion (averaged subendocardial and subepicardial torsion). Furthermore, subendocardial, subepicardial and global peak recoil

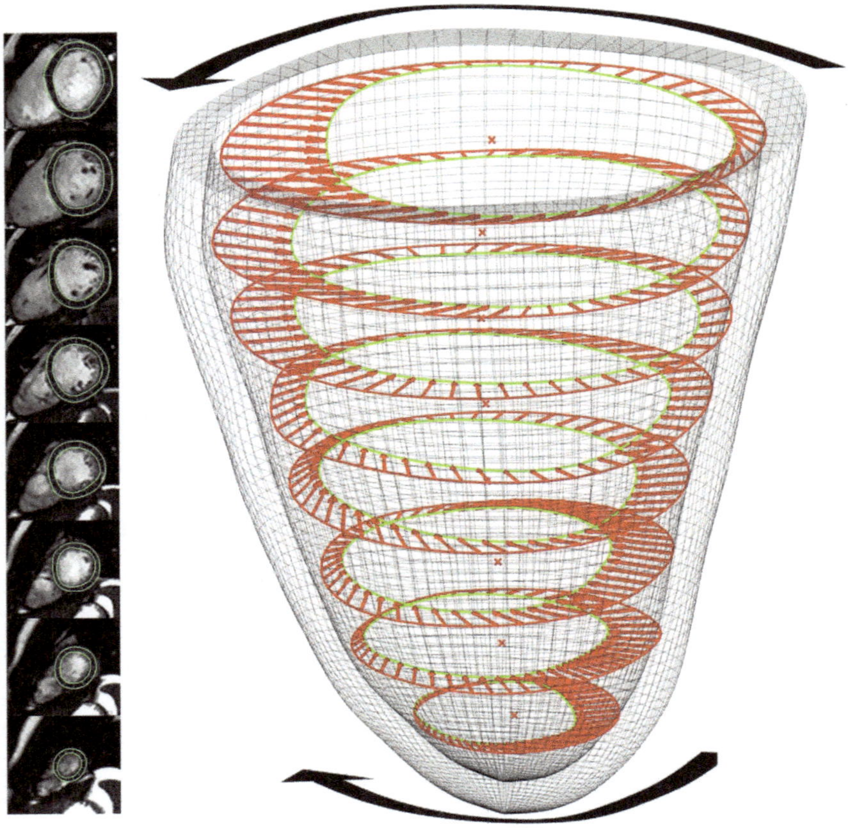

Figure 1. 3 D model of LV rotational displacement. Rotation between time points (angular difference between red and green contours) is computed in each slice, and it is then linearly interpolated between slices. The 3D ventricular model is automatically fitted to the contours [48] and is used here only for illustration purposes, and not for the definition of the location of the most apical and basal points.

rates were calculated from the maximum slope ($-d\theta/dt$) of the diastolic limb of the torsion-time curve (**Figure 2**).

Statistical Analysis

Statistical analysis was performed using Microsoft Excel and IBM SPSS Statistics version 22 for Macintosh. Data are expressed as mean (± standard deviation). Differences of torsion and peak recoil rate calculated between models 1–4 were assessed by the Friedman test. Pairwise comparisons between variables at rest and with increasing levels of dobutamine were evaluated using the Wilcoxon test. All statistical tests with p values <0.05 were considered statistically significant.

Two independent observers analysed all cases to assess inter-observer variability (JTK & AS). Intra-observer variability was derived from the repeated analysis by the first observer (JTK) after four weeks. The intra- and inter-observer variability were assessed by intraclass correlation coefficients (ICC) using a model of absolute agreement. Agreement was considered excellent when ICC>0.74, good when ICC = 0.60–0.74, fair when ICC = 0.40–0.59, and poor when ICC<0.4 [24]. Furthermore, Bland Altman analysis [25] and coefficients of variation (CoV) were calculated. The CoV was defined as the standard deviation of the differences divided by the mean [26].

Results

The image quality was sufficient to perform CMR-FT in all subjects and for all slices at rest and during dobutamine stress. CMR-FT post-processing took 10 to 12 minutes for a LV short-axis stack on average including adjustments if necessary. Participant demographics are summarised in **table 1**.

Haemodynamic response to dobutamine

There were no side effects to dobutamine exposure. There was a significant increase of cardiac output, mean blood pressure and ejection fraction between rest and both levels of dobutamine as well as between 10 and 20 $\mu g \cdot kg^{-1} \cdot min^{-1}$ of dobutamine. Stroke volume increased significantly between rest and both levels of dobutamine, whilst no further increase was observed between 10 and 20 $\mu g \cdot kg^{-1} \cdot min^{-1}$ of dobutamine (**table 2**).

Torsion and recoil rate at rest

Inter-slice distances used for torsion calculation were 2.9±0.4 cm (model 1), 5.8±0.7 cm (model 2) and 4.4±0.5 cm (model 3 and 4). There was no significant difference of endocardial, epicardial or global torsion and endocardial and global recoil rate between the models 1–4 at rest. Results are displayed in **table 3**. There was a significant difference ($p = 0.02$) of epicardial recoil rate between model 2 (0–100%) and model 4 (0–75%).

Torsion and recoil rate during dobutamine stress

Table 4 summarises torsion and recoil rate parameters at rest and during dobutamine stress as calculated by the different models. The mean inter-slice distance during dobutamine exposure was slightly lower compared with rest due to increased

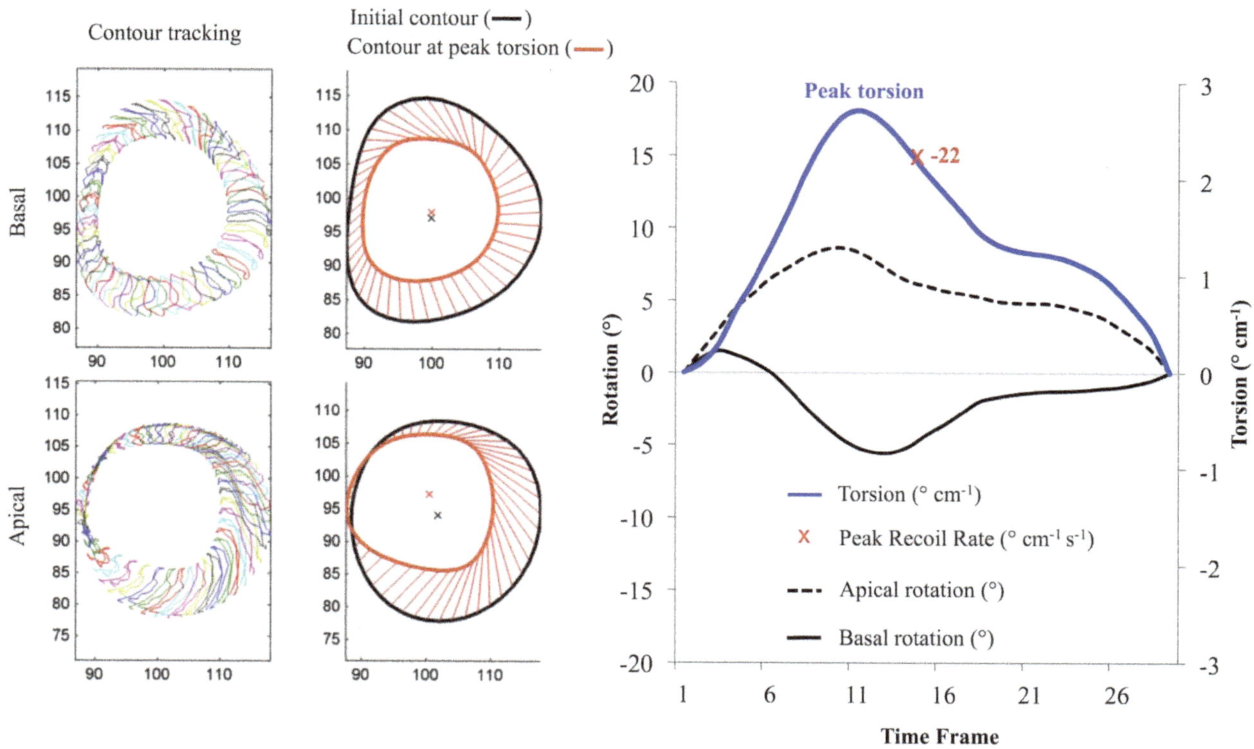

Figure 2. Evaluation of rotation. Rotational displacement (degrees) of 48 voxels was tracked throughout the cardiac cycle (**left**). Left ventricular torsion (° cm^{-1}) was calculated as the difference in counter-clockwise (positive) apical rotation and clockwise (negative) rotation at the base, divided by the inter-slice distance (**right**).

longitudinal shortening with stress. The inter-slices distances were 2.8±0.3 cm (model 1), 5.6±0.6 cm (model 2) and 4.2±0.4 cm (model 3 and 4) for measurements during 10 and 20 $\mu g \cdot kg^{-1} \cdot min^{-1}$ of dobutamine.

Model 1 (25–75%) was the only approach that revealed significantly increased torsion and recoil rate (subendocardial, subepicardial and global) between rest and both levels of dobutamine as well as between 10 and 20 $\mu g \cdot kg^{-1} \cdot min^{-1}$ of dobutamine except there was no significant difference of subepicardial torsion ($p = 0.33$) and global torsion ($p = 0.06$) between rest and 10 $\mu g \cdot kg^{-1} \cdot min^{-1}$ of dobutamine (**Figure 4**). The increase of torsion during dobutamine stress was more pronounced on the subendocardial as compared to the subepicarial level. All other models showed only partly significant results or trends towards increased torsion and recoil rates as outlined in **table 4**.

Reproducibility

Bland Altman analysis, ICC and CoV are displayed in **table 5**. There was no difference in reproducibility between rest and dobutamine stimulation. ICC for model 1 (25–75%) and model 3 (25–100%) consistently showed values above 0.85. The model 2 (0–100%) and 4 (0–75%) showed slightly higher inter-observer variability for subendocardial torsion with ICC of 0.78 and 0.79, respectively.

Discussion

Myocardial twisting and untwisting represent fundamental mechanisms of LV systolic and diastolic function. It has been suggested that even up to 40% of stroke volume is produced from systolic twisting forces [27]. The subsequent fast untwisting during early diastole is a major indicator of the restoring forces that contribute to rapid diastolic filling [28,29]. In a clinical context, a simple, quick and robust quantification of LV twisting and untwisting motion is therefore desirable. The present study applied CMR-FT to assess both systolic torsion and diastolic recoil directly from routine SSFP cine images to capture these phenomena and demonstrates several important findings. CMR-FT based quantification of myocardial twisting motion as assessed with torsion and diastolic recoil is feasible and reproducible. Furthermore, we were able to show that CMR-FT allows discrimination of both systolic torsion and diastolic recoil at rest and dobutamine stress when using standardized analyses based on rotation measurements at 25% and 75% LV distance.

Feasibility of CMR-FT derived torsion

The presented approach used a complete LV rotational model to define exact apical and basal slice positions by assessing rotational profiles of all short-axis slices of a short-axis stack with subsequent linear interpolation of inter-slice rotation between adjacent slices. This approach appears suitable since several studies revealed strict linear progression of rotation from base to apex [10,12,14]. Previous reports have shown that the amount of LV rotation is highly dependent on the site of measurements at apical and basal levels. This needs to be taken into account when calculating the simple twist angle [10]. We therefore applied torsion (twist normalized to inter-slice distance) to quantify the myocardial twisting motion since this technique is supposed to be less influenced by the variation in rotation as compared to the simple twist definition (difference in apical and basal rotation) [30]. The results of our study indicate, that in fact CMR-FT

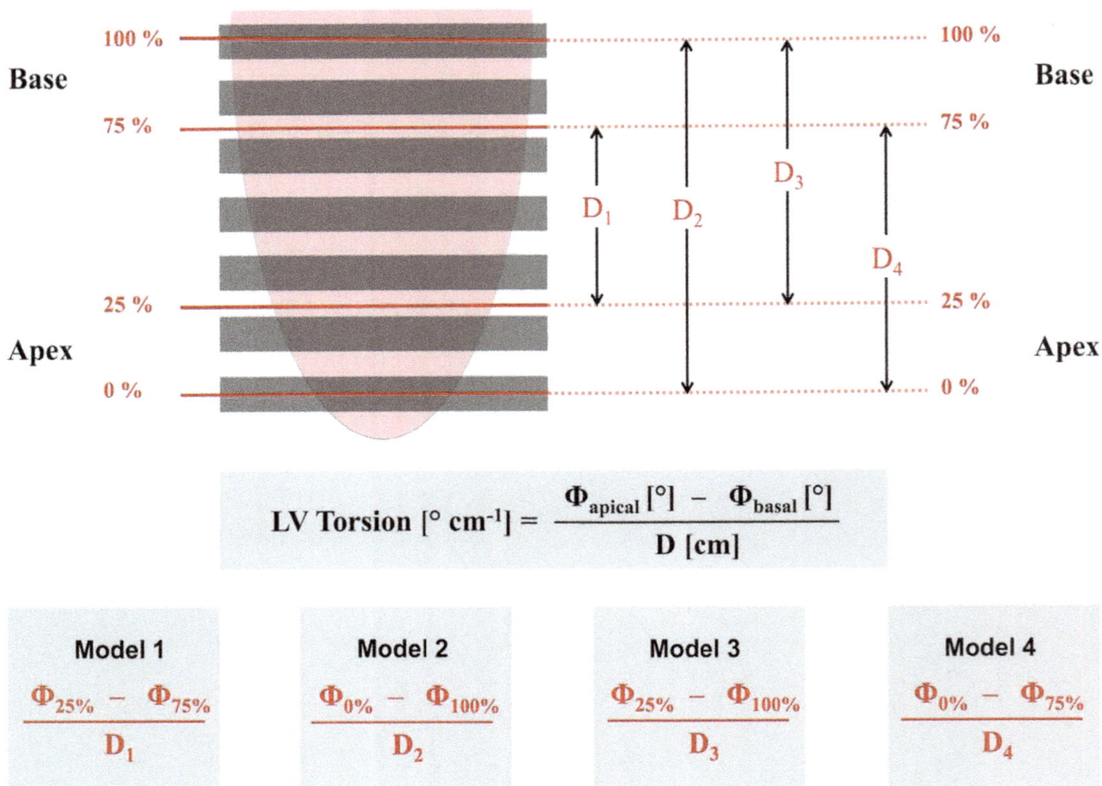

Figure 3. Definitions to calculate torsion. CMR feature tracking was performed in all slices of a short-axis stack. Four models (1–4) to calculate torsion were evaluated. Left ventricular (LV) torsion was calculated as the difference in counter-clockwise apical rotation (ϕ_{apex}) and clockwise rotation at the base (ϕ_{base}), divided by the inter-slice distance (D). The rotation of points at 0% ($\phi_{0\%}$) and 100% ($\phi_{100\%}$) distance correspond to the most apical and most basal levels. The rotation of points at 25% ($\phi_{25\%}$) and 75% ($\phi_{75\%}$) distance correspond to points that are typically located in between slices (linearly interpolated from adjacent slices). This approach allows generating constant distances (D_1-D_4) between corresponding apical and basal slices independently of varying cardiac anatomy.

quantification of torsion at rest is not that dependant on measurement positions since we have not detected any significant differences between the four examined models that used rotation from different standardized LV levels serving for the calculation of torsion. However, differences in recoil rate were more pronounced. Hence, quantification of recoil rate might be more dependent on the exact slice position as compared to quantification of torsion. This is particularly important when quantification of diastolic function is required which underpins the need for a method allowing a uniform slice selection at standardized LV levels. It is important to note that our methodology allows accurate, specific assessments of LV torsion and diastolic recoil at different levels throughout the myocardial wall which could be particularly valuable in the assessment of myocardial diseases that predominantly affect the endocardial layer such as subendocardial myocardial infarction, cardiac amyloid or endomyocardial fibrosis.

Table 1. Subject characteristics.

Demographics	Healthy volunteers
Study population	N = 10
Gender (f/m)	5/5
Age (y)	40.6 (23–51)
LV-EDV (ml/m^2)	51.0 (7.5)
LV-ESV (ml/m^2)	21.7 (5.1)
LV-CI (l/min/m^2)	2.0 (0.4)
LV-EF (%)	57.9 (5.6)

Continuous variable are expressed as mean (standard deviation), age is expressed as median (range).
f: female, m: male, EDV: end-diastolic volume, ESV: end-systolic volume, CI: cardiac index, EF: ejection fraction.

Table 2. Volumetric and hemodynamic response to 10 and 20 µg kg^{-1}min^{-1} of dobutamine.

Parameter	Level of dobutamine (µg kg^{-1} min^{-1})			P value		
	Rest	10	20	Rest vs. 10	Rest vs. 20	10 vs. 20
LV-CI (l/min/m^2)	2.0 (0.4)	3.3 (0.8)	4.2 (0.6)	**<0.01**	**<0.01**	**<0.01**
LV-EDV (ml/m^2)	51.0 (7.5)	52.7 (9.1)	43.8 (15.4)	0.33	**<0.05**	**<0.01**
LV-ESV (ml/m^2)	21.7 (5.1)	14.4 (5.9)	11.4 (4.6)	**<0.01**	**<0.01**	**<0.01**
LV-SV (ml/m^2)	29.4 (4.1)	38.3 (7.4)	37.3 (6.5)	**<0.01**	**<0.01**	0.24
LV-EF (%)	57.9 (5.6)	72.9 (9.5)	77.0 (5.7)	**<0.01**	**<0.01**	**<0.05**
Mean BP (mmHg)	91.5 (10.2)	98.6 (10.4)	102.9 (10.7)	**<0.01**	**<0.05**	**<0.05**
Heart Rate	69.3 (10.3)	85.2 (16.6)	112.8 (11.9)	**<0.01**	**<0.01**	**<0.01**

Bold p values indicate a significance level <0.05.
BP: blood pressure, other abbreviations as in table 1.

Reproducibility of CMR-FT derived torsion

CMR-FT represents a relatively novel approach to quantify myocardial deformation. Previous CMR-FT studies primarily focused on ventricular strain measurements. The reported amount of reproducibility and repeatability varies between studies with most studies reporting reasonable reproducibility of global strain levels [19,31,32,33]. Therefore, intra- and inter-observer variability for torsion and recoil rate needs to be taken into special consideration. In order to maximise reproducibility all measurements were repeated three times and corresponding averaged rotational profiles were included in the calculation of torsion. As a result, all torsion and recoil rate parameters were highly reproducible on an intra-observer and inter-observer level. We found slightly lower reproducibility of model 2 (0–100%) and model 4 (0–75%) as compared to model 1 (25–75%) or model 3 (25–100%). Both, model 2 and model 4, involve rotational measurements taken from the most apical slice included in the calculation of torsion. As described in previous reports, reproducibility for CMR-FT derived strain parameters was lower at apical myocardial levels than at mid-ventricular or basal levels [34]. Our study shows that this holds true for apical and basal rotation assessment with CMR-FT and emphasises to rather include apical rotation from a slice position at 25% LV distance instead of using the most apical slice of a short-axis stack.

Torsion as a function of dobutamine exposure

Previous studies investigated the effect of inotropic stimulation with dobutamine on LV torsion in a canine model and found increased torsion paralleled by accelerated recoil rate [35,36]. The findings were confirmed in a human model using echocardiographic speckle tracking [37]. The authors found that subepicardial torsion remained unchanged during low dose dobutamine infusion and increased with higher doses of dobutamine. In contrast, subendocardial torsion already increased during low dose dobutamine infusion [37]. In the present study, we showed that model 1 (25–75%) using the shortest distance between apical and basal slices, consistently revealed significant increases of subendocardial and global torsion as well as accelerated recoil rate (subendocardial, subepicardial and global) with increasing levels of dobutamine. Conversely, subepicardial torsion only increased with the application of an intermediate dose of dobutamine, which is in accordance with the published findings by Akagawa et al. [37]. The other models using either the most apical or basal slice did not reliably differentiate torsion and recoil rate between rest and pharmacological stress and only showed non-significant trends towards increased torsion and recoil rates. This is most likely explained by through-plane motion causing loss of tracked features from the imaging plane. This might be particularly pronounced in the very apical and basal LV slices since longitudinal shortening is increased during dobutamine stress and may explain the need to

Table 3. Torsion and recoil rate.

	Model 1 (25–75%)	Model 2 (0–100%)	Model 3 (25–100%)	Model 4 (0–75%)	P value
Torsion Endo (°/cm)	3.0 (1.9)	3.6 (1.6)	3.6 (1.7)	3.4 (2.0)	0.72
Torsion Epi (°/cm)	2.3 (1.3)	2.7 (0.9)	2.6 (1.4)	2.6 (0.8)	0.37
Global Torsion (°/cm)	2.7 (1.5)	3.2 (1.2)	3.1 (1.5)	3.0 (1.3)	0.56
Recoil Rate Endo (°/cm/s)	−34.2 (10.3)	−46.2 (18.3)	−42.2 (9.7)	−45.5 (24.7)	0.56
Recoil Rate Epi (°/cm/s)	−26.1 (14.6)	−26.4 (9.3)	−24.8 (12.5)	−31.4 (10.6)*	**0.048**
Global Recoil Rate (°/cm/s)	−30.1 (11.1)	−36.3 (12.7)	−33.5 (9.1)	−38.5 (16.4)	0.29

Baseline values for torsion and recoil rate in comparison between the four models.
Variables are given as mean (SD)
***p = 0.022 vs. Model 2**
Bold p values indicate a significance level <0.05.
Endo: subendocardial, Epi: subepicardial, Global: average of subendocardial and subepicardial, rest: measurement at rest, 10: level of 10 µg kg^{-1} min^{-1} of dobutamine, 20: level of 20 µg kg^{-1} min^{-1} of dobutamine.

Table 4. Comparison of torsion and recoil rate between rest and stimulation with dobutamine.

		Level of dobutamine (μg $kg^{-1}min^{-1}$)			P value		
		rest	10	20	Rest vs. 10	Rest vs. 20	10 vs. 20
Model 1 (25–75%)	**Torsion Endo (°/cm)**	3.0 (1.9)	4.6 (2.5)	6.0 (2.4)	**0.02**	**<0.01**	**0.02**
	Torsion Epi (°/cm)	2.3 (1.3)	2.7 (1.5)	4.1 (2.2)	0.33	**0.01**	**0.03**
	Global Torsion (°/cm)	2.7 (1.5)	3.6 (2.0)	5.1 (2.2)	0.06	**<0.01**	**0.01**
	Recoil Rate Endo (°/cm/s)	−34.2 (10.3)	−53.6 (14.8)	−79.1 (35.1)	**0.01**	**<0.01**	**0.04**
	Recoil Rate Epi (°/cm/s)	−26.1 (14.6)	−40.3 (19.2)	−58.6 (32.3)	**0.02**	**<0.01**	**0.04**
	Global Recoil Rate (°/cm/s)	−30.1 (11.1)	−46.9 (15.0)	−68.9 (32.3)	**<0.01**	**<0.01**	**0.03**
Model 2 (0–100%)	**Torsion Endo (°/cm)**	3.6 (1.6)	5.2 (2.5)	5.8 (2.5)	0.14	0.09	0.51
	Torsion Epi (°/cm)	2.7 (0.9)	3.8 (2.0)	3.9 (1.8)	0.29	0.06	0.45
	Global Torsion (°/cm)	3.2 (1.2)	4.5 (2.2)	4.8 (1.9)	0.17	0.07	0.51
	Recoil Rate Endo (°/cm/s)	−46.2 (18.3)	−72.7 (37.9)	−82.6 (32.9)	0.17	0.047	0.33
	Recoil Rate Epi (°/cm/s)	−26.4 (9.3)	−49.0 (34.0)	−55.5 (28.0)	0.047	**<0.01**	0.39
	Global Recoil Rate (°/cm/s)	−36.3 (12.7)	−60.8 (34.7)	−69.1 (28.3)	0.11	**0.02**	0.39
Model 3 (25–100%)	**Torsion Endo (°/cm)**	3.6 (1.7)	4.8 (2.6)	6.1 (3.0)	0.07	**<0.01**	0.09
	Torsion Epi (°/cm)	2.6 (1.4)	2.9 (1.4)	3.9 (2.1)	0.51	**0.02**	**0.03**
	Global Torsion (°/cm)	3.1 (1.5)	3.8 (2.0)	5.0 (2.4)	0.07	**<0.01**	**0.02**
	Recoil Rate Endo (°/cm/s)	−42.2 (9.7)	−62.9 (29.7)	−69.5 (25.0)	**0.02**	**0.02**	0.45
	Recoil Rate Epi (°/cm/s)	−24.8 (12.5)	−37.8 (18.5)	−48.3 (25.3)	**0.02**	**0.01**	0.07
	Global Recoil Rate (°/cm/s)	−33.5 (9.1)	−50.4 (23.6)	−58.9 (24.6)	**0.01**	**0.01**	0.33
Model 4 (0–75%)	**Torsion Endo (°/cm)**	3.4 (2.0)	5.4 (2.5)	5.5 (3.0)	0.17	0.11	0.96
	Torsion Epi (°/cm)	2.6 (0.8)	4.0 (2.3)	4.1 (1.7)	0.24	**0.02**	0.20
	Global Torsion (°/cm)	3.0 (1.3)	4.7 (2.3)	4.8 (1.8)	0.14	**0.047**	0.88
	Recoil Rate Endo (°/cm/s)	−45.5 (24.7)	−69.8 (39.4)	−99.5 (45.6)	0.24	**0.01**	0.11
	Recoil Rate Epi (°/cm/s)	−31.4 (10.6)	−55.0 (34.7)	−70.4 (38.4)	0.06	**<0.01**	0.14
	Global Recoil Rate (°/cm/s)	−38.5 (16.4)	−62.4 (36.4)	−84.9 (38.9)	0.09	**0.01**	0.11

Bold p values indicate a significance level <0.05. Abbreviations as in table 3.

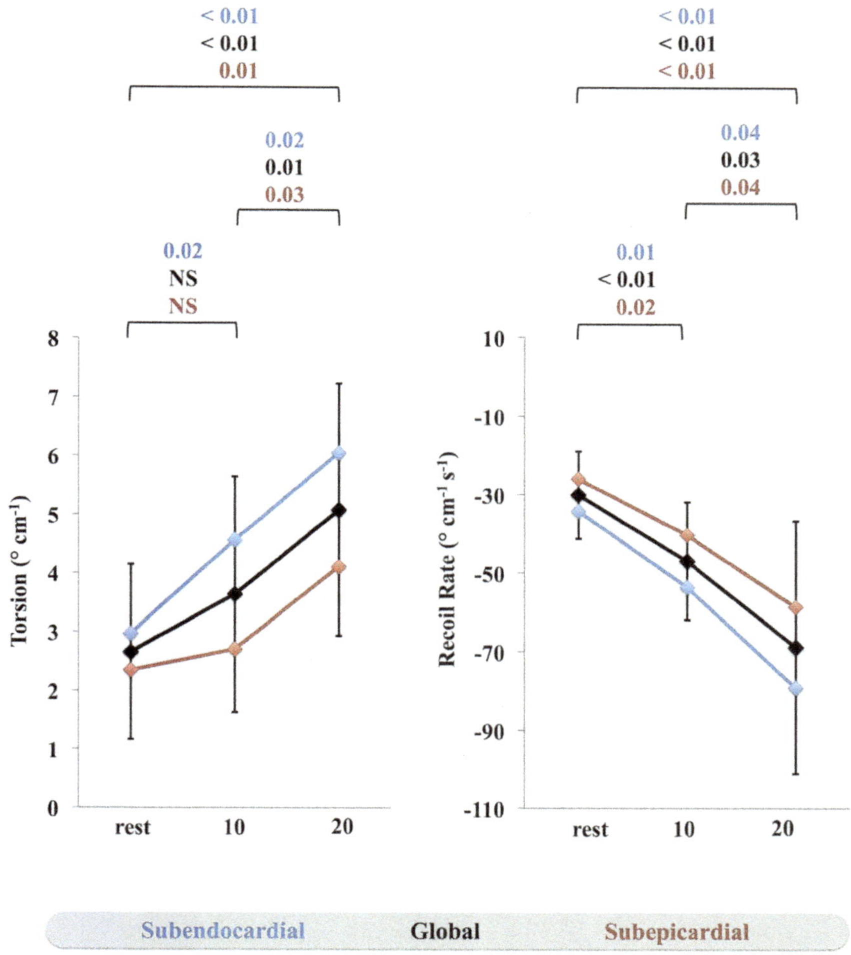

Figure 4. Torsion and recoil rate during dobutamine stress. Torsion and recoil rate (blue: subendocardial; red: subepicardial, black: global) as derived using model 1 (25–75%) in comparison between rest and increasing levels of dobutamine. A p-value <0.05 was considered statistically significant.

measure torsion from positions a bit farer away from the apex and the base.

CMR-FT in the context of existing methods to calculate torsion

Previously described CMR based modalities for the study of myocardial twisting and untwisting motion include myocardial tagging [10,38], tissue phase mapping [39] and displacement encoding with stimulated echoes (DENSE) [40]. Although accelerated techniques have been reported for myocardial tagging [41,42], all mentioned approaches commonly require additional sequence acquisitions and are usually associated with time-consuming post-processing both limiting their clinical applicability. In contrast, CMR-FT allows direct quantification of myocardial motion from standard SSFP images, which are widely available since they are generally part of every clinical CMR volumetric examination. From a clinical perspective, evaluation of myocardial torsion using CMR-FT has the potential to be integrated into a given clinical CMR protocol. Speckle-tracking echocardiography is another technique that has proved feasible for the quantification of myocardial rotation [8,10,43]. Speckle tracking echocardiography is widely available and benefits from high temporal resolution but suffers from limited image quality especially occasionally poor acoustic windows [23]. In general echocardiography does not allow a reliable and uniform selection of apical and basal slices in individual subjects, which has proved to be crucial for a robust quantification of myocardial twisting motion as expressed by our data and in previous reports [10]. Furthermore it is challenging to quantify torsion (twist per length) with speckle-tracking echocardiography, since the assessment of the inter-slice distance between apical and basal slices is generally not possible. Speckle-tracking echocardiography is therefore limited to the simple twist definition, which is even more dependent on the exact slice locations and difficult to reproduce in longitudinal studies [30]. Notwithstanding these considerations, several echocardiography speckle tracking based studies have shown the feasibility of twisting and untwisting motion quantification in various heart diseases. These involve conditions with a predominant diastolic involvement such as heart failure with preserved ejection fraction [17], diseases with predominant systolic involvement such as ischemic cardiomyopathy [44] and also diseases that equally affect systole and diastole such as hypertrophic cardiomyopathy [45] or cardiac amyloidosis [46]. Whether or not such assessments could also be derived from CMR-FT torsion and diastolic recoil measurements need to be investigated with future research studies.

Table 5. Reproducibility for all four models to calculate torsion and diastolic recoil rate.

		Model 1 (25–75%)			Model 2 (0–100%)			Model 3 (25–100%)			Model 4 (0–75%)		
		Mean Difference (SD)	ICC (95%CI)	CoV (%)	Mean Difference (SD)	ICC (95%CI)	CoV (%)	Mean Difference (SD)	ICC (95%CI)	CoV (%)	Mean Difference (SD)	ICC (95%CI)	CoV (%)
Intra-observer	**Torsion Endo (°/cm)**	0.02 (1.36)	0.92 (0.83–0.96)	30.14	−0.06 (0.79)	0.97 (0.94–0.99)	16.09	−0.16 (0.83)	0.97 (0.95–0.99)	16.91	0.00 (1.04)	0.96 (0.91–0.98)	21.80
	Torsion Epi (°/cm)	−0.02 (0.91)	0.94 (0.87–0.97)	29.81	0.05 (0.42)	0.99 (0.97–0.99)	12.23	0.03 (0.51)	0.98 (0.95–0.99)	16.50	−0.02 (0.61)	0.97 (0.94–0.99)	16.99
	Global Torsion (°/cm)	0.00 (1.05)	0.93 (0.86–0.97)	27.65	−0.01 (0.50)	0.98 (0.96–0.99)	12.07	−0.06 (0.49)	0.99 (0.97–0.99)	12.14	−0.01 (0.66)	0.97 (0.94–0.99)	15.81
	Recoil Rate Endo (°/cm/s)	6.48 (15.24)	0.92 (0.82–0.96)	25.88	0.98 (23.49)	0.91 (0.81–0.96)	34.73	−2.82 (10.88)	0.95 (0.90–0.98)	19.17	−0.56 (31.59)	0.88 (0.75–0.95)	44.29
	Recoil Rate Epi (°/cm/s)	−0.44 (9.74)	0.96 (0.92–0.98)	23.50	−0.81 (11.72)	0.95 (0.90–0.98)	27.11	−1.64 (7.51)	0.96 (0.92–0.98)	20.79	−3.80 (16.43)	0.93 (0.85–0.97)	32.63
	Global Recoil Rate (°/cm/s)	3.02 (9.68)	0.96 (0.92–0.98)	19.30	0.09 (15.77)	0.94 (0.87–0.97)	28.44	−2.23 (7.89)	0.96 (0.92–0.98)	16.97	−2.18 (21.34)	0.91 (0.82–0.96)	35.08
Inter-observer	**Torsion Endo (°/cm)**	0.07 (1.58)	0.89 (0.77–0.95)	35.30	0.94 (1.33)	0.85 (0.54–0.94)	30.35	0.52 (1.18)	0.94 (0.85–0.97)	25.84	0.62 (1.89)	0.80 (0.59–0.91)	42.31
	Torsion Epi (°/cm)	−0.15 (0.74)	0.96 (0.92–0.98)	23.55	0.35 (0.78)	0.94 (0.85–0.97)	23.73	0.21 (0.50)	0.98 (0.94–0.99)	16.54	0.14 (1.03)	0.93 (0.85–0.97)	29.61
	Global Torsion (°/cm)	−0.04 (1.07)	0.93 (0.86–0.97)	28.04	0.64 (0.97)	0.89 (0.68–0.96)	25.33	0.37 (0.70)	0.96 (0.91–0.99)	18.44	0.38 (1.35)	0.86 (0.71–0.93)	33.78
	Recoil Rate Endo (°/cm/s)	8.09 (17.07)	0.90 (0.76–0.95)	28.60	−9.31 (17.17)	0.91 (0.77–0.96)	27.47	−0.70 (8.61)	0.97 (0.94–0.99)	14.89	−7.01 (25.30)	0.89 (0.76–0.95)	37.15
	Recoil Rate Epi (°/cm/s)	−0.05 (9.42)	0.96 (0.93–0.98)	22.63	−5.35 (12.64)	0.93 (0.85–0.97)	30.85	−2.35 (7.02)	0.97 (0.93–0.98)	19.61	−6.42 (16.56)	0.92 (0.82–0.96)	33.77
	Global Recoil Rate (°/cm/s)	4.02 (10.76)	0.95 (0.90–0.98)	21.24	−7.33 (10.86)	0.95 (0.82–0.98)	21.00	−1.52 (6.02)	0.98 (0.96–0.99)	12.86	−6.71 (17.38)	0.92 (0.83–0.96)	29.67

ICC: Intraclass-correlation coefficient; CoV: coefficient of variation; SD: standard deviation; CI: confidence interval. Other abbreviations as in table 3.

Regarding longitudinal assessments, previous studies applied myocardial tagging to investigate the inter-study reproducibility for quantitative analysis of torsion and recoil rate and found good reproducibility for torsion whilst peak recoil rate was only poorly reproducible [38]. In fact, the study of recoil rate may require a more strict definition of measurement positions at apical and basal levels. This may be challenging using myocardial tagging, since this is usually performed at 3 LV levels only (apical, mid-ventricular and basal) and therefore subject to manual planning of slice positions. In contrast, we have now introduced a CMR-FT based technique that allows a uniform and exact definition of apical and basal slice positions independent of different heart sizes. Future work will need to address whether this approach positively impacts on inter-study reproducibility of torsion and of recoil rate in particular.

Limitations

The sample size of this feasibility study was relatively small. Notwithstanding this fact the results demonstrate feasibility and good reproducibility for torsion and diastolic recoil quantification with CMR-FT from routine cine images. Ideally we would have compared our results to myocardial tagging representing the reference standard for such acquisitions. However, given the necessity to obtain a whole SSFP short-axis stack at rest and with different levels of dobutamine we felt that the acquisition of an equal number of tagged images would have resulted in scanning times difficult to tolerate during dobutamine stimulation.

A general limitation of CMR based quantification of myocardial twisting motion is the current lack of standardized methods. Future studies will need to compare CMR-FT derived torsion and recoil rate with parameters from myocardial tagging using equal computation (twist per length) [38] or alternative computational methods e.g. the circumferential-longitudinal shear angle [11,12] which has not been addressed in the present study. However, there is evidence to suggest that twisting mechanics as assessed by torsion (twist per length) and shear angle deliver somewhat similar results [15]. The individual merits of both methods remain to be addressed in future investigations. A further limitation of both, conventional myocardial tagging and CMR-FT is the two-dimensional acquisition technique. We developed a pseudo three-dimensional mesh of myocardial torsion based on linear interpolation. However, this method does not compensate for through plane motion. Previous studies compared 2D and 3D derived torsion measured by myocardial tagging [47] and found that through plane motion did not significantly impact on 2D torsion since both methods showed reasonable agreement. The authors concluded to rather use the faster and easier 2D method for calculation of LV torsion. If this also holds true for 2D derived torsion from CMR-FT remains to be addressed in future investigations.

The clinical applicability of CMR-FT derived torsion and diastolic recoil assessment will depend on the speed of the analysis. At the present time the result files originating from CMR-FT are analysed using an in-house module for MATLAB. Future software developments will need to incorporate both post-processing steps in a single application to further minimize post-processing time.

Finally the current work aimed to determine the feasibility and reproducibility to quantify torsion and recoil rate from CMR-FT in a collective of healthy volunteers at rest and during dobutamine stress. Future research needs to prospectively validate this novel technique in pathologies such as coronary artery disease, heart failure or valvular disease.

Conclusions

CMR-FT allows derivation of myocardial torsion directly from standard SSFP cine images. Torsion and recoil rate calculated from apical and basal slices with 25–75% distance consistently discriminated between rest and increasing levels of dobutamine. Reproducibility was good to excellent for all torsion and recoil rate parameters, but was especially high when using an apical level at 25% LV distance instead of the most apical slice. When using CMR-FT to quantify myocardial torsion, it is therefore suggested to select apical and basal slices at standardized 25% and 75% levels. The analysis of myocardial torsion and recoil motion based on CMR-FT may have potential clinical and research applications when exact quantification of systolic and diastolic function is required. Future validation studies in larger cohorts should follow to establish the clinical utility and the prognostic implications of this technique.

Author Contributions

Conceived and designed the experiments: JTK PL AS. Performed the experiments: JTK PL STH SK BB AS. Analyzed the data: JTK PL AS. Contributed reagents/materials/analysis tools: MS JMS MF WS CUB JL GH. Wrote the paper: JTK PL AS.

References

1. Murray CJ, Lopez AD (1997) Alternative projections of mortality and disability by cause 1990–2020: Global Burden of Disease Study. Lancet 349: 1498–1504.
2. Owan TE, Hodge DO, Herges RM, Jacobsen SJ, Roger VL, et al. (2006) Trends in prevalence and outcome of heart failure with preserved ejection fraction. The New England journal of medicine 355: 251–259.
3. Karamitsos TD, Francis JM, Myerson S, Selvanayagam JB, Neubauer S (2009) The role of cardiovascular magnetic resonance imaging in heart failure. Journal of the American College of Cardiology 54: 1407–1424.
4. Kowallick JT, Edelmann F, Lotz J, Lamata P, Schuster A (2014) Imaging Diastolic Dysfunction with Cardiovascular Magnetic Resonance. Journal of Cardiology and Therapy 1: 58–64.
5. Pennell DJ (2010) Cardiovascular magnetic resonance. Circulation 121: 692–705.
6. Delhaas T, Kotte J, van der Toorn A, Snoep G, Prinzen FW, et al. (2004) Increase in left ventricular torsion-to-shortening ratio in children with valvular aortic stenosis. Magnetic resonance in medicine: official journal of the Society of Magnetic Resonance in Medicine/Society of Magnetic Resonance in Medicine 51: 135–139.
7. Dong SJ, Hees PS, Siu CO, Weiss JL, Shapiro EP (2001) MRI assessment of LV relaxation by untwisting rate: a new isovolumic phase measure of tau. American journal of physiology Heart and circulatory physiology 281: H2002–2009.
8. Opdahl A, Remme EW, Helle-Valle T, Edvardsen T, Smiseth OA (2012) Myocardial relaxation, restoring forces, and early-diastolic load are independent determinants of left ventricular untwisting rate. Circulation 126: 1441–1451.
9. Swoboda PP, Larghat A, Zaman A, Fairbairn TA, Motwani M, et al. (2014) Reproducibility of myocardial strain and left ventricular twist measured using complementary spatial modulation of magnetization. Journal of magnetic resonance imaging: JMRI 39: 887–894.
10. Goffinet C, Chenot F, Robert A, Pouleur AC, le Polain de Waroux JB, et al. (2009) Assessment of subendocardial vs. subepicardial left ventricular rotation and twist using two-dimensional speckle tracking echocardiography: comparison with tagged cardiac magnetic resonance. European heart journal 30: 608–617.
11. Russel IK, Gotte MJ, Kuijer JP, Marcus JT (2008) Regional assessment of left ventricular torsion by CMR tagging. Journal of cardiovascular magnetic resonance: official journal of the Society for Cardiovascular Magnetic Resonance 10: 26.
12. Buchalter MB, Weiss JL, Rogers WJ, Zerhouni EA, Weisfeldt ML, et al. (1990) Noninvasive quantification of left ventricular rotational deformation in normal humans using magnetic resonance imaging myocardial tagging. Circulation 81: 1236–1244.
13. Sorger JM, Wyman BT, Faris OP, Hunter WC, McVeigh ER (2003) Torsion of the left ventricle during pacing with MRI tagging. Journal of cardiovascular magnetic resonance: official journal of the Society for Cardiovascular Magnetic Resonance 5: 521–530.
14. Yoneyama K, Gjesdal O, Choi EY, Wu CO, Hundley WG, et al. (2012) Age, sex, and hypertension-related remodeling influences left ventricular torsion assessed by tagged cardiac magnetic resonance in asymptomatic individuals: the multi-ethnic study of atherosclerosis. Circulation 126: 2481–2490.

15. Donekal S, Venkatesh BA, Liu YC, Liu CY, Yoneyama K, et al. (2014) Interstitial Fibrosis, Left Ventricular Remodeling, and Myocardial Mechanical Behavior in a Population-Based Multiethnic Cohort: The Multi-Ethnic Study of Atherosclerosis (MESA) Study. Circulation Cardiovascular imaging 7: 292–302.
16. Park SJ, Miyazaki C, Bruce CJ, Ommen S, Miller FA, et al. (2008) Left ventricular torsion by two-dimensional speckle tracking echocardiography in patients with diastolic dysfunction and normal ejection fraction. Journal of the American Society of Echocardiography: official publication of the American Society of Echocardiography 21: 1129–1137.
17. Wang J, Khoury DS, Yue Y, Torre-Amione G, Nagueh SF (2008) Preserved left ventricular twist and circumferential deformation, but depressed longitudinal and radial deformation in patients with diastolic heart failure. European heart journal 29: 1283–1289.
18. Abozguia K, Nallur-Shivu G, Phan TT, Ahmed I, Kalra R, et al. (2010) Left ventricular strain and untwist in hypertrophic cardiomyopathy: relation to exercise capacity. American heart journal 159: 825–832.
19. Hor KN, Gottliebson WM, Carson C, Wash E, Cnota J, et al. (2010) Comparison of magnetic resonance feature tracking for strain calculation with harmonic phase imaging analysis. JACC Cardiovascular imaging 3: 144–151.
20. Kowallick JT, Kutty S, Edelmann F, Chiribiri A, Villa A, et al. (2014) Quantification of left atrial strain and strain rate using Cardiovascular Magnetic Resonance myocardial feature tracking: a feasibility study. Journal of cardiovascular magnetic resonance: official journal of the Society for Cardiovascular Magnetic Resonance 16: 60.
21. Morton G, Schuster A, Jogiya R, Kutty S, Beerbaum P, et al. (2012) Inter-study reproducibility of cardiovascular magnetic resonance myocardial feature tracking. Journal of cardiovascular magnetic resonance: official journal of the Society for Cardiovascular Magnetic Resonance 14: 43.
22. Schuster A, Paul M, Bettencourt N, Morton G, Chiribiri A, et al. (2013) Cardiovascular magnetic resonance myocardial feature tracking for quantitative viability assessment in ischemic cardiomyopathy. International journal of cardiology 166: 413–420.
23. Nagel E, Lehmkuhl HB, Bocksch W, Klein C, Vogel U, et al. (1999) Noninvasive diagnosis of ischemia-induced wall motion abnormalities with the use of high-dose dobutamine stress MRI: comparison with dobutamine stress echocardiography. Circulation 99: 763–770.
24. Oppo K, Leen E, Angerson WJ, Cooke TG, McArdle CS (1998) Doppler perfusion index: an interobserver and intraobserver reproducibility study. Radiology 208: 453–457.
25. Bland JM, Altman DG (1986) Statistical methods for assessing agreement between two methods of clinical measurement. Lancet 1: 307–310.
26. Grothues F, Smith GC, Moon JC, Bellenger NG, Collins P, et al. (2002) Comparison of interstudy reproducibility of cardiovascular magnetic resonance with two-dimensional echocardiography in normal subjects and in patients with heart failure or left ventricular hypertrophy. The American journal of cardiology 90: 29–34.
27. Esch BT, Warburton DE (2009) Left ventricular torsion and recoil: implications for exercise performance and cardiovascular disease. Journal of applied physiology 106: 362–369.
28. Burns AT, La Gerche A, Prior DL, Macisaac AI (2009) Left ventricular untwisting is an important determinant of early diastolic function. JACC Cardiovascular imaging 2: 709–716.
29. Moon MR, Ingels NB, Jr., Daughters GT, 2nd, Stinson EB, Hansen DE, et al. (1994) Alterations in left ventricular twist mechanics with inotropic stimulation and volume loading in human subjects. Circulation 89: 142–150.
30. Young AA, Cowan BR (2012) Evaluation of left ventricular torsion by cardiovascular magnetic resonance. Journal of cardiovascular magnetic resonance: official journal of the Society for Cardiovascular Magnetic Resonance 14: 49.
31. Schuster A, Kutty S, Padiyath A, Parish V, Gribben P, et al. (2011) Cardiovascular magnetic resonance myocardial feature tracking detects quantitative wall motion during dobutamine stress. Journal of cardiovascular magnetic resonance: official journal of the Society for Cardiovascular Magnetic Resonance 13: 58.
32. Schuster A, Morton G, Hussain ST, Jogiya R, Kutty S, et al. (2013) The intra-observer reproducibility of cardiovascular magnetic resonance myocardial feature tracking strain assessment is independent of field strength. European journal of radiology 82: 296–301.
33. Singh A, Steadman CD, Khan JN, Horsfield MA, Bekele S, et al. (2014) Intertechnique agreement and interstudy reproducibility of strain and diastolic strain rate at 1.5 and 3 tesla: A comparison of feature-tracking and tagging in patients with aortic stenosis. Journal of magnetic resonance imaging: JMRI.
34. Wu L, Germans T, Guclu A, Heymans MW, Allaart CP, et al. (2014) Feature tracking compared with tissue tagging measurements of segmental strain by cardiovascular magnetic resonance. Journal of cardiovascular magnetic resonance: official journal of the Society for Cardiovascular Magnetic Resonance 16: 10.
35. Buchalter MB, Rademakers FE, Weiss JL, Rogers WJ, Weisfeldt ML, et al. (1994) Rotational deformation of the canine left ventricle measured by magnetic resonance tagging: effects of catecholamines, ischaemia, and pacing. Cardiovascular research 28: 629–635.
36. Rademakers FE, Buchalter MB, Rogers WJ, Zerhouni EA, Weisfeldt ML, et al. (1992) Dissociation between left ventricular untwisting and filling. Accentuation by catecholamines. Circulation 85: 1572–1581.
37. Akagawa E, Murata K, Tanaka N, Yamada H, Miura T, et al. (2007) Augmentation of left ventricular apical endocardial rotation with inotropic stimulation contributes to increased left ventricular torsion and radial strain in normal subjects: quantitative assessment utilizing a novel automated tissue tracking technique. Circulation journal: official journal of the Japanese Circulation Society 71: 661–668.
38. Donekal S, Ambale-Venkatesh B, Berkowitz S, Wu CO, Choi EY, et al. (2013) Inter-study reproducibility of cardiovascular magnetic resonance tagging. Journal of cardiovascular magnetic resonance: official journal of the Society for Cardiovascular Magnetic Resonance 15: 37.
39. Codreanu I, Robson MD, Golding SJ, Jung BA, Clarke K, et al. (2010) Longitudinally and circumferentially directed movements of the left ventricle studied by cardiovascular magnetic resonance phase contrast velocity mapping. Journal of cardiovascular magnetic resonance: official journal of the Society for Cardiovascular Magnetic Resonance 12: 48.
40. Haggerty CM, Kramer SP, Binkley CM, Powell DK, Mattingly AC, et al. (2013) Reproducibility of cine displacement encoding with stimulated echoes (DENSE) cardiovascular magnetic resonance for measuring left ventricular strains, torsion, and synchrony in mice. Journal of cardiovascular magnetic resonance: official journal of the Society for Cardiovascular Magnetic Resonance 15: 71.
41. Reyhan M, Ennis DB (2013) Quantitative assessment of systolic and diastolic left ventricular twist using Fourier Analysis of Stimulated echoes (FAST) and CSPAMM. Journal of magnetic resonance imaging: JMRI 37: 678–683.
42. Reyhan M, Natsuaki Y, Ennis DB (2012) Fourier analysis of STimulated echoes (FAST) for the quantitative analysis of left ventricular twist. Journal of magnetic resonance imaging: JMRI 35: 587–593.
43. Notomi Y, Lysyansky P, Setser RM, Shiota T, Popovic ZB, et al. (2005) Measurement of ventricular torsion by two-dimensional ultrasound speckle tracking imaging. Journal of the American College of Cardiology 45: 2034–2041.
44. Bansal M, Leano RL, Marwick TH (2008) Clinical assessment of left ventricular systolic torsion: effects of myocardial infarction and ischemia. Journal of the American Society of Echocardiography: official publication of the American Society of Echocardiography 21: 887–894.
45. Notomi Y, Martin-Miklovic MG, Oryszak SJ, Shiota T, Deserranno D, et al. (2006) Enhanced ventricular untwisting during exercise: a mechanistic manifestation of elastic recoil described by Doppler tissue imaging. Circulation 113: 2524–2533.
46. Karabay CY, Kocabay G (2011) Left ventricular torsion by two-dimensional speckle tracking echocardiography in patient with a-type amyloid heart disease. Journal of the American Society of Echocardiography: official publication of the American Society of Echocardiography 24: 818 e815–819.
47. Russel IK, Tecelao SR, Kuijer JP, Heethaar RM, Marcus JT (2009) Comparison of 2D and 3D calculation of left ventricular torsion as circumferential-longitudinal shear angle using cardiovascular magnetic resonance tagging. Journal of cardiovascular magnetic resonance: official journal of the Society for Cardiovascular Magnetic Resonance 11: 8.
48. Lamata P, Sinclair M, Kerfoot E, Lee A, Crozier A, et al. (2014) An automatic service for the personalization of ventricular cardiac meshes. Journal of the Royal Society, Interface/the Royal Society 11: 20131023.

Retreatment and Outcomes of Recurrent Intracranial Vertebral Artery Dissecting Aneurysms after Stent Assisted Coiling: A Single Center Experience

Ying Song, Yang Wang, Chuanhui Li, Yanmin Wang, Shiqing Mu, Xinjian Yang*

Department of Interventional Neuroradiology, Beijing Neurosurgical Institute and Beijing Tiantan Hospital, Capital Medical University, Beijing, China

Abstract

Background and purpose: The retreatment of recurrent intracranial vertebral artery dissecting aneurysms (VADAs) after stent assisted coiling (SAC) has not yet been studied. The purpose of this study was to evaluate the strategies and outcomes for retreatment of recurrent VADAs after SAC.

Methods: Between September 2009 and November 2013, six consecutive patients presenting with recurrent intracranial VADAs after SAC were enrolled in this study. They were all male with age ranging from 29 to 54 years (mean age, 46.2 years). The procedures of treatments and angiographic and clinical follow-up were reviewed retrospectively. Retreatment modalities were selected individually according to the characteristics of recurrence. The outcomes of retreatment were evaluated by angiographic and clinical follow-up.

Results: Six patients with recurrent intracranial VADAs after SAC were retreated, with second SAC in three patients, coil embolization, double overlapping stents placement and endovascular occlusion with aneurysm trapping in one patient, respectively. Immediate angiographic outcomes of retreatment were: complete occlusion in three patients, nearly complete occlusion in two patients, and contrast medium retention in dissecting aneurysm in one patient. All cases were technically successful. No complications related to endovascular procedures occurred. Angiographic follow-up was available in all five patients treated with second SAC or double overlapping stents, which was complete occlusion in four patients, obliteration of parent artery in one patient, showing no recurrence at 4–11 months (mean: 8.6 months). Clinical follow-up was performed in all six patients at 11–51 months after initial endovascular treatment and at 9–43 months after retreatment. The mRS of last clinical follow-up was excellent in five patients and mild disability in only one patient.

Conclusions: Endovascular retreatment is feasible and effective for recurrent intracranial VADAs after SAC. Individualized strategies of retreatment should be enacted according to the characteristics and reasons for the recurrence.

Editor: Jinglu Ai, St Michael's Hospital, University of Toronto, Canada

Funding: This work was supported by the National Science Foundation of China (grant nos. 81220108007, 81171079 and 81471167) and Special Research Project for Capital Health Development (grant No. 2014-1-1071). The funders had no role in study design, data collection and analysis, decision to publish, or preparation of the manuscript.

Competing Interests: The authors have declared that no competing interests exist.

* Email: yang-xj@163.net

Introduction

Intracranial vertebral artery dissecting aneurysms (VADAs) have been increasingly recognized as a cause of subarachnoid hemorrhage (SAH) and posterior circulation ischemia with high morbidity and mortality, especially in young and middle-aged people [1–4]. In recent years, endovascular treatment has become one of the major modalities of treatment for these lesions, including deconstructive (proximal occlusion, endovascular occlusion with or without aneurysm trapping) and reconstructive treatment (stent assisted coiling, SAC, stent only) [5–6]. Endovascular occlusion with or without aneurysm trapping of dissected segment of the parent artery is deemed as the most reliable technique to prevent re-bleeding, but not applicable for VADAs involving the posterior inferior cerebellar artery (PICA) origin, bilateral vertebral artery (VA), predominant VA and the basilar artery [7]. SAC has become a vital option for the endovascular treatment for VADAs, which not only allows preserving the parent artery, but also occludes the dissecting aneurysm [8–13]. With the increasing number of cases being treated, recurrence after SAC is gradually seen, [4,14–17] and some patients with recurrent intracranial VADAs need retreatment. However, the retreatment and outcomes of recurrent intracranial VADAs after SAC have rarely been studied [19,20].

The present study is to retrospectively analyze the reasons of recurrence, evaluate the strategies and outcomes of retreatment for recurrent intracranial VADAs after SAC in order to improve the efficacy of endovascular treatment for intracranial VADAs. We especially pay attention to the outcomes of retreatment. We wonder if recurrence will happen again after retreatment as seen post initial endovascular treatment. To our best knowledge, it is the first report about the retreatment and follow-up outcomes of recurrent VADAs after SAC.

Methods

Patients

The retrospective study was approved by Ethics Committee at Beijng Tiantan Hospital affiliated to the Capital Medical University of China. Written Informed consents were obtained from patients or their family members.

Between September 2009 and November 2013, 112 consecutive patients presenting with intracranial veterbrobasilar dissecting aneurysms (VBDAs) underwent endovascular treatment including endovascular occlusion with or without aneurysm trapping, SAC and stent only, at our institution. 72 patients were treated with SAC. Angiographic follow-ups were available in 59 patients. Recurrence was confirmed by angiographic follow-up in 10 patients. Retreatment needed to be performed in six patients with VADAs, which is the focus of our study.

All 6 patients were male, with age ranging from 29 to 54 years (mean age, 46.2 years). The lesions were located in the left VA (cases 2, 5), right VA (cases 1, 3, 4, 6), and involving PICA (cases 1, 3, 4). MR showed intramural hematoma (cases 1–6), intimal flap (cases 4, 5) and mass effect (cases 3, 6). Angiographic signs included fusiform dilation (cases 1, 2, 4, 6); pearl and string sign (case 3) and double lumen sign (case 5). The clinical status on admission was evaluated by the modified Rankin Scale (mRS). Demographic, angiographic and clinical characteristics of these six patients are shown in Table 1.

Initial SAC and follow-up

All procedures were performed with patients under general anesthesia. After femoral sheath placement, systemic heparinization was started with a loading dose of 3000 IU of heparin and was maintained with a dose of 1000 IU on an hourly basis. Through the guiding catheters, proper shaped microcatheters were introduced over microguidewires and navigated into the dissecting aneurysms. Stents were deployed after the microcatheter used for coiling was in position and the first coil was deployed but not detached (jailing technique). Bare coils were used including Guglielmi detachable coils (Stryker Neurovascular, Fremont, California, USA), NXT coils (Covidien/ev3, Irvine, California, USA), Complex and HyperSoft coils (Microvention Terumo, Tustin, California, USA). Enterprise stent (Cordis Codman and Shurtleff Inc, Raynham, Massachusetts, USA) was used in all six patients. Five patients (cases 1–5) were treated using a single stent assisted coiling procedure, and one patient (case 6) was treated with three overlapping stents and coils. Patients received 100 mg of aspirin orally and 75 mg of clopidogrel daily for three days preoperatively and for one month postoperatively, then aspirin monotherapy was continued for 6 months after the endovascular procedure.

The extent of occlusion of dissecting aneurysms was defined as follows: complete occlusion where the entire dissecting aneurysm sac was occluded; nearly complete occlusion where most of the dissecting aneurysm sac was occluded but a small portion of the sac opacified with contrast medium; and partial occlusion where the dissecting aneurysm sac was opacified [7].

Angiographic recurrence was defined as a substantial increase in the contrast medium–filled portion of the dissecting aneurysm compared with a control angiogram taken immediately after the initial treatment [4]. Recurrences were divided into recanalization and regrowth. Recanalization means opening of the previously embolized dissecting aneurysms, which has the same size, but the coils have been moved away from the original site due to blood flow and consequent compaction. Regrowth signifies that the dissecting aneurysm has become larger and the coil mass is no longer sufficient to obliterate it [20]. Extent of occlusion and criteria of recurrence were evaluated by three neuroradiologists at our institution.

The immediate angiographic outcomes of initial treatment were complete occlusion (cases 2, 6), nearly complete occlusion (cases 1, 3), and partial occlusion (cases 4, 5). Recurrence was confirmed by angiographic follow-up at 2 to 8 months (mean: 5.2 months). According to the angiographic characteristics, recurrence was manifested as recanalization in two patients (cases 3, 5), regrowth in four patients (cases 1, 2, 4, 6).

The symptoms of recurrence were headache in four patients (cases 1, 2, 4, 5), sudden dyspnea in one patient (case 6). There were no obvious symptoms before recurrence seen on angiographic follow-up in one of the patient (case 3). Initial endovascular treatment results, recurrence type, time, symptom and mRS are showed in Table 2.

Retreatment of recurrent VADAs and follow up

The indications for retreatment must meet one of the following criteria: 1) symptoms related to SAH or posterior circulation ischemia; 2) recanalization more than 20% of the original

Table 1. Demographic, angiographic and clinical characteristics on admission.

Patient NO.	Age(yrs)/sex	Initial symptom	MRI findings	DSA findings		mRS
				Angiographic sign	lesion site	
1	43/M	IVH, SAH	IMH	fusiform dilation	right VA involving PICA	2
2	49/M	headache	IMH	fusiform dilation	left VA distal to PICA	2
3	29/M	dizziness, hemiplegia	ME, IMH	pearl and string sign	right VA involving PICA	1
4	49/M	headache, dizziness	IMH,IF	fusiform dilation	right VA involving PICA	1
5	53/M	headache, dizziness	IMH, IF	double lumen sign	left VA proximal to PICA	2
6	54/M	headache, dysphagia	ME, IMH	fusiform dilation	right VA distal to PICA	3

IVH = intraventricular hemorrhage; SAH = subarachnoid hemorrhage; VA = vertebral artery; PICA = posterior inferior cerebellar artery; IMH = intramural hematoma; IF = Intimal flap; ME = Mass effect.

Table 2. Initial endovascular treatment results and angiographic and clinical follow-up.

Patient NO.	Initial treatment modality	Stent type, size (mm×mm) (number)	Immediate angiographic outcomes	Angiographic FU		Clinical FU	
				Recurrence type	time (mons)	Recurrence symptom	mRS
1	SAC	EN, 4.5×28 (1)	NC	regrowth	8	headache	1
2	SAC	EN, 4.5×22 (1)	CO	regrowth	7	headache	1
3	SAC	EN, 4.5×28 (1)	NC	recanalization	3	no	0
4	SAC	EN, 4.5×37 (1)	PO	regrowth	6	headache	1
5	SAC	EN, 4.5×37 (1)	PO	recanalization	5	headache	1
6	Multi-stents assisted coiling	EN, 4.5×28 (2), 4.5×22 (1)	CO	regrowth	2	dyspnea	5

SAC = stent assisted coiling; FU = follow up; EN = Enterprise; CO = complete occlusion; NC = nearly complete; PO = partial occlusion.

dissecting aneurysms and 3) obvious regrowth. Retreatment modalities were selected individually according to the characteristics of recurrence which included SAC, double overlapping stents placement, coil embolization and endovascular occlusion with aneurysm trapping. Angiographic follow-up were performed between 4 and 11 months. Clinical follow-up by telephone or out-patient interview was conducted up to November 2013. The clinical status was evaluated by mRS.

Results

In three patients (cases 1, 2, 4), the recurrence was manifested as regrowth in parent arteries on the opposite side and in a different location from the original dissecting aneurysm (case 1, Fig. 1 E), from distal to the original dissecting aneurysm (case 2) or as enlargement of the original dissecting aneurysm (case 4). We believed the recurrence was due to stent malapposition with inadequate radial force against vessel wall and inability for the flow to divert. So, retreatment with a second stent assisted coiling was performed in these 3 patients (Fig. 1 F). Immediate angiographic outcomes of retreatment were: complete occlusion in one case (case 1) and nearly complete occlusion in 2 cases (cases 2, 4).

In case 3, recurrence was shown as recanalization of previously embolized dissecting aneurysms (Fig. 2 E). The volume of dissecting aneurysm did not enlarged continuously. The reason of recurrence was due to flow disruption and consequent coil compaction, which was similar to recurrence of the sac aneurysm. So, in this case, we performed coil embolization for the recanalization. Complete occlusion was achieved as seen on immediate angiography.

In case 5, recurrent VADA was a fusiform dilation. Because of the worry of coil protrusion into the parent artery, we only deployed two Enterprise stents in an overlapping fashion trying to heal the dissection by increasing the flow diversion. Immediate angiographic outcome of the retreatment was contrast medium retention in dissecting aneurysm.

In case 6, a huge dissecting aneurysm accompanying an "onion skin" like thrombus causes obvious mass effect to the brain stem. Initial treatment was performed using three overlapping stents assisted coiling. Patient presented with sudden dyspnea after two months. He required emergent intubation for airway protection. His respiration was dependent of breathing machine. An immediate digital subtraction angiography revealed regrowth of coiled dissecting aneurysm (Fig. 3 G). Endovascular occlusion with aneurysm trapping was performed as the retreatment modality. Immediate contrast angiography showed complete occlusion of the parent artery (Fig. 3 H). Collateral blood flow could be seen from contralateral VA (Figure 3 I) and left posterior communicating artery (Figure 3 J).

All procedures were technically successful. No complications related to endovascular procedures.

Angiographic follow-ups were available in all five patients treated with second SAC or double overlapping stents between 4 to 11 months after retreatment. Clinical follow-ups were performed in all six patients at 11–51 months after initial endovascular treatment, and at 9–43 months after retreatment. Angiographic follow-ups after retreatment were as followed: complete occlusion in four patients (cases 1, 2, 3, 4), obliteration of parent artery in one patient (case 5), showing no recurrence at 4–11 months (mean: 8.6 months). The mRS improved from 1 to 0 in four patients (cases 1, 2, 4, 5), from mRS 5 to 2 in one patient (case 6). Case 3 maintained mRS = 0 before and after retreatment. The last clinical follow-up, measured by mRS was excellent in five patients (cases 1–5), mild disability in only one patient (case 6).

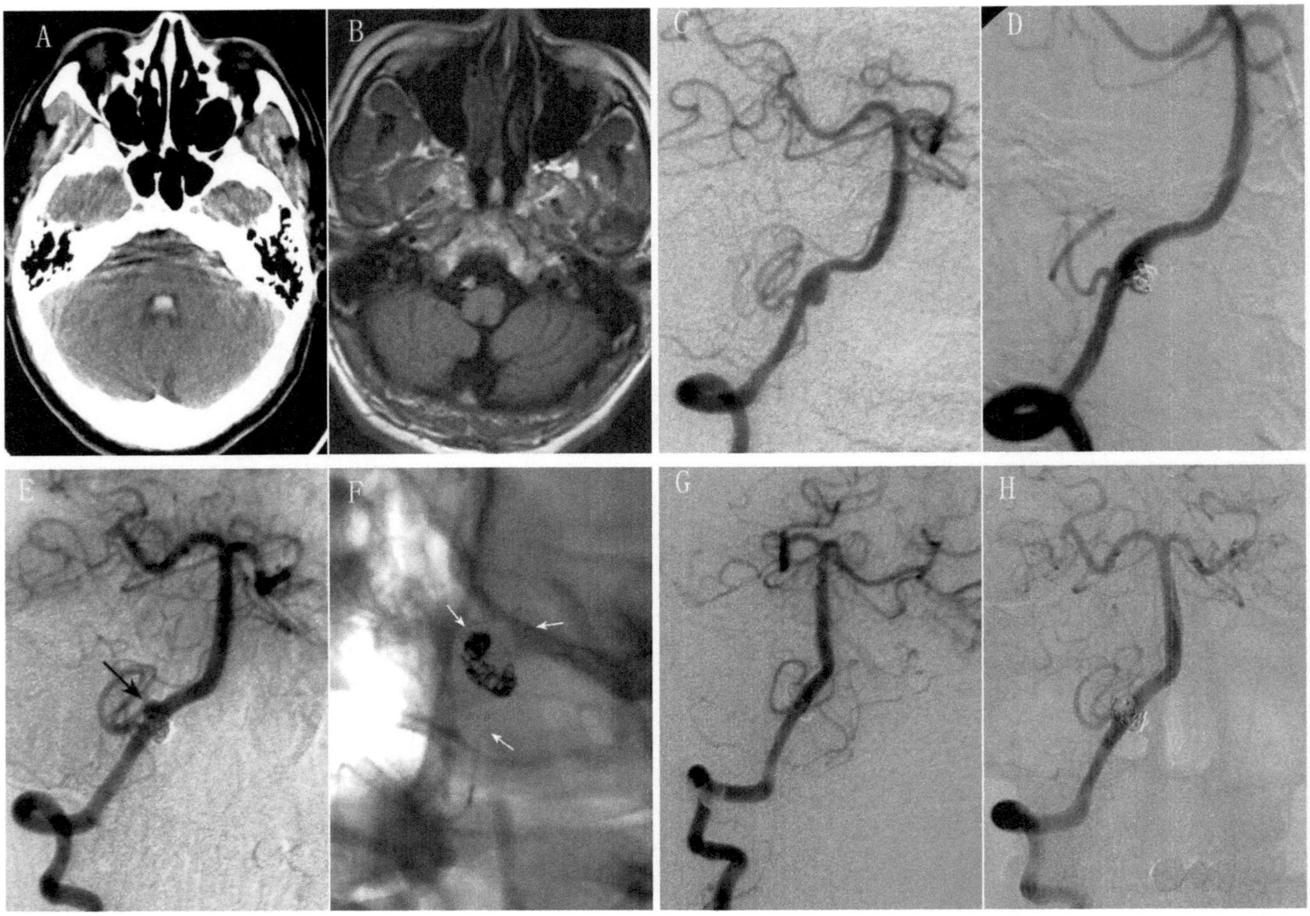

Figure 1. Retreatment with a second stent assisted coiling was performed for recurrent intracranial VADA after SAC. A 43-year old male presented with severe headache. CT scan showed subarachnoid hemorrhage and intraventricular hemorrhage (A). MR imaging showed intramural hematoma (B). Right vertebral angiograms of oblique view showed a dissecting aneurysm involving PICA (C). SAC were performed with near complete occlusion (D). Follow up angiography after eight months revealed regrowth of dissecting aneurysm on the opposite side and in a different location from the original dissecting aneurysm (black arrow) (E). Retreatment by SAC (white arrows) (F) was performed with complete occlusion (G). Follow up angiography after ten months of retreatment showed not only complete occlusion of dissecting aneurysm, but also patency of parent artery (H).

Retreatment results, angiographic and clinical follow-ups are shown in Table 3.

Representative cases are provided in figures 1–3. Other three cases are provided in figures S1, S2, S3.

Discussion

As reconstructive endovascular modality, SAC of intracranial VADAs has been proven effective and feasible, especially when deconstructive treatment is contraindicated [7–9,15]. Due to maintenance of patency of the parent artery, recurrence is a risk factor which influenced the prognosis of patients with intracranial VADAs after SAC [2,11]. There have been some small case reports and case series about recurrence of intracranial VADAs after SAC [4,14–16]. Post-treatment recurrence may be more dangerous in dissecting aneurysms than in berry aneurysms [4]. However, the retreatment and outcomes after recurrence have not been specifically studied. In our retrospective study, six recurrent intracranial VADAs after SAC were retreated with different endovascular modalities and followed up angiographically and clinically. From this case series, we tried to analyze the reasons and characteristics of recurrence, evaluate the strategies and outcomes of retreatment for recurrent VADAs after SAC.

Reasons of recurrence

Recurrence has posed a great challenge to reconstructive endovascular treatment of intracranial VADAs [4,14–16]. There is a 13–33% recurrence rate after endovascular treatment of VBDAs [4,15,16,20]. On follow up angiography for 97 VBDAs in 89 patients after endovascular treatment, Kim et al. found that PICA origin involvement was the only independent risk factor for recurrence [4]. Persistent blood flow through the unprotected remnant dissecting aneurysm toward the PICA was believed to be the reason of recurrence. Differing from deconstructive treatment that obliterates the parent artery, SAC, as a reconstructive treatment modality, maintains the blood flow of parent artery increasing the possibility of recurrence.

Combined with related references and the experience gained from our case series we considered the recurrence probably due to the following reasons:

(1) The stent did not cover the dissected length of the vessel completely [14]. Pathological research revealed that Internal

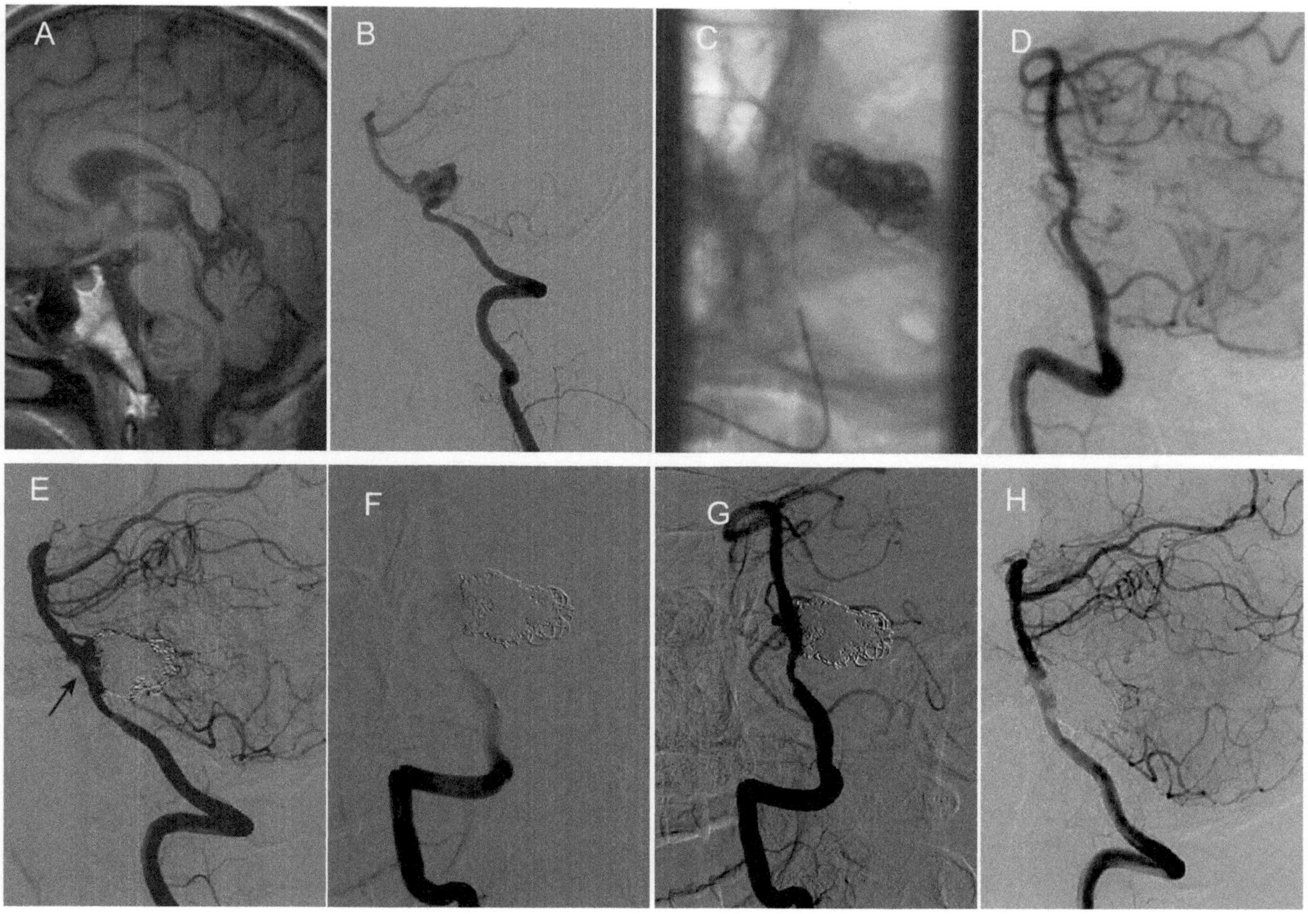

Figure 2. Retreatment with coil embolization was performed for recurrent intracranial VADA after SAC. A 29-year old male presented with dizziness and hemiplegia. Sagittal view of MR imaging showed intramural hematoma and compression to brain stem (A). Right vertebral angiograms showed a dissecting aneurysm involving PICA (B). SAC (C) were performed with nearly complete occlusion (D). Follow up angiography after three months revealed recanalization of the dissecting aneurysm (black arrow) (E). Retreatment was performed by coil embolization (F, G). Follow up angiography after 7 months of retreatment showed complete occlusion of right vertebral dissecting aneurysm (H).

Elastic Lamina (IEL) ruptures were longer than expected from angiographic results [18]. Among the total length of both intimal tears and medial defects, the mean length of proximal lesions from the center of the adventitial rupture was longer than that of distal lesions. With the increase of blood flow, from the defects of the intima, dissecting aneurysms can grow continuously. Although DSA still represents the gold standard in diagnostic imaging, Flat panel CTA such as Vaso CT, Dyna CT or Innova CT, MRI, MRA and HR-MRI have also demonstrated to be of value during initial treatment for a better understanding of the diseased segment of the parent vessel which should be covered with stents [27,28].

(2) Radial force of the Entreprise stent was insufficient. Self Expandable Stents (SES), have been broadly used in endovascular treatment of intracranial VADAs because of their flexibility [4,9,14–16]. Radial force against the vessel wall can promote the healing of the dissection. Meanwhile, SES can remodel the true lumen compressed by the dissecting aneurysm and the radial force may be less than the force of the blood flow within the pseudoaneurysms. Consequently, these types of stents may not attach or tack up the intimal flap to the parent vessel wall nor close the entrance of dissection.

Nowadays, no ideal stent seems to satisfy the demand of reconstructive endovascular treatment of intracranial VADAs. Because of the high porosity of the Entreprise stent, which is approximately 80% to 85% free metal to artery ratio, this self expandable stent can preserve the patency of perforating arteries, but the ability to divert the blood flow still poor in order to avoid recurrence [14]. These intracranial stents are not specifically designed to alter intra-aneurysmal hemodynamics. It is also difficult to navigate the tortuous vessels by using balloon expandable stents [21]. Newly developed flow diverters including Pipeline embolization device (PED) (Covidien/ev3 Irvine, CA, USA), SILK (BALT Extrusion, France) and the new Flow Re-direction Endoluminal Device FRED (MicroVention Inc. Tustin, CA, USA) devices, which have far less porosity than conventional neurovascular stents, may play a role in reconstructive treatment of intracranial dissecting aneurysms, by demonstrating favorable long-term clinical and angiographic outcomes with the ability to maintain parent artery and side-branch patency. There have been some severe complications previously reported such as rebleeding, side branch occlusion in posterior circulation dissecting aneurysms [13,22,23].To our knowledge, flow diverters have not been approved yet by the FDA for the treatment of vertebrobasilar dissecting aneurysms. There are few ongoing studies where the use of newest flow diverters is evaluated in the posterior circulation

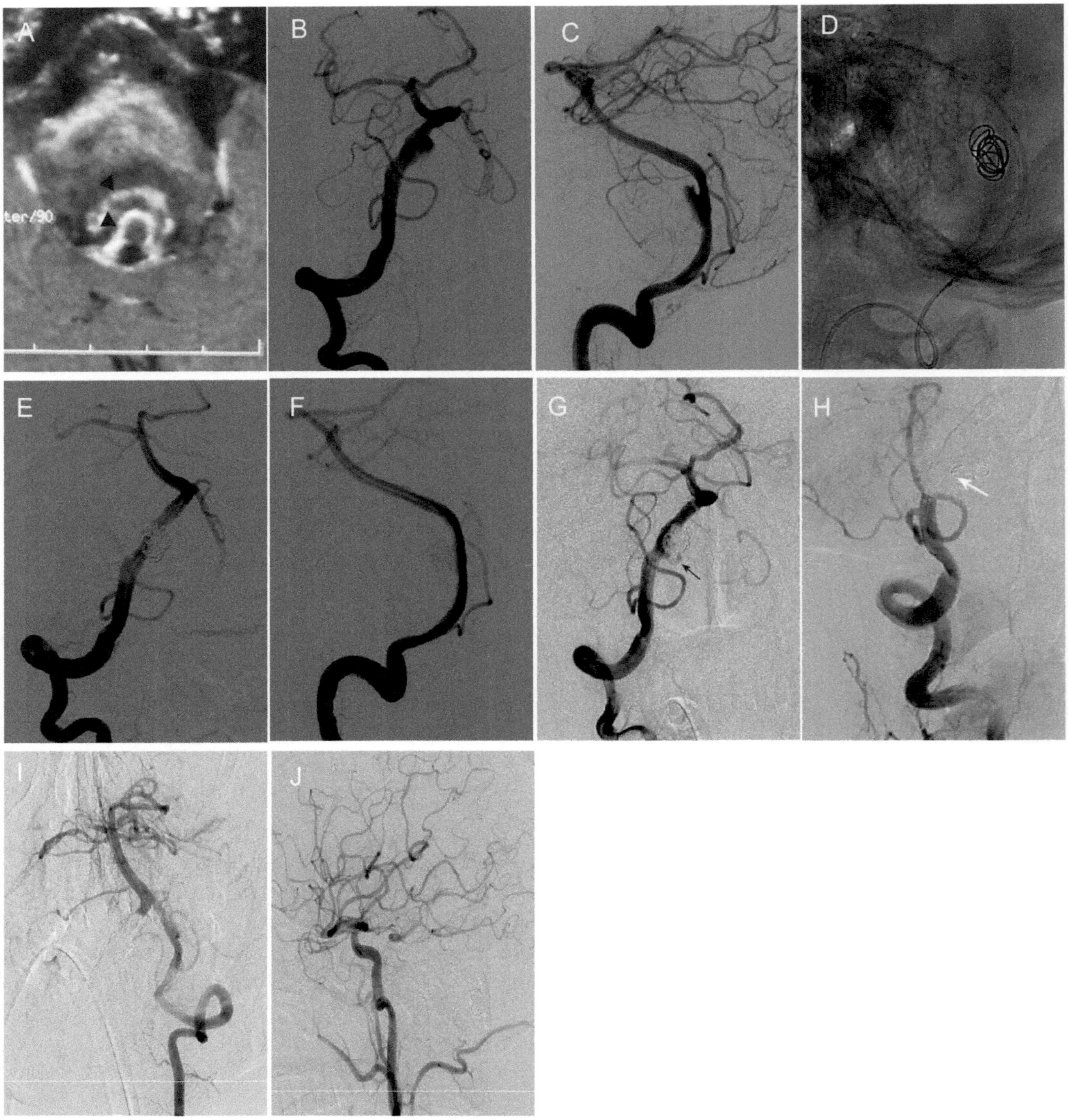

Figure 3 Retreatment with endovascular occlusion with aneurysm trapping was performed for recurrent huge intracranial VADA after multiple stents assisted coiling. A 54-year old male presented with headache and dysphagia. MR imaging showed huge onion skin-like thrombus (black arrowhead), intramural hematoma and compression to brain stem (A). Right vertebral angiograms of frontal (B) and lateral (C) view showed a dissecting aneurysm. Multiple stents assisted coiling (D) were performed with complete occlusion (E, F). Follow up angiography (G) after three months revealed regrowth of original dissecting aneurysm (black arrow). Retreatment by endovascular occlusion with aneurysm trapping (white arrow) (H) was performed. Collateral blood flow could be seen from contralateral VA (I) and left posterior communicating artery (J).

and there are also few recent case series published in the literature showing some potential good outcomes [24]. Flow diverters are not made widely available in our country for the moment.

(3) Incomplete occlusion of intracranial aneurysms resulted in recurrence. Dense coil packing is crucial to decrease the rate of recurrence. But for dissecting aneurysm with irregular shape and complex geometry, plus fragile vessel wall, and without definite aneurysm neck, it is difficult and challenging to perform complete occlusion [20]. Persistent blood flow into dissecting aneurysm, not completely obliterated, will result in recurrence of the dissecting aneurysms.

Table 3. Retreatment results and angiographic and clinical follow-up.

Patient NO.	Retreatment methods	Stent type, size (mm×mm) (number)	Immediate angiographic outcomes	Re-angiographic FU		Clinical FU	
				outcomes	time(mons)	time(mons)	mRS
1	SAC	EN 4.5×22 (1)	CO	CO	10	51	0
2	SAC	EN 4.5×22 (1)	NC	CO	4	46	0
3	coiling	—	CO	CO	7	33	0
4	SAC	EN 4.5×28 (1)	NC	CO	11	19	0
5	DS	EN 4.5×28 (2)	CMR	PAO	11	18	0
6	EOWAT	—	CO	—	—	11	2

DS = double stents; EOWAT = endovascular occlusion with aneurysm trapping; CMR = contrast medium retention; PAO = parent artery occlusion.

In other words, in treating VADAs using SAC procedure if the flow diversion property of the stent and the packing density of the coils are not enough to reduce or exclude the blood flow from the dissecting aneurysm the recurrence of intracranial VADAs will occur.

Strategies and outcomes of retreatment

With the development of intracranial stents, more and more intracranial VADAs are being treated with reconstructive endovascular modality based on increasing favorable results [8–13]. Meanwhile, the recurrence and retreatment should be evaluated. Retreatment modality of recurrent intracranial VADAs is determined by several factors including initial treatment modality, recurrence symptoms, recurrence types, neurovascular materials and the preference of the operators [16,17,19,20]. In theory, reconstructive procedures are more reasonable than deconstructive ones because we cannot predict the destiny of collateral vessels for the rest of the patient's life. The prognosis is better with the preservation of the parent vessel [15]. However, for hemorrhagic recurrence, parent artery occlusion, which is deemed to be the most reliable option, can decrease the possibility of recurrence [4]. For recurrent intracranial VADAs which did not allowed for occlusion of the parent artery, reconstructive endovascular retreatment will be considered first [20]. In our case series, 5 (cases 1–5) of the 6 patients were retreated with reconstructive retreatment. Clinical follow-up was excellent in all five cases. The Enterprise stent used in our procedures is a self-expandable stent with high porosity. The flow diversion and radial force of a single stent were limited. Overlapping multiple stents technique has been shown to divert more blood flow from the dissecting aneurysm sac than a single stent by decreasing stent porosity, further straightening the parent artery, increasing stent thickness and subsequent neointimal endothelial formation [7,25,26]. In our study, retreatment with a second stent assisted coiling was performed in 3 patients (cases 1, 2, 4). The results suggest that retreatment with a second stent and better coiling, which improved radial force against vessel wall, decreased porosity, repaired the intimal flap, increased blood flow diversion, improved coil density and can gain a favorable result. Although angiographic follow up after 11 months revealed obliteration of the parent artery, in patient (case 5) there were no neurologic deficits. We analyzed that the mechanism was probably due to slow in-stent thrombosis and subsequent occlusion [16,22].

Adequate flow diversion and dense packing are equally significant to avoid recurrence. But there are still several intracranial VADAs with unfavorable outcomes even after being treated by reconstructive endovascular techniques where adequate flow diversion and complete occlusion are seen because of the complexity and flow dynamics changes in dissecting aneurysms. In case 6, although three overlapping stents were deployed to try to remodel the blood flow and to achieve a complete occlusion in the initial treatment, recurrence still couldn't be avoided probably due to the severe deconstruction of the vessel wall. High resolution MR showed a huge VADA involving onion skin-like thrombus inside that aneurysm (Fig. 3 A). Because of severe recurrence symptom (sudden dyspnea) and regrowth of the original dissecting aneurysm we selected deconstructive endovascular retreatment modality for this patient. The improvement of clinical status on follow up showed that the retreatment modality was appropriate and effective for this kind of recurrent dissecting aneurysm.

In general, individualized strategies of retreatment should be done based on the initial treatment modalities and the characteristics of recurrence. We are optimistic about the retreatment of recurrent intracranial VADAs after SAC, based on our positive outcomes. But large case series and long-term follow up are necessary to draw a definite conclusion.

Conclusions

Endovascular retreatment is feasible and effective for recurrent intracranial VADAs after SAC. Individualized strategies of retreatment should be enacted according to the reasons and characteristics of recurrence. But only proper design studies and large population data with proper follow-ups will help us to drive to that conclusion.

Supporting Information

Figure S1 Case 2. A 49-year-old male was admitted with headache. DSA showed a left vertebral artery dissecting aneurysm distal to the origin of left PICA (1-1, 1-2). SAC were performed with complete occlusion (2-1, 2-2). Follow up angiography after seven months revealed regrowth of dissecting aneurysm from distal to the original dissecting aneurysm (3). Retreatment by stent assisted coiling (4) was performed with near complete occlusion (5-1, 5-2). Follow up angiography after 4 months of retreatment showed complete occlusion of recurrent dissecting aneurysm (6-1, 6-2). Follow up CTA after 22 months of retreatment showed no recurrence (7).

Figure S2 Case 4. A 49-year old male presented with headache and dizziness. MR imaging showed intramural hematoma and intimal flap (1-1, 1-2). Right vertebral angiograms showed a dissecting aneurysm involving PICA (2-1, 2-2, 2-3). SAC (3) were performed with partial occlusion (4-1, 4-2). Follow up angiography after six months revealed regrowth of the dissecting aneurysm (5-1, 5-2, 5-3). Retreatment by stent assisted coiling (6) was performed with near complete occlusion (7). Follow up angiography after 11 months of retreatment showed complete occlusion of recurrent dissecting aneurysm (8-1, 8-2).

Figure S3 Case 5. A 53-year old male presented with headache and dizziness. MR imaging showed intramural hematoma and intimal flap (1-1, 1-2). Left vertebral angiograms showed a dissecting aneurysm (2-1, 2-2). SAC (3) were performed with partial occlusion (4). Follow up angiography after five months revealed recanalization of the dissecting aneurysm (5-1, 5-2, 5-3). Retreatment by double stent (6) was performed with contrast medium retention (7-1, 7-2). Angiographic follow up after 11 months revealed obliteration of the parent artery (8-1, 8-2, 8-3).

Author Contributions

Conceived and designed the experiments: YS X-JY. Performed the experiments: YS Yang Wang C-HL Yanmin Wang S-QM. Analyzed the data: YS C-HL Yang Wang. Contributed reagents/materials/analysis tools: YS C-HL Yang Wang. Wrote the paper: YS. Revised the article: X-JY S-QM.

References

1. Jin SC, Kwon DH, Choi CG, Ahn JS, Kwun BD (2009) Endovascular strategies for vertebrobasilar dissecting aneurysms. AJNR Am J Neuroradiol 30: 1518–1523.
2. Park KW, Park JS, Hwang SC, Im SB, Shin WH, et al. (2008) Vertebral artery dissection: natural history, clinical features and therapeutic considerations. J Korean Neurosurg Soc 44: 109–115.
3. Mizutani T, Aruga T, Kirino T, Miki Y, Saito I, et al. (1995) Recurrent subarachnoid hemorrhage from untreated ruptured vertebrobasilar dissecting aneurysms. Neurosurgery 36: 905–913.
4. Kim BM, Shin YS, Kim SH, Suh SH, Ihn YK, et al. (2011) Incidence and risk factors of recurrence after endovascular treatment of intracranial vertebrobasilar dissecting aneurysms. Stroke 42: 2425–2430.
5. Peluso JPP, van Rooij WJ, Sluzewski M, Beute GN, Majoie CB (2008) Endovascular treatment of symptomatic intradural vertebral dissecting aneurysms. AJNR Am J Neuroradiol 29: 102–106.
6. Rho MH, Park HJ, Chung EC, Choi YJ, Lee SY, et al. (2013) Various techniques of stent-assisted coil embolization of wide-necked or fusiform artherosclerotic and dissecting unruptured vertebrobasilar artery aneurysms for reducing recanalization: mid-term results. Acta Neurochir 155: 2009–2017.
7. Suh SH, Kim BM, Park SI, Kim DI, Shin YS, et al. (2009) Stent-assisted coil embolization followed by a stent-within-a-stent technique for ruptured dissecting aneurysms of the intracranial vertebrobasilar artery. J Neurosurg 111:48–52.
8. Lylyk P, Ceratto R, Hurvitz D, Basso A (1998) Treatment of a vertebral dissecting aneurysm with stents and coils: technical case report. Neurosurgery 43:385–388.
9. Lylyk P, Cohen JE, Ceratto R, Ferrario A, Miranda C (2001) Combined endovascular treatment of dissecting vertebral artery aneurysms by using stents and coils. J Neurosurg 94:427–432.
10. Irie K, Negoro M, Hayakawa M, Eayashi J, Kanno T (2003) Stent assisted coil embolization: the treatment of wide-necked, dissecting, and fusiform aneurysms. Interventional Neuroradiology 9: 255–261.
11. Naito I, Takatama S, Shimaguchi H, Iwai T (2004) Endovascular treatment of vertebral artery dissecting aneurysms using stents. Interventional Neuroradiology 10 (Suppl1): 181–186.
12. Irie K, Negoro M, Hayakawa M, Hayashi J, Kanno T (2003) Treatment of a spontaneous intracranial dissecting aneurysm with stent-assisted coil embolization. Neuroradiology 45: 825–829.
13. van Oel LI, van Rooij WJ, Sluzewski M, Beute GN, Lohle PNM,et al.(2013) Reconstructive endovascular treatment of fusiform and dissecting basilar trunk aneurysms with flow diverters, stents, and coils. AJNR Am J Neuroradiol 34: 589–595.
14. MacKay CI, Han PP, Albuquerque FC, McDougall CG (2003) Recurrence of a vertebral artery dissecting pseudoaneurysm after successful stent-supported coil embolization: case report. Neurosurgery 53: 754–760.
15. Ahn JY, Han IB, Kim TG, Yoon PH, Lee YJ, et al. (2006) Endovascular treatment of intracranial vertebral artery dissections with stent placement or stent assisted coiling. AJNR Am J Neuroradiol 27: 1514–1520.
16. Wakhloo AK, Mandell J, Gounis MJ, Brooks C, Linfante I, et al. (2008) Stent-assisted reconstructive endovascular repair of cranial fusiform atherosclerotic and dissecting aneurysms: Long-term clinical and angiographic follow-up. Stroke 39: 3288–3296.
17. Ono H, Nakatomi H, Tsutsumi K, Inoue T, Teraoka A, et al. (2013) Symptomatic recurrence of intracranial arterial dissections: Follow-up study of 143 consecutive cases and pathological investigation. Stroke 44: 126–131.
18. Ro A, Kageyama N (2013) Pathomorphometry of ruptured intracranial vertebral arterial dissection: adventitial rupture, dilated lesion, intimal tear, and medial defect. J Neurosurg 119:221–227.
19. Dorfer C, Gruber A, Standhardt H, Bavinzski G, Knosp E (2012) Management of residual and recurrent aneurysms after initial endovascular treatment. Neurosurgery 70: 537–554.
20. Islak C (2013) The retreatment: Indications, technique and results. European Journal of Radiology 82:1659–1664.
21. Lee DH, Yoon WK, Baik MW, Kim H (2013) The difference of each angiographic finding after multiple stent according to stent type in bilateral vertebral artery dissection. J Cerebrovasc Endovasc Neurosurg 15: 229–234.
22. Faria MB, Castro RN, Lundquist J, Scrivano E, Ceratto R, et al. (2011) The role of the pipeline embolization device for the treatment of dissecting intracranial aneurysms. AJNR Am J Neuroradiol 32: 2192–2195
23. Yeung TW, Lai V, Lau HY, Poon WL, Tan CB, et al. (2012) with the Pipeline embolization device in the management of unruptured dissecting aneurysms of the intracranial vertebral artery. J Neurosurg 116:882–887.
24. Phillips TJ, Wenderoth JD, Pharouros CC, Rice H, Singh TP, et al. (2012) Safety of the Pipeline Embolization Device in treatment of posterior circulation aneurysms. AJNR Am J Neuroradiol 33: 1225–1231.
25. Kim BM, Suh SH, Park SI, Shin YS, Chung EC, et al. (2008) Management and clinical outcome of acute basilar artery dissection. AJNR Am J Neuroradiol 29:1937–1941.
26. Mehta B, Burke T, Kole M, Bydon A, Seyfried D, et al. (2003) Stent-within-a-Stent Technique for the Treatment of Dissecting Vertebral Artery Aneurysms. AJNR Am J Neuradiol 24:1814–1818.
27. Santos-Franco JA, Zenteno M, Lee A (2008) Dissecting aneurysms of the vertebrobasilar system: A comprehensive review on natural history and treatment options. Neurosurg Rev 31:131–140.
28. Wang Y, Lou X, Li Y, Sui B, Sun S, et al. (2014) Imaging investigation of intracranial arterial dissecting aneurysms by using 3T high-resolution MRI and DSA: from the interventional neuroradiologists' view. Acta Neurochir 156:515–525.

Optimal Brain MRI Protocol for New Neurological Complaint

William A. Mehan Jr., R. Gilberto González*, Bradley R. Buchbinder, John W. Chen, William A. Copen, Rajiv Gupta, Joshua A. Hirsch, George J. Hunter, Scott Hunter, Jason M. Johnson, Hillary R. Kelly, Mykol Larvie, Michael H. Lev, Stuart R. Pomerantz, Otto Rapalino, Sandra Rincon, Javier M. Romero, Pamela W. Schaefer, Vinil Shah

Neuroradiology Division, Massachusetts General Hospital, Harvard Medical School, Boston, Massachusetts, United States of America

Abstract

Background/Purpose: Patients with neurologic complaints are imaged with MRI protocols that may include many pulse sequences. It has not been documented which sequences are essential. We assessed the diagnostic accuracy of a limited number of sequences in patients with new neurologic complaints.

Methods: 996 consecutive brain MRI studies from patients with new neurological complaints were divided into 2 groups. In group 1, reviewers used a 3-sequence set that included sagittal T1-weighted, axial T2-weighted fluid-attenuated inversion recovery, and axial diffusion-weighted images. Subsequently, another group of studies were reviewed using axial susceptibility-weighted images in addition to the 3 sequences. The reference standard was the study's official report. Discrepancies between the limited sequence review and the reference standard including Level I findings (that may require immediate change in patient management) were identified.

Results: There were 84 major findings in 497 studies in group 1 with 21 not identified in the limited sequence evaluations: 12 enhancing lesions and 3 vascular abnormalities identified on MR angiography. The 3-sequence set did not reveal microhemorrhagic foci in 15 of 19 studies. There were 117 major findings in 499 studies in group 2 with 19 not identified on the 4-sequence set: 17 enhancing lesions and 2 vascular lesions identified on angiography. All 87 Level I findings were identified using limited sequence (56 acute infarcts, 16 hemorrhages, and 15 mass lesions).

Conclusion: A 4-pulse sequence brain MRI study is sufficient to evaluate patients with a new neurological complaint except when contrast or angiography is indicated.

Editor: Jan Kassubek, University of Ulm, Germany

Funding: The authors have no support or funding to report.

Competing Interests: The authors have declared that no competing interests exist.

* Email: rggonzalez@mgh.harvard.edu

Introduction

Diagnostic medical imaging is one of the major driving forces behind rising healthcare expenditures. Between 2000 and 2006, Medicare spending on imaging services more than doubled, increasing to $14 billion[1]. The volume of brain MR studies performed may continue to rise in the future due to the expansion of health care insurance under the Patient Protection and Affordable Care Act (PPACA) and as a result of an aging population. At our institution, patients with various neurologic complaints are often imaged with MRI protocols that may involve a large number of pulse sequences, resulting in long scan times. There have been major advances in MRI hardware and software technology since the days of the first nuclear magnetic resonance (NMR) images in 1974. These advancements have provided us with an array of available MR sequences to choose from for our neuroimaging protocols. Long scan times related to multiple sequence acquisitions likely result in patient inconvenience and discomfort. It is unclear whether the multiple MR sequences performed are necessary and which of the sequences add value to the interpretation of the study. Optimizing the number of sequences in a routine screening brain MR protocol could improve efficiency as well as increase patient compliance and satisfaction by reducing scan time. Our goal was to investigate the diagnostic accuracy of brain MRI protocols containing a limited number of basic sequences in the evaluation of patients with new neurologic complaints.

Methods

Patient Selection

This retrospective study was approved by the Partners Human Research Committee, our hospital's Institutional Review Board

Table 1. Patient Demographics and MRI Findings Group 1.

Parameter	**Group 1 (n = 497)**	**Group 2 (n = 499)**
Age (years)	**mean 54.3 (range 0.5–98)**	**mean 51.3 (range 0.5–93)**
Male:Female (%)	**43:57**	**38:62**
Significant MRI Findings	84	117 (23.4%)
Acute/subacute infarction	39 (46.4%)	67 (57.3%)
Intracranial hemorrhages	9 (10.7%)	7 (6.0%)
Posterior reversible encephalopathy syndrome (PRES)	2 (2.4%)	4 (3.4%)
Vascular lesions*	4 (4.8%)	4 (3.4%)
Cavernous malformations	4 (4.8%)	1(0.9%)
Active demyelinating lesions	3 (3.6%)	2(1.7%)
Hydrocephalus	1 (1.2%)	3 (2.6%)
Metastases	5 (6.0%)	9 (7.7%)
Meningiomas or schwannomas	8 (9.5%)	7 (6.0%)
Mass lesions**	4 (4.8%)	11 (9.4%)
Infectious/Inflammatory lesions	3 (3.6%)	2(1.7%)
Cortical dysplasia	2 (2.4%)	0
Major discrepancies	21	19 (16.2%)
Enhancing lesions***	12 (57.1%)	17 (89.5%)
Punctate acute/subacute infarcts	4 (19.0%)	0
Cortical dysplasias	2(9.5%)	0
Vascular lesions	3 (14.3%)	2 (10.5%)
Microhemorrhage discrepancies		
Microhemorrhages	Group 1 (n = 19)	Group 2 (n = 28)
Discrepancies	15 (77.8%)	0

* Venous sinus thrombosis, ICA dissection, arterial thrombus, absent vertebrobasilar flow voids, MCA branch thrombosis
** Cerebellar mass, brainstem mass, optic nerve sheath mass, thalamic masses, lobar masses, pituitary/sellar masses, corpus callosal mass, clival mass, colloid cysts
***Included probable metastases, probable primary tumors, inflammatory/demyelinating lesions, and indeterminate punctate enhancing foci

(IRB). Consent was not obtained and patient records/information was anonymized and de-identified prior to analysis.

We performed a retrospective study of consecutive brain MR examinations performed at our institution, a major urban academic medical center, between February 20, 2010 and April 21, 2010. Studies included patients of all ages who underwent brain MR imaging for the evaluation of new neurologic complaints for which there was no established diagnosis stated on the radiology requisition. We included studies referred from the emergency department, inpatient and outpatient settings. Both intravenous contrast- enhanced and unenhanced studies were included as were studies that contained MR angiogram (MRA) and MR venogram (MRV) sequences. Image review commenced in June 2012, at least 24 months after the examinations were performed. Exclusion criteria were MR studies performed for follow-up evaluation of pre-existing neurological conditions (e.g. serial neuro-oncology studies) and specialized MR protocols (e.g. pituitary, orbits, brainstem and internal auditory canal studies).

All MRI examinations were performed on either 1.5T (Tesla) or 3T MR systems (GE Healthcare Clinical Systems, Wauwatosa, WI, USA; Siemens Medical Solutions, Erlangen, Germany). A total of 9 MRI scanners were used during the period that was reviewed. Eight scanners had field strengths of 1.5T. Six were manufactured by General Electric; 3 were located within the hospital and 3 were located at free standing imaging centers. Two 1.5T MRI scanners were manufactured by Siemens and were located within the hospital. Additionally, a single Siemens 3T scanner was located within the hospital. All MR images in the study were reviewed on a PACS system (Agfa Impax 5.3, Agfa Healthcare, Mortsel, Belgium).

Study Interpretation

The total number of consecutive MRI studies was partitioned into two separate data sets (group 1, MR studies from February 20, 2010 through March 23, 2010; group 2, MR studies from March 24, 2010 through April 21, 2010).

The group 1 neuroradiologists reviewed a three-sequence abbreviated image set composed of sagittal T1-weighted images, axial T2-weighted FLAIR images, and images derived from a single diffusion-weighted imaging sequence, which included images with and without diffusion gradients, as well as derived apparent diffusion coefficient maps. The neuroradiologists interpreted those three MRI sequences while blinded to both the additional MRI sequences that were acquired, and to the official radiologic report. For each case, a group 1 neuroradiologist formulated an impression based on the three limited sequences and then subsequently compared it to the unblinded impression in the reference official radiologic report. For any discrepancy between the two interpretations, the neuroradiologist was instructed to revisit the limited MR sequences and determine

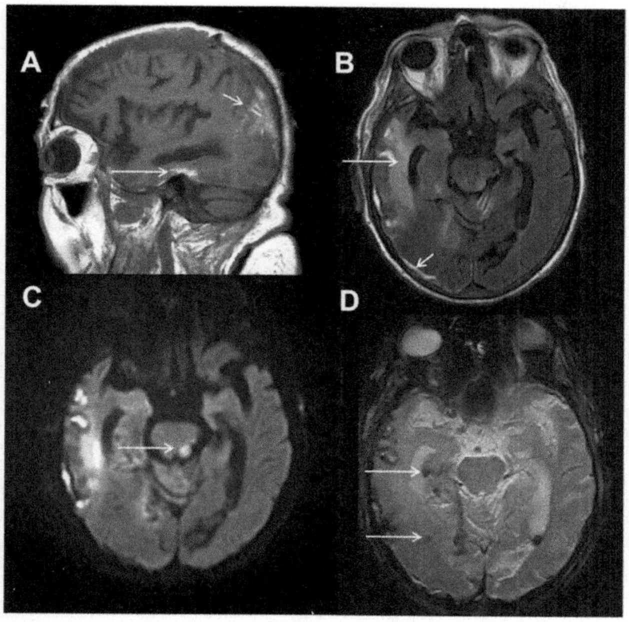

Figure 1. Intracranial hemorrhages and diffuse axonal injury. 83 year old female status post fall. Sagittal T1-weighted image (A) shows hyperintense signal involving the lateral right temporal lobe consistent with cortical contusion and subacute blood products (white arrow). Axial T2-weighted FLAIR image (B) depicts edema in the right temporal lobe from traumatic contusion (long white arrow) and a subdural hemorrhage overlying the lateral right temporal and occipital lobes (short white arrow). Axial diffusion weighted trace image (C) shows a focus of restricted diffusion within the left dorsolateral midbrain compatible with non-hemorrhagic diffuse axonal injury (white arrow). Axial gradient recalled echo image (D) shows a punctate focus of susceptibility effect within the right temporal lobe compatible with hemorrhagic diffuse axonal injury (white arrow).

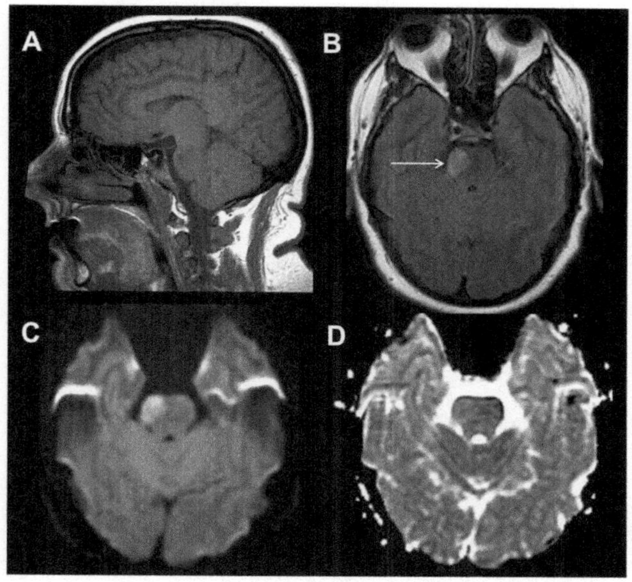

Figure 2. Brainstem mass lesion. 38 year old female with transient left sided weakness. Sagittal T1-weighted image (A) shows a subtle hypointense lesion within the pons. Axial T2-weighted FLAIR image (B) demonstrates a hyperintense, expansile mass-like lesion within the right mid pons (white arrow). Axial diffusion weighted trace (C) and apparent diffusion coefficient images (D) reveal slightly increased diffusivity within the lesion compatible with a demyelinating lesion, neoplasm, or subacute infarction.

whether, in retrospect, the discrepant findings could have been made on the limited sequences, but were missed due to perceptual error.

The second phase of the study involved a different set of staff neuroradiologists with experience ranging from 2 to 20 years. The group 2 neuroradiologists reviewed a four-sequence abbreviated image set composed of the three basic sequences that were reviewed by the group 1 neuroradiologists, with the addition of an axial magnetic susceptibility sensitive sequence (either T2* gradient recalled echo (GRE), or susceptibility weighted imaging (SWI), including susceptibility weighted angiography (SWAN)). The neuroradiologists interpreted those four MRI sequences while blinded to both the additional MRI sequences that were acquired, and to the official radiologic report. For each case, a group 2 neuroradiologist formulated an impression based on the four limited sequences and then subsequently compared it to the unblinded impression in the official radiologic report, (the reference standard). For any discrepancy between the two interpretations, the neuroradiologist revisited the limited MR sequences and determined whether, in retrospect, the discrepant findings could have been appreciated on the limited sequences, but were missed due to perceptual error.

The limited sequence interpretations by the neuroradiologists in groups 1 and 2 were performed on the same PACS workstations as the original interpretations, and they are located in the same interpretation areas as in the original clinical interpretation. The only history that was permitted to the new study reviewer was the limited one provided with the original request for imaging. The neuroradiologists in groups 1 and 2 were allowed to review previous MRI studies when available, but only the limited MRI sequences on the prior study could be reviewed when formulating an impression. Readers in both groups were not permitted to review post-contrast, MRA, or MRV images, if these were acquired.

In order to eliminate recall bias, the assignment of MRI cases to each neuroradiologist was reviewed. If any case had been previously reviewed by the neuroradiologist to which the case was assigned, then the case was reassigned to an additional neuroradiologist (RGG) who reviewed the case with the same instructions.

We designated findings and discrepancies as major if they were likely to have a significant impact on patient management. Level 1 findings were designated as those requiring immediate communication at our institution: acute infarction, intracranial hemorrhage and unexpected mass lesion. The following imaging findings were also designated as major: subacute infarctions; posterior reversible encephalopathy syndrome (PRES); vascular malformations; malformations of cortical development (including focal cortical dysplasia); hydrocephalus; parenchymal lesions suspicious for infection, inflammatory disease, primary or secondary CNS neoplasm; and other mass lesions. Abnormalities of the major intracranial flow voids including arterial dissection, venous sinus thrombosis and intra-arterial thrombus were also considered major abnormalities. Acute/subacute infarctions required observation of decreased diffusivity in DWI sequences. Microhemorrhages (punctate parenchymal foci of susceptibility effect) were

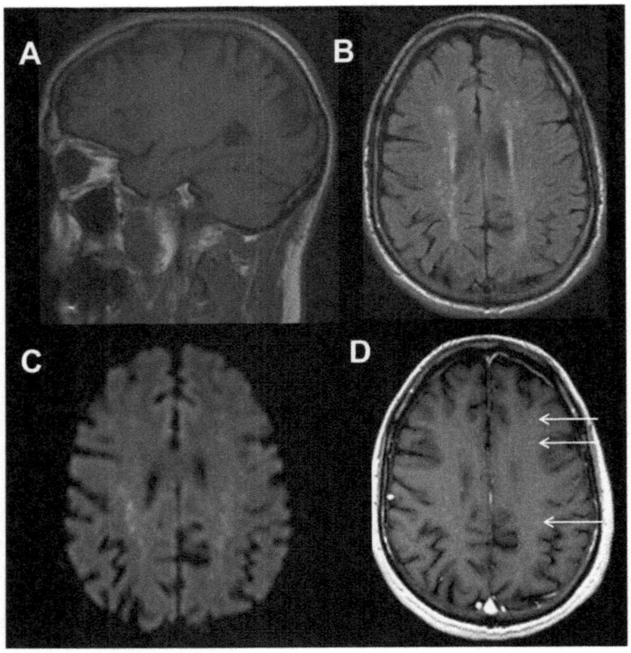

Figure 3. Foci of enhancement in a 57 year old male with ataxia. Sagittal T1-weighted image (A) shows no definite abnormality. Axial T2-weighted FLAIR image (B) demonstrates multiple punctate hyperintense foci involving the deep and periventricular white matter of the bilateral cerebral hemispheres with corresponding restricted diffusion on the axial diffusion weighted trace (C) image. Axial T1-weighted post contrast image (D) reveals numerous punctate foci of enhancement corresponding to the deep and periventricular white matter lesions (white arrows). In this patient, the differential diagnosis included intravascular lymphoma, granulomatous disease, neurosarcoidosis, and vasculitis.

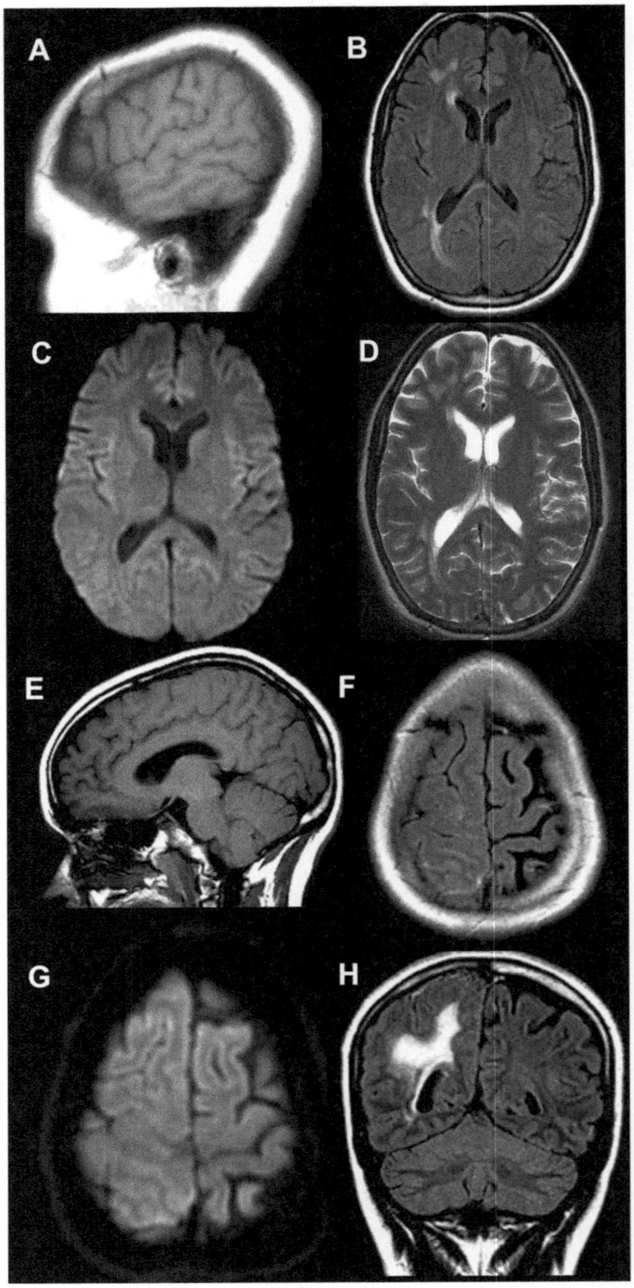

Figure 4. 22 year old female with right frontal hemispheric dysplasia. Sagittal T1-weighted image (A) shows no definite abnormality. Axial FLAIR image (B) demonstrates subtle enlargement of the right hemisphere with focal areas of signal hyperintensity within the subcortical white matter of the right frontal and parietal lobes but without corresponding restricted diffusion on the axial diffusion weighted trace (C) image. Additionally noted is ipsilateral ventricular enlargement. Pachygyria was also demonstrated within the right frontal and parietal lobes, better demonstrated on more superior axial FLAIR images. Axial T2-weighted image (D) also demonstrates these findings. Sagittal T1-weighted image (E) shows no definite abnormality. Axial FLAIR image (F) demonstrates asymmetric cortical thickening, gyral enlargement within the right frontal and parietal lobes without restricted diffusion on the axial diffusion weighted trace (G) image, consistent with pachygyria. Coronal FLAIR image (H) reveals asymmetric cortical thickening, abnormal sulcation and white matter signal hyperintensity in the right parietal lobe. The group 1 reader described the right frontal lobe signal abnormality, but did not diagnose the full extent of the hemispheric abnormality. These findings are more apparent on the coronal FLAIR sequence, not available to the reader.

considered potentially important findings. Other typically incidental findings were designated as non-major.

Statistical Analysis

A descriptive analysis of the data from groups 1 and 2 was performed.

Results

Out of a total of ~3750 brain MRI studies, 998 brain MRI studies met our eligibility criteria. The first 497 studies were placed in group 1, and the remaining 499 in group 2.

In group 1, 84 major findings were identified (16.9% of studies, Table 1). All 41 level 1 findings (28 acute infarcts, 9 hemorrhages, and 4 mass lesions) were identified on the limited sequences. Examples of cases with accurately interpreted major findings included traumatic brain injury with multi-compartment intracranial hemorrhages (Figure 1) and neoplasms (Figure 2). Of these 84 major findings, there were 21 discrepancies between the interpretation based on the abbreviated MRI protocol, and the official interpretation from the radiologic report, yielding an error rate of 25.0%.

The most common discrepant major findings were enhancing intracranial lesions (12 cases) (Figure 3). There were 4 small acute or subacute infarctions that were missed by two of the group 1 readers. All of these abnormalities were identified on the diffusion MR sequences when the readers re-examined these studies. Thus,

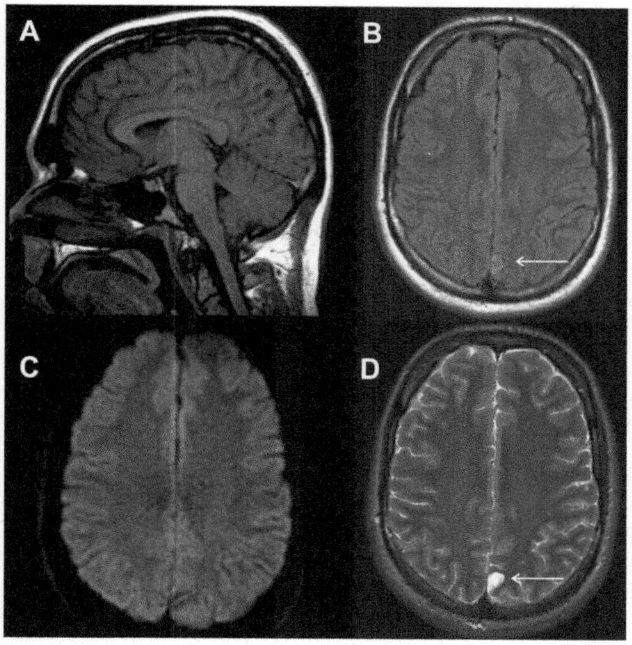

Figure 5. Cortical dysplasia versus dysembryoplastic neuroepithelial tumor in an 18 year old male with seizures. Sagittal T1-weighted image (A) shows no definite abnormality. Axial T2-weighted FLAIR image (B) demonstrates a subtle focal area of signal hyperintensity within the cortex and subcortical white matter of the left parafalcine parietal lobe(white arrow) with no corresponding restricted diffusion on the axial diffusion weighted trace (C) image. Axial T2-weighted image (D) again demonstrates the hyperintense lesion within the cortex and subcortical white matter of the left parafalcine parietal lobe (white arrow), which is compatible with cortical dysplasia or dysembryoplastic neuroepithelial tumor. This finding is subtle and was not seen prospectively when using the limited sequences. However, the lesion can be seen on the FLAIR images in retrospect. Furthermore, for seizure patients, additional sequences, including isotropic multiplanar sequences, could be added that would help in identifying subtle abnormalities.

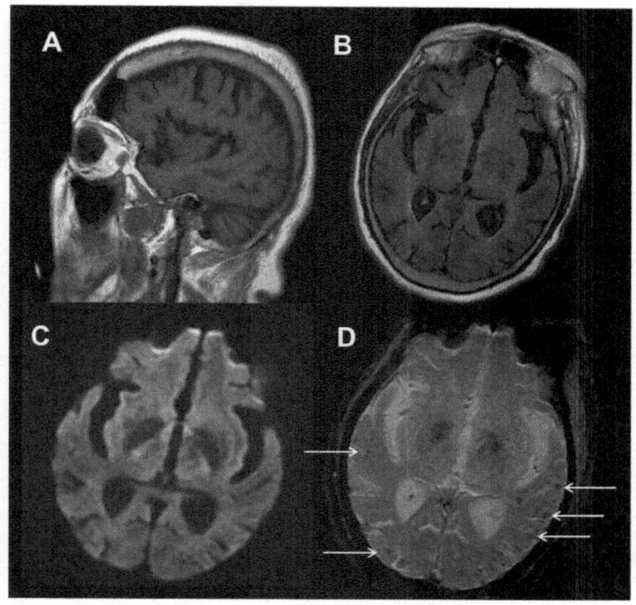

Figure 6. Cerebral amyloid angiopathy in a 78 year old female with altered mental status. Sagittal T1-weighted image (A) shows age appropriate parenchymal volume loss. Axial FLAIR image (B) demonstrates a small number of nonspecific hyperintense foci that are not unusual in a patient of this age. The axial diffusion weighted image (C) demonstrates no evidence of acute ischemia. Sequences A-C (group 1 sequences) show no definite abnormality that would explain the patient's symptoms. Axial gradient recalled echo image (D) reveals multiple punctate foci of susceptibility effect (white arrows) involving peripheral grey-white matter junctions, consistent with chronic micro-hemorrhages, which was not identified by the group 1 reader. This sequence alone (in addition to the other 3 sequences) provides the information needed to make the diagnosis of cerebral amyloid angiopathy.

these discrepancies were due to perceptual error. The diagnosis of cortical dysplasia was not made in 2 studies by group 1 readers. Abnormalities on the limited sequences were identified (Figure 4), but the diagnosis was not suggested. In the other case, a small non-enhancing lesion was only observed upon repeat review of the study (Figures 5).

There were 3 vascular abnormalities that were not identified on the abbreviated sequences; 2 cases of middle cerebral artery branch (MCA) thrombus in patients with concurrent acute infarctions and a case of transverse sinus thrombosis. The cases of MCA branch occlusion were not visualized on the 3-sequence series, although the acute infarctions in the MCA distribution were identified. The group 1 reader who did not identify the venous thrombosis reported that they would not have seen this lesion without an MR venogram.

In group 1, there were 19 cases that had evidence of probable microhemorrhage (3.8%). Out of these 19 cases, 15 were not identified by group 1 readers on the abbreviated MR sequences (77.8%) (Figure 6).

In the group 2 evaluation, there were 117 major findings in the 499 MR studies (23.4%, Table 2). Examples of cases with accurately detected major findings included early infarctions (Figures 7, 8, and 9) and neoplasms (Figure 10). Of these, 19 major findings were not identified on the abbreviated 4-sequence MRI series resulting in an error rate of 16.2%. Enhancing parenchymal lesions were the most commonly missed major findings (17 cases). The other major discrepancies were vascular lesions; one case of ICA dissection (Figure 11) and one case of vertebrobasilar arterial occlusion (Figure 12). In both of these cases, the readers reported that the absence of the flow voids was not identifiable without the aid of a non-inversion recovery T2-weighted sequence or MR angiogram (Figures 11D-F and 12E-G). There were 28 cases with probable microhemorrhages in the group 2 data set. All of these were identified by the group 2 readers.

Discussion

Since the introduction of MRI for the clinical evaluation of brain pathology, a large number of pulse sequences have been developed, and those with the highest clinical value have been extensively evaluated. However, there is little documented research on the optimal set of MRI sequences for the evaluation of patients with specific clinical presentations. In this evaluation of MRI used in patients with a new neurological complaint, we found that a limited-sequence imaging protocol can identify nearly all significant brain abnormalities with the major exceptions of small,

Table 2. Patient Demographics and MRI Findings Group 2.

Parameter	Group 2 (n = 499)
Age (years)	**mean 51.3 (range 0.5–93)**
Male:Female (%)	**38:62**
Significant MRI Findings	117
Acute/subacute infarction	67 (57.3%)
Intracranial hemorrhages	7 (6.0%)
Posterior reversible encephalopathy syndrome (PRES)	4 (3.4%)
Vascular lesions*	4 (3.4%)
Cavernous malformations	1(0.9%)
Active demyelinating lesions	2(1.7%)
Hydrocephalus	3 (2.6%)
Metastases	9 (7.7%)
Meningiomas or schwannomas	7 (6.0%)
Mass lesions**	11 (9.4%)
Infectious/Inflammatory lesions	2(1.7%)
Cortical dysplasia	0
Major discrepancies	19
Enhancing lesions***	17 (89.5%)
Punctate acute/subacute infarcts	0
Cortical dysplasias	0
Vascular lesions	2 (10.5%)
Microhemorrhage discrepancies	
Microhemorrhages	Group 2 (n = 28)
Discrepancies	0

* Venous sinus thrombosis, ICA dissection, arterial thrombus, absent vertebrobasilar flow voids, MCA branch thrombosis
** Cerebellar mass, brainstem mass, optic nerve sheath mass, thalamic masses, lobar masses, pituitary/sellar masses, corpus callosal mass, clival mass, colloid cysts
***Included probable metastases, probable primary tumors, inflammatory/demyelinating lesions, and indeterminate punctate enhancing foci

contrast-enhancing lesions and vascular lesions that are revealed by MR angiography. The 4-sequence protocol was superior to the 3-sequence protocol due to improved detection of probable microhemorrhages, and we conclude that it is sufficiently robust for the routine evaluation of patients who have new neurological symptoms and do not have a clear clinical indication for the use of contrast (e.g. history of a primary non-CNS malignancy or suspicion of demyelinating/inflammatory disorders) or direct evaluation of the cerebral vasculature (e.g. vascular risk factors with high suspicion for acute ischemia).

The T2-weighted FLAIR sequence has been shown to be the single most sensitive sequence for the detection of brain pathology [1–16]. Saleh et al. demonstrated in 1026 consecutive outpatient MRI studies that this sequence alone had positive and negative predictive values of 96.1% and 98.4%, respectively, for lesions detectable by a complete MRI protocol that included contrast enhancement [17]. The data presented here are fully consistent with this work. However, the T2-weighted FLAIR sequence is not sensitive in detecting small enhancing lesions, small structural lesions, early ischemia, and microhemorrhages, and it cannot be relied upon as the only sequence. The use of diffusion MRI and susceptibility sequences are excellent supplemental sequences for the detection of the latter two types of abnormalities.

Cerebral microhemorrhages are a common finding, but have indeterminate prognostic and therapeutic significance [18]. Using the 3-sequence protocol, 78% of cases with probable cerebral microhemorrhages were undetected by readers viewing the T1, T2-weighted FLAIR and diffusion sequences. This is similar to prior reports [19,20]. All probable microhemorrhages were correctly identified by readers who were able to view an axial susceptibility sequence as part of the 4 sequence protocol. This finding is consistent with the known superiority of susceptibility-weighted sequences in identifying small foci of susceptibility effect [18–23].

The use of the 3-sequence protocol resulted in lack of detection of 25% of major abnormalities, with over half of these being enhancing lesions. An improved detection rate was manifest with the 4-sequence protocol, with a lack of detection of 16% of major findings, but 90% of these were enhancing lesions. Enhancing lesions included meningiomas, active inflammatory/demyelinating lesions, metastases and probable primary brain tumors, as well as indeterminate punctate areas of parenchymal enhancement. Our findings suggest that intravenous gadolinium-based contrast should be administered in patients with a history of malignancy or suspected demyelinating/inflammatory disorders.

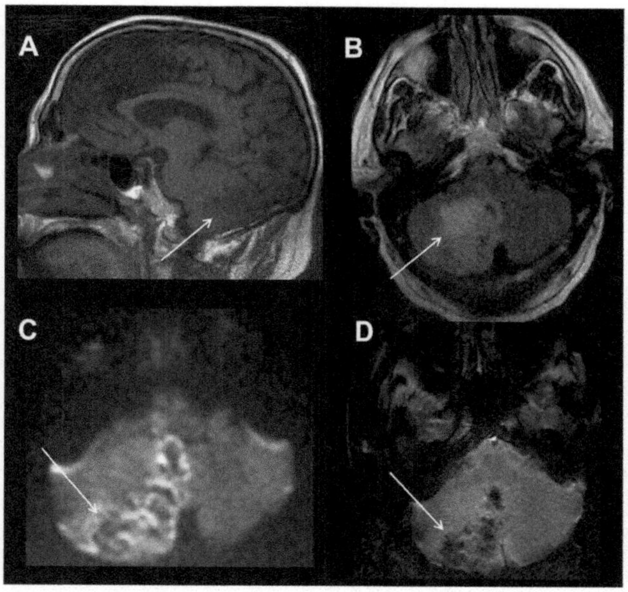

Figure 7. Hemorrhagic acute cerebellar infarction in a 79 year old male with a focal neurological deficit. Sagittal T1-weighted image (A) shows hypointense signal within the right inferior cerebellar hemisphere (white arrow). Axial T2-weighted FLAIR image (B) demonstrates geographic hyperintense signal and mass effect within the right inferior cerebellar hemisphere (white arrow). Axial diffusion weighted trace image (C) shows restricted diffusion in the right cerebellar hemisphere compatible with infarction (white arrow) as well as areas of hypointensity reflecting hemorrhage. Axial gradient recalled echo image shows susceptibility effect within the right cerebellar hemisphere, which is consistent with hemorrhage (white arrow).

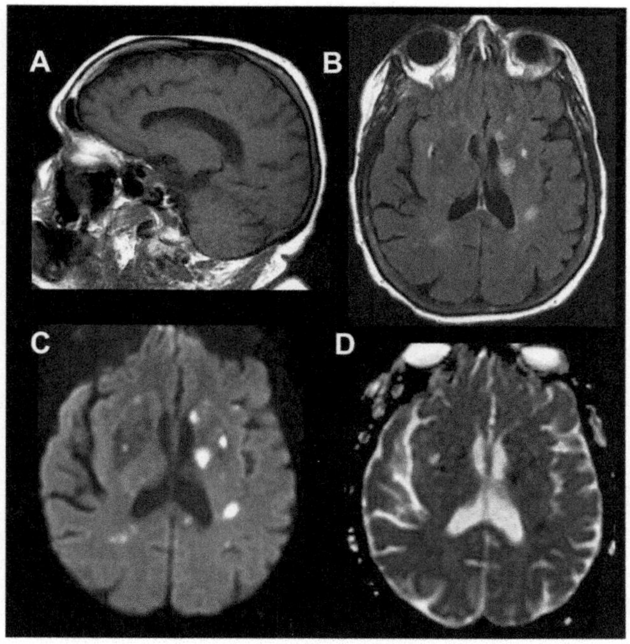

Figure 8. Acute infarctions in a 77 year old female with altered mental status. A 77-year-old woman underwent MRI examination because of altered mental status. Her complete examination included 12 pulse sequences, but all significant abnormalities are apparent in images derived from the three pulse sequences that comprised the abbreviated examination described in phase 1 of this study. A sagittal T1-weighted image (A) reveals no apparent abnormality. Axial T2-weighted FLAIR images (B) demonstrate multiple small hyperintense lesions in deep gray matter and white matter structures. The lesions are markedly hyperintense in diffusion-weighted images (C) and apparent diffusion coefficient maps derived from the DWI sequence (D) show restricted diffusion within the lesions, confirming that they are ischemic infarcts.

Several significant vascular lesions were not identified on the 3- or 4-sequence protocols, even upon revisiting the study, but were identified on MRA or MRV. Two of the missed vascular abnormalities in group 1 were occlusions in MCA branches. In cases where arterial dissection, vascular thrombosis or occlusion is clinically suspected, a vascular imaging sequence such as an MRA or MRV may add considerable value (Figures 11D-F and 12E-G).

One case of cortical dysplasia in group 1 was not initially identified, but the dysplasia was discernible in retrospect (Figure 5). The finding is subtle but visible on FLAIR images, and more obvious on T2 images. In these patients with a history of seizures, additional sequences could be added to the protocol for diagnostic imaging, including the use of high resolution, isotropic multiplanar sequences that would aid in identifying the structural abnormalities that may often be subtle.

The limited 4-sequence MRI protocol should increase efficiency and reduce scan length. The amount of time saved using the 4-sequence protocol is difficult to precisely calculate due to the variable pre-scan preparation times; however, we estimate that the time saved ranges from 5 to 25 minutes per study compared to our standard protocols. Further efficiencies in study acquisition may be possible through optimization of the limited sequence parameters. Also, substantial time savings in the interpretation of the 4-sequence MRI studies are expected since there will be fewer images per study for the neuroradiologist to review.

The 4-sequence MRI protocol will only be efficient and of value if the limited sequences allow the neuroradiologist to make a correct diagnosis with a limited rate of patient recall for additional sequences. The data in our study suggest that the patient recall rate will be very low and on the order of "misses" using the standard protocol.

A proper review of the patient's history should allow the neuroradiologist to tailor the MRI sequences to be performed for any given indication. The limited 4-sequence MRI screening protocol is only appropriate for the patient with new neurological complaints without an existing diagnosis. For example, a patient with known metastatic cancer will receive a contrast-enhanced MRI study. For patients undergoing the limited screening protocol, unexpected findings may be detected that warrant work-up with additional MR sequences. In these cases, we envision a hybrid solution. A large number of cases are monitored in 'real-time' by the neuroradiologist, which allows for immediate tailoring of the examination based on the findings on the limited sequences. Current technology even permits the neuroradiologist to remotely monitor cases and tailor them off-site. However, there will be some cases that cannot be monitored and such patients may require additional sequences to be performed at another time.

This study has several limitations. It has a retrospective design, although effort was made to minimize bias by analyzing consecutive cases. Despite our diligent attempt to minimize bias, results should be interpreted with caution as they have not yet been validated in a prospective fashion or using active clinical

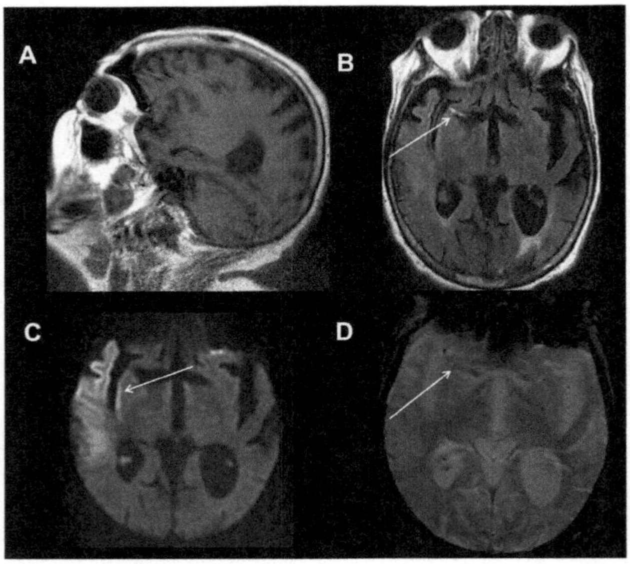

Figure 9. Acute stroke in a 78 year old female with altered mental status. Sagittal T1-weighted image of the right temporal lobe/ insula (A) is normal. Axial T2-weighted FLAIR image (B) shows hyperintense signal within the M1 segment of the right middle cerebral artery (MCA), suggesting slow flow or clot (white arrow). Axial diffusion weighted image (DWI) (C) shows restricted diffusion within the right temporal lobe and insula, diagnostic of acute stroke to this region (white arrow). Axial gradient recalled echo (GRE) susceptibility image (D) shows subtle linear susceptibility effect within the right MCA, consistent with recent passage of embolic material (white arrow).

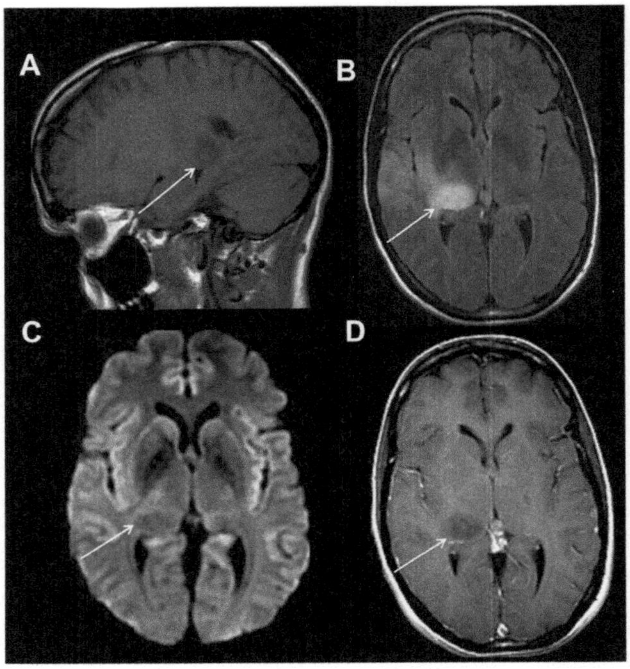

Figure 10. Right thalamic neoplasm identified in a 48 year old female with seizures. Limited pre-contrast set of imaging sequences are sufficient to clearly identify an expansile lesion within the pulvinar of the right thalamus; a finding requiring immediate communication for action (Level I) (white arrows). It is hypointense on sagittal T1-weighted image (A) and has associated hyperintensity on axial T2-weighted FLAIR extending into the adjacent insular-opercular region (B). Even within the confines of the limited set of sequences, neoplastic differential considerations are still able to be favored over acute ischemia as no evidence of restricted diffusion is seen on diffusion-weighted imaging (DWI) sequences; specifically low signal on DWI trace images (C) and elevated diffusivity on Apparent-Diffusion-Coefficient images (not shown). Post-contrast imaging, not initially available to the readers within the limited set of review sequences, demonstrated no abnormal enhancement (D).

cases. A prospective study is currently being designed to confirm the findings described here. An additional limitation is that the impressions from each original MRI interpretation were used as the reference standard. There may have been findings on brain MRI that were mentioned only in the body of a report and not in the impression. This most notably occurred in patients with probable microhemorrhages. Another limitation is that the original MRI interpretations were performed in the true clinical setting where the neuroradiologist may have been interrupted or distracted by phone calls, teaching and consultations, which is different than the clinical research conditions under which the group 1 and 2 neuroradiologists reviewed the cases. However, the group 1 and 2 neuroradiologsists interpreted their cases using the same PACS workstations in the same clinical work areas as those of the original interpretations and, therefore, were subject to similar disturbances and distractions. In addition, for the original clinical interpretations, the readers also had access to the full medical record that is readily accessible at the workstation, as well as the ability to contact the referring the physician for further information. Thus the reading of the limited sequences was more restricted than the original reading, thus providing an added measure of assurance on the validity of the results. The heterogeneity of our institutions MRI scanners, which had different manufacturers and field strengths, may be considered as another limitation. Bearing that in mind, the national installed base of clinical magnets has far greater heterogeneity than our institutions and one might argue that these studies cannot reflect the diversity of clinical practice. Additionally, this paper describes an effort to limit the number of sequences required for routine performance and is not making any comment with respect to interpretation times. Finally, the readers were primarily experienced neuroradiologists, which is not necessarily true for all those interpreting brain MRIs. We have not attempted to validate error rates utilizing this protocol amongst general radiologists or other specialists.

Conclusions

A four-sequence MRI protocol that includes sagittal T1 weighted images, axial T2-weighted FLAIR images, axial diffusion-weighted images, and T2*-weighted images reliably detects nearly all non-enhancing brain MRI findings in patients without a known history of a neurologic disease undergoing evaluation for a new neurologic complaint. If a patient has persistent unexplained symptoms, an additional MRI study including post-contrast and high-resolution imaging should reveal abnormalities characterized by blood brain barrier breakdown or small structural lesions. Clinical information suggesting a vascular lesion should be evaluated using an angiographic or venographic sequence.

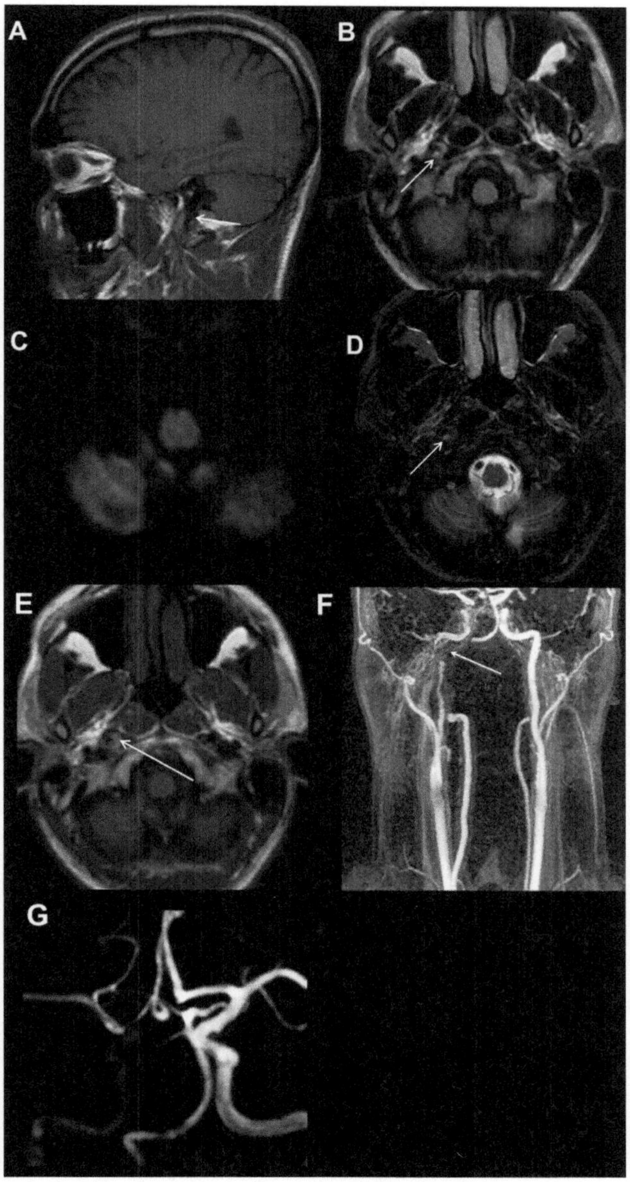

Figure 11. Internal carotid artery dissection in a 41 year old male with headache. The dissection was not identified on the limited 3 sequence review. Sagittal T1-weighted image (A) shows narrowing of the distal cervical portion of the right internal carotid artery with T1 hyperintense intramural hematoma (white arrow). Axial FLAIR image (B) demonstrates loss of the normal right internal carotid artery flow void (white arrow), which is more conspicuous on the axial T2-weighted image (D). Axial diffusion weighted trace image (C) shows no restricted diffusion in the region of the right internal carotid artery. Axial pre-contrast T1-weighted image (E) demonstrates an eccentric T1 hyperintense intramural hematoma (white arrow) in the distal cervical right internal carotid artery. MR angiography maximum intensity projection images reveal irregular critical narrowing (white arrow) of the distal cervical right ICA (F) and asymmetrical flow-related signal in the right intracranial ICA (G).

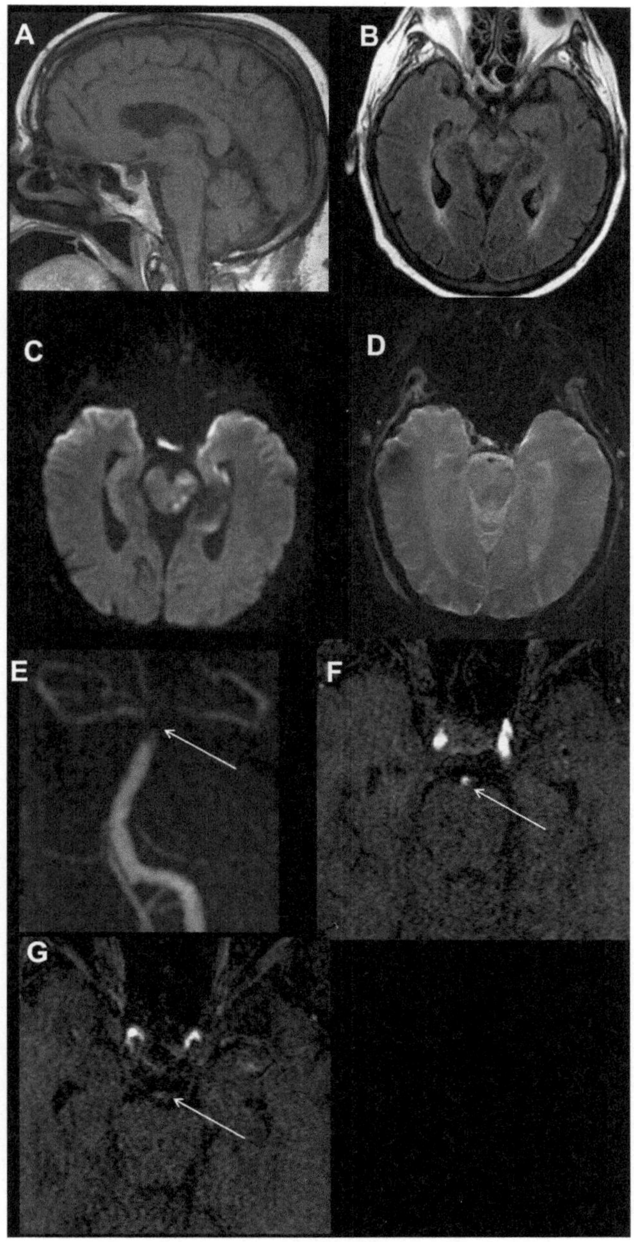

Figure 12. 72-year-old female with altered mental status and ischemic stroke. On the 4-sequence MRI protocol (A-D), the axial FLAIR image (B) demonstrates multifocal ill-defined areas of signal hyperintensity within the midbrain with corresponding restricted diffusion on the axial diffusion weighted trace image (C), consistent with infarctions. Additional foci of infarction were seen in the left occipital lobe, left mesial temporal lobe, both thalami and the cerebellum (images not shown). No definite abnormality is seen on the sagittal T1-weighted image (A) or axial T2* image (D). MR angiography was also requested. MRA maximum intensity projection image (E) reveals thrombus with the distal basilar (white arrow) and proximal posterior cerebral arteries, which is confirmed on the axial source MR angiography images (F, G) (white arrow). Even in retrospect, this finding was not apparent on any of the sequences included in the 4-sequence MRI protocol. MRA imaging adds significant value in cases with clinical suspicion for vascular occlusion or thrombosis.

Author Contributions

Conceived and designed the experiments: WAM RGG. Performed the experiments: WAM RGG BRB JWC WAC RG JAH GJH SH JMJ HRK ML MHL SRP OR SR JMR PWS VS. Analyzed the data: WAM RGG BRB JWC WAC RG JAH GJH SH JMJ HRK ML MHL SRP OR SR JMR PWS VS. Wrote the paper: WAM RGG BRB JWC WAC RG JAH GJH SH JMJ HRK ML MHL SRP OR SR JMR PWS VS.

References

1. Hashemi RH, Bradley WG Jr, Chen DY, Jordan JE, Queralt JA, et al. (1995) Suspected multiple sclerosis: MR imaging with a thin-section fast FLAIR pulse sequence. Radiology 196: 505–510.
2. Brant-Zawadzki M, Atkinson D, Detrick M, Bradley WG, Scidmore G (1996) Fluid-attenuated inversion recovery (FLAIR) for assessment of cerebral infarction. Initial clinical experience in 50 patients. Stroke 27: 1187–1191.
3. Ashikaga R, Araki Y, Ishida O (1997) MRI of head injury using FLAIR. Neuroradiology 39: 239–242.
4. Noguchi K, Ogawa T, Seto H, Inugami A, Hadeishi H, et al. (1997) Subacute and chronic subarachnoid hemorrhage: diagnosis with fluid-attenuated inversion-recovery MR imaging. Radiology 203: 257–262.
5. Thurnher MM, Thurnher SA, Fleischmann D, Steuer A, Rieger A, et al. (1997) Comparison of T2-weighted and fluid-attenuated inversion-recovery fast spin-echo MR sequences in intracerebral AIDS-associated disease. AJNR Am J - Neuroradiol 18: 1601–1609.
6. Demaerel P, Bosmans H, Caerts B, Herpels V, Vercruysse J, et al. (1998) Fast FLAIR MRI in childhood white-matter abnormalities. Neuroradiology 40: 355–358.
7. Maubon AJ, Pothin A, Ferru JM, Berger VM, Daures JP, et al. (1998) Unselected brain 0.5-T MR imaging: comparison of lesion detection and characterization with three T2-weighted sequences. Radiology 208: 671–678.
8. Aprile I, Iaiza F, Lavaroni A, Budai R, Dolso P, et al. (1999) Analysis of cystic intracranial lesions performed with fluid-attenuated inversion recovery MR imaging. AJNR Am J Neuroradiol 20: 1259–1267.
9. Bakshi R, Kamran S, Kinkel PR, Bates VE, Mechtler LL, et al. (1999) Fluid-attenuated inversion-recovery MR imaging in acute and subacute cerebral intraventricular hemorrhage. AJNR Am J Neuroradiol 20: 629–636.
10. Meiners LC, van Gils AD, De Kort G, Van Der Graaf Y, Jansen GH, et al. (1999) Fast fluid-attenuated inversion recovery (FLAIR) compared with T2-weighted spin-echo in the magnetic resonance diagnosis of mesial temporal sclerosis. Invest Radiol 34: 134–142.
11. Palmer S, Bradley WG, Chen DY, Patel S (1999) Subcallosal striations: early findings of multiple sclerosis on sagittal, thin-section, fast FLAIR MR images. Radiology 210: 149–153.
12. Taillibert S, Oppenheim C, Baulac M, Dormont D, Marsault C, et al. (1999) Yield of fluid-attenuated inversion recovery in drug-resistant focal epilepsy with noninformative conventional magnetic resonance imaging. Eur Neurol 41: 64–72.
13. Casey SO, Sampaio RC, Michel E, Truwit CL (2000) Posterior reversible encephalopathy syndrome: utility of fluid-attenuated inversion recovery MR imaging in the detection of cortical and subcortical lesions. AJNR Am J Neuroradiol 21: 1199–1206.
14. Essig M, Wenz F, Schoenberg SO, Debus J, Knopp MV, et al. (2000) Arteriovenous malformations: assessment of gliotic and ischemic changes with fluid-attenuated inversion-recovery MRI. Invest Radiol 35: 689–694.
15. Herskovits EH, Itoh R, Melhem ER (2001) Accuracy for detection of simulated lesions: comparison of fluid-attenuated inversion-recovery, proton density–weighted, and T2-weighted synthetic brain MR imaging. AJR Am J Roentgenol 176: 1313–1318.
16. Maeda M, Yamamoto T, Daimon S, Sakuma H, Takeda K (2001) Arterial hyperintensity on fast fluid-attenuated inversion recovery images: a subtle finding for hyperacute stroke undetected by diffusion-weighted MR imaging. AJNR Am J Neuroradiol 22: 632–636.
17. Saleh A, Wenserski F, Cohnen M, Furst G, Godehardt E, et al. (2004) Exclusion of brain lesions: is MR contrast medium required after a negative fluid-attenuated inversion recovery sequence? Br J Radiol 77: 183–188.
18. Koennecke HC (2006) Cerebral microbleeds on MRI: prevalence, associations, and potential clinical implications. Neurology 66: 165–171.
19. Lin DD, Filippi CG, Steever AB, Zimmerman RD (2001) Detection of intracranial hemorrhage: comparison between gradient-echo images and b(0) images obtained from diffusion-weighted echo-planar sequences. AJNR Am J Neuroradiol 22: 1275–1281.
20. Lam WW, So NM, Wong KS, Rainer T (2003) B0 images obtained from diffusion-weighted echo planar sequences for the detection of intracerebral bleeds. J Neuroimaging 13: 99–105.
21. Atlas SW, Mark AS, Grossman RI, Gomori JM (1988) Intracranial hemorrhage: gradient-echo MR imaging at 1.5 T. Comparison with spin-echo imaging and clinical applications. Radiology 168: 803–807.
22. Chan S, Kartha K, Yoon SS, Desmond DW, Hilal SK (1996) Multifocal hypointense cerebral lesions on gradient-echo MR are associated with chronic hypertension. AJNR Am J Neuroradiol 17: 1821–1827.
23. Tsushima Y, Aoki J, Endo K (2003) Brain microhemorrhages detected on T2*-weighted gradient-echo MR images. AJNR Am J Neuroradiol 24: 88–96.

Quantitative Spatial and Temporal Analysis of Fluorescein Angiography Dynamics in the Eye

Flora Hui[1], Christine T. O. Nguyen[1], Phillip A. Bedggood[1], Zheng He[1], Rebecca L. Fish[2], Rachel Gurrell[2], Algis J. Vingrys[1], Bang V. Bui[1]*

1 Department of Optometry and Vision Sciences, The University of Melbourne, Parkville, Victoria, Australia, 2 Neusentis, Pfizer Research and Development, Grant Park Science Park, Cambridge, United Kingdom

Abstract

Purpose: We describe a novel approach to analyze fluorescein angiography to investigate fluorescein flow dynamics in the rat posterior retina as well as identify abnormal areas following laser photocoagulation.

Methods: Experiments were undertaken in adult Long Evans rats. Using a rodent retinal camera, videos were acquired at 30 frames per second for 30 seconds following intravenous introduction of sodium fluorescein in a group of control animals (n = 14). Videos were image registered and analyzed using principle components analysis across all pixels in the field. This returns fluorescence intensity profiles from which, the half-rise (time to 50% brightness), half-fall (time for 50% decay) back to an offset (plateau level of fluorescence). We applied this analysis to video fluorescein angiography data collected 30 minutes following laser photocoagulation in a separate group of rats (n = 7).

Results: Pixel-by-pixel analysis of video angiography clearly delineates differences in the temporal profiles of arteries, veins and capillaries in the posterior retina. We find no difference in half-rise, half-fall or offset amongst the four quadrants (inferior, nasal, superior, temporal). We also found little difference with eccentricity. By expressing the parameters at each pixel as a function of the number of standard deviation from the average of the entire field, we could clearly identify the spatial extent of the laser injury.

Conclusions: This simple registration and analysis provides a way to monitor the size of vascular injury, to highlight areas of subtle vascular leakage and to quantify vascular dynamics not possible using current fluorescein angiography approaches. This can be applied in both laboratory and clinical settings for *in vivo* dynamic fluorescent imaging of vasculature.

Editor: Alfred S. Lewin, University of Florida, United States of America

Funding: RLF and RG are employees of Pfizer Neusentis and Pfizer Global Research and Development. CTN, PAB, AJV and BVB are employees of University of Melbourne, supported by Australia Research Council Linkage Project Grant (LP100200129). FH received an Australian postgraduate award. BVB received an Australia Research Council Future Fellowship (FT130100388). The funders had no role in study design, data collection and analysis, decision to publish, or preparation of the manuscript.

Competing Interests: RLF and RG are employees of the commercial funder of this research (Pfizer Neusentis and Pfizer Global Research and Development).

* Email: bvb@unimelb.edu.au

Introduction

The retina is the only place in the body that allows non-invasive, direct *in vivo* visualization of neuronal tissue and vasculature. Retinal imaging is an important laboratory and clinical tool for the study of ophthalmic disease [1] and increasingly retinal blood vessel changes are shown to help stratify the severity of systemic disease [2]. Retinal imaging can be undertaken with or without the aid of a contrast agent. The addition of a contrast agent such as sodium fluorescein provides additional information regarding the integrity of the retinal vasculature. Since the early 1900s intravenous injection of sodium fluorescein has been shown to temporarily highlight retinal vessels [3,4], thus improving *in vivo* assessment of the retinal circulation and blood-retinal-barrier integrity [5–7]. It has since been adopted as a clinical tool for a host of conditions including glaucoma, diabetes, vascular occlusion, neovascularization and inflammatory disease [4,8–10]. In particular, the recent development of ultra wide-field fluorescein angiography has allowed for easier detection of peripheral blood-retinal-barrier disruption [8,11,12]. Pre-clinically, fluorescein angiography has also been utilized in studies of vascular disease, angiogenesis and blood-neural-barrier compromise [13–16].

The standard approach to fluorescein angiography is to take a series of photographs at various times (several seconds to minutes) following fluorescein delivery to demonstrate choroidal, arterial and venous filling and clearance. These images are used to identify areas of vascular non-perfusion or retained fluorescence, which may highlight vascular compromise as indicated by fluorescein leakage. The intermittent recording and lack of accurate timing

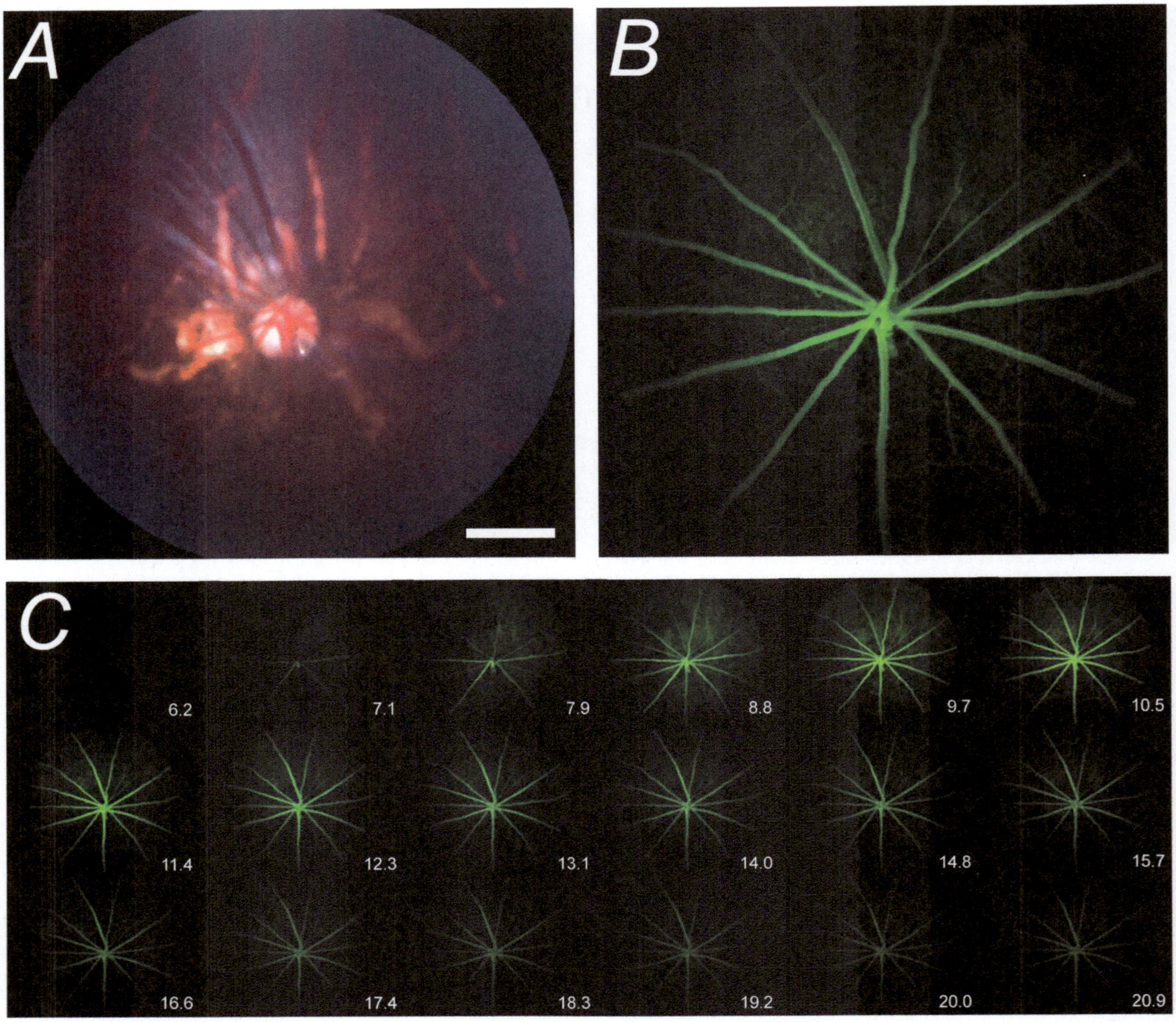

Figure 1. Video fluorescein angiography in rat retina. A–B. Representative bright-field image and its corresponding fluorescein image 10 seconds post fluorescein administration. **C.** Montage demonstrating the fluorescein transit through the retinal blood vessels for times between 6.2 and 20.9 seconds after the start of fluorescein infusion. Montage shows every 20th frame taken from **Video S1**. White bar in Panel A represents 500 μm.

however, limits the analysis of fluorescein images to a qualitative assessment, almost a binary outcome. Thus the sensitivity to detect subtle changes, including differentiating vascular leakage from angiogenesis, is hampered. Video angiography provides the potential for quantitative analysis of more subtle differences in filling and leakage that may occur with vascular changes in disease [17–19]. To date, most studies that analyze video angiography have only examined the time it takes for fluorescein to appear in particular regions of interest [20–22]. Whilst this is useful, it does not provide insight to the degree and extent to which the vasculature in any given location may be altered. A method was developed by Hipwell et al [23], to analyze the entire image in human fluorescein angiograms. Although the analysis was limited to identifying the time to reach maximal fluorescence, it demonstrated the potential that analysis of the whole image has in assessing retinal vascular disease.

Here we describe a novel means to quantitatively measure fluorescein angiography profiles. Combining systematic fluorescein delivery, video angiography and a precise analysis, the spatial and temporal characteristics of rodent fluorescein angiography dynamics can be quantified. To test the robustness of the analysis method, we used the approach to identify areas of altered fluorescein angiography dynamics following acute focal laser photocoagulation injury on a separate cohort of rodents.

Materials and Methods

All experimental methods and animal care procedures conformed to the Association of Research in Vision and Ophthalmology, the National Health and Medical Research Council of Australia's guidelines for animal care and experimentation [24] and was approved by the University of Melbourne Animal Ethics Committee (1111991.1).

General animal preparation

Experiments were performed on adult, *Long-Evans* rats (n = 14, 336±11 g) housed in a temperature and light controlled (20°C, < 50 lux, 12 hour light/dark cycle on at 8 am) animal facility. Normal rat chow (AIN93G) and water were available *ad libitum.*

General anesthesia was induced with an intramuscular injection of ketamine and xylazine (60 mg/kg and 5 mg/kg respectively, Troy Laboratories Pty Ltd, Smithfield, NSW, Australia) prior to surgery and imaging. Corneal anesthesia and mydriasis were achieved with topical proxymetacaine (0.5% Alcaine, Alcon Laboratories, Frenchs Forest, NSW, Australia) and tropicamide (0.5% Mydriacyl, Alcon Laboratories) respectively. A custom-made water heating pad and immersion heater ensured body temperature was maintained at 37°C (Tempette Junior TE-8J, Techne, New Jersey, USA).

Fluorescein angiography and blood pressure monitoring

For intravenous delivery of sodium fluorescein, a femoral vein cannulation was performed using polyethylene tubing (inner diameter 0.28 mm, outer diameter 0.61 mm, Microtube Extrusions, NSW, Australia). Blood pressure was continuously monitored with a Powerlab system (ML110G, ADInstruments, NSW, Australia) and LabChart software (ADInstruments, Australia) via a femoral artery cannula. A bolus of sodium fluorescein (1%, 100 µl/kg) was intravenously delivered at 1.05 ml/min for 4 seconds with a syringe pump (Harvard Standard Pump 22, Serial #28974, Harvard Apparatus, MA, USA). Images of the posterior pole were taken from the start of fluorescein infusion with the Micron III rodent fundus camera (Phoenix Research Labs, CA, USA) with a 435–469 nm excitation filter and 520–530 nm barrier filter at 30 frames/sec using Streampix software (NorPix Inc., Quebec, Canada) for 30 seconds. Data were converted into tiff image stacks for offline analysis (Figure 1).

Laser-induced blood-retinal-barrier disruption

Retinal tissue injury was induced by Nd: YAG focal laser photocoagulation (532 nm, 1.34 mW.s, 0.5 s, 100 µm diameter) in four sectors of the retina to produce disruption of the blood-retinal-barrier. This laser power was insufficient to disrupt Bruch's membrane, the layer separating the retinal pigment epithelium from the choroid, as no bubbling of the tissue or hemorrhaging was evident. This was confirmed using optical coherence tomography (Micron III, Phoenix Research Labs). Imaging was undertaken 30 minutes post-injury with fluorescein angiography. Post-laser imaging was extended to 60 seconds to capture the fluorescein leakage to greater extent. It is worth noting that whilst the use of laser photocoagulation to induce extravascular leakage mainly affects areas between the large blood vessels, the analysis method can also be applied to changes in fluorescein dynamics occurring within the arteries and veins.

Fluorescence profile analysis methods

Image registration. All images were registered using custom written MATLAB scripts (R2013a, The MathWorks Inc., Massachusetts, USA; see Files S1–S8) via cross-correlation to a reference image, chosen to be when all vessels were filled with fluorescein (~15 seconds from the start of fluorescein infusion). A simple x/y translation correction was sufficient to eliminate most image movement associated with animal breathing and small eye movements. Rigid and affine registration approaches provided little additional advantage. Minor contributions from rotation, scale and shear remained at times, however we found that attempting to correct these often produce more variability and significantly extended computation time. Instead, it was more practical to ameliorate small residual motion artifacts by PCA motion artifacts were ameliorated by PCA filtering as described below.

Principal component analysis (PCA) filtering. Custom software written in MATLAB (see Files S1–S8) was used to quantitatively assess intensity profiles for each pixel. Pilot studies showed that a 30 second acquisition epoch fully captured the fluorescence transit in normal eyes, with the profile showing asymptotic behavior by 25 seconds (see Figure 2). Following image registration, PCA was used to smooth the data and remove artifacts associated with any remnant movement that was not corrected by translational image registration. In brief, PCA is a mathematical procedure of pattern recognition. It takes a data set made up of observations (in this case, image pixels) that can be described by several dependent variables (in this case, image frames) and represents the data by a new set of orthogonal variables called principal components [25,26]. The first component accounts for the maximal amount of variance in the data, which for our usage is equivalent to finding the shape of the intensity profile that best fits the greatest number of pixels analyzed. If this component is removed, the second principal component explains the maximal remaining variance, and so forth. PCA extracts the most important information from the data and thus simplifies the data set. Two principal components were found to be sufficient to explain at least 95% of the variance in each of our image sequences in the control cohort, rendering the smoothed curves shown in Figure 2.

Extracted intensity profile parameters. Following PCA, the intensity profile at each pixel was determined. Parameters could then be extracted to describe the fluorescence dynamics including the half-rise, the time to reach 50% fluorescence; offset amplitude, the remnant fluorescence taken as an average of the

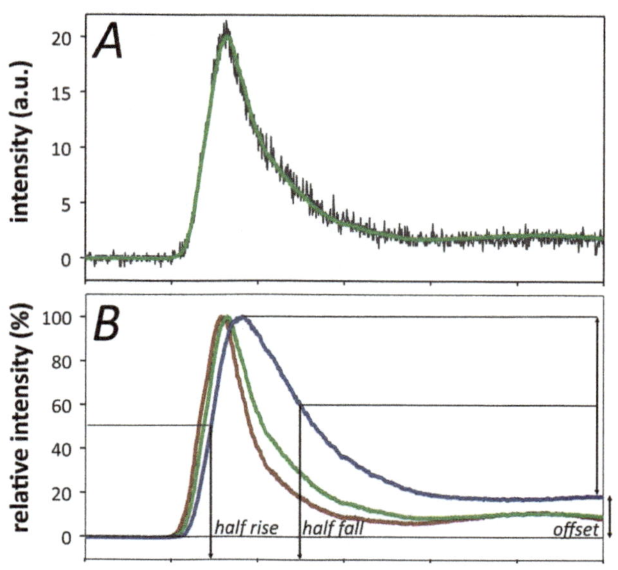

Figure 2. Video fluorescein dynamics in rat retinal vessels. A. Representative intensity profile for an individual pixel before (grey trace) and after PCA (green trace). **B.** Representative normalized fluorescein intensity profile as a function of time in an artery (red), vein (blue) and capillary/choroid (green). Parameters used to analyze fluorescence profiles include the half-rise, half-fall and offset amplitude.

last second of recording, expressed relative to the peak intensity; and the half-fall, the time to 50% decay between the peak and offset amplitude (see Figures 2, 3 and 4). Whilst PCA is excellent for imaged fields showing normal variance, it is less suited to fields with high variance such as those with focal laser injury. Thus for laser-injury data, a three-point moving median filter was applied to the data instead. Estimates of half-rise, half-fall and offset for the laser-injury data were then derived from the intensity profiles at each pixel.

Blood vessel tracing. To analyze the blood vessel types separately, manual tracing was used to segment the major retinal arteries and veins from the rest of the fundus, which was taken to be the capillaries and choroid (see Figure 4B). Optic nerve fluorescence was masked from analysis. Whilst not employed in this study a robust automatic blood vessel segmentation algorithm would speed up analysis. However, automatic vessel segmentation should not impact the results of individual pixel data shown in this study. The retina was divided into four quadrants, corresponding to the superior, nasal, temporal and inferior retina. First, differences in fluorescein angiography dynamics between blood vessel types were considered. Second, to consider changes in dynamics that may occur with distance from the optic nerve head, the images were further divided into 2 zones by drawing two annuli: the first, inner zone with a 640 μm radius; the second, outer zone with a 1280 μm radius, centered on the optic nerve head (see Figure 5 inset).

Identification of abnormal pixels. To identify abnormal pixels that fill or decay slower, one can compare against a baseline image sequence or a control cohort. Alternatively, quantification can be undertaken within the same image sequence, which has the advantage that no baseline sequence is needed and variability associated with measurements between sessions or between animals can be minimized. To achieve this, the half-fall and offset amplitude were used for comparisons. The half-fall and offset amplitude were chosen as we hypothesized that these parameters would be more affected by laser injury which can induce blood-retinal-barrier disruption and vascular leakage of fluorescein. It is worth noting that despite extending post-laser sequences out to 60 seconds, half-fall could not be identified in some pixels (see Figure 6D). In those cases, the half-fall time was recorded as 60 seconds. Similar to a Grubbs' test for outliers, Equation 1 was used to identify for each pixel the number of standard deviations away from the mean; where x = half-fall or offset amplitude for a single pixel, μ = average half-fall/offset for that eye, σ = standard deviation for that eye. The number of standard deviations from the mean represents probabilities that a highlighted pixel randomly falls outside the normal range, which can be between 1 and 4 SD (see Figure 7).

$$\textit{Number of SD from mean} = (x - \mu) / \sigma \qquad (1)$$

Statistical analysis

All data are shown as group mean ±SEM. Parameters were compared using two-way ANOVA to assess for differences in the quadrants and eccentricity comparisons with Tukey's multiple comparisons test for post-hoc analysis. Statistical significance is indicated when $p < 0.05$.

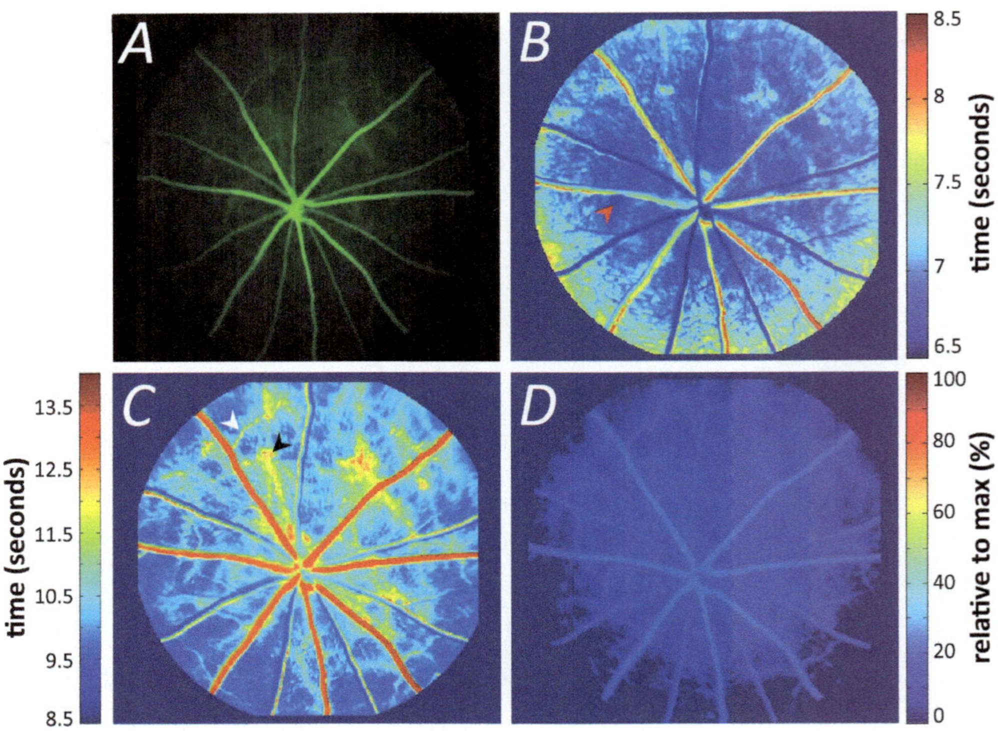

Figure 3. Pixel-by-pixel analysis of retinal video fluorescein angiography. (**A**). The half-rise (**B**) and half-fall (**C**) parameters of the same retina. Warmer colors indicate increasing delay in the parameter. Arrowheads indicate areas of early choroidal filling (red), delayed fluorescein clearance due to secondary venules (white) and delayed choroidal clearance (black). The offset amplitude (**D**) expressed relative to maximum fluorescence (%).

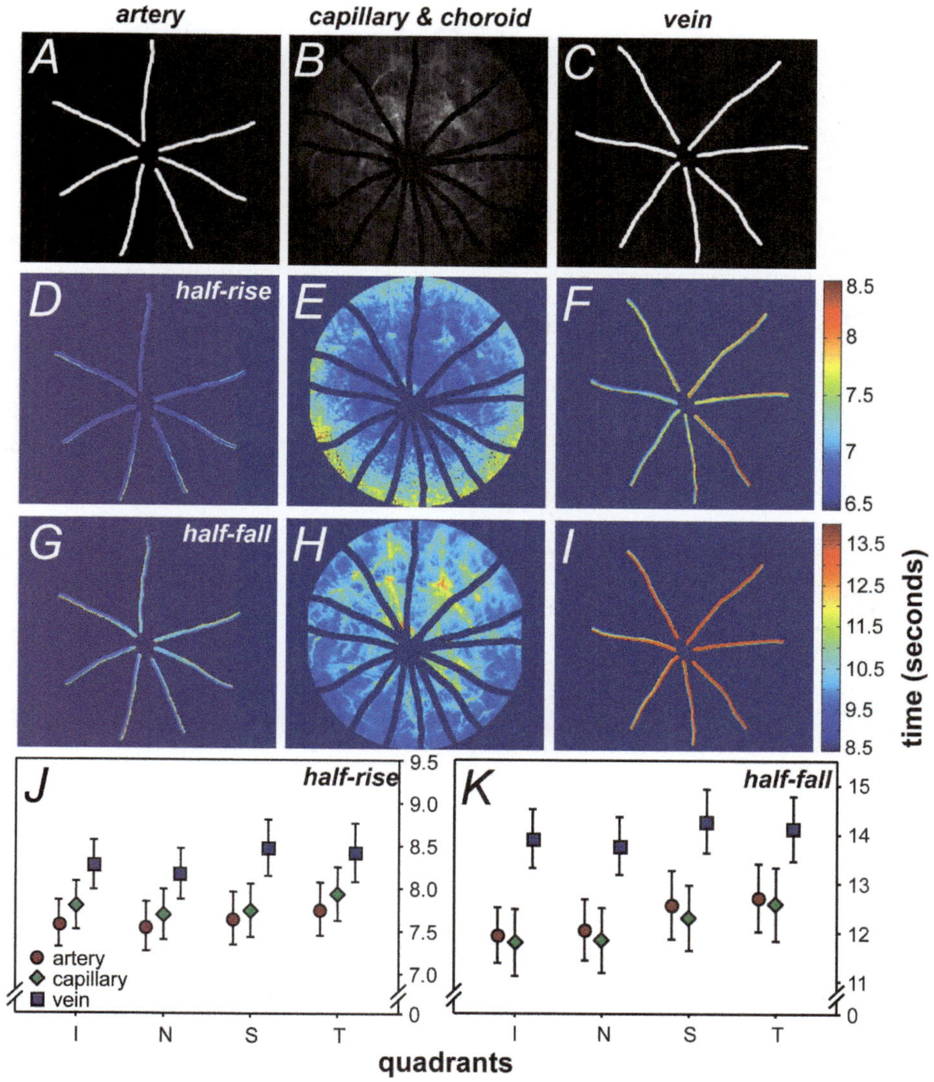

Figure 4. Segmentation of pixel-by-pixel analysis by blood vessel type. A–C. Development of the mask via manual vessel tracing: artery, capillary/choroid and vein respectively. **D–F.** Representative images of the half-rise of each pixel. **G–I.** Representative images of the half-fall of each pixel. **J–K.** Group average of the half-rise and fall respectively, across the four quadrants of the retina shows fluorescein filling in the order of arteries, capillaries and veins followed by their decay. Significant differences in rise ($p = 0.01$) and fall ($p < 0.001$) were found between vessel types (two-way ANOVA). Data shown is mean ±SEM, $n = 14$.

Results

Dynamic fluorescein angiography

Compared to *en face* fundus images taken under broad-spectrum light (Figure 1A), the presence of fluorescein acts as a contrast medium that improves the resolution of both major and minor retinal vessels (Figure 1B). Dynamic angiography provides clear delineation of the arterial and venous phases of fluorescein filling as well as their relative decay kinetics (please see Video S1). Figure 1C shows a montage of every 20th frame over the course of the same fluorescein angiogram sequence.

Pixel-by-pixel analysis reveals spatial profiles in the dynamics of fluorescein onset and offset

Figure 2A shows the difference in the intensity profiles for a representative pixel chosen in an area outside of the major retinal vessels, before and after PCA. The raw data (grey trace) contains inherent variability, which can be due to remnant image movement and background noise. By utilizing PCA, this noise can be reduced (green trace) without alteration of the underlying fluorescein angiography dynamics. Figure 2B shows a representative intensity profile taken from 3 individual pixels from an artery, vein and a capillary/choroidal area away from a major vessel. As the choroidal vasculature directly underlies the retinal vasculature, the capillary fluorescence profile also contains contributions from the choroid. This can be particularly evident in areas where there are breaks in the pigmentation of the retina.

Following fluorescein administration, the dye appears in the separate blood vessel types at a similar time (Figure 2B). Fluorescence then quickly reaches its peak intensity before decaying more slowly. After 25 seconds, fluorescence is relatively stable with the veins retaining greater fluorescence than the arteries and capillaries/choroid.

To explore fluorescein angiography dynamics of the posterior retina, the pixel-by-pixel analysis method was developed, allowing

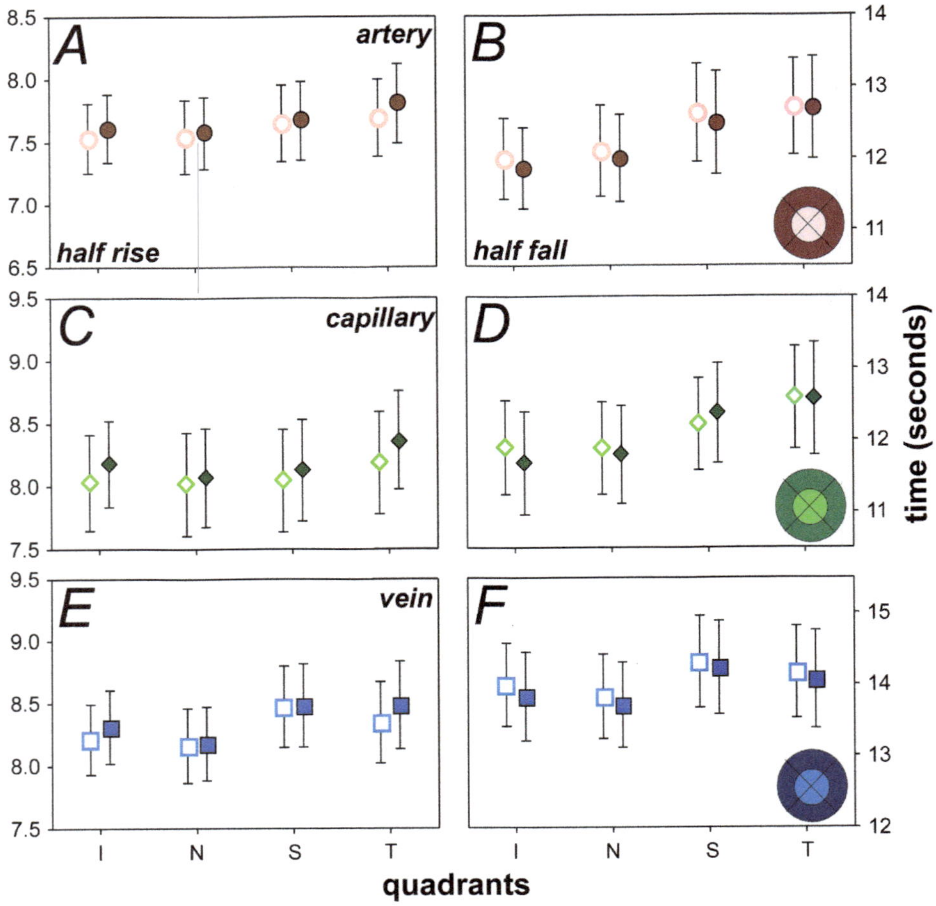

Figure 5. Half-rise and half-fall characteristics across two eccentricity zones. Group averaged comparison of changes to half-rise and half-fall time in arteries (**A–B**), capillaries (**C–D**) and veins (**E–F**). Inset shows how the retina was divided into 4 sectors with two eccentricity zones forming the inner (light shade) and outer zones (dark shade). Unfilled markers represent the inner zone and filled markers show the outer zone. Data shown is mean ±SEM, n = 14.

both spatial and temporal changes in retina blood vessels to be simultaneously analyzed (Figure 3). Figure 3B shows that the half-rise of the arteries occurs first but can be difficult to differentiate as their half rise times are only slightly faster (~0.1 ms to 0.3 ms) than the surrounding areas of capillaries and choroid. This indicates that arteries and capillaries have similar half-rise times and that veins are slower by about 1 second in the rat, compared with arteries (warmer colors in Figure 3B). The differences between the various vessel types become more apparent with the half-fall as shown in Figure 3C. In particular the arteries show a rapid decay but the veins show a substantially slower decay to half brightness. It is also apparent that particular areas between the major vessels fill and decay more slowly (arrow heads in Figure 3C). We believe that this may arise due to the presence of secondary venules (white arrow head) and delayed choroidal filling (black arrow head) due to the watershed zones in the choroidal vascular bed as described by Hayreh [27]. After 30 seconds, fluorescence reaches asymptotic levels with the veins retaining greater fluorescence than the rest of the retina (Figure 3D).

To quantify differences between blood vessel types, large arteries and veins were segmented by manual tracing (Figure 4A–C) and analyzed separately from the rest of the fundus image. Figure 4D–F and 4G–I show the half-rise and half-fall, respectively in a representative animal. Figure 4J–K shows the comparison in half-rise and half-fall between blood vessel types in the four retinal quadrants. Significant differences were found between blood vessel types for half-rise ($F_{2,156} = 5.79$, $p<0.01$) and half-fall ($F_{2,156} = 10.10$, $p<0.001$) but not between quadrants. On average, veins showed a slower half-rise (8.3±0.1 s, 95% confidence limits: 6.1–10.6 s) compared to arteries (7.6±0.1 s, 5.5–9.8 s) and capillaries (7.8±0.1 s, 5.6–10.0 s). This is consistent with data reported in previous studies [28–30]. A greater difference in half-fall was apparent (Figure 4K), as veins were much slower to decay (13.9±0.3 s, 9.5–18.5 s) compared with arteries (11.9±0.3 s, 7.6–17.0 s) and capillaries (11.8±0.3 s, 7.2–17.1 s).

To consider changes to fluorescence dynamics with eccentricity, pixels were averaged in two eccentricity zones forming an inner (640 µm radius) and outer zone (1280 µm radius) as shown in the inset of Figure 5. No significant differences were found with eccentricity for the half-rise (Figure 5A,C,E) and half-fall (Figure 5B,D,F) for all vessel types. Smaller pixel bins were also used in a separate analysis; i.e. instead of 640 µm radius zones, 200 µm zones were used, but no significant change with eccentricity was apparent (data not shown). Differences in fluorescein dynamics may become apparent if we were able to image further into the periphery with the camera. By centering on the optic nerve we are limited to a ~3 mm diameter area of the posterior pole.

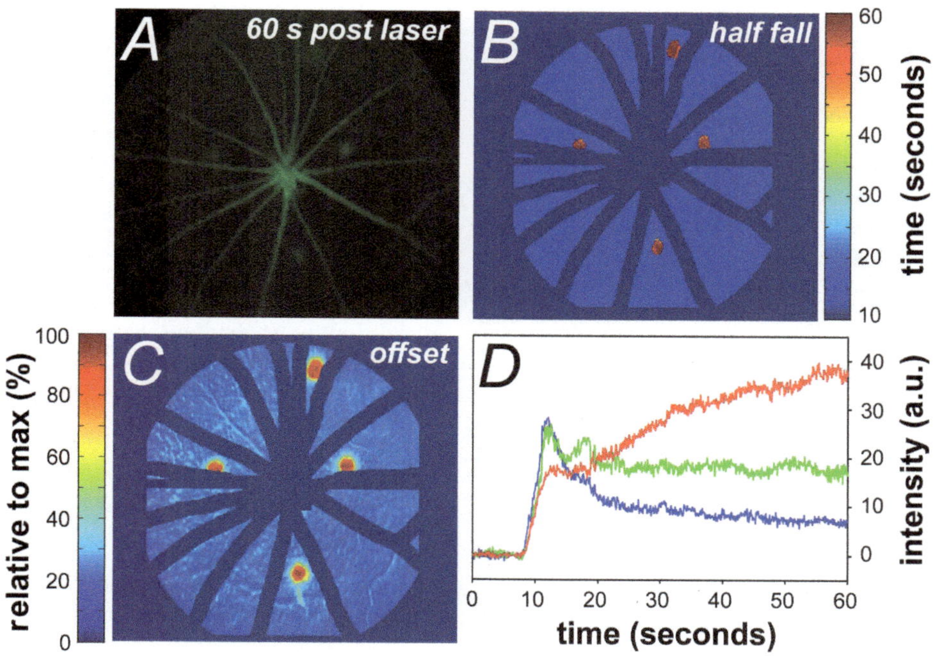

Figure 6. Video Fluorescein dynamics following laser injury. A. Fluorescein angiogram leakage 60 seconds post dye delivery. **B**. Pixel-by-pixel analysis highlights areas of prolonged half-fall in laser-injured retina. **C**. Analysis of offset amplitude highlights the extent of elevated offset post-laser injury. **D**. Representative intensity profiles of two pixels within a laser-burned region highlighting the diversity in fluorescence dynamics. The red trace demonstrates continuous increase in fluorescence; green trace shows minimal fluorescence decay plotted against a representative intensity profile in the control cohort (blue trace). Data expressed in raw intensity with arbitrary units, colours of trace correlate to the relative offset of the pixel.

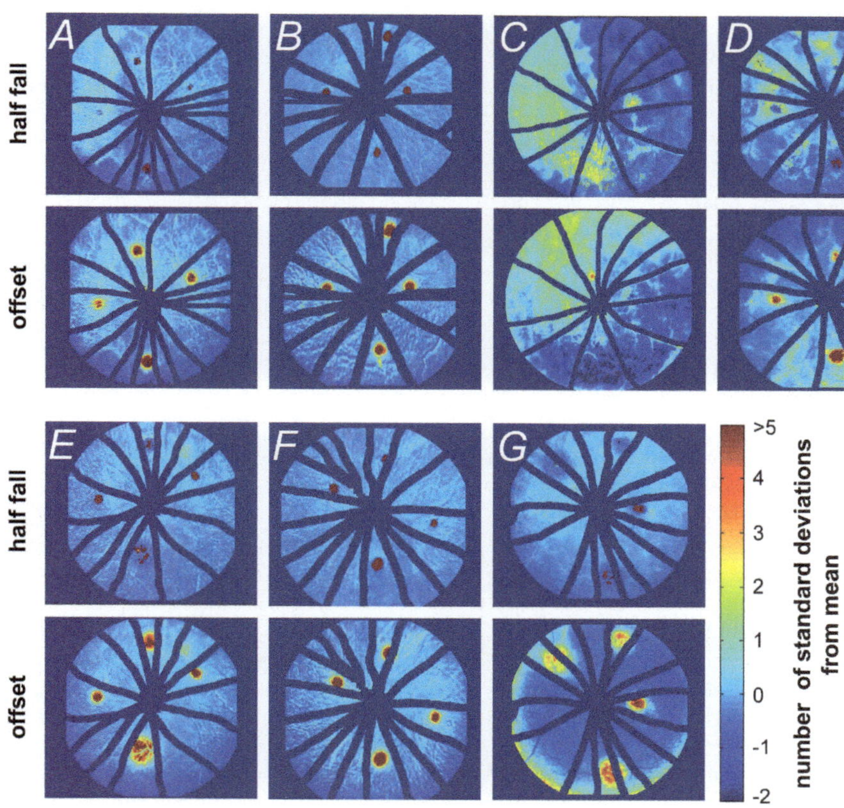

Figure 7. Half-fall and offset characteristics following laser injury in rat retina. Retinal probability maps identifying the areas of abnormal half-fall (1st and 3rd rows) and offset amplitude (2nd and 4th rows) in relation to the number of standard deviations from the mean of the whole image, n = 7 eyes. Panels A to G represent each of the 7 laser-injured retinas.

Fluorescein retention and changes to angiography dynamics identified by pixel-by-pixel analysis

For validation, the analysis method was implemented in a cohort of animals that had undergone laser photocoagulation to cause disruption to the blood retinal barrier. Thirty minutes after the retina had been laser injured; fluorescein angiography was performed in 7 eyes. Although prolonged fluorescence can be detected from the fluorescein angiogram at a particular time point (Figure 6A), the size and severity of the abnormal fluorescence cannot easily be quantified. The pixel-by-pixel half-fall (Figure 6B) and offset (Figure 6C) analysis clearly highlights the size and extent of the four laser lesions compared to their surrounding capillary/background areas (the large retinal vessels and immediate surroundings have been masked). In these particular areas some pixels do not fall in fluorescence (red trace in Figure 6D), whereas others show an elevated offset (green trace in Figure 6D) when compared with the dynamics of a pixel from the surrounding retina (blue trace in Figure 6D).

This analysis method is able to highlight the diversity of fluorescein angiography dynamics in various areas of the retina. Figure 7 shows individual probability maps for half-fall (1st and 3rd rows) and offset (2nd and 4th rows) for each of the 7 eyes that had undergone laser injury. The half-fall maps help to differentiate those areas where fluorescence continues to increase or show minimal decay compared with the rest of the retina. On the other hand, the offset indicates all areas of the retina where there is excess fluorescence. These types of maps can be used to return global indices of abnormal fluorescence, to facilitate monitoring across longitudinal trials.

Discussion

Fluorescein angiography is a useful tool for *in vivo* assessment of the blood-retinal-barrier both in clinic and laboratory experiments. Building on previous studies that have utilized dynamic analysis on contrast enhanced imaging [17,23,29,31]; our pixel-by-pixel dynamic analysis method returns a suite of parameters that allows quantification of fluorescein dynamics across the entire image. This analysis method reliably delineates arteries and veins from the surrounding retina, determines the rate of fluorescence decay and locates areas of abnormality.

Laboratory studies largely deliver fluorescein via subcutaneous or intraperitoneal injection to identify blood-retinal-barrier compromise [13,15,32,33]. Whilst this is an easy method of dye administration, it provides limited temporal information. Although intravenous fluorescein delivery is widely used clinically, as well as in some laboratories, its analysis is largely confined to a qualitative appraisal of areas of abnormal fluorescence (similar to our 'offset' parameter but without spatial quantification of the lesion). Regardless, a major problem with all methods of fluorescein delivery is that the extent of fluorescence is not static. Indeed, in areas of injury the fluorescence profile may not fit the canonical form (see Figure 6D). A good example of this problem is in the interpretation of the 'offset' in the laser injury, where pixels showing increased fluorescence could reflect injury at that site or could reflect the spreading of fluorescein from adjacent areas. Thus the size of the lesion is critically dependent on the timing of image acquisition. Without accurate timing, temporal changes in fluorescein can hamper quantification. Our analysis provides the half-fall to complement the offset, as it differentiates between those pixels that demonstrate a continuous increase in brightness, compared with those that show slow or minimal decay (compare upper and lower panels in Figure 7G). This may prove to be a more robust index for quantification of the spatial extent of injury in longitudinal studies or therapeutic interventions.

We have used the laser model here to demonstrate the utility of our analysis in terms of the derived half-fall and offset parameters. It is worth mentioning that our approach is also sensitive to small differences in the half-rise, particularly that between arteries, veins and capillaries. Previous studies have employed the arterio-venous transit time (or mean circulation time) as an index of blood flow velocity [28]. Our pixel-by-pixel approach can return information about local delays in circulation dynamics.

Previous studies have either manually segmented or employed an automated method to count microaneurysms in diabetic fluorescein angiograms as a means to monitor disease progression [34,35]. Again care must be taken with such static quantitative approaches, given the temporal changes in the signal to noise ratio of fluorescein associated with the quenching of fluorescence, binding to albumin, dye dilution and leakage [36]. Our approach attempts to deal with these potential limitations by statistically segmenting pixels that show abnormal temporal characteristics. In this way it avoids confounds associated with differences in absolute fluorescein brightness and issues associated with the dimming of the image periphery as found with any optical imaging system.

The sensitivity of the approach to detect subtle changes relies on several experimental procedures that help to minimize sources of error. It is important that the delivery of fluorescein is standardized. In this study, a syringe pump was used to standardize the rate and volume of fluorescein delivery into the femoral vein. The size and length of cannula tubing was matched between animals to ensure that there was no difference in resistance. Furthermore, all lines were primed to have fluorescein 3 cm from the tip of the intravenous cannula prior to fluorescein infusion. Although at the time of experimentation the starting of the syringe pump and video recording could not be automated, the same operator was responsible for all recordings and thus inter-experimenter variability was kept to a minimum. In future, variability would decrease further with simultaneous triggering of the pump and image recording.

Blood pressure should be monitored during angiography as changes in this parameter can contribute to changes in circulation dynamics. Blood pressure was continuously monitored throughout this study via a femoral artery cannulation and returned stable recordings (mean blood pressure: 116.1 ± 7.5 mmHg), which is similar to that previously reported for anaesthetized rats [37–39].

Image stability is also important to facilitate accurate pixel analysis. Whilst image registration and PCA helps to remove most eye movements and movement associated with breathing, the best approach is to ensure adequate depth of anesthesia. All animals in this study were measured at a similar time following the onset of anesthesia, approximately 1 hour after injection, due to surgery prior to imaging. Our preliminary experiments show that the current image registration and analysis approach works with 10–15 minutes of anesthesia induction (data not shown). Additionally, animals were lightly secured to the imaging platform via a neck strap, which helps to dampen breathing related movements. In this regard further improvement could be gained by using ear bars.

Despite these limitations, pilot data undertaken in 3 animals suggest that parameters returned from our analysis approach are reproducible. When fluorescein angiography is repeated 30 minutes apart, we find that half-rise (Arteries 0.02 ± 0.03 s; veins 0.3 ± 0.2 s, capillaries/choroid 0.2 ± 0.2 s) and half-fall (Arteries 1.1 ± 0.6 s; veins 0.7 ± 0.4 s, capillaries/choroid 0.9 ± 0.5 s), in the inferior quadrant inner eccentricity zone show very little difference.

Our study was acute in nature; however, the procedure can be adapted to longitudinal investigations. In particular, our temporary surgical cannulation of femoral vein can be replaced by chronic procedures (indwelling femoral cannulas for fluorescein injection and blood pressure monitoring) or less invasive approaches. For example, a tail vein injection allows for repeated fluorescein delivery along with non-invasive tail cuff sphygmomanometry.

Conclusions

Pixel-by-pixel analysis of video fluorescein angiography has clear advantages over conventional, static angiography in allowing the quantification of fluorescence dynamics across the entire image and automated, objective identification of areas exhibiting abnormal fluorescein flow. This approach can be used for longitudinal studies to allow quantification of disease progression and treatment efficacy in vascular diseases such as diabetes, choroidal neovascularization and retinopathy of prematurity. The simplicity of the analysis means that it can be easily applied to video angiography acquired in clinical or laboratory settings using any number of contrast-enhancing dyes such as lucifer yellow and indocyanine green. Future studies may elucidate its value in human fluorescein angiography.

Supporting Information

Video S1 Video fluorescein angiography of the rat posterior retina. Images were acquired at 30 Hz over 30 seconds.

File S1 Matlab code to register a tiff stack.

File S2 Matlab code to perform principle component analysis on a tiff stack.

File S3 Matlab code to read in the trace masking the major blood vessels.

File S4 Matlab code to fit the intensity profiles.

File S5 Matlab code bin.m bins an image.

File S6 Matlab code circle.m adds a circle to a plotted figure.

File S7 Matlab code find_com.m finds teh centre of mass of a matrix.

File S8 Matlab code fitThisPixel.m finds the intensity profile parameters.

Author Contributions

Conceived and designed the experiments: FH CTON RLF RG AJV BVB. Performed the experiments: FH CTON ZH BVB. Analyzed the data: FH CTON PB BVB. Contributed reagents/materials/analysis tools: FH PB. Wrote the paper: FH CTON PB ZH RLF RG AJV BVB.

References

1. Patton N, Aslam TM, MacGillivray T, Deary IJ, Dhillon B, et al. (2006) Retinal image analysis: concepts, applications and potential. Progress in retinal and eye research 25: 99–127.
2. Wong TY, Klein R, Couper DJ, Cooper LS, Shahar E, et al. (2001) Retinal microvascular abnormalities and incident stroke: the Atherosclerosis Risk in Communities Study. Lancet 358: 1134–1140.
3. Abelsdorff G, Wessely K (1909) Vergleichend physiologische Untersuchungen über den Flüssigkeitswechsel des Auges in der Wirbeltierreihe: I. Vögel. Arch Augenheilk 64: 65–125.
4. Richard G (1990) Fluorescein angiography: Textbook and atlas. New York: Thieme Medical Publishers Inc.
5. Comander J, Loewenstein J, Sobrin L (2011) Diagnostic testing and disease monitoring in birdshot chorioretinopathy. Seminars in ophthalmology 26: 329–336.
6. Hill DW (1970) Fluorescein angiography in fundus diagnosis. British medical bulletin 26: 161–165.
7. Kohner EM, Dollery CT (1970) Fluorescein angiography of the fundus in diabetic retinopathy. British medical bulletin 26: 166–170.
8. Patel M, Kiss S (2014) Ultra-wide-field fluorescein angiography in retinal disease. Curr Opin Ophthalmol 25: 213–220.
9. Ffytche TJ, Shilling JS, Chisholm IH, Federman JL (1980) Indications for fluorescein angiography in disease of the ocular fundus: a review. J R Soc Med 73: 362–365.
10. Arend O, Plange N, Sponsel WE, Remky A (2004) Pathogenetic aspects of the glaucomatous optic neuropathy: fluorescein angiographic findings in patients with primary open angle glaucoma. Brain Res Bull 62: 517–524.
11. Kong M, Lee MY, Ham DI (2012) Ultrawide-field fluorescein angiography for evaluation of diabetic retinopathy. Korean J Ophthalmol 26: 428–431.
12. Hong BK, Nazari Khanamiri H, Rao NA (2013) Role of ultra-widefield fluorescein angiography in the management of uveitis. Can J Ophthalmol 48: 489–493.
13. Guthrie MJ, Osswald CR, Valio NL, Mieler WF, Kang-Mieler JJ (2014) Objective area measurement technique for choroidal neovascularization from fluorescein angiography. Microvasc Res 91: 1–7.
14. Sun C, Li XX, He XJ, Zhang Q, Tao Y (2013) Neuroprotective effect of minocycline in a rat model of branch retinal vein occlusion. Exp Eye Res 113: 105–116.
15. Kowalczuk L, Touchard E, Omri S, Jonet L, Klein C, et al. (2011) Placental growth factor contributes to micro-vascular abnormalization and blood-retinal barrier breakdown in diabetic retinopathy. PLoS One 6: e17462.
16. Ieki Y, Nishiwaki H, Miura S, Hirata Y, Sakata I, et al. (2002) Quantitative evaluation for blood-retinal barrier breakdown in experimental retinal vein occlusion produced by photodynamic thrombosis using a new photosensitizer. Curr Eye Res 25: 317–323.
17. Clermont AC, Bursell SE (2007) Retinal blood flow in diabetes. Microcirculation 14: 49–61.
18. David NJ, Norton EW, Gass JD, Beauchamp J (1967) Fluorescein angiography in central retinal artery occlusion. Arch Ophthalmol 77: 619–629.
19. Scott DJ, Dollery CT, Hill DW, Hodge JV, Fraser R (1963) Fluorescein Studies of the Retinal Circulation in Diabetics. Br J Ophthalmol 47: 588–589.
20. Koyama T, Matsuo N, Shimizu K, Mihara M, Tsuchida Y, et al. (1990) Retinal circulation times in quantitative fluorescein angiography. Graefes Arch Clin Exp Ophthalmol 228: 442–446.
21. Arend O, Remky A, Plange N, Martin BJ, Harris A (2002) Capillary density and retinal diameter measurements and their impact on altered retinal circulation in glaucoma: a digital fluorescein angiographic study. Br J Ophthalmol 86: 429–433.
22. Wolf S, Jung F, Kiesewetter H, Korber N, Reim M (1989) Video fluorescein angiography: method and clinical application. Graefes Arch Clin Exp Ophthalmol 227: 145–151.
23. Hipwell JH, Manivannan A, Vieira P, Sharp PF, Forrester JV (1998) Quantifying changes in retinal circulation: the generation of parametric images from fluorescein angiograms. Physiol Meas 19: 165–180.
24. NH&MRC (2013) Australian code for the care and use of animals for scientific purposes. In: NH&MRC, editor. 8th ed. Australia.
25. Abdi H, Williams LJ (2010) Principal component analysis Wiley Interdisciplinary Reviews: Computational Statistics Volume 2, Issue 4. Wiley Interdisciplinary Reviews: Computational Statistics. pp.433–459.
26. Hotelling H (1933) Analysis of a complex of statistical variables into principal components. Journal of Educational Psychology 24: 417–441.
27. Hayreh SS (1990) In vivo choroidal circulation and its watershed zones. Eye (Lond) 4 (Pt 2): 273–289.
28. Leskova W, Watts MN, Carter PR, Eshaq RS, Harris NR (2013) Measurement of retinal blood flow rate in diabetic rats: disparity between techniques due to redistribution of flow. Invest Ophthalmol Vis Sci 54: 2992–2999.
29. Prager O, Chassidim Y, Klein C, Levi H, Shelef I, et al. (2010) Dynamic in vivo imaging of cerebral blood flow and blood-brain barrier permeability. Neuroimage 49: 337–344.
30. Hickam JB, Frayser R (1966) Studies of Retinal Circulation in Man - Observations on Vessel Diameter Arteriovenous Oxygen Difference and Mean Circulation Time. Circulation 33: 302–&.

31. Canas RV, Liatsis P (2012) Interactive retinal blood flow estimation from fluorescein angiograms. Proceedings of the Institution of Mechanical Engineers Part C-Journal of Mechanical Engineering Science 226: 2521–2537.
32. Nagai N, Lundh von Leithner P, Izumi-Nagai K, Hosking B, Chang B, et al. (2014) Spontaneous CNV in a novel mutant mouse is associated with early VEGF-A driven angiogenesis and late stage focal edema, neural cell loss and dysfunction. Invest Ophthalmol Vis Sci.
33. Lee J, Park DY, Park do Y, Park I, Chang W, et al. (2014) Angiopoietin-1 suppresses choroidal neovascularization and vascular leakage. Invest Ophthalmol Vis Sci 55: 2191–2199.
34. Spencer T, Phillips RP, Sharp PF, Forrester JV (1992) Automated detection and quantification of microaneurysms in fluorescein angiograms. Graefes Arch Clin Exp Ophthalmol 230: 36–41.
35. Spencer T, Olson JA, McHardy KC, Sharp PF, Forrester JV (1996) An image-processing strategy for the segmentation and quantification of microaneurysms in fluorescein angiograms of the ocular fundus. Comput Biomed Res 29: 284–302.
36. Nichols JJ, King-Smith PE, Hinel EA, Thangavelu M, Nichols KK (2012) The use of fluorescent quenching in studying the contribution of evaporation to tear thinning. Invest Ophthalmol Vis Sci 53: 5426–5432.
37. Lim JK, Nguyen CT, He Z, Vingrys AJ, Bui BV (2014) The Effect of Ageing on Ocular Blood Flow, Oxygen Tension and Retinal Function during and after Intraocular Pressure Elevation. PLoS One 9: e98393.
38. Vidt DG, Bredemeyer A, Sapirstein E, Sapirstein LA (1959) Effect of ether anesthesia on the cardiac output, blood pressure, and distribution of blood flow in the albino rat. Circ Res 7: 759–764.
39. Bunag RD, Butterfield J (1982) Tail-cuff blood pressure measurement without external preheating in awake rats. Hypertension 4: 898–903.

Neutrophil/Lymphocyte Ratio Is Associated with Non-Calcified Plaque Burden in Patients with Coronary Artery Disease

Lennart Nilsson[1,2]*, Wouter G. Wieringa[4], Gabija Pundziute[4], Marcus Gjerde[1,2], Jan Engvall[1,3], Eva Swahn[1,2], Lena Jonasson[1,2]

1 Department of Medical and Health Sciences, Linköping University, Linköping, Sweden, **2** Department of Cardiology, Linköping University, Linköping, Sweden, **3** Department of Clinical Physiology, Linköping University, Linköping, Sweden, **4** University of Groningen, University Medical Center Groningen, Department of Cardiology, Groningen, The Netherlands

Abstract

Background: Elevations in soluble markers of inflammation and changes in leukocyte subset distribution are frequently reported in patients with coronary artery disease (CAD). Lately, the neutrophil/lymphocyte ratio has emerged as a potential marker of both CAD severity and cardiovascular prognosis.

Objectives: The aim of the study was to investigate whether neutrophil/lymphocyte ratio and other immune-inflammatory markers were related to plaque burden, as assessed by coronary computed tomography angiography (CCTA), in patients with CAD.

Methods: Twenty patients with non-ST-elevation acute coronary syndrome (NSTE-ACS) and 30 patients with stable angina (SA) underwent CCTA at two occasions, immediately prior to coronary angiography and after three months. Atherosclerotic plaques were classified as calcified, mixed and non-calcified. Blood samples were drawn at both occasions. Leukocyte subsets were analyzed by white blood cell differential counts and flow cytometry. Levels of C-reactive protein (CRP) and interleukin(IL)-6 were measured in plasma. Blood analyses were also performed in 37 healthy controls.

Results: Plaque variables did not change over 3 months, total plaque burden being similar in NSTE-ACS and SA. However, non-calcified/total plaque ratio was higher in NSTE-ACS, 0.25(0.09–0.44) vs 0.11(0.00–0.25), $p<0.05$. At admission, levels of monocytes, neutrophils, neutrophil/lymphocyte ratios, CD4+ T cells, CRP and IL-6 were significantly elevated, while levels of NK cells were reduced, in both patient groups as compared to controls. After 3 months, levels of monocytes, neutrophils, neutrophil/lymphocyte ratios and CD4+ T cells remained elevated in patients. Neutrophil/lymphocyte ratios and neutrophil counts correlated significantly with numbers of non-calcified plaques and also with non-calcified/total plaque ratio ($r=0.403$, $p=0.010$ and $r=0.382$, $p=0.024$, respectively), but not with total plaque burden.

Conclusions: Among immune-inflammatory markers in NSTE-ACS and SA patients, neutrophil counts and neutrophil/lymphocyte ratios were significantly correlated with non-calcified plaques. Data suggest that these easily measured biomarkers reflect the burden of vulnerable plaques in CAD.

Editor: Carmine Pizzi, University of Bologna, Italy

Funding: The authors have no support or funding to report.

Competing Interests: The authors have declared that no competing interests exist.

* Email: lennart.nilsson@liu.se

Introduction

Coronary artery disease (CAD) is the leading cause of death in the western world. Although multifactorial in its origin, inflammatory and immunological events are considered to play central roles in initiation and progression of atherosclerotic plaques [1]. Indeed, elevations in soluble markers of inflammation as well as changes in leukocyte subset distribution are frequently reported in patients with CAD [2–5]. However, studies on relationships between markers of inflammation and severity of CAD have yielded disparate results [6–9].

In recent years, several studies have demonstrated the important role of neutrophils in all stages of atherosclerosis and plaque destabilization leading to acute coronary syndromes (ACS) [10]. Accordingly, neutrophil infiltration has been detected in very early stages of atherosclerosis as well as in shoulder regions of plaques prone to rupture [11,12]. Circulating neutrophil counts and neutrophil/lymphocyte ratios are emerging markers of the presence and severity of CAD [13–15]. Furthermore, they are independent predictors of mortality and cardiovascular events in high-risk groups and a broad range of CAD patients [14,16–19].

CAD severity is not only a question about the extent of obstructive stenosis, but the risk of plaque rupture and ACS largely depends on plaque composition [20]. Coronary computed tomography angiography (CCTA) is a non-invasive method allowing accurate assessment of CAD [21]. In contrast to invasive coronary angiography (ICA), CCTA provides information about the vessel wall and composition of plaques in addition to degree of stenosis. CCTA may therefore provide valuable information about the burden of CAD with prognostic implications as well as assessing the morphological aspects of the disease process [22–24]. The identification of circulating immune-inflammatory markers that are associated with the atherosclerotic disease process in coronary arteries may provide additive information. The aim of the study was to investigate if neutrophil counts, neutrophil/lymphocyte ratio or other immune-inflammatory markers were related to plaque burden, as assessed by CCTA in patients with stable angina (SA) and ACS.

Methods

Study design and population

This study is a single-center, prospective, pilot study. The study population consisted of 30 patients with SA, 20 patients with non-ST-elevation acute coronary syndrome (NSTE-ACS), and 37 healthy control subjects. In order to assess coronary atherosclerosis the patients underwent CCTA prior to ICA and revascularization (percutaneous coronary intervention (PCI) or coronary artery bypass grafting). A follow-up CCTA was performed at three months following revascularization in order to reevaluate the plaque burden and plaque composition. Blood samples were collected at baseline (prior to CCTA and ICA), and at three months follow-up. Inclusion criteria were as follows: 1) patients with planned ICA due to SA, defined as clinically probable angina pectoris and positive exercise test or myocardial perfusion imaging; 2) NSTE-ACS, defined as unstable angina or non-ST-elevation myocardial infarction, according to universally accepted definitions [25,26]. The exclusion criteria were: 1) inability to perform CCTA (contraindications to betablockers or nitroglycerine, allergy to contrast medium, pregnancy, permanent atrial fibrillation); 2) renal dysfunction (creatinine >150 μmol/L) or risk factors for contrast induced acute kidney injury (treatment with metformin, high dose diuretics); 3) known factors influencing immunological and inflammatory markers (active immunologic or inflammatory disease, infection with fever or use of antibiotics during the last 30 days, immunosuppressive treatment); and 4) major trauma, surgery or PCI in the last 30 days. The control subjects, randomly invited from the Swedish Population Register and representative for hospital recruitment area, were clinically healthy and received no medication.

Ethical Considerations

The study protocol was approved by the Regional Ethical Review Board in Linköping and written informed consent was obtained from all study participants. The study was conducted in accordance with the ethical guidelines set forth in the Declaration of Helsinki.

Coronary computed tomography angiography: image acquisition

Patients underwent CCTA within twenty-four hours after inclusion using a 16-slice multi-slice CT scanner or a 64-slice dual-source CT scanner (Sensation or Somatom Definition, Siemens Healthcare, Forchheim, Germany). During CTA acquisition non-ionic contrast medium was administered (Iomeron 400, Bracco, Altana, Pharma, Konstanz, Germany). Beta-blocker treatment (orally or intravenously) and nitroglycerine was administered to achieve optimal image quality. In order to reduce radiation exposure, electrocardiogram-gated current modulation was used in all patients. The following scan parameters were used: 1. For the 16-slice multi-slice scanner: 16×0.75 mm collimation, gantry rotation time of 375 ms, temporal resolution of 188 ms, tube voltage 100 or 120 kV, and maximal tube current of 650 mAs; 2. For the 64-slice dual-source CT scanner: 64×2×0.6 mm collimation, gantry rotation time of 330 ms, temporal resolution of 83 ms, tube voltage 100 or 120 kV, and maximal tube current of 560 mAs. Upon completion of the scan, images were reconstructed, if possible in several phases of the R-R interval, to obtain motion-free images of the coronary arteries.

Coronary computed tomography angiography: image analysis

Evaluation of CCTA images was performed on a remote workstation with dedicated software (QAngio CT, Medis Medical Imaging Systems, Leiden, the Netherlands) [27], side by side in consensus by two experienced observers blinded to baseline patient characteristics and ICA results. A predefined window and level setting (window 900 HU, level 250 HU) was used for analysis of lumen and plaque [28]. Coronary segments were differentiated into seventeen segments, according to a modified American Heart Association classification [29]. Segments of insufficient quality for evaluation were scored as non-evaluable and excluded from analysis. The CT scan was considered unevaluable if 2 vessels had 3 or more segments that were non-evaluable. Presence of plaques was visually assessed. Coronary atherosclerosis was defined as tissue structures >1 mm2 within or adjacent to the coronary artery lumen but distinctive from surrounding pericardial or epicardial tissue. Per segment, one coronary plaque was selected. The degree of luminal narrowing of the coronary artery was quantified visually, based on comparison of the luminal diameter of the plaque containing segment to the luminal diameter of the most normal-appearing site immediately proximal to the plaque. Plaques with ≥50% luminal narrowing were classified as obstructive. In addition, plaque composition was assessed. Three types of plaques were classified: 1) Non-calcified plaque (plaques with lower density compared to contrast-enhanced lumen), 2) calcified plaque (plaques with high density structures compared to contrast-enhanced lumen), or 3) mixed plaque (non-calcified and calcified constituents in single plaque) [30]. The number of any plaques (total plaque burden), as well as plaques with different features was calculated per patient.

Invasive coronary angiography: image acquisition and analysis

Since the assessment of degree of stenosis with 16-slice CCTA is only moderately accurate, ICA was used to assess the obstructive plaque burden. ICA of left and right coronary arteries was performed in multiple views by using the transfemoral approach. Coronary segments were scored in the same manner as on CCTA images, and a diameter stenosis of ≥50% was classified as obstructive. Digital angiograms were analyzed off-line with dedicated software (Coronary Artery Analysis System 9, Pie Medical Imaging, Maastricht, The Netherlands). All segments > 1.5 mm in diameter with a <100% diameter stenosis were measured on the angiograms. The contrast-filled non-tapered catheter tip was used for calibration. The proximal and distal reference vessel diameters and minimal lumen diameter of the

Table 1. Baseline clinical and biochemical characteristics of patients and controls.

	SA	NSTE-ACS	Controls	P-value
	N = 30	N = 20	N = 37	
Age (years)	64±9	67±10	64±8	NS
Female	4 (13)	5 (25)	9 (24)	NS
Waist circumference (cm)	102±11	99±13	95±9	0.003$^{\psi}$
Current or previous smoker	22 (73)	15 (75)	1 (3)	<0.001$^{\psi\gamma}$
Hypertension	21 (70)	7 (35)	0	<0.001$^{\psi\gamma}$, 0.015$^{\Phi}$
Diabetes mellitus	4 (13)	1 (5)	0	0.022$^{\psi}$
History of MI	6 (20)	2 (10)	0	0.004$^{\psi}$
Statin treatment	24 (80)	6 (30)	0	<0.001$^{\psi\gamma\Phi}$
Plasma cholesterol (mmol/L)	5.1±1.0	5.4±1.3	5.5±1.1	NS
Plasma LDL-cholesterol (mmol/L)	2.9±0.8	3.2±1.2	3.4±0.9	0.013$^{\psi}$
Plasma HDL-cholesterol (mmol/L)	1.2±0.2	1.3±0.4	1.4±0.4	0.010$^{\psi}$
Triglycerides (mmol/L)	1.4 (1.1,2.1)	1.4 (1.2,1.7)	1.1 (0.9,1.6)	0.018$^{\psi}$, 0.038$^{\gamma}$

The data are presented as mean ±SD, median (25th, 75th percentile), or numbers (%). SA = stable angina; ACS = acute coronary syndrome; MI = myocardial infarction; LDL = low density lipoprotein, HDL = high density lipoprotein. NS = non-significant (p≥0.05). For comparisons between groups, p-values indicating significant differences are denoted by ψ (controls vs SA), γ (controls vs NSTE-ACS) and Φ (SA vs NSTE-ACS), respectively.

suspected lesion were recorded. The percentage of diameter stenosis was calculated.

Blood sampling, biochemical analysis and flow cytometry

Venous blood samples were collected in vacutainer tubes (using sodium heparin as anticoagulant). Baseline blood samples of NSTE-ACS patients were received within 24 hours of hospital admission. For all CAD patients, the samples at baseline and at three months were collected prior to CCTA and ICA. Samples were centrifuged within 30 minutes to separate plasma, which then was stored immediately at −70°C until analyzed. White blood cell differential counts were determined in whole blood by Cell-Dyn Sapphire™ (Abbot Diagnostics). Leukocyte subset distributions were analyzed in whole blood by flow cytometry as previously described [31,32]. Briefly, monoclonal antibodies against CD3, CD4, CD8, CD19, CD16 and CD56 were purchased from BD Biosciences, San José, CA, US. The antibodies were marked with one of 3 fluorochromes: fluorescein isothiocyanate, phycoerythrin and peridinin chlorophyll protein. The cells were identified by combinations as follows: CD3/CD4/CD8 (T helper cells and cytotoxic T cells), CD19 (B cells) and CD3/CD16/CD56 (NK cells). Whole blood and antibodies were incubated for 15 minutes at room temperature, thereafter erythrocytes were lysed with FACS™ Lysing Solution (BD Biosciences) for 15 minutes at room temperature. Samples were analyzed on a FACSCanto II (BD Biosciences) equipped with 3 lasers, a blue 488 nm, a red 633 nm and a violet 405 nm. Analysis of samples was stopped when 10 000 cells were collected in the lymphocyte gate. Data were analyzed and subpopulations gated with FACSDiva™ 6.1.2 software (BD Biosciences). C-reactive protein (CRP) was measured in serum using a highly sensitive latex-enhanced turbidimetric immunoassay (Roche Diagnostics GmbH, Vienna, Austria) with a lower limit of detection of 0.03 mg/L. IL-6 levels in plasma were measured using an ELISA (R&D Systems Europe, Abingdon, United Kingdom) with a lower limit of detection of 0.48 pg/mL.

Statistical analysis

Categorical variables are presented as numbers (percentages) and were compared between groups using chi-square or Fisher's exact tests. When normally distributed, continuous variables are expressed as mean ±SD and were compared using one-way ANOVA and Students t-test for independent samples. When non-Gaussian distributed, continuous variables are presented as medians with 25th and 75th percentiles and were compared using the nonparametric Kruskal-Wallis test and Mann-Whitney-U test. Wilcoxon signed-rank test was used for paired comparisons. Bivariate correlations were performed to assess the associations between continuous variables using Spearman's correlation coefficient. A p-value of <0.05 was considered statistically significant. Statistical analyses were performed using SPSS version 20 (Chicago, IL, USA) and STATA version 11.0 (College Station, TX, USA).

Results

Study population

During the study period from March 2006 till January 2009 a total of 64 patients were initially included in the study. Fourteen patients were excluded from analysis: 11 patients did not complete any CCTA examination and in 3 patients the CCTA was of non-diagnostic quality. Baseline clinical characteristics of all patients are listed in Table 1. Revascularization was performed in 22 of 30 SA patients (8 PCI and 14 CABG) and in 13 of 20 NSTE-ACS patients (9 PCI and 4 CABG) within the first two months after study inclusion. All CAD patients were treated with statin therapy after admission.

Coronary computed tomography angiography

Data of the baseline CCTAs are summarized in Table 2. A 16-slice CCTA was used in 10 and a 64-slice CCTA in 40 of the 50 patients. Typical CCTA images of coronary plaques are shown in Figure 1. The total plaque burden (i.e. the total number of any plaque) did not differ between SA and NSTE-ACS patients neither did plaque characteristics differ significantly between the patient groups. However, there was a trend towards more calcified plaques in SA patients, whereas NSTE-ACS patients tended to have more non-calcified plaques. As a measure of vulnerable plaques, the ratio between non-calcified plaques and total plaques was calculated. This ratio was significantly higher in ACS patients as compared to SA patients.

Follow-up CCTA at 3 months was available in 41 patients (26 SA and 15 NSTE-ACS patients), 9 performed by a 16-slice CCTA and 32 by a 64-slice CCTA. There were no differences in total plaque burden or plaque characteristics between baseline and 3 months. Total plaque burden and non-calcified plaque/total plaque ratio were 9 (5, 11) and 0.16 (0.00, 0.26), respectively, in SA patients, and 8 (3, 10) and 0.25 (0.09, 0.44), respectively, in NSTE-ACS patients, at 3 months.

Invasive coronary angiography

The findings on ICA are presented in Table 2. There was no difference in the number of coronary artery segments with obstructive lesions in SA patients as compared to NSTE-ACS patients. Strong positive correlations were found between the number of obstructive stenosis on ICA and total plaque burden as well as number of non-calcified plaques on CCTA ($r = 0.694$, $p < 0.001$, and $r = 0.398$, $p = 0.004$, respectively). On the other hand, the non-calcified plaque/total plaque ratio was not associated with the number of obstructive lesions on ICA ($r = 0.163$, NS).

Immune-inflammatory markers

At admission, levels of leukocytes, neutrophils, monocytes, neutrophil/lymphocyte ratios, CD4+ T cells, and plasma levels of CRP and IL-6 were significantly elevated, while levels of NK cells were reduced, in SA and NSTE-ACS patients as compared to controls (Table 3). Plasma CRP in SA and NSTE-ACS patients declined over time reaching similar levels as control subjects at 3 months (0.9 (0.3, 2.8), 0.7 (0.3, 1.9) and 0.7 (0.4, 1.2) ng/mL, respectively, NS). Similarly, plasma IL-6 in SA and NSTE-ACS patients did not differ significantly from controls at follow-up (2.4 (1.1, 2.9), 1.7 (1.2, 3.1) and 1.4 (1.0, 2.2) ng/mL, respectively, NS).

At 3 months, neutrophil counts were still significantly higher in SA and NSTE-ACS patients as compared to control subjects (4.0 ± 1.6, 4.0 ± 1.4 and $3.0 \pm 1.0 \times 10^9$/L, respectively, $p = 0.006$), as were the neutrophil/lymphocyte ratios (2.0 ± 0.8, 2.2 ± 0.7 and 1.5 ± 0.7, respectively, $p = 0.030$). Also, levels of monocytes and CD4+ T cells remained unchanged at 3 months whereas NK cell levels increased (data not shown). Of note, SA and NSTE-ACS patients did not differ significantly in any immune-inflammatory markers at 3 months.

Correlations of coronary computed tomography angiography and invasive coronary angiography with immune-inflammatory markers

Neutrophil/lymphocyte ratios and neutrophil counts correlated with numbers of non-calcified plaques ($r = 0.302$, $p = 0.028$ and $r = 0.327$, $p = 0.017$) and also with non-calcified plaque/total plaque ratio ($r = 0.403$, $p = 0.010$ and $r = 0.382$, $p = 0.024$, respectively), but not with total plaque burden on CCTA (Figure 2). Furthermore, neutrophil/lymphocyte ratios and neutrophil counts did not correlate with number of obstructive lesions on ICA. Other leukocyte subsets did not show any correlations with any of the plaque variables, neither did CRP or IL-6 (data not shown).

Discussion

This study investigated associations between immune-inflammatory markers and plaque burden, as assessed by CCTA in patients with stable and unstable conditions of CAD. The main finding of this study was the consistent and significant correlation of neutrophil counts and neutrophil/lymphocyte ratios with numbers of non-calcified plaques and non-calcified plaque/total plaque ratio, but not with total plaque burden.

Neutrophils and neutrophil/lymphocyte ratios were significantly higher in both SA and NSTE-ACS patients as compared to controls, not only at admission but also at 3 months. The contribution of immune cells such as monocytes/macrophages and T cells to atherosclerosis and plaque progression has been firmly established over the years [33]. Howere, while being the most abundant white blood cell in the circulation, circulation, neutrophils are rarely detected in atherosclerotic plaques and therefore have attracted less attention. Nevertheless, over the past couple of years numerous studies have lent support to an important role of neutrophils in all stages of atherosclerosis [10]. Neutrophil count and neutrophil/lymphocyte ratio are

Table 2. Baseline coronary computed tomography angiography and invasive coronary angiography.

	SA; N = 30	NSTE-ACS; N = 20	P-value
CCTA characteristics at admission			
Number of segments	15 (15,16)	16 (15,16)	NS
Total plaque burden	9 (6,11)	8 (6,10)	NS
Non-calcified plaque	1 (0,2)	2 (1,4)	NS
Mixed plaque	3 (1,5)	4 (1,6)	NS
Calcified plaque	3 (2,5)	2 (0,3)	NS
Non-calcified & mixed plaque	4 (3,7)	6 (2,8)	NS
Ratio non-calcified plaque/plaque burden	0.13 (0.00,0.25)	0.25 (0.10,0.44)	0.049
ICA characteristics at admission			
Number of segments	15 (15,16)	16 (15,16)	NS
Segments with significant stenosis (>50%)	3 (2,6)	2 (1,4)	NS
Segments without significant stenosis	12 (9,14)	14 (11,15)	NS

The data are presented as median (25th, 75th percentile). CCTA = coronary computed tomography angiography; ICA = invasive coronary angiography; SA = stable angina; ACS = acute coronary syndrome. NS = non-significant ($p \geq 0.05$).

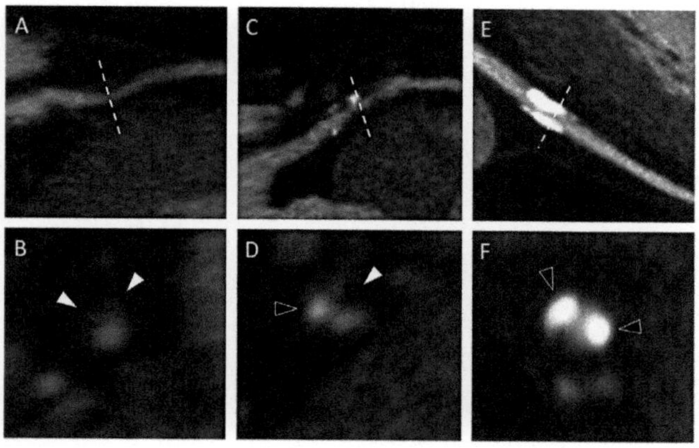

Figure 1. Different plaque compositions as seen by CCTA. The different types of coronary plaque are shown in longitudinal views, with cross-sectional views at the level of the dotted line. A non-calcified plaque is shown on the left (A and B), with white arrowheads pointing at the non-calcified plaque component. A mixed plaque is shown in the middle (C and D), with a white arrowhead indicating the non-calcified plaque component and a black arrowhead indicating the calcified component. A large calcified plaque is shown on the right side (E and F), with black arrowhead indicating the calcifications.

emerging markers of presence and severity of CAD [13–15,34]. They are both independent predictors of mortality and future cardiovascular events in healthy populations, high-risk groups and a broad range of CAD patients [14,16–19,35,36].

Neutrophil counts and neutrophil/lymphocyte ratios have been associated with the presence, severity and progression of coronary atherosclerosis as assessed by various modes of coronary imaging [14,15,37]. In a large cohort study of 3005 consecutive patients undergoing ICA for various indications, neutrophil count and neutrophil/lymphocyte ratio correlated significantly with the number of diseased vessels [14]. Moreover, a higher neutrophil/lymphocyte ratio was associated with higher coronary calcium scores measured by multidetector CT in 849 clinically healthy individuals participating in a health promotion program [37]. However, neither ICA nor coronary calcium score, provide any information about the plaque composition. Correlations of neutrophil counts and neutrophil/lymphocyte ratios with plaque composition on CCTA have not previously been performed.

By using CCTA it has been possible to show that plaque morphology is an independent predictor of prognosis [22,24,38]. Several studies have found that non-calcified plaques are associated with worse outcomes [23,39–40]. Among 3,499 consecutive symptomatic SA patients who underwent CCTA, 1,102 subjects with non-obstructive CAD were prospectively followed for a mean of 78 months. The death rate of these patients was 3.1%, increasing incrementally from calcified plaque (1.4%) to mixed plaque (3.3%) to non-calcified plaque (9.6%) [23]. Our present data indicate that the absolute neutrophil count as well as the neutrophil/lymphocyte ratio, obtained by a white blood cell differential test, reflects the burden of high-risk plaques, rather than the crude number of plaques. Combining these easily available biomarkers and CCTA may be of supplemental value in the identification of patients with vulnerable atherosclerotic plaques. It opens up the potential for early selective treatment and prevention of future myocardial damage.

The increased levels of CD4+ T cells and dynamic changes of NK cells in the patient population of the present study have been described recently [32,41]. However, we did not find any association between these cell subsets and CCTA plaque characteristics. Neither were there any relationships between the well-established inflammatory markers, CRP and IL-6, and the CCTA findings. Only one previous CCTA study has investigated immune cells in relation to plaque burden and plaque composition. Kashiwagi et al found that an increased level of the proinflammatory CD14+ CD16+ monocyte subset, but not the total number of monocytes or CRP, is related to the presence of vulnerable plaques in patients with stable angina pectoris [42]. Unfortunately, we did not measure monocyte subsets, but the lack of association between total number of monocytes, CRP and the presence of vulnerable plaques on CCTA was also found in our study.

A few studies have been performed in search of associations between other inflammatory markers and CCTA characteristics [43,44]. Bamberg et al determined the association between several

Table 3. Baseline leukocyte subsets and plasma cytokines of patients and controls.

	SA	NSTE-ACS	Controls	P-value
	N = 30	N = 20	N = 37	
Leukocytes (x10^9/L)	7.1±2.2	7.7±2.3	5.5±1.4	$<0.001^{\psi\gamma}$
Neutrophils (x10^9/L)	4.1±1.5	4.5±1.7	3.0±1.0	$<0.001^{\psi\gamma}$
Monocytes (x10^9/L)	0.6±0.2	0.6±0.3	0.4±0.1	$<0.001^{\psi\gamma}$
Lymphocytes (x10^9/L)	2.2±1.0	2.4±0.9	2.0±0.6	NS
CD19+ cells, % of lymphocytes	10 (7,12)	10 (8,15)	10 (7,14)	NS
CD4+ cells, % of lymphocytes	49 (42,54)	50 (44,54)	39 (33,48)	0.005^{ψ}, 0.001^{γ}
CD8+ cells, % of lymphocytes	25 (20,31)	25 (17,31)	23 (19,29)	NS
NK cells, % of lymphocytes	12 (9,18)	12 (7,15)	18 (11,28)	$0.023^{\psi\gamma}$
Neutrophil/lymphocyte ratio	2.1 (1.4,2.4)	2.0 (1.5,2.5)	1.5 (1.2,1.9)	0.012^{ψ}, 0.027^{γ}
Plasma IL-6, pg/mL	3.1 (2.0,5.7)	4.9 (2.9,8.0)	1.4 (1.0,2.2)	$<0.001^{\psi\gamma}$
Plasma CRP, mg/L	1.2 (0.3,3.2)	3.2 (2.2,5.0)	0.7 (0.4,1.2)	0.023^{Φ}, $<0.001^{\gamma}$

The data are presented as mean ±SD or median (25th, 75th percentile). SA = stable angina; NSTE-ACS = non-ST-elevation acute coronary syndrome; CD19+ cells, B cells; CD4+ cells, T helper cells; CD8+ cell, cytotoxic T cell; NK = Natural killer; IL = interleukin; CRP = C-reactive protein. NS = non-significant (p≥0.05). For comparisons between groups, p-values indicating significant differences are denoted by ψ (controls vs SA), γ (controls vs NSTE-ACS) and Φ (SA vs NSTE-ACS), respectively.

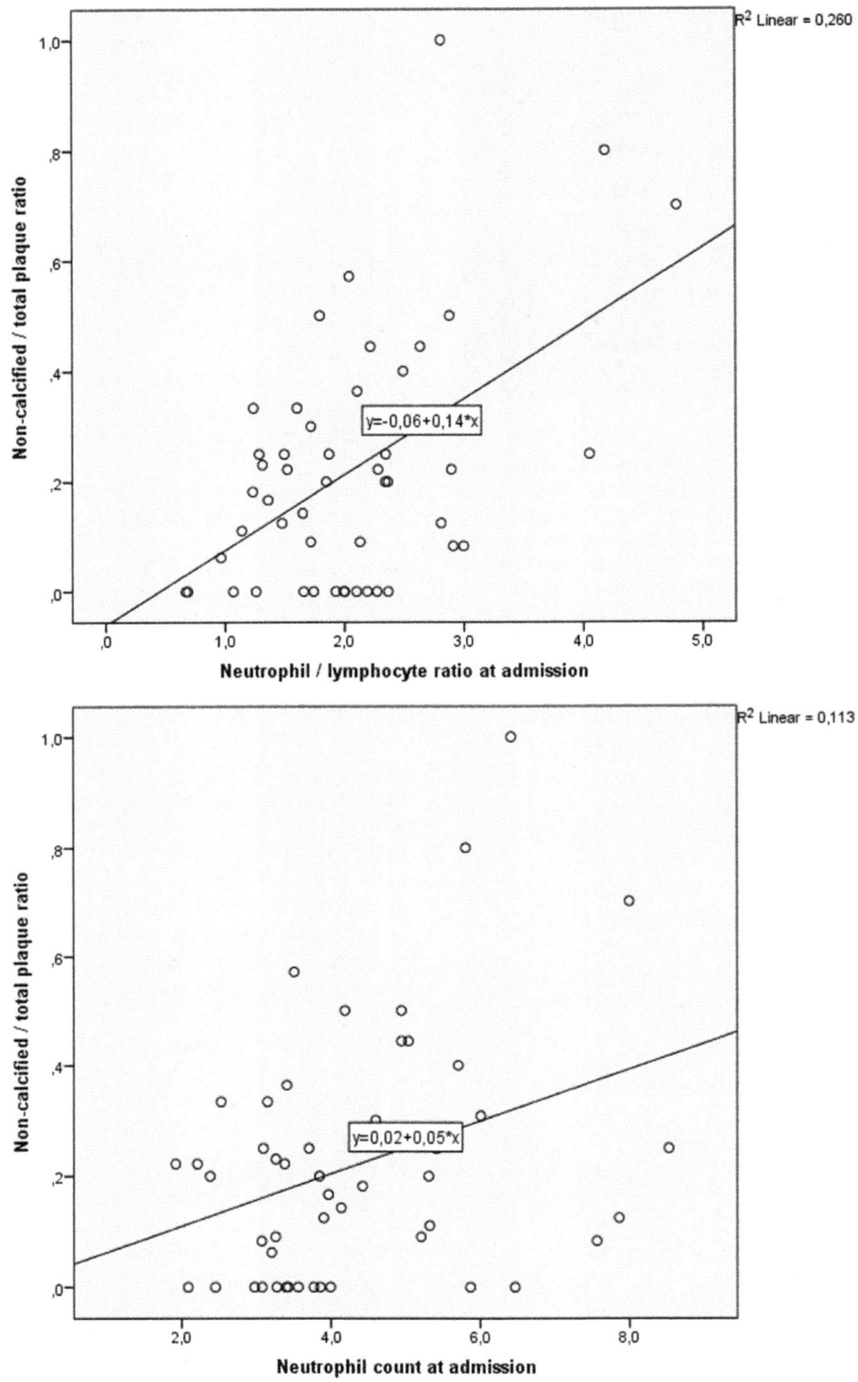

Figure 2. Neutrophils and coronary plaques on CCTA. Scatterplots demonstrating the associations between non-calcified/total plaque ratio on baseline CCTA and neutrophil/lymphocyte ratio and neutrophil counts at admission. Neutrophil counts are given as $\times 10^9$/L.

plasma biomarkers and coronary plaque burden assessed by CCTA in 313 patients with acute chest pain who ultimately had no evidence of ACS [43]. Only 25% of study individuals were on statins and those with prior CAD were excluded. Interestingly, they found higher levels of CRP and oxidized LDL cholesterol and lower levels of adiponectin in patients with exclusively non-calcified plaques as compared to those with any calcified plaque or no plaque at all. In our study, 60% of all patients were on statin treatment at the time of inclusion. This may explain the absence of correlations between CRP and plaque characteristics, since statins are known to markedly reduce CRP levels [45]. Another study by Harada et al included 178 non-ACS acute chest pain patients, who underwent CCTA examination [44]. In contrast to the study by Bamberg et al, they found an association between CRP and the presence of calcified rather than non-calcified plaques.

This study has some major limitations. First, the size of the study population was small. On the other hand, we included both SA and ACS patients, who were examined by CCTA and blood sample analysis prior to ICA and revascularization as well as in the stabilized phase at 3 months. Secondly, this study was performed between 2006 and 2009, first using a 16-slice and later a 64-slice CCTA. The 16-slice CCTA is less accurate than the 64-slice CCTA in measuring degree of stenosis and plaque composition. However, we did use ICA as well to assess obstructive and non-obstructive plaque burden and CCTA was performed twice in a majority of patients yielding identical results. Thus, in order not to reduce the size of the study population, all study patients irrespective of CT-scanner used were included in the data analysis.

To conclude, both neutrophil counts and neutrophil/lymphocyte ratio were significantly correlated with non-calcified plaque burden and non-calcified plaque/total plaque ratio. The results highlight the potential utility of these easily measured cellular markers in the risk assessment and monitoring of CAD patients.

Acknowledgments

The authors thank Elisabeth Logander, RN, for coordinating patient logistics, Petter Quick, RN, and the radiology technicians at CMIV for performing CCTA, and Karin Backteman, PhD, for performing flow cytometri.

Author Contributions

Conceived and designed the experiments: LN MG JE ES LJ. Performed the experiments: LN WW GP MG LJ. Analyzed the data: LN WW GP MG JE ES LJ. Contributed reagents/materials/analysis tools: LN GP JE LJ. Wrote the paper: LN WW GP JE ES LJ.

References

1. Hansson GK (2005) Inflammation, atherosclerosis, and coronary artery disease. N Engl J Med 352: 1685–95.
2. Pai JK, Pischon T, Ma J, Manson JE, Hankinson SE, et al. (2004) Inflammatory markers and the risk of coronary heart disease in men and women. N Engl J Med 351: 2599–610.
3. Nijm J, Wikby A, Tompa A, Olsson AG, Jonasson L (2005) Circulating levels of proinflammatory cytokines and neutrophil-platelet aggregates in patients with coronary artery disease. Am J Cardiol 95(4): 452–6.
4. Jonasson L, Backteman K, Ernerudh J (2005) Loss of natural killer cell activity in patients with coronary artery disease. Atherosclerosis 183(2): 316–21.
5. Packard RR, Libby P (2008) Inflammation in atherosclerosis: from vascular biology to biomarker discovery and risk prediction. Clin Chem 54(1): 24–38.
6. Abdelmouttaleb I, Danchin N, Ilardo C, Aimone-Gastin I, Angioï M, et al. (1999) C-Reactive protein and coronary artery disease: additional evidence of the implication of an inflammatoryprocess in acute coronary syndromes. Am Heart J 137(2): 346–51.
7. Rifai N, Joubran R, Yu H, Asmi M, Jouma M (1999) Inflammatory markers in men with angiographically documented coronary heart disease. Clin Chem 45(11): 1967–73.
8. Bamberg F, Truong QA, Koenig W, Schlett CL, Nasir K, et al. (2012) Differential associations between blood biomarkers of inflammation, oxidation, and lipid metabolism with varying forms of coronary atherosclerotic plaque as quantified by coronary CT angiography. Int J Cardiovasc Imaging 28: 183–92.
9. Harada K, Amano T, Uetani T, Yoshida T, Kato B, et al. (2013) Association of inflammatory markers with the morphology and extent of coronary plaque as evaluated by 64-slice multidetector computed tomography in patients with stable coronary artery disease. Int J Cardiovasc Imaging 29: 1149–58.
10. Soehnlein O (2012) Multiple roles for neutrophils in atherosclerosis. Circ Res 110(6): 875–88.
11. Drechsler M, Megens RT, van Zandvoort M, Weber C, Soehnlein O (2010) Hyperlipidemia-triggered neutrophilia promotes early atherosclerosis. Circulation 122(18): 1837–45.
12. Rotzius P, Thams S, Soehnlein O, Kenne E, Tseng CN, et al. (2010) Distinct infiltration of neutrophils in lesion shoulders in ApoE-/- mice. Am J Pathol 177(1): 493–500.
13. Kawaguchi H, Mori T, Kawano T, Kono S, Sasaki J, et al. (1996) Band neutrophil count and the presence and severity of coronary atherosclerosis. Am Heart J 132(1 Pt 1): 9–12.
14. Arbel Y, Finkelstein A, Halkin A, Birati EY, Revivo M, et al. (2012) Neutrophil/lymphocyte ratio is related to the severity of coronary artery disease and clinical outcome in patients undergoing angiography. Atherosclerosis 225: 456–60.
15. Kalay N, Dogdu O, Koc F, Yarlioglues M, Ardic I, et al. (2012) Hematologic parameters and angiographic progression of coronary atherosclerosis. Angiology 63: 213–7.
16. Duffy BK, Gurm HS, Rajagopal V, Gupta R, Ellis SG, et al. (2006) Usefulness of an elevated neutrophil to lymphocyte ratio in predicting long-term mortality after percutaneous coronary intervention. Am J Cardiol 97(7): 993–6.
17. Papa A, Emdin M, Passino C, Michelassi C, Battaglia D, et al. (2008) Predictive value of elevated neutrophil-lymphocyte ratio on cardiac mortality in patients with stable coronary artery disease. Clin Chim Acta 395: 27–31.
18. Guasti L, Dentali F, Castiglioni L, Maroni L, Marino F, et al. (2011) Neutrophils and clinical outcomes in patients with acute coronary syndromes and/or cardiac revascularisation. A systematic review on more than 34,000 subjects. Thromb Haemost 106(4): 591–9.
19. Azab B, Chainani V, Shah N, McGinn JT (2013) Neutrophil-lymphocyte ratio as a predictor of major adverse cardiac events among diabetic population: a 4-year follow-up study. Angiology 64(6): 456–65.
20. Kolodgie FD, Burke AP, Farb A, Gold HK, Yuan J, et al. (2001) The thin-cap fibroatheroma: A type of vulnerable plaque: The major precursor lesion to acute coronary syndromes. Curr Opin Cardiol 16: 285–92.
21. Voros S, Rinehart S, Qian Z, Joshi P, Vazquez G, et al. (2011) Coronary atherosclerosis imaging by coronary CT angiography: Current status, correlation with intravascular interrogation and meta-analysis. JACC Cardiovasc Imaging 4: 537–48.
22. Russo V, Zavalloni A, Bacchi Reggiani ML, Buttazzi K, Gostoli V, et al. (2010) Incremental prognostic value of coronary CT angiography in patients with suspected coronary artery disease. Circ Cardiovasc Imaging 3: 351–9.
23. Ahmadi N, Nabavi V, Hajsadeghi F, Flores F, French WJ, et al. (2011) Mortality incidence of patients with non-obstructive coronary artery disease diagnosed by computed tomography angiography. Am J Cardiol 107: 10–16.
24. Pundziute G, Schuijf JD, Jukema JW, Boersma E, de Roos A, et al. (2007) Prognostic value of multislice computed tomography coronary angiography in patients with known or suspected coronary artery disease. J Am Coll Cardiol 49: 62–70.
25. The Joint European Society of Cardiology/American College of Cardiology Committee for the redefinition of myocardial infarction (2000) Myocardial infarction redefined - a consensus document of The Joint European Society of Cardiology/American College of Cardiology Committee for the redefinition of myocardial infarction. Eur Heart J 21(18): 1502–13.
26. Luepker RV, Apple FS, Christenson RH, Crow RS, Fortmann SP, et al. (2003) Case definitions for acute coronary heart disease in epidemiology and clinical research studies. Circulation 108(20): 2543–9.
27. Boogers MJ, Schuijf JD, Kitslaar PH, van Werkhoven JM, de Graaf FR, et al. (2010) Automated quantification of stenosis severity on 64-slice CT: A comparison with quantitative coronary angiography. JACC Cardiovasc Imaging 3: 699–709.
28. Leber AW, Knez A, Becker A, Becker C, von Ziegler F, et al. (2004) Accuracy of multidetector spiral computed tomography in identifying and differentiating the composition of coronary atherosclerotic plaques: A comparative study with intracoronary ultrasound. J Am Coll Cardiol 43: 1241–7.
29. Austen WG, Edwards JE, Frye RL, Gensini GG, Gott VL, et al. (1975) A reporting system on patients evaluated for coronary artery disease. report of the ad hoc committee for grading of coronary artery disease, council on cardiovascular surgery, american heart association. Circulation 51: 5–40.
30. Kitagawa T, Yamamoto H, Horiguchi J, Ohhashi N, Tadehara F, et al. (2009) Characterization of noncalcified coronary plaques and identification of culprit lesions in patients with acute coronary syndrome by 64-slice computed tomography. JACC Cardiovasc Imaging 2: 153–60.
31. Backteman K, Ernerudh J (2007) Biological and methodological variation of lymphocyte subsets in blood of human adults. J Immunol Methods 322: 20–7.
32. Bergstrom I, Backteman K, Lundberg A, Ernerudh J, Jonasson L (2012) Persistent accumulation of interferon-gamma-producing CD8+CD56+ T cells in blood from patients with coronary artery disease. Atherosclerosis 224: 515–20.
33. Galkina E, Ley K (2009) Immune and inflammatory mechanisms of atherosclerosis. Annu Rev Immunol 27: 165–97.
34. Wheeler JG, Mussolino ME, Gillum RF, Danesh J (2004) Associations between differential leucocyte count and incident coronary heart disease: 1764 incident cases from seven prospective studies of 30,374 individuals. Eur Heart J 25(15): 1287–92.
35. Rana JS, Boekholdt SM, Ridker PM, Jukema JW, Luben R, et al. (2007) Differential leucocyte count and the risk of future coronary artery disease in healthy men and women: the EPIC-Norfolk Prospective Population Study. J Intern Med 262(6): 678–89.
36. Madjid M, Awan I, Willerson JT, Casscells SW (2004) Leukocyte count and coronary heart disease: implications for risk assessment. J Am Coll Cardiol 44(10): 1945–56.
37. Park BJ, Shim JY, Lee HR, Lee JH, Jung DH, et al. (2011) Relationship of neutrophil-lymphocyte ratio with arterial stiffness and coronary calcium score. Clin Chim Acta 412: 925–9.
38. Hadamitzky M, Freissmuth B, Meyer T, Hein F, Kastrati A, et al. (2009) Prognostic value of coronary computed tomographic angiography for prediction

of cardiac events in patients with suspected coronary artery disease. JACC Cardiovasc Imaging 2: 404–11.
39. van Werkhoven JM, Schuijf JD, Gaemperli O, Jukema JW, Kroft LJ, et al. (2009) Incremental prognostic value of multi-slice computed tomography coronary angiography over coronary artery calcium scoring in patients with suspected coronary artery disease. Eur Heart J 30: 2622–9.
40. Gaemperli O, Valenta I, Schepis T, Husmann L, Scheffel H, et al. (2008) Coronary 64-slice CT angiography predicts outcome in patients with known or suspected coronary artery disease. Eur Radiol 18: 1162–73.
41. Backteman K, Ernerudh J, Jonasson L (2014) Natural killer (NK) cell deficit in coronary artery disease: no aberrations in phenotype but sustained reduction of NK cells is associated with low-grade inflammation. Clin Exp Immunol 175(1): 104–12.
42. Kashiwagi M, Imanishi T, Tsujioka H, Ikejima H, Kuroi A, et al. (2010) Association of monocyte subsets with vulnerability characteristics of coronary plaques as assessed by 64-slice multidetector computed tomography in patients with stable angina pectoris. Atherosclerosis 212(1): 171–6.
43. Bamberg F, Truong QA, Koenig W, Schlett CL, Nasir K, et al. (2012) Differential associations between blood biomarkers of inflammation, oxidation, and lipid metabolism with varying forms of coronary atherosclerotic plaque as quantified by coronary CT angiography. Int J Cardiovasc Imaging 28: 183–92.
44. Harada K, Amano T, Uetani T, Yoshida T, Kato B, et al. (2013) Association of inflammatory markers with the morphology and extent of coronary plaque as evaluated by 64-slice multidetector computed tomography in patients with stable coronary artery disease. Int J Cardiovasc Imaging 29: 1149–58.
45. Jialal I, Stein D, Balis D, Grundy SM, Adams-Huet B, et al. (2001) Effect of hydroxymethyl glutaryl coenzyme a reductase inhibitor therapy on high sensitive C-reactive protein levels. Circulation 103(15): 1933–5.

23

Comparison of NOGA Endocardial Mapping and Cardiac Magnetic Resonance Imaging for Determining Infarct Size and Infarct Transmurality for Intramyocardial Injection Therapy Using Experimental Data

Noemi Pavo[1], Andras Jakab[2], Maximilian Y. Emmert[3,4,5], Georg Strebinger[1], Petra Wolint[3,4,5], Matthias Zimmermann[6], Hendrik Jan Ankersmit[6,7], Simon P. Hoerstrup[3,4,5], Gerald Maurer[1], Mariann Gyöngyösi[1]*

1 Department of Cardiology, Medical University of Vienna, Vienna, Austria, **2** Department of Biomedical Imaging and Image-guided Therapy, Medical University of Vienna, Vienna, Austria, **3** Swiss Centre for Regenerative Medicine, University of Zürich, Zürich, Switzerland, **4** Division of Surgical Research, University Hospital of Zürich, Zürich, Switzerland, **5** Clinic for Cardiovascular Surgery, University Hospital of Zürich, Zürich, Switzerland, **6** Department of Thoracic Surgery, Medical University of Vienna, Vienna, Austria, **7** Christian Doppler Laboratory for Cardiac and Thoracic Diagnosis and Regeneration, Vienna, Austria

Abstract

Objectives: We compared the accuracy of NOGA endocardial mapping for delineating transmural and non-transmural infarction to the results of cardiac magnetic resonance imaging (cMRI) with late gadolinium enhancement (LE) for guiding intramyocardial reparative substance delivery using data from experimental myocardial infarction studies.

Methods: Sixty domestic pigs underwent diagnostic NOGA endocardial mapping and cMRI-LE 60 days after induction of closed-chest reperfused myocardial infarction. The infarct size was determined by LE of cMRI and by delineation of the infarct core on the unipolar voltage polar map. The sizes of the transmural and non-transmural infarctions were calculated from the cMRI transmurality map using signal intensity (SI) cut-offs of>75% and>25% and from NOGA bipolar maps using bipolar voltage cut-off values of <0.8 mV and <1.9 mV. Linear regression analysis and Bland-Altman plots were used to determine correlations and systematic differences between the two images. The overlapping ratios of the transmural and non-transmural infarcted areas were calculated.

Results: Infarct size as determined by 2D NOGA unipolar voltage polar mapping correlated with the 3D cMRI-LE findings ($r=0.504$, $p<0.001$) with a mean difference of 2.82% in the left ventricular (LV) surface between the two images. Polar maps of transmural cMRI and bipolar maps of NOGA showed significant association for determining of the extent of transmural infarction ($r=0.727$, $p<0.001$, overlap ratio of $81.6\pm11.1\%$) and non-transmural infarction ($r=0.555$, $p<0.001$, overlap ratio of $70.6\pm18.5\%$). NOGA overestimated the transmural scar size (6.81% of the LV surface) but slightly underestimated the size of the non-transmural infarction (−3.04% of the LV surface).

Conclusions: By combining unipolar and bipolar voltage maps, NOGA endocardial mapping is useful for accurate delineation of the targeted zone for intramyocardial therapy and is comparable to cMRI-LE. This may be useful in patients with contraindications for cMRI who require targeted intramyocardial regenerative therapy.

Editor: Joshua M. Hare, University of Miami Miller School of Medicine, United States of America

Funding: This study was sponsored by the Christian Doppler Laboratory for Cardiac and Thoracic Diagnosis and Regeneration, Vienna, Austria; by the Ludwig Boltzmann Institute Cluster of Cardiovascular Diseases; and by the Swiss Centre for Regenerative Medicine, University of Zurich, Zurich, Switzerland. The funders had no role in study design, data collection and analysis, decision to publish, or preparation of the manuscript.

Competing Interests: The authors have declared that no competing interests exist.

* Email: mariann.gyongyosi@meduniwien.ac.at

Introduction

The border zone of myocardial infarction (MI) represents myocardial areas with decreased viability and reduced wall motion capacity. Perfusion and transport of cell-death waste products, such as oxygen radicals and other metabolic substances, is impaired due to the close proximity to the non-perfused infarcted area, and this may account for the functional decline. These areas are targeted by cardiac regenerative therapies because regenerative cells delivered to these areas may survive and help restore cardiac function.

Compared to intracoronary or intravenous delivery, intramyocardial delivery of regenerative drugs, genes, or cells into the border zone of chronic myocardial ischemia results in higher retention of the applied substances, which may result in more effective therapy [1–4]. However, accurate real-time localization of this area for application of intramyocardial regenerative therapy remains a challenge. Cardiac magnetic resonance imaging (cMRI) with late gadolinium enhancement (LE) is the gold standard for assessing myocardial infarct size, infarct transmurality, and left ventricular (LV) function and for assessing the efficacy of cardiac therapies [5,6]. Identification of subendocardial or non-transmural infarcted areas using cMRI-LE would be ideal for guiding targeted intramyocardial regenerative therapy. However, cMRI is an off-line imaging modality, and there is a delay between diagnostic imaging and application of the therapy. Further, cMRI is contraindicated for patients with cMRI-non-compatible pacemakers or implantable defibrillators.

Three-dimensional (3D) NOGA endocardial mapping and electromagnetic guided percutaneous intramyocardial therapy is the method that is currently used for real-time (on-table) assessment of myocardial viability and for delineation of the infarct and infarct border zone [7–10]. The accuracy and reproducibility of NOGA maps for evaluating myocardial viability have been established [11–15], and this 3D imaging method has been compared with other 3D imaging methods such as myocardial scintigraphy, positron emission tomography, and cMRI [16–20]. Furthermore, histology, echocardiography, and other methods have confirmed that NOGA mapping can be used to correctly assess the size and severity of myocardial necrosis [21]. In order to assess the accuracy of the point-to-point sampling method of NOGA mapping, several research groups have developed fusion software for constructing hybrid images of cMRI and NOGA CARTO mapping [22–29]. These reports on a limited number of patients confirmed that there is good correlation between the two 3D images regarding the location and size of the infarction. However, the reports noted that NOGA mapping does not show good correlation with cMRI-LE in terms of the delineation of non-transmural areas. Moreover, the aim of these multimodality images was to find a focus for arrhythmogen substrates for ablation therapy to treat reentry tachycardias using unipolar and bipolar voltage electrocardiograms.

Here we focused on the accuracy of NOGA mapping to delineate transmural and non-transmural infarction by comparing it with cMRI-LE imaging. We investigated whether NOGA mapping is suitable for guiding intramyocardial drug or cell delivery using data from experimental myocardial infarction studies. We chose to use an animal model of closed chest reperfused MI. This is very similar to human primary percutaneous coronary intervention in acute MI, which simulates post-infarction left ventricular dysfunction.

We hypothesized that real-time, on-table 3D endocardial mapping using the NOGA system can accurately delineate the zone of decreased viability and non-transmural scars that is the target area for percutaneous intramyocardial therapy. Here we show that there is a significant correlation between the two images in terms of infarct size and the sizes of the transmural and non-transmural infarction, with high degree of overlap between endocardial mapping and cMRI-derived infarcted areas.

Materials and Methods

Experimental chronic left ventricular dysfunction post MI

Closed-chest reperfused acute MI was induced in 60 female farm pigs by percutaneous occlusion of the mid left anterior descending coronary artery. Sixty days later, the pigs underwent cMRI-LE images to confirm chronic myocardial infarction. Additional NOGA endocardial mapping was then performed 2 ± 1 days later, just before the animals were euthanized, aiming to search for correlations between the two images.

Briefly, all pigs were sedated with ketamine hydrochloride (12 mg/kg), xylazine (1 mg/kg), and atropine (0.04 mg/kg) intramuscularly. The pigs were intubated intratracheally and anesthetized with isoflurane (1.5–2.5 vol%), O_2 (1.6–1.8 vol%), and N_2O (0.5 vol%). O_2 saturation, blood pressure, and electrocardiography were monitored continuously. After an arteriotomy of the right femoral artery, a 6F introducer sheath (Terumo Medical Corporation, Somerset, NJ, USA) was inserted. Heparin (200 IU/kg) was administered followed by selective angiography of the left coronary artery tree. A balloon catheter (3.0 mm in diameter, 9 mm long; Maverick, Boston Scientific Corp, Natick, MA, USA) was advanced into the left anterior descending coronary artery (LAD). After the origin of the second major diagonal branch, the mid LAD was occluded by inflation of the balloon at 5 atmospheres for 90 minutes, followed by deflation of the balloon to allow opening of the infarct-related artery and reperfusion of the ischemia-affected myocardium. The pigs were then allowed to recover from the anesthesia.

This study was carried out in strict accordance with the recommendations in the Guide for the Care and Use of Laboratory Animals of the National Institutes of Health. The protocol was approved by the Experimental Animal Care and Use Committee at the Faculty of Animal Science of the University of Kaposvar (Hungary) (Permit Numbers: 246/002/SOM2006/11/11 and 246/002/SOM2006/08/11). All procedures were performed under general anesthesia, and all efforts were made to minimize the suffering of the animals.

NOGA electroanatomical mapping of the LV

The electromechanical maps of the pigs were obtained 62 ± 1 days after induction of acute MI. The principles and procedures of NOGA electroanatomical mapping have been described previously [7–10]. Briefly, the external reference patch, which contains a tip sensor, was taped onto the experimental animal's back below its heart. A 7 F introducer sheath was introduced into the left femoral artery, followed by administration of 5000 IU of unfractionated heparin. To begin the navigation process, a fully deflected NogaStar (Johnson & Johnson, Diamond Bar, CA) mapping catheter was introduced through the femoral sheath and was advanced inside the aorta under fluoroscopic guidance. Before entering the LV chamber, the mapping catheter was bent and then introduced through the aortic valve. As soon as the tail of the catheter was inside the LV, the catheter tip was straightened and orientated towards the apex. The first few endocardial points in different regions of the LV (apical point, outflow tract, and lateral and posterior points) were sampled to initiate a three-dimensional silhouette of the heart, which was then updated in real time with every new mapping point which facilitated further electromagnetic navigation with limited use of fluoroscopy.

At least four points were acquired in each of twelve myocardial segments. During the mapping process, simultaneous unipolar and bipolar electrocardiograms were recorded as well as the 3D location and orientation of the catheter tip of several sites within the LV cavity. The electrophysiological and mechanical data were integrated to create a color-coded 3D reconstruction of the LV chamber to facilitate assessment of the regional viability. The stability of the catheter-to-wall contact was evaluated at every location in real time, and only stable location points were accepted to create the 3D maps [9,10]. When constructing the NOGA maps, care was taken to correctly define the apex and the heart axis.

Using the movement of the catheter tip in the LV cavity, the end-diastolic, end-systolic volumes and global ejection fraction were calculated automatically. The average heart rate was calculated during the electroanatomical mapping procedure.

Evaluation of the NOGA maps

ImageJ for Windows (U.S. National Institutes of Health [NIH], Bethesda, Maryland, USA) was used to determine the relative size of the area of interest. The 3D unipolar (UPV) and bipolar (BiPV) voltages of each measuring point were displayed as two-dimensional polar maps (bull's eye format). The same discriminatory threshold values were used for all NOGA maps: <5 mV for non-viable infarcted area, 5–15 mV for infarct border zone and> 15 mV for normal viability in unipolar maps and <0.8 mV for transmural, 0.8–1.9 mV for non-transmural infarction and> 1.9 mV for normal myocardium in bipolar maps. These cut-off values are represented by the color-coding of the NOGA images and facilitate the identification of areas with reduced UPVs and BiPVs (Table 1, Fig. 1). As a next step, in order to validate the discriminatory threshold values for bipolar NOGA maps, we determined the correlation between MRI-based infarct area measurements and different discriminatory bipolar cut-off values. Specifically, we exported the raw images of the NOGA transmurality data (i.e. the bipolar recordings) into the image processing pipeline of Matlab R2010 for Windows, converted the image RGB (red-green-blue) color values into voltage values, and cropped the image to the cMRI-LE infarct area. Using 100 threshold steps (from 0.5 to 1.5 mV), we iteratively exported the NOGA-based transmurality areas to the cMRI transmurality maps and determined the correlation coefficient between the two images using different thresholds (25, 30, 50, 60, and 75% transmurality) (Fig. 2A).

In order to determine the BiPV cut-off that provides the best fit to the size of transmural and non-transmural cMRI-LE areas, we also tested 0.5–1.5 mV and 1.0–2.0 mV BiPV cut-offs (Fig. 3). The fibrous ring and cardiac valves, represented as red zones at the outer edge of the bull's eye NOGA maps, were excluded from analysis as they contained low UPVs and BiPVs that were indicative of non-contractile collagen structures [9,10].

The relative size of the infarct core, border areas, and normal myocardium was determined from the color-coded unipolar voltage polar map, and the sizes of the transmural and non-transmural infarction were delineated on the bipolar maps (Figs. 4 and 5). The demarcation and measurement of these areas on the NOGA maps was carried out by a researcher who was blinded to the results of the cMRI-LE.

cMRI-LE acquisitions

Cardiac magnetic resonance (cMRI) images were acquired on a 1.5 T Siemens Avanto Syngo B17 clinical scanner (Erlangen, Germany) with a phased-array coil and a vector ECG system. Functional (dynamic) images were acquired using a retrospective ECG-gated (HR: 80–100 beats/minute), steady-state free precession (SSFP - TRUFISP sequence) technique in short-axis and long-axis sections of the heart using 1.2-ms echo time (TE), 40-ms repetition time (TR), 25 phases, 50° flip angle, 360-mm field-of-view, 8-mm slice thickness, and a 256×256 image matrix. For quantitative measurement of infarct extent and transmurality, delayed enhancement diastolic phase short-axis images were obtained after injection of 0.05 mmol/kg of contrast medium using an inversion recovery prepared gradient-echo sequence. LE images were obtained 10 minutes after gadolinium contrast agent injection.

Analysis and visualization of cMRI images

In all cases, care was taken to include the entire heart volume from the apex to the level of the great vessels, and the entire left ventricle was included in the MRI analysis. Analysis was consistently restricted to slices between the apex and the basis on which the left ventricle myocardium is seen in 360 degrees. Image analysis was performed using Segment for Windows software (version 1.9; Medviso AB, Lund, Sweden) [30]. The extent and transmurality of the infarct was semi-automatically quantified on the 10-minute LE images using the "2SD" approach. During this procedure, hyperintense image pixels were tagged as infarcted if their signal intensity (SI) was greater than the mean value plus 2 standard deviations of the normal-appearing LV myocardium. Signal intensity was derived from the absolute value of the voxel intensity data, which were stored in the DICOM files from the cMRI-LE acquisitions.

The 3D infarct volume was determined both in absolute units and as a percentage of the total LV myocardium volume (Fig. 1). The entire LV was imaged by both NOGA and cMRI-LE in order to obtain an accurate volume measurement. The non-contractile mitral valve areas, which are clearly visible in both images, were excluded from the quantitative analysis of infarct size and transmurality.

Polar plots were derived from the infarct segmentations using segmental transmurality data. The corresponding bull's eye maps were processed to achieve the same apex, heart axis, and orientation as for NOGA maps.

For these visualizations, viability data from 8 apico-basal slices and 32 wall sectors per slice were interpolated and smoothed. The linear borders of 17 segments were overlaid on the images

Table 1. NOGA endocardial unipolar and bipolar map-derived cut-off values.

Cut-off value	Color on the NOGA map	Definition
Unipolar voltage map		
>15 mV	Blue, violet	Normal tissue
5–15 mV	Yellow, green	Border zone of infarction
<5 mV	Red	Area of myocardial infarction
Bipolar voltage map		
>1.9 mV	Blue, violet	Normal tissue
0.8–1.9 mV	Yellow, green	Non-transmural infarction
<0.8 mV	Red	Transmural infarction

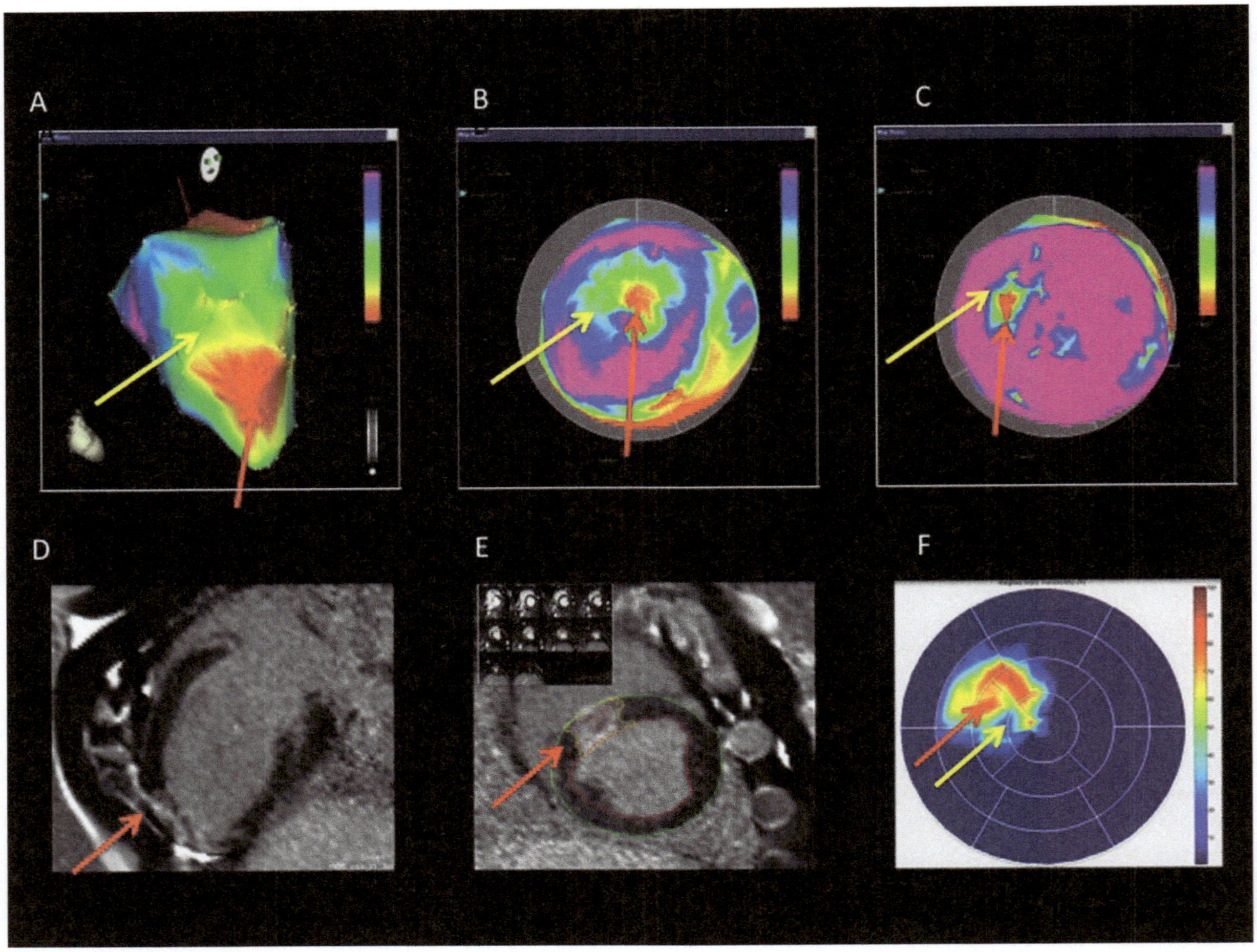

Figure 1. NOGA endocardial mapping and cardiac magnetic resonance imaging (cMRI) of a pig with chronic myocardial ischemia. A. 3D NOGA mapping showing anterior, anteroseptal, and apical myocardial infarction. Red indicates the infarct core (red arrow), the surrounding green-yellow area shows the border zone of infarction (yellow arrow). B. The corresponding unipolar voltage polar map. The color-coding is the same as in A. C. The bipolar voltage polar map of the same pig. Red indicates the transmural infarction (red arrow); yellow-green indicates the non-transmural infarction (yellow arrow), and blue-pink indicates normal myocardium. D. cMRI with late enhancement reveals the myocardial scar (red arrow). Long axis image. E. cMRI late enhancement short axis images with myocardial infarction (red arrow). Quantitative size of infarction was assessed by dividing of the myocardium to 8 slices from heart basis to apex (left upper corner). F. A cMRI transmurality polar map shows the transmural infarction (red arrow) with a surrounding area of non-transmural infarction (yellow arrow).

graphically to help interpret the images using "classical" segmental nomenclature, while the interpolated data originated from 32 sections per slice. The endo- and epicardial borders were segmented, and a segmental model was fitted on the left ventricle model (32 sections per slice). Using the standard transmurality analysis feature of the Segment software (Medviso Inc., Lund, Sweden), the midline was calculated for each section of the LV myocardium. The transmurality of the infarct is given as the radial projection of the segmented scar volume on the midline, summed for each section.

By applying two-dimensional planimetry to the polar plots, we performed two distinct measurements of the transmurality of the infarct. The extents of the transmural or non-transmural infarct and normal areas were defined as the percentage of sectors in which the SI was>75% (infarct core), 51–75% (border zone of infarction), 25–50% (non-transmural infarction), or <25% (normal) [22]. Alternatively, SI>60% was defined as transmural infarct, 31–60% as non-transmural infarct, and <30% as a normal area [21]. To calculate the areas, we used the raw transmurality data from 32 sections per slice, as noted above. All MRI area measurements are reported as the percentage of segments in the threshold range divided by the total number of segments.

Dynamic MR images were analyzed for myocardial wall movement and functional parameters. We carried out semi-automatic segmentation of the LV endocardial and epicardial borders while the end-diastolic volume (EDV), end-systolic volume (ESV), global LV ejection fraction (EF), and cardiac output (CO) were calculated automatically on short-axis images.

Overlap ratio

The overlap ratio between the cMRI and NOGA bipolar transmurality maps was calculated as follows [28] (Fig. 6):

(NOGA bipolar map overlap area + cMRI transmural map overlap area)/(NOGA bipolar low voltage area + cMRI transmurality area)

For the overlap ratio of the transmural, non-transmural and the combined transmural and non-transmural (not normal) areas the following cut-off values were used:

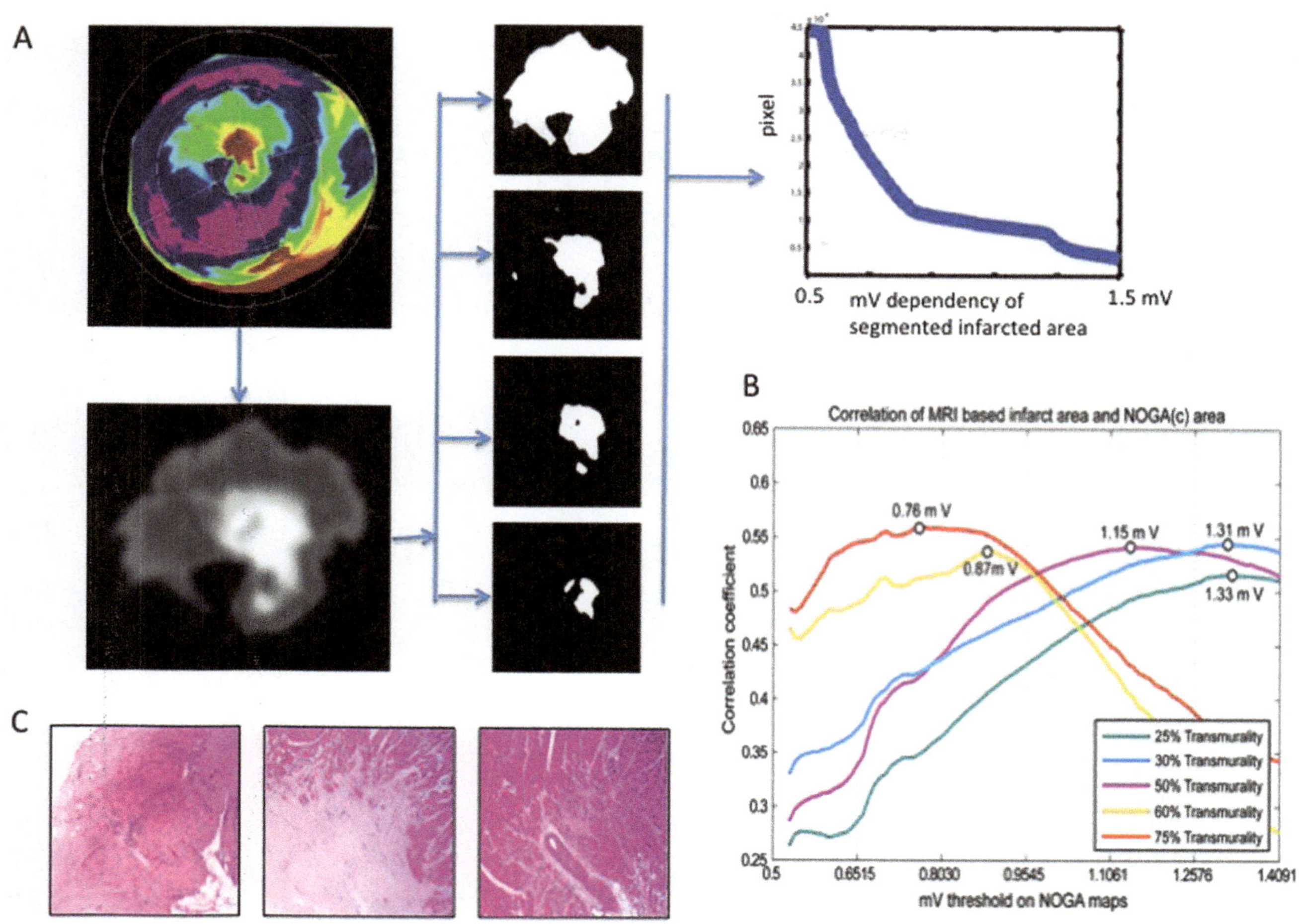

Figure 2. Magnet resonance imaging- (MRI-) derived NOGA bipolar threshold values for infarct transmurality. A. Iterative thresholding of voltage maps (left panel). The original NOGA maps were cropped to infarct areas, converted to a mV scale, then iteratively thresholded using 100 steps from 0.5 to 1.5 mV. The middle panel shows examples of the iterative thresholding process. The right panel shows the association between the area of infarction and the applied mV threshold. B. Voltage-threshold dependence of the correlation between NOGA maps and areas on an MRI. The maximum correlation coefficient is shown for each line plot. C. Histological correlations of transmural (left) and non-transmural (middle) infarctions and normal heart tissue (right). Samples were taken from areas with bipolar voltage values <0.8 mV, between 0.8–1.9 mV, and>1.9 mV with corresponding cMRI-LE transmurality values of>75%, 50%, and <25%, respectively. Magnification: 2x.

- Transmurality overlap ratio: between a NOGA bipolar map area with BipV <0.8 mV and a cMRI transmurality area with SI>75%;
- Non-transmural areas overlap ratio: between a NOGA bipolar map area with BipV 0.8-1.9 mV and a cMRI transmurality area with SI 25–75%;
- Combined transmural and non-transmural (not normal) area overlap ratio: between a NOGA bipolar map area with BipV <1.9 mV and a cMRI transmurality area with SI>25% (Figs. 4 and 5).

Overlap>60% was considered good accuracy [28], and 50–60% overlap was considered moderate accuracy (arbitrary value).

Histology

Myocardial samples were collected from transmural and non-transmural infarctions and from normal heart tissue. These were areas with bipolar voltage values <0.8 mV, from 0.8–1.9 mV, and>1.9 mV with corresponding cMRI-LE transmurality values of>75%, 50%, and <25%, respectively. The samples were stored in 4.5% buffered formalin for at least 24 h and embedded in paraffin. Sections were cut into 4- to 6-µM thick slices and stained with hematoxylin-eosin.

Statistical analysis

Continuous variables are presented as mean values ± standard deviation. The correlation between NOGA- and cMRI-derived parameters (infarct size, transmural and non-transmural infarct size) was calculated by linear regression analysis using Pearson Product Moment Correlation and Bland-Altman plots. Linear regression and Bland-Altman analysis was performed using Matlab R2010 software for Windows. During the iterative fitting of the linear function, a "least absolute residual" robust regression approach was used [31]. For interpretation of the correlations between 2 images the standardized nomenclature was used: if the correlation coefficient is greater than 0.5 is large, 0.5–0.3 is moderate, and 0.3–0.1 is a small correlation [32].

In order to choose the correct BiPV cut-off values for determining the transmural and non-transmural scars, all UPVs were also correlated with the corresponding BiPVs using linear regression analysis. Using a 5 mV UPV value as the cut-off for viability/non-viability, receiver operator curve (ROC) analysis was

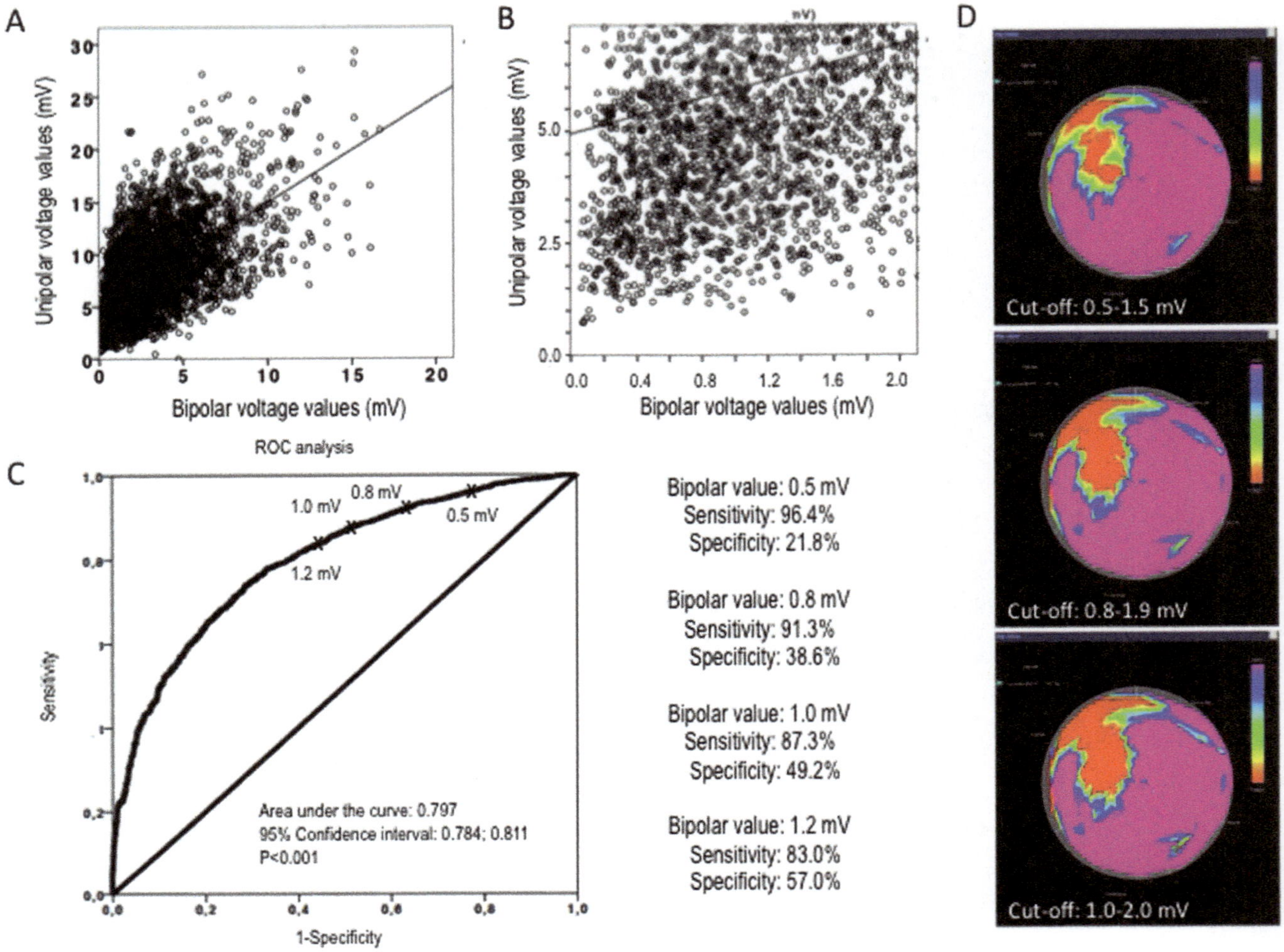

Figure 3. Determination of the bipolar voltage (BiPV) cut-off value for calculating the transmural and non-transmural infarct size using unipolar voltage values. A. Linear correlation between unipolar and bipolar voltage values. B. Part of the correlation showing the non-viable range defined as unipolar voltage values <5 mV. C. Receiver operator characteristics curve for determination of different bipolar voltage cut-off values. D. Display of bipolar maps using different cut-offs.

performed, and the sensitivity, specificity of different BiPV values, and the area under the curve, with 95% confidence intervals, were calculated.

For all statistical analyses, a p-value <0.05 was considered statistically significant.

Results

There were no complications during the NOGA and cMRI-LE procedures that required additional medication or cardiopulmonary resuscitation.

Correlation of NOGA threshold values with MRI-based transmurality

Depending on the threshold values applied to the NOGA bipolar voltage maps, the correlations between the different cut-offs of the two images were r = 0.27–0.57. The 75% MRI transmurality areas showed the best correlation with the NOGA-based areas using a cut-off of 0.76 mV, while the 60% transmurality areas correlated best with NOGA maps using a 0.87 mV threshold. The validation experiment resulted in a cut-off value of 1.3 mV for 25% transmurality. In order to exclude non-transmural ischemia, we used the usual value of 1.9 mV for normal, non-infarcted areas (Figure 2B). Notably, these cut-offs correlated well with the histological findings (Fig. 2C), confirming the proprietary diagnosis of transmural and non-transmural areas.

cMRI and NOGA mapping results

The cMRI-LE and NOGA endocardial mapping results are summarized in Tables 2 and 3. NOGA mapping and cMRI-LE showed similar results for LV volumes and global EF. Heart rates were slightly higher during the NOGA procedure, probably due to the longer procedure time.

The NOGA endocardial maps contained a mean of 202±31 (range: 152–295) mapping points per animal, with a mapping point distribution of 16.8±5.5 points per segment of the 12-segment view. The mapping points were connected automatically if the distance between points was less than 15 mm. The mean time for the NOGA procedure was 35±9 min.

The BiPV values correlated significantly with the UPV values (Fig. 3). ROC analysis showed that a BiPV value of 0.8 mV as the non-transmural cut-off value had a sensitivity>90% and low but acceptable specificity. Display of the bipolar maps with different cut-offs revealed small differences between the images, with a

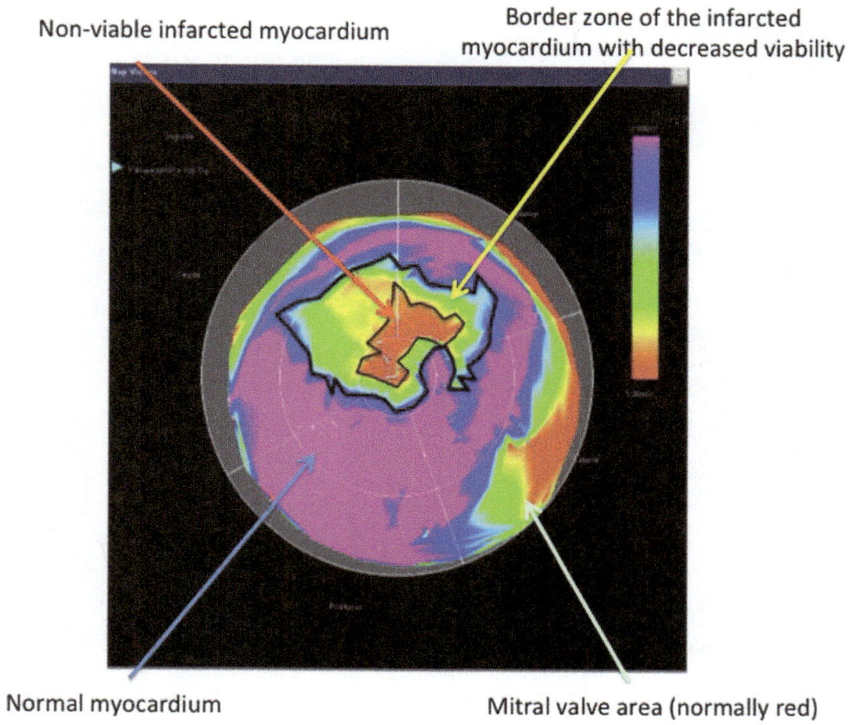

Figure 4. Schematic illustration of the planimetric calculation of the size of the infarct core and the size of the border zone of the infarction with decreased viability in the NOGA endocardial mapping. Red indicates the infarct core, and green-yellow indicates the surrounding area that has decreased viability.

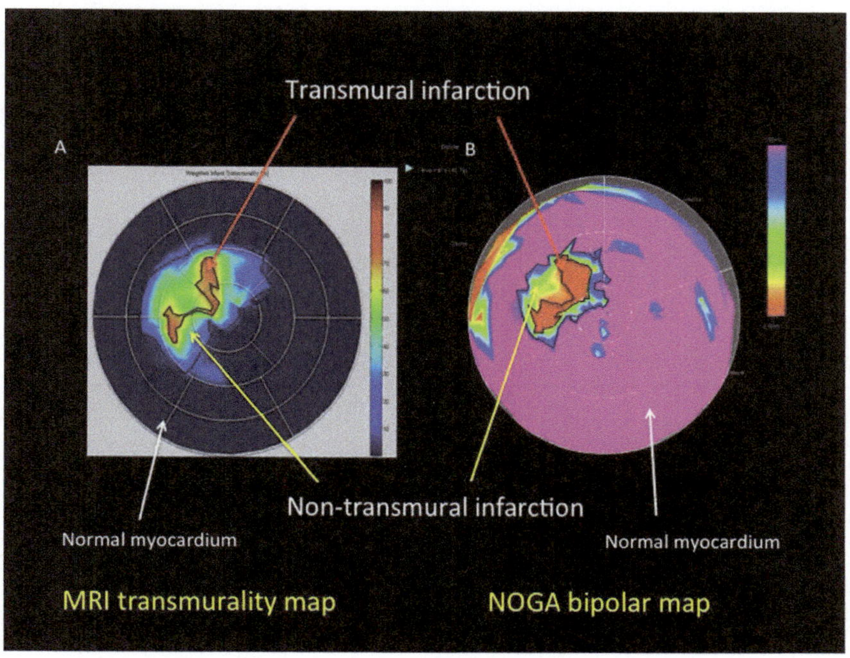

Figure 5. Schematic illustration of the planimetric calculation of the transmural and non-transmural infarct sizes as shown in polar maps from cardiac magnetic resonance imaging (cMRI) and NOGA endocardial mapping. A. Planimetric calculations of the sizes of the transmural and non-transmural infarction by cMRI. B. Planimetric calculations of the sizes of the transmural and non-transmural infarction in a NOGA bipolar voltage map.

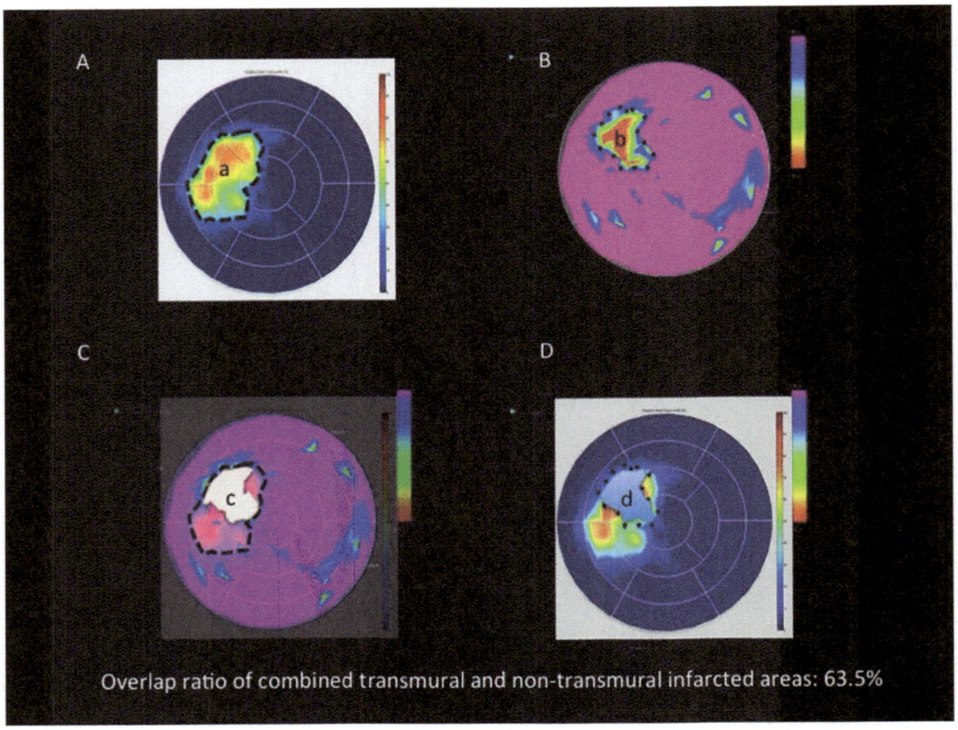

Figure 6. Calculation of the overlapping ratio of the transmural plus the non-transmural infarction by cardiac magnetic resonance imaging (cMRI) and NOGA endocardial mapping. A. cMRI transmurality polar map. B. NOGA bipolar polar map. C and D. Overlap of the cMRI and NOGA polar maps. a: The size of the transmural and non-transmural infarction by cMRI; b: the size of transmural and non-transmural infarction by NOGA bipolar mapping; c: overlap of the NOGA bipolar infarct shape on a cMRI polar map; d: overlap of the cMRI infarct shape on a NOGA bipolar map. The overlapping ratio was calculated as follows: (c+d)/(a+b).

transmural infarct size of 12.5±8.7% using a 0.5-mV cut-off value, 14.1±6.2% using a 0.8-mV cut-off value, and 16.8±5.3% using a 1-mV BiPV cut-off value, with no statistically significant differences between the 3 area measurements. Based on the best overlap ratio between the two images, a BiPV cut-off of 0.8–1.9 mV was used for further analysis.

The unipolar voltage map-derived scar size (UPV<5 mV) showed a moderate association with the transmural scar size as determined by bipolar maps (BiPV<0.8 mV) ($r=0.385$, $p=0.002$). There was better concordance between the border zone of infarction (UPV 5–15 mV) and non-transmural scars (BiPV 0.8–1.9 mV) ($r=0.457$, $p<0.001$). The total size of the ischemic area showed good correlation between the two maps ($r=0.575$, $p<0.001$).

Correlation of infarct size as determined by cMRI-LE and NOGA mapping

There was a significant correlation ($r=0.504$, $p<0.001$) between the infarct size as determined using the NOGA unipolar voltage polar map and the size determined by cMRI-LE. The Bland-Altman plot showed that NOGA mapping resulted in a systematically higher infarct size compared to cMRI-LE, with a mean difference between the two images of 2.82±7.43% in the LV surface (Fig. 7).

Table 2. Endocardial NOGA mapping results.

NOGA electromechanical mapping	Value (mean ±SD) (n = 60)
End-diastolic volume	108±12 mL
End-systolic volume	67.1±9.6 mL
Stroke volume	41.3±11.6 mL
Left ventricular ejection fraction	38.7±7.6%
Heart rate	110±7 bpm
Relative size of the infarct core (area of unipolar voltage <5 mV)	19.5±8.1%
Size of the area of border zone of the infarction (area of unipolar voltage 5–10 mV)	20.4±9.7%
Size of the transmural infarction (area of bipolar voltage <0.8 mV)	14.1±6.2%
Size of the non-transmural infarction (area of bipolar voltage 0.8–1.9 mV)	11.6±5.6%

Table 3. Results of cardiac magnetic resonance (cMRI) with late enhancement.

cMRI	Value (mean ±SD) (n = 60)
End-diastolic volume	106±22 mL
End-systolic volume	67.8±22 mL
Stroke volume	38.2±8.4 mL
Left ventricular ejection fraction	37.6±8.9%
Heart rate	102±11 bpm
Cardiac output	4.2±1.1 L/min
Cardiac index	3.7±0.9 L/min/m^2
Left ventricular myocardial mass	108±15 g
Left ventricular myocardial volume	103±14 mL
Relative infarct size of left ventricular myocardial mass	16.9±6.3%
Volume of myocardial infarction	15.7±6.5 mL
0%–30%–60%–100% SI for transmurality	
Size of transmural infarction if SI>60%	10.4±5.1%
Size of non-transmural infarction if SI = 31–60%	8.4±3.9%
Size of non-infarcted tissue if SI<30%	81.2±6.7%
0%–25%–50%–75%–100% SI for transmurality	
Size of transmural infarction if SI>75%	6.4±5.6%
Size of border zone of transmural infarction if SI = 51–75%	7.5±4.3%
Size of non-transmural infarction if SI = 25–50%	6.7±2.9%
Size of non-infarcted tissue if SI<25%	79.4±7.6%

SI: signal intensity.

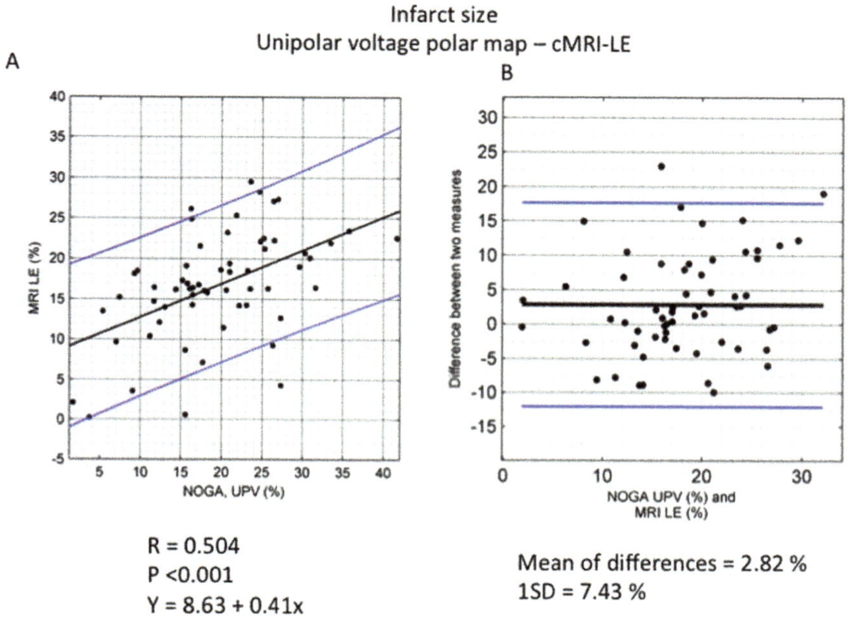

Figure 7. Correlation between NOGA endocardial mapping and cardiac magnetic resonance imaging (cMRI) and statistical analysis of the determination of infarct size. A. Regression equation between the size of the infarct core as determined on a unipolar voltage map (UPV) and as determined using late enhancement cMRI. B. Bland-Altman plot of the size of the infarct core as determined on a unipolar voltage map and the size as determined using late enhancement cMRI. Mean (black line) ±2SD (blue line).

Correlation of transmural infarct size as determined by cMRI and NOGA mapping

Using SI>75% and NOGA BipV <0.8 mV, the correlation between the two images was r = 0.727 (p<0.001) for the size of the transmural infarction. NOGA bipolar mapping resulted in a larger transmural infarction size than did cMRI-LE, with a mean difference of 6.81±4.39%) in the LV surface.

Using cut-offs for infarct transmurality of SI>60% and NOGA BipV<0.8 mV, the correlation was slightly lower (r = 0.576, p< 0.001), with a mean difference between the two images of 2.14%±5.62% of LV surface.

Correlation between cMRI and NOGA mapping regarding non-transmural infarct size

Using SI = 51–75% and NOGA BipV 0.8–1.9 mV to define non-transmural infarction, the correlation between the two images was r = 0.555 (p<0.001). NOGA bipolar mapping resulted in a smaller area of non-transmural infarction, with a mean difference of 3.04±5.92% between the two images (Fig. 8).

Using SI = 31–60% and NOGA BipV 0.8–1.9 mV as cut-offs for non-transmural infarction, the correlation was slightly higher (r = 0.657, p<0.001), with a mean difference between the two images of 3.23±4.56% of LV surface.

Overlap ratio

The overlap ratio was 81.6±11.1% and 70.6±18.5% for delineation of the transmural and non-transmural infarction size on the cMRI and NOGA images, respectively. None of the images showed an overlapping accuracy below 60% regarding transmural infarction. Regarding non-transmurality, two of the 60 animals (3.3%) showed an overlapping ratio between 50% and 60%, which was considered moderate agreement between the two imaging methods.

The overlap ratio of the combined transmural and non-transmural infarction was 70.2±12.2%.

Discussion

Our results indicate that NOGA electroanatomical mapping is accurate enough to guide targeted intramyocardial therapy if both unipolar and bipolar maps are used. The results of NOGA were comparable to those of cMRI-LE, regarding the extent of the transmural and non-transmural scars and viable and reduced viability myocardial areas.

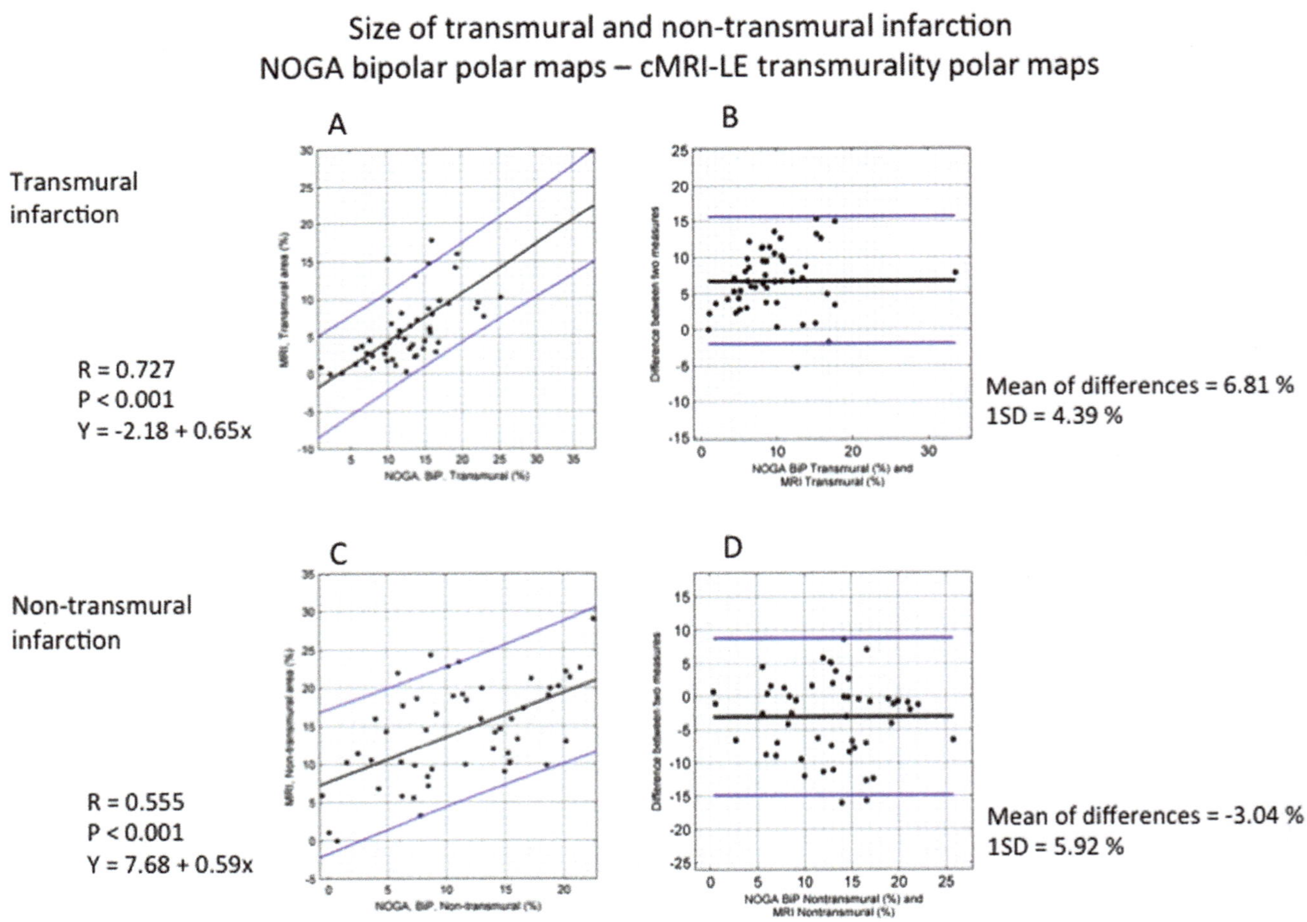

Figure 8. Correlation between NOGA endocardial mapping and cardiac magnetic resonance imaging (cMRI) and statistical analysis of the determinations of transmural and non-transmural infarction. A. Regression equation between the size of the transmural infarction as determined on a bipolar voltage map and the size as determined using cMRI. B. Bland-Altman plot of the size of the transmural infarction as determined on a bipolar voltage map and the size as determined using cMRI. Mean (black line) ±2SD (blue line). C. Regression equation between the size of the non-transmural infarction as determined on a bipolar voltage map and the size as determined using cMRI. D. Bland-Altman plot of the size of the non-transmural infarction as determined on a bipolar voltage map and the size as determined using cMRI. Mean (black line) ±2SD (blue line).

The main difference between the two 3D images is that different sampling methods are used to construct them. The NOGA 3D LV shape is constructed by point-to-point measurements, which is in contrast with the other 3D methods, such as cMRI-LE, which have a spatial resolution of 1.4 mm per voxel. For map construction, a 15-mm point-to-point distance was used by endocardial mapping, while an in-plane resolution of 1–2 mm with an 8-mm slice thickness was utilized for cMRI-LE analysis. Accordingly, the accuracy of the NOGA map depends mainly on the number of gathered and measured points and on the quality of the acquired points used to construct the 3D map. Difficulties in reaching some regions with the mapping catheter due to LV cavity structures such as the papillary muscles or the occurrence of ventricular arrhythmias due to touching vulnerable ischemic areas might lead to insufficient sampling, resulting in incomplete mapping. Nevertheless, unipolar voltage mapping overestimated the infarct size by just 2.82% of the entire LV endocardial surface, and bipolar mapping overestimated the transmural scar by just 6.82% of the LV. These estimates are acceptable for performing intramyocardial procedures safely and accurately. The overestimation of the infarct size and transmural scar as compared to cMRI-LE might result from the quantitative comparison of 2D NOGA polar maps and 3D cMRI-LE and 2D transmurality cMRI-LE images. According to our results, both the unipolar and bipolar voltage maps showed wider zones of interest than on cMRI, which may raise the risk of injecting reparative substances into normal myocardium. The intramyocardial injections are oriented into the non-transmural infarct or into areas with decreased viability. Different cut-offs are suggested for viability and transmurality thresholds in the literature; there are no universally agreed-upon definitions for these terms. Of course, the operators should try to make sure that the intramyocardial injections are made into the correct area, but an injection may be made into the "normal" myocardium if stronger cut-off criteria for non-normal territory are used. However, regenerative cells or other material delivered into the lane neighboring the non-transmural infarction have a good chance of being retained, being functional, and migrating or penetrating into the ischemic area, so a wider zone might result in more effective and safe treatment.

The sizes of the unipolar voltage scar and border zone differed from the sizes of transmural and non-transmural infarction as determined on the bipolar maps. Although the total size of the unhealthy areas on the unipolar and bipolar polar maps showed good correlation, the size of the infarction and border area determined on the unipolar maps was systematically larger than the size of the transmural and non-transmural regions on the bipolar maps. This is not surprising, because an infarct area contains heterogeneously viable myocytes that can be apoptotic or hibernating. Accordingly, the infarct core and the border area (i.e. the extent of infarction) do not necessarily overlap the transmural and non-transmural infarction (i.e. the infarction severity) because the infarct core may include transmural and non-transmural necrotic areas.

The unipolar voltage values represent a summation of the action potentials of the surrounding endocardial surface areas, while the bipolar voltage values represent the amplified difference between the tip of the unipolar electrode and the additional proximal electrode placed within the catheter. Accordingly, a non-transmural infarction with severe endocardial (but not epicardial) necrosis may appear to be an infarct core in the unipolar map. This might explain the differences between the unipolar and bipolar NOGA maps, and between the NOGA maps and other 3D images that measure infarct size. Nevertheless, using both (uni- and bipolar) maps of the NOGA images, information about both the extent and the severity of infarction are available real-time, on-table during a procedure, in contrast to off-line images such as cMRI-LE or myocardial single photon emission computed tomography.

Additionally, to set the correct and right cut-off values of the NOGA maps is of great importance. Several authors used several different cut-off values for definition of viability using the unipolar voltage maps, while the usage of bipolar maps is less common, probably due to the small range of not normal values (0–1.9 mV of interest) suggesting less precise differentiations. We have measured the transmural and non-transmural scars on the cMRI-LE image using two different SI cut-offs, because a SI between 25% and 50% suggests a false positive non-transmural infarction. When the cMRI transmurality threshold is lowered to 60% from 75% and to 31–60% from 51–75%, the size of the transmural and non-transmural infarct areas increase, and the correlations are slightly lower and higher, respectively. The SI of 30% and 60% for cut-off of non-transmural and transmural scars gave a better correlation with slight overestimation of the non-transmural scar by 3.23% of the LV. Since the endocardial injections should target non-transmural infarct areas, higher correlation between the two images in that region is desirable.

Comparison of our results with literature data

The need to localize the arrhythmogenic focus for ablation during catheter-based electrophysiological procedure prompted several research groups to develop hybrid software that analyzes the 3D images of both NOGA maps and cMRI-LE. Fusion of cMRI with electroanatomical mapping of the LV proved to be successful with a registration error of 3.8±0.6 mm [22], with visual mismatches between the NOGA scars and LE in cMRI, particularly in patients with inferior infarction [22]. To enhance the accuracy of the electroanatomical mapping relative to cMRI-LE for the determination of myocardial scars with a presumed arrhythmogenic focus, different cut-off values were tested: 1.5 mV for non-transmural scars and 0.5 mV for dense scars [22]; 1.0 mV [28], 1.3 mV [23], 1.54 mV [24], 1.55 mV [26], and 1.9 mV [27] for bipolar maps; and 5.8 mV [23], 6.52 mV [24], 6.9 mV [18], 6.78 mV [26], 6.7 mV [27], and 5.1 mV [28] for unipolar maps. This reflects the uncertainty of finding the arrhythmogenic focus with electroanatomical mapping alone and emphasizes the visual mismatch between the two images in certain cases. In contrast with these studies, the sample size in our animal study was much larger (n = 60), but we did not use fusion software. Instead, we compared the 2D maps of the NOGA images with the 3D LE and 2D transmurality map of the cMRI. Nevertheless, we did not search for a single focus but rather for an area with reduced viability.

Limitations

We did not use local linear shortening maps of the NOGA for delineating of the hibernating myocardium characterized by preserved viability and decreased segmental wall motion [12], because of the lower accuracy of the local linear shortening map and higher discordance with cMRI [9] regarding the segmental wall motion abnormalities. We overlaid the two images in order to determine the overlapping accuracies, while other research groups used 3D fusion software. Accordingly, our method has several shortcomings in the technique used. The study reports comparisons of 2D transmurality cMRIs and NOGA bipolar maps as well as comparisons of the 2D projection of the NOGA-derived infarct size and the 3D cMRI-LE-derived infarct size. However, both imaging modalities for quantitatively determining infarct size use standardized image processing functions of the software and are widely used.

We are aware that there are ongoing efforts to fuse 3D NOGA endocardial maps and cardiac MRIs to determine the similarities of infarct location and extent. Although numerous percutaneous intramyocardial therapy studies are currently underway with the aim of determining the optimal injection location, currently there is no commercially available 3D MRI-NOGA fusion software. The comparisons of cMRI and NOGA polar maps published previously lack some of the refinements we used, such as comparison of the transmurality map with the bipolar map and calculation of the overlapping ratio.

Unfortunately, we could not perform 3D volumetric co-registration of the compared modalities, as currently we do not have an image-processing tool with which to conduct such a comparison. The spatial correspondence was ensured by (1) similar selection of the basal and apical slice positions and (2) similar orientation of the bull's eye maps. The definition of sector orientation was based on manual selection of the right ventricular insertion point (sector 0) on the most basal MRI slice of the left ventricular myocardium. A real value of the fusion of the off-line cMRI-LE and on-table NOGA endocardial mapping would be the real-time display of the actual catheter position and location of the intramyocardial therapy on the reconstructed hybrid (cMRI and NOGA) image; which software is currently not available.

We have included the NOGA-derived volumetric measurements. The similarities between the NOGA-derived and cMRI-derived end-diastolic and end-systolic volume and calculated stroke volume and ejection fraction (Tables 2 and 3) ensure the acquisition of the entire LV map of the NOGA procedure and also ensure that the two images are comparable.

The use of 2SD method of cMRI-LE might overestimate the infarct size, as compared with the 5SD or "full width at half maximum" (FWHM) method. In our experience, it has not been the case that the 5SD method better reflects the infarct size compared to the 2SD approach, and there are data in the literature that show a higher correlation coefficient for the 2SD approach than the 5SD approach [33]. The FWHM method might correlate better with post-mortem measurements, but this approach has not yet been implemented into the software we used for our data analysis. Based on the different sampling modes and standardized segmentation of both MRI (17 segments divided into 6 basal, 6 mid and 5 apical segments) and NOGA (9 segments divided into 4 basal, 4 mid and 1 apex segments), direct comparison of segmental mean values to search for a mathematical cut-off for unipolar and bipolar values based on MRI cut-off values would require extensive digital processing and adaptation of both images. However, we correlated the unipolar and bipolar voltage values and calculated different bipolar voltage cut-offs using ROC analysis. Additionally, we have determined the optimal bipolar cut-offs using iterative thresholding and calculated the transmural and non-transmural infarct areas using 3 cut-offs and compared these results with those of the cMRI-LE data. However, we did not search unipolar voltage threshold values based on cMRI-LE images because voltage maps correspond to myocardial viability and cMRI is not the first-choice imaging method for viability assessment. Extensive research has been performed to establish cut-offs for viable, non-viable, and hibernating myocardium using imaging technologies such as myocardial scintigraphy and positron emission tomography [9]. We used these literature-based cut-off values to calculate infarct size.

Conclusions

Our results demonstrate the usefulness of unipolar and bipolar maps generated using real-time electroanatomical mapping for targeted intramyocardial regenerative therapy. NOGA mapping showed good concordance with the off-line gold standard, cMRI-LE imaging. NOGA mapping may be useful in patients with contraindications for cMRI who require targeted intramyocardial regenerative therapy.

Author Contributions

Conceived and designed the experiments: NP AJ ME SH MG. Performed the experiments: NP AJ ME SH MG. Analyzed the data: NP AJ ME GS PW MZ HJA GM MG. Contributed reagents/materials/analysis tools: AJ PW GS MZ. Wrote the paper: NP MG.

References

1. Freyman T, Polin G, Osman H, Crary J, Lu M, et al. (2006) A quantitative, randomized study evaluating three methods of mesenchymal stem cell delivery following myocardial infarction. Eur Heart J 27: 1114–22.
2. Perin EC, Silva GV, Assad JAR, Vela D, Buja LM, et al. (2008) Comparison of intracoronary and transendocardial delivery of allogeneic mesenchymal cells in a canine model of acute myocardial infarction. J Mol Cell Cardiol 44: 486–495.
3. Dib N, Khawaja H, Varner S, McCarthy M, Campbell A (2011) Cell therapy for cardiovascular disease: a comparison of methods of delivery. J Cardiovasc Transl Res. 4: 177–81.
4. Vrtovec B, Poglajen G, Lezaic L, Sever M, Socan A, et al. (2013). Comparison of transendocardial and intracoronary CD34+ cell transplantation in patients with nonischemic dilated cardiomyopathy. Circulation 128(11 Suppl 1): S42–9.
5. Constantine G, Shan K, Flamm SD, Sivananthan MU (2004) Role of MRI in clinical cardiology. Lancet 363: 2162–71.
6. Poon M, Fuster V, Fayad Z (2002) Cardiac magnetic resonance imaging: a "one-stop-shop" evaluation of myocardial dysfunction. Curr Opin Cardiol 17: 663–70.
7. Ben-Haim SA, Osadchy D, Schuster I, Gepstein L, Hayam G, et al. (1996) Nonfluoroscopic, in vivo navigation and mapping technology. Nat Med 2: 1393–5.
8. Gepstein L, Hayam G, Shpun S, Ben-Haim SA (1997) Hemodynamic evaluation of the heart with a nonfluoroscopic electromechanical mapping technique. Circulation 96: 3672–80.
9. Gyöngyösi M, Dib N (2011) Diagnostic and prognostic value of 3D NOGA mapping in ischemic heart disease. Nat Rev Cardiol 8: 393–404.
10. Psaltis PJ Worthley SG (2009) Endoventricular electromechanical mapping—the diagnostic and therapeutic utility of the NOGA XP Cardiac Navigation System. J Cardiovasc Transl Res 2: 48–62.
11. Kornowski R, Hong MK, Leon MB (1998) Comparison between left ventricular electromechanical mapping and radionuclide perfusion imaging for detection of myocardial viability. Circulation 98: 1837–41.
12. Gyöngyösi, M. Khorsand A, Sochor H, Sperker W, Strehblow C, et al. (2005) Characterization of hibernating myocardium with NOGA electroanatomic endocardial mapping. Am J Cardiol 95: 722–8.
13. Gyöngyösi M, Sochor H, Khorsand A, Gepstein L, Glogar D (2001) Online myocardial viability assessment in the catheterization laboratory via NOGA electroanatomic mapping: quantitative comparison with thallium-201 uptake. Circulation 104: 1005–11.
14. Callans DJ, Ren JF, Michele J, Marchlinski FE, Dillon SM (1999) Electroanatomic left ventricular mapping in the porcine model of healed anterior myocardial infarction. Correlation with intracardiac echocardiography and pathological analysis. Circulation 100: 1744–50.
15. Fuchs S, Hendel RC, Baim DS, Moses JW, Pierre A, et al. (2001) Comparison of endocardial electromechanical mapping with radionuclide perfusion imaging to assess myocardial viability and severity of myocardial ischemia in angina pectoris. Am J Cardiol 87: 874–80.
16. Keck A, Hertting K, Schwartz Y, Kitzing R, Weber M, et al. (2002) Electromechanical mapping for determination of myocardial contractility and viability. A comparison with echocardiography, myocardial single-photon emission computed tomography, and positron emission tomography. J Am Coll Cardiol 40: 1067–74.
17. Sheehan FH, Bolson EL, McDonald JA, Reisman M, Koch KC, et al. (2002) Method for three-dimensional data registration from disparate imaging modalities in the NOGA Myocardial Viability Trial. IEEE Trans Med Imaging 21: 1264–70.
18. Perin EC, Silva GV, Sarmento-Leite R, Sousa AL, Howell M, et al. (2002) Assessing myocardial viability and infarct transmurality with left ventricular

electromechanical mapping in patients with stable coronary artery disease: validation by delayed-enhancement magnetic resonance imaging. Circulation 106: 957–61.
19. Wiggers H, Bøtker HE, Søgaard P, Kaltoft A, Hermansen F, et al. (2003) Electromechanical mapping versus positron emission tomography and single photon emission computed tomography for the detection of myocardial viability in patients with ischemic cardiomyopathy. J Am Coll Cardiol 41: 843–8.
20. Graf S, Gyöngyösi M, Khorsand A, Nekolla SG, Pirich C, et al. (2004) Electromechanical properties of the perfusion/metabolism mismatch: comparison of nonfluoroscopic electroanatomic mapping with ^{18}F-FDG PET imaging. J Nucl Med 45: 1611–8.
21. Wolf T, Gepstein L, Dror U, Hayam G, Shofti R, et al. (2001) Detailed endocardial mapping accurately predicts the transmural extent of myocardial infarction. J Am Coll Cardiol 37: 1590–7.
22. Wijnmaalen AP, van der Geest RJ, van Huls van Taxis CF, Siebelink HM, et al. (2011) Head-to-head comparison of contrast-enhanced magnetic resonance imaging and electroanatomical voltage mapping to assess post-infarct scar characteristics in patients with ventricular tachycardias: real-time image integration and reversed registration. Eur Heart J 32: 104–14.
23. Desjardins B, Crawford T, Good E, Oral H, Chugh A, et al. (2009) Infarct architecture and characteristics on delayed enhanced magnetic resonance imaging and electroanatomic mapping in patients with postinfarction ventricular arrhythmia. Heart Rhythm 6: 644–51.
24. Codreanu A, Odille F, Aliot E, Marie PY, Magnin-Poull I, et al. (2008) Electroanatomic characterization of post-infarct scars comparison with 3-dimensional myocardial scar reconstruction based on magnetic resonance imaging. J Am Coll Cardiol 52: 839–842.
25. Gupta S, Desjardins B, Baman T, Ilg K, Good E, et al. (2012) Delayed-enhanced MR scar imaging and intraprocedural registration into an electroanatomical mapping system in post-infarction patients. JACC Cardiovasc Imaging 5: 207–10.
26. Desjardins B, Yokokawa M, Good E, Crawford T, Latchamsetty R, et al. (2013) Characteristics of intramural scar in patients with nonischemic cardiomyopathy and relation to intramural ventricular arrhythmias. Circ Arrhythm Electrophysiol 6: 891–7.
27. Spears DA, Suszko AM, Dalvi R, Crean AM, Ivanov J, et al. (2012) Relationship of bipolar and unipolar electrogram voltage to scar transmurality and composition derived by magnetic resonance imaging in patients with nonischemic cardiomyopathy undergoing VT ablation. Heart Rhythm 9: 1837–46.
28. Tokuda M, Tedrow UB, Inada K, Reichlin T, Michaud GF, et al. (2013) Direct comparison of adjacent endocardial and epicardial electrograms: implications for substrate mapping. J Am Heart Assoc. 2: e000215.
29. van Slochteren FJ, Teske AJ, van der Spoel TI, Koudstaal S, Doevendans PA, et al. (2012) Advanced measurement techniques of regional myocardial function to assess the effects of cardiac regenerative therapy in different models of ischaemic cardiomyopathy. Eur Heart J Cardiovasc Imaging 13: 808–18.
30. Heiberg E, Sjögren J, Ugander M, Carlsson M, Engblom H, et al. (2010) Design and validation of Segment–freely available software for cardiovascular image analysis. BMC Medical Imaging 10: 1–13.
31. Holland PW, Welsch RE (1977) Robust Regression Using Iteratively Reweighted Least-Squares. Communications in Statistics: Theory and Methods, A6, pp.813–827.
32. Cohen J (1988) Statistical power analysis for the behavioral sciences (2nd ed.). Hillsdale, NJ: Lawrence Earlbaum Associates
33. Amado LC, Gerber BL, Gupta SN, Rettmann DW, Szarf G, et al. (2004) Accurate and objective infarct sizing by contrast-enhanced magnetic resonance imaging in a canine myocardial infarction model. J Am Coll Cardiol 44: 2383–9.

24

Mapping of Autogenous Saphenous Veins as an Imaging Adjunct to Peripheral MR Angiography in Patients with Peripheral Arterial Occlusive Disease and Peripheral Bypass Grafting: Prospective Comparison with Ultrasound and Intraoperative Findings

Ann-Marie Bintu Munda Jah-Kabba[1], Guido Matthias Kukuk[1], Dariusch Reza Hadizadeh[1], Frank Träber[1], Arne Koscielny[2], Mustapha Sundifu Kabba[2], Frauke Verrel[2], Hans Heinz Schild[1], Winfried Albert Willinek[1]*

1 University of Bonn, Dept. of Radiology, Germany, **2** University of Bonn, Dept. of Surgery, Germany

Abstract

Background: Mapping of the great saphenous vein is very important for planning of peripheral and coronary bypass surgery. This study investigated mapping of the great saphenous vein as an adjunct to peripheral MR angiography using a blood pool contrast agent in patients who were referred for evaluation of peripheral arterial occlusive disease and bypass surgery.

Methods: 38 patients with peripheral arterial occlusive disease (21 men; mean age: 71 years, range, 44–88 years) underwent peripheral MR angiography using the blood pool contrast agent Gadofosveset trisodium. Apart from primary arterial assessment images were evaluated in order to determine great saphenous vein diameters at three levels: below the saphenofemoral junction, mid thigh and 10 cm above the knee joint (usability: diameter range: >3 and <10 mm at one level and >3.5 and <10 mm at a neighboring level). Duplex ultrasound was performed by an independent examiner providing diameter measurements at the same levels. Additionally, vessel usability was determined intraoperatively by the vascular surgeon during subsequent bypass surgery.

Results: Mean venous diameters for MR angiography/duplex ultrasound were $5.4\pm2.6/5.5\pm2.8$ mm (level 1), $4.7\pm2.7/4.6\pm2.9$ mm (level 2) and $4.4\pm2.2/4.5\pm2.3$ mm (level 3), respectively, without significant differences between the modalities ($P=0.207/0.806/0.518$). Subsequent surgery was performed in 27/38 patients. A suitable saphenous vein was diagnosed in 25 and non-usability was diagnosed in 2 of the 27 patients based on MR angiography/duplex ultrasound, respectively. Usability was confirmed by intraoperative assessment in all of the 24 patients that received a venous bypass graft in subsequent bypass surgery. In 1 case, in which the great saphenous vein was assessed as useable by both MR angiography and duplex ultrasound, it was not used during subsequent bypass surgery due to the patients clinical condition and comorbidities.

Conclusion: Simultaneous mapping of the great saphenous vein as an imaging adjunct to peripheral MR angiography with a blood pool contrast agent is an alternative to additive duplex ultrasound in patients undergoing subsequent peripheral bypass grafting.

Editor: Alberto Aliseda, University of Washington, United States of America

Funding: These authors have no support or funding to report.

Competing Interests: The authors have read the journals policy and have the following conflicts: Winfried Willinek has/had speakers bureau appointments with Bracco, Bayer AG, Lantheus Medical Imaging, Koninklijke Philips Electronics and General Electric Company. He is/was on the advisory board of Bayer AG, Lantheus Medical Imaging and General Electric Company.

* Email: Winfried.Willinek@ukb.uni-bonn.de

Introduction

The first bypass surgery with an autologous saphenous vein was carried out by Jean Kunlin in 1948 [1]. Nowadays bypass grafting has been fully established as a standard surgical treatment option in peripheral arterial occlusive disease (PAOD). An autologous saphenous vein is generally regarded as the material of choice for a femorodistal bypass [2]–[4], since it provides the best patency rates [4] and its anatomic position, its length and its wall strength make it suitable to be used as an arterial bypass graft [5]. This is particularly true if it is of good quality i.e. wide enough in diameter

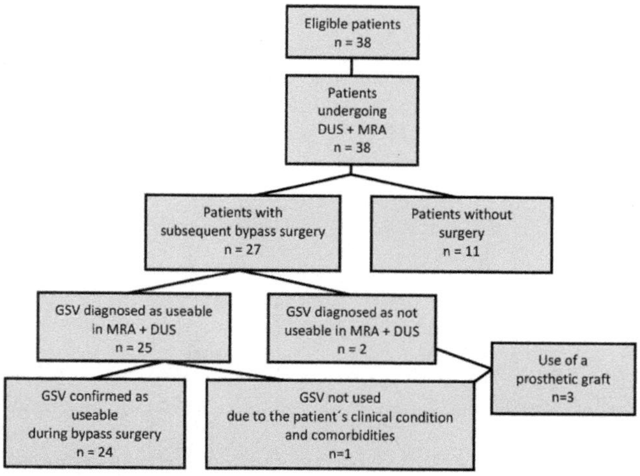

Figure 1. Flowchart portraying the study design.

as well as free of varicosities, thrombotic segments and too many tributaries [6].

Since the 1970 s, the preoperative assessment of the saphenous vein regarding its anatomic configuration, venous abnormalities and pathologic changes has been proven successful in evaluating its suitability as a bypass graft in arterial reconstructions [7], [8]. In the 1980 s, the use of phlebography [9] was challenged by B-mode ultrasound [10], [11] being a procedure which is not invasive, prevents confusion concerning the discrimination of deep and superficial veins and last but not least renders more accurate information about the venous diameters [12], [13].

The advantages of the preoperative saphenous vein mapping, i.e. reduction in morbidity, operation time and hospital stay [13], have been evaluated in several studies on coronary artery grafts [14], [15] as well as peripheral bypass surgery [16], [17].

The major quantitative parameter which has to be determined during venous mapping and has been identified as the predominant technical factor in predicting primary patency, primary assisted patency and secondary patency is the internal venous diameter [4]. In this context the superiority of veins having a larger diameter (>3.5 mm) over narrow ones (<3 mm) is well established [4], [18]. However, Wengerter et al. demonstrated that grafts having a diameter of 3.5 mm as well as grafts which have a diameter of 3.0 mm and are at the same time not longer than 45 mm, present similar patency rates compared to grafts which have a diameter of at least 4.0 mm [19]. This highlights the point that the decisive factor for the short- and long-term success of the bypass surgery is the suitability of the venous conduit, which may be even more important than the quality of the arteries.

B-mode ultrasound has been established as the gold standard in the preoperative mapping of the great saphenous vein (GSV) [20]. However, this noninvasive procedure is highly operator dependent, very time consuming, especially in patients who have already undergone venous surgery, and has technical limitations in patients with edema, obesity and ulcerations.

Contrast-enhanced magnetic resonance angiography (CE-MRA) is considered an alternative to digital subtraction angiography (DSA) in the diagnosis and assessment of patients with peripheral arterial occlusive disease [21], [22] and increasingly replaces DSA in the imaging of the arterial vascular system [23]. However, spatial resolution is limited with standard extracellular Gadolinium chelates during "first pass" imaging. Recently, a contrast agent, with a reversible albumin binding and an extended intravascular retention and contrast enhancement [24], a "blood pool contrast agent (BPCA)", was approved by the U.S. Food and Drug Administration (FDA). During "first pass" it offers an image quality which, depending on the dose, is at least as good as that of standard extracellular contrast agents [25]–[27]. In addition to first pass MR angiography, blood pool contrast agents allow contrast enhancement during an "equilibrium phase" (i.e. steady state) due to the lack of a relevant extravasation of the contrast agent into the interstitial space. Providing an imaging window of up to 60 minutes [28], the equilibrium phase facilitates the acquisition of much higher spatial resolution images without a significant loss of vessel-to-background contrast [28]–[30]. Steady state MRA with the blood pool contrast agent Gadofosveset trisodium in patients with peripheral arterial occlusive disease was found to render better results than first pass imaging alone [31] and leads – as an add-on – to the simultaneous visualization of the venous system [30]. The additional visualization of veins to that of arteries is inherent to steady state MRA and requires neither a second contrast administration nor any other change of examination parameters. As early as in 1998, Grist et al. indicated the benefits which might be drawn from the simultaneous visualization of arteries and veins in the steady state imaging with Gadofosveset [29]. Today, preliminary data supports the hypothesis that this approach allows for MR-venography as an add-on to the MRA of the arterial system [32]–[34]. Gadofosveset-enhanced MR-imaging has already been proven successful in the detection of thromboembolic processes. Deep venous thrombosis [35] as well as collateral pathways in patients suffering from a massive thromboembolic occlusion of the central veins were reliably detected; the latter could even be achieved in a way better than conventional X-ray-based phlebography [30].

The basis of this work was the hypothesis that peripheral MRA in the steady state using a blood pool contrast agent to image the size and quality of great saphenous veins would be a useful adjunct to arterial phase MRA to improve the performance of peripheral bypass surgery in patients with PAOD. Thus, the purpose of this study was to prospectively determine the accuracy of high-spatial-resolution steady-state MR angiography using the blood pool contrast agent Gadofosveset trisodium in comparison to color-coded duplex ultrasound (DUS) as the standard of reference in order to assess the usability of autologous saphenous veins for subsequent peripheral bypass surgery. Results were correlated with intraoperative findings.

Methods

Ethics Statement

The study protocol was approved by the institutional ethic committee of the University Hospital Bonn, Germany (approval number: 132/07). All patients provided written informed consent.

Patients

This prospective, intraindividual comparative study included 38 consecutive patients (mean age, 71 years; range, 44–88 years) (21 men, 17 women) (table 1) with peripheral arterial occlusive disease who underwent 3D-enhanced MR angiography in preparation for or evaluation of a peripheral (femoropopliteal, popliteocrural or femorocrural) bypass surgery (figure 1).

Clinical inclusion criteria were PAOD stage IIb-IV (Fontaine classification) and indication for MRA. Exclusion criteria were contraindications for 3D contrast-enhanced MR angiography (e.g. allergy, metallic implants that are incompatible with MR imaging including pacemakers). The indication for MRA was defined clinically by the vascular surgeons. Every patient who was enrolled

Table 1. Clinical and demographic characteristics of the study population.

	PAOD stage II b	PAOD stage III	PAOD stage IV
number of patients	13	9	16
age range - years	57–78	45–88	56–85
male sex - no.	7	3	11

All patients were of white ethnicity.

into the study also underwent DUS. 3D contrast-enhanced MR angiographic and ultrasound examinations were carried out in random order. MR-angiographic venous mapping was performed as an adjunct to the BPCA-MRA which was done in order to assess arterial occlusive disease. A possible surgical intervention was not delayed for any patient because of his or her participation in this study.

MR Angiography

MR imaging was performed as previously described [31]: A 1.5-T whole–body imager (Achieva; Philips Healthcare) (maximum gradient amplitude, 33 mT/m; slew rate, 200 T/m/sec) was used to acquire three-dimensional contrast-enhanced MR angiographic sequences of the vasculature. While images of the lower legs were obtained using a commercially available flexible four-channel phased-array coil (Philips Healthcare, Best, the Netherlands), an

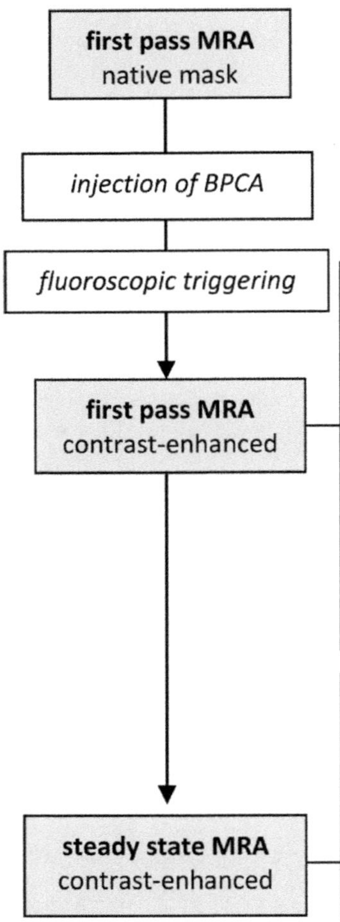

First pass MRA, contrast-enhanced:

	pelvis	upper legs	lower legs
repetition time msec	2.7	2.8	4.8
echo time msec	0.89	0.94	1.36
flip angle (degrees)	25	25	25
field of view (mm)	451	451	451
rectangular field of view (%)	100	100	100
slab thickness (mm)	104	90	88
image matrix	384 x 285	336 x 252	400 x 300
partition	65	60	80
k space acquisition order	CENTRA	CENTRA	CENTRA
acquired voxel (mm)	1.48 x 2.33 x 1.60	1.34 x 2.11 x 1.50	1.13 x 1.77 x 1.10
reconstructed voxel (mm)	1.04 x 1.04 x 1.60	0.88 x 0.88 x 1.50	0.88 x 0.88 x 1.10
acquisition time	12.6	13.4	35.9

Steady state MRA, contrast-enhanced:

	pelvis	upper legs	lower legs
repetition time msec	4.8	4.9	5.8
echo time msec	1.42	1.44	1.68
flip angle (degrees)	25	25	25
field of view (mm)	451	451	451
rectangular field of view (%)	100	100	100
slab thickness (mm)	135	94.05	83.3
image matrix	400 x 300	416 x 312	464 x 348
partition	90	95	170
k space acquisition order	linear	linear	linear
acquired voxel (mm)	1.13 x. 1.48 x 1.50	1.08 x 1.42 x0.99	0.97 x 0.97 x 0.49
reconstructed voxel (mm)	0.88 x 0.88 x 1.50	0.88 x 0.88 x 0.88	0.52 x 0.52 x 0.49
acquisition time	100	110	174

Figure 2. MR-angiographic protocol. Sequence flow of the combined first-pass and steady-state MR angiographic protocol and technical parameters of T1-weighted gradient-echo sequences for first-pass and steady-state MR angiography.

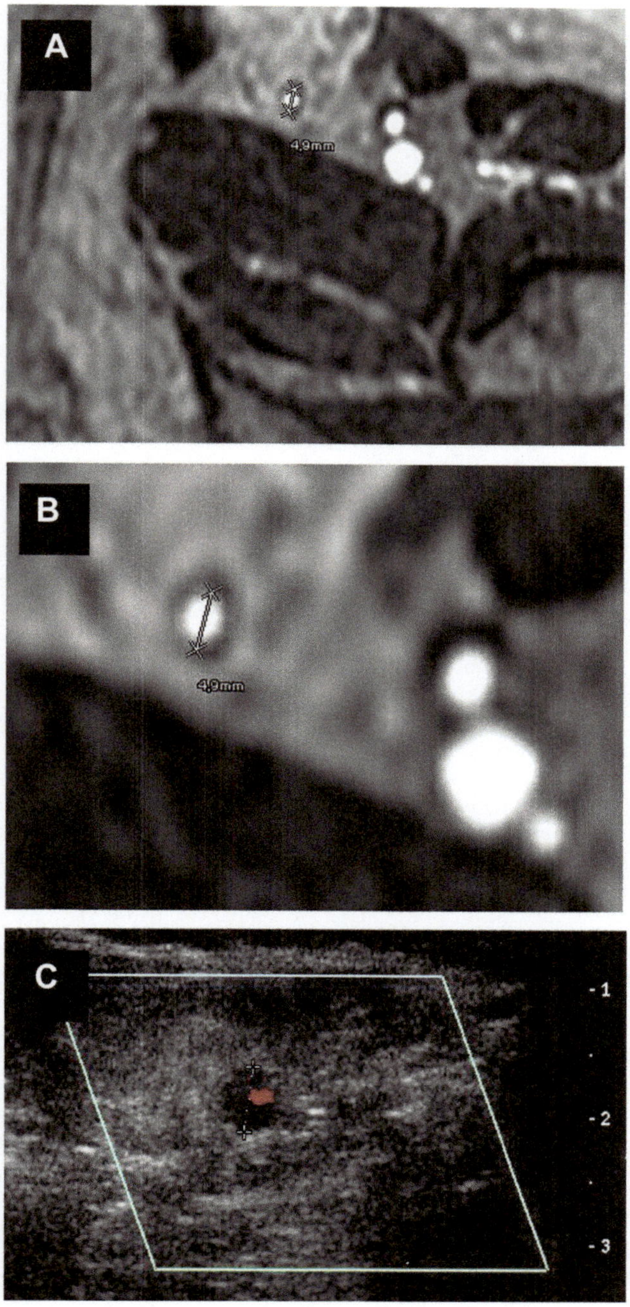

Figure 3. MR-angiographic and duplex sonographic images of the great saphenous vein. Magnetic resonance imaging (BPCA-MRA) and color-coded duplex sonography in the proximal level of the left GSV of a 63 year old female patient who suffered from PAOD stage III and was referred to the radiological department for assessment of the arterial status prior to a proposed bypass surgery. (a, b) Axial multiplanar reformat of contrast-enhanced T1-weighted gradient-echo images during the steady-state. (c) Axial color-coded duplex sonography.

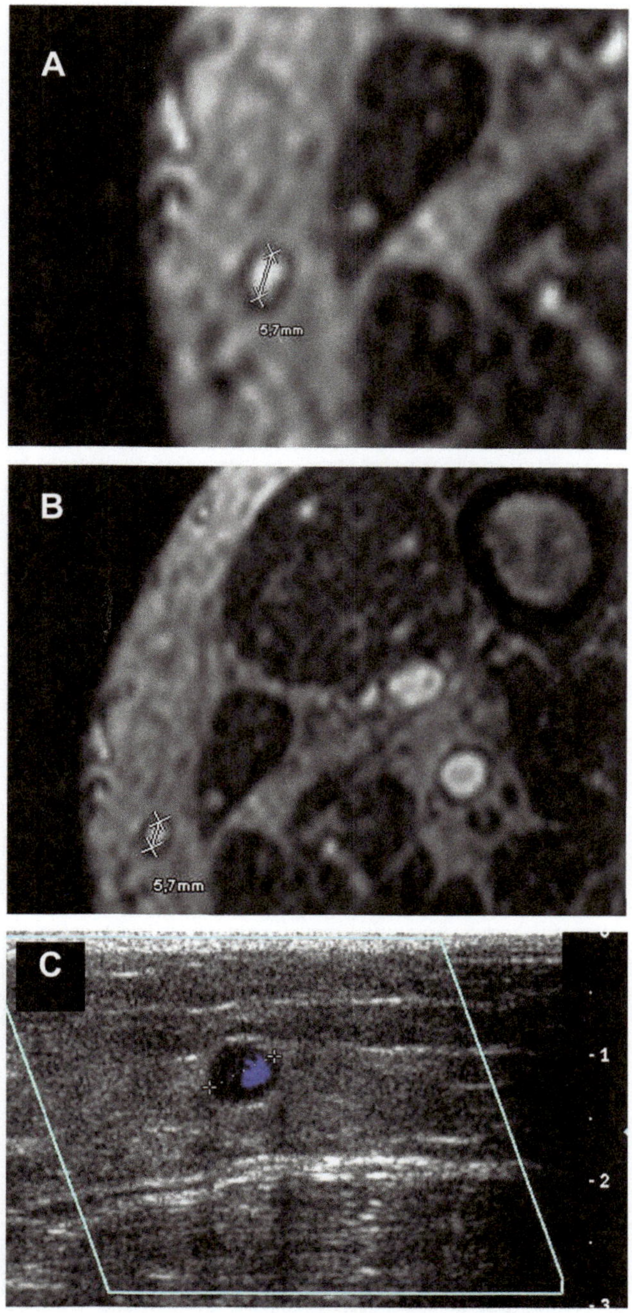

Figure 4. MR-angiographic and duplex sonographic images of the great saphenous vein. Magnetic resonance imaging (BPCA-MRA) and color-coded duplex sonography in the distal level of the left GSV in a 69 year old male patient with PAOD stage IV. (a, b) Axial multiplanar reformat of contrast-enhanced T1-weighted gradient-echo images during the steady-state. (c) Axial color-coded duplex sonography.

integrated body coil served for image acquisition of the upper legs and pelvic region. Using a biphasic injection protocol, Gadofosveset trisodium was administered with an automatic power injector (Spectris; Medrad Europe, Beek, the Netherlands) at a flow rate of 1.2 ml/sec followed by a 25 ml saline flush at a flow rate of 0.6 ml/sec. As soon as the contrast medium was detected at the level of the common iliac arteries by means of fluoroscopic triggering, the acquisition of first pass images was started. The imaging protocol as well as technical parameters of the T1-weighted gradient-echo sequences that were used for first-pass and steady-state MR angiography are shown in figure 2 [31], [35]. Steady-state imaging followed first-pass imaging 4 minutes after contrast injection [36].

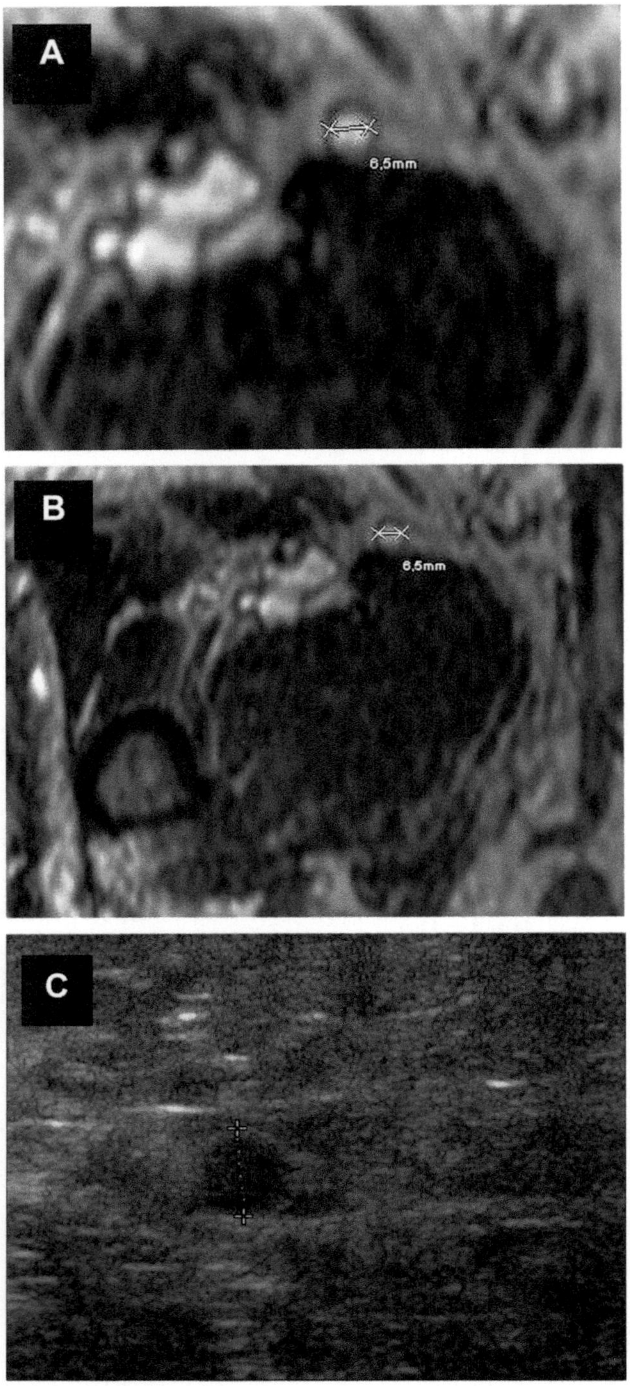

Figure 5. MR-angiographic and duplex sonographic images of the great saphenous vein. Magnetic resonance imaging (BPCA-MRA) and color-coded duplex sonography in the proximal level of the left GSV of a 69 year old male patient who suffered from ulcerations of the lower leg. (a, b) Axial multiplanar reformat of contrast-enhanced T1-weighted gradient-echo images during the steady-state. (c) Axial color-coded duplex sonography.

Contrast Agent

Gadofosveset trisodium (Vasovist, Bayer Healthcare, Leverkusen, Germany; discontinued, now available in the US and Canada as Ablavar, Lantheus Medical Imaging, N. Billerica, MA) was the first intravascular contrast agent approved for use with MRA in the European Union, Switzerland, Turkey, Canada and Australia [37]. In 2008 it became the first contrast agent specifically approved for MR angiography in the US and Canada by the FDA in order to investigate aortoiliac occlusive disease. Due to an additional diphenylcyclohexyl group, this gadolinium-based contrast agent strongly but reversibly binds to human serum albumin resulting in a higher relaxivity (r1 = 19 L *mmol^{-1} sec^{-1} at 1.5 T and 37°C in plasma) and an extended plasma half-life as compared to standard Gadolinium-containing contrast agents. A dose of 0.03 mmol/kg has been proven safe and effective for imaging of peripheral vascular disease [38] and was applied in all patients in our study.

Image analysis of MR Angiography

The maximum venous vessel diameter of the GSV (area of enhancing vessel lumen) was measured on cross-sectional images perpendicular to the flow axis by one radiologist (10 years of experience in vascular radiology) on multiplanar reformats of steady-state MR angiograms on a post-processing workstation (Viewforum; Philips Healthcare, Best, Netherlands) (figure 3–5). Each vein was measured at three levels: at the level just below the groin, at the level of the mid-thigh and 10 cm above the knee joint. To account for both the influence of the graft diameter on the patency rate and the influence of the graft length on the minimal diameter regarded as useable, [4] we decided to rate veins suitable which offered a diameter of at least 3.5 mm at one level and simultaneously a diameter of at least 3.0 mm at a neighboring level. In accordance to clinical practice we defined an upper limit of 10 mm. Nodular varicosities as well as other venous pathologies like thrombosis were exclusion criteria for use in bypass surgery. In order to minimize intraindividual measuring variability, three independent measurements were noted in each of the defined points and the mean was taken for comparison. Moreover a fixed magnification factor of 4 was applied. The reader was blinded regarding the patients names, clinical histories and the results of other diagnostic procedures, including color-coded duplex sonography.

Color-coded duplex sonography

Examinations were performed with the patient in supine position. A HD 11 ultrasound system (Philips Healthcare, Best, the Netherlands) with a 5–10 MHz ultrasonographic transducer was used to visualize the saphenous vein in transverse scans. Starting from the groin, the main trunk was tracked distally to the knee joint. Analogously to the MR angiographic image analysis, three independent measurements were taken from the cross-sectional scan at each level (figure 3–5) and the mean value was calculated. The reader of the DUS was blinded with regard to the results of the MRA.

Intraoperative Evaluation

The preparation of the GSV was carried out through an inguinal incision and a few auxiliary incisions along the saphenous vein. The vein was dissected and measured with a ruler as seen in figure 6. Branches were ligated, the vein was cut to size if necessary and anastomosed at its proximal and distal ends. Absolute values were not compared statistically because measurements were performed on dissected veins that are not in the same physiological condition as in vivo.

Statistical analysis

Students t-test for paired samples was used to test the differences between the diameters measured by DUS and MR angiography

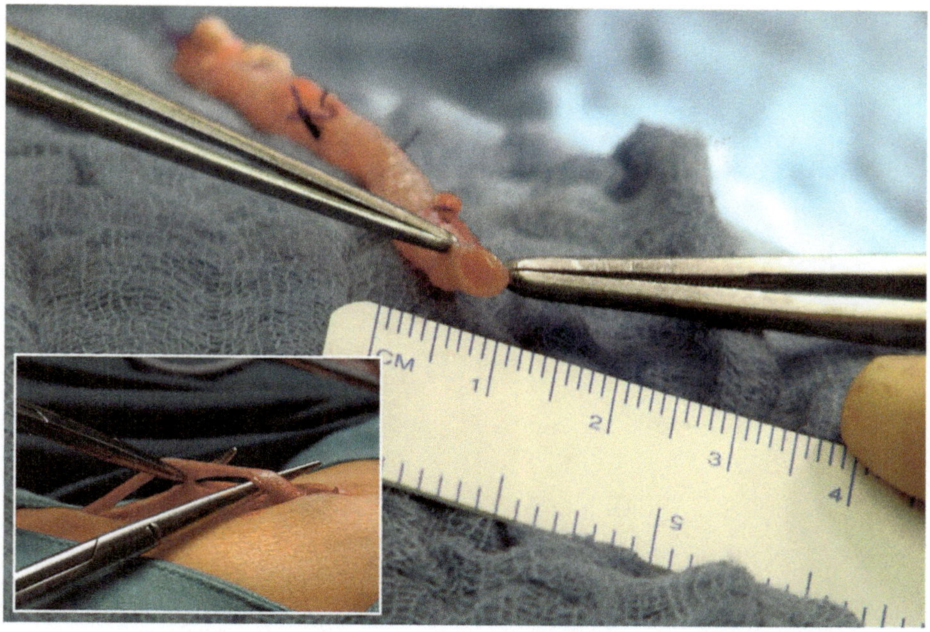

Figure 6. Intraoperative measurement of the dissected great saphenous vein.

based on a venous segment level. A *P* value of less than 0.050 was considered to indicate statistical significance. Correlation between the MR-tomographic and sonographic data was analyzed using Pearsons correlation coefficient. All statistical analyses were performed with the Statistical package for Social Sciences (SPSS) version 17.0 (SPSS, Chicago, Il, USA).

Results

3D steady-state MR angiography was successfully completed in 38 patients (76 assessable legs). Legs, which offered no measureable saphenous vein due to stripping of the saphenous vein (14/76), amputation at the level of mid-thigh (1/76) and absent definability in MRA as well as in sonography (no available level for comparison) (3/76) were excluded. Finally a total of 58 veins were available for intraindividual comparison at level 1, 54 veins for comparison at level 2, and 49 veins for comparison at level 3. The difference between the number of measurements available at the different levels is due to the fact that in some cases a segment (i.a. a level) of the vein was not included in the scanned volume (5/13) or certain levels were not clearly definable in MRA and/or DUS (8/13). All segments containing the measuring points were satisfactorily displayed on steady-state MR angiography as well as with DUS. Altogether, 161 comparative measurements were performed (Table S1).

Mean venous diameters in MRA/DUS for level 1, 2 and 3 were 5.4±2.6 mm/5.5±2.8 mm, 4.7±2.7 mm/4.6±2.9 mm and 4.4±2.2 mm/4.5±2.3 mm respectively, without significant differences between the two modalities ($P = 0.207/0.806/0.518$, df = 57/53/48) (figure 7). The venous diameters measured were higher on steady-state MR angiography than on color-coded duplex sonography in 54 out of 161 measurements (33.54%) (overestimation) and lower on 82 out of 161 measurement (50.93%) (underestimation). In 25 out of 161 measurements (15.53%) the two methods yielded identical values. The mean values of the positive and negative differences (MRA-DUS) are 0,52±0,67 mm and −0,45±0,59 mm, respectively, with an overall mean of differences (MRA-DUS) of −0,06±0,72 mm.

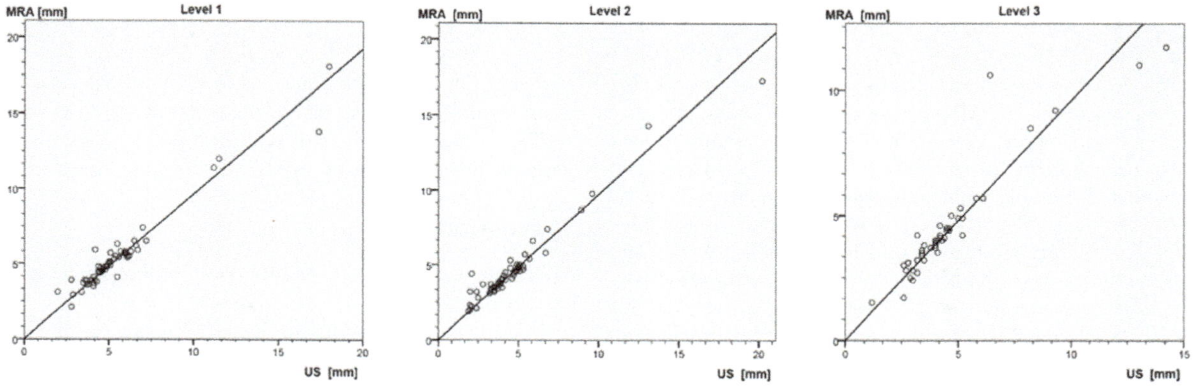

Figure 7. Correlation between MR-angiographic (MRA) and duplex sonographic (DUS) values in the three levels. Pearson correlation coefficients R^2: level 1: 0.989; level 2: 0.986, level 3: 0.973.

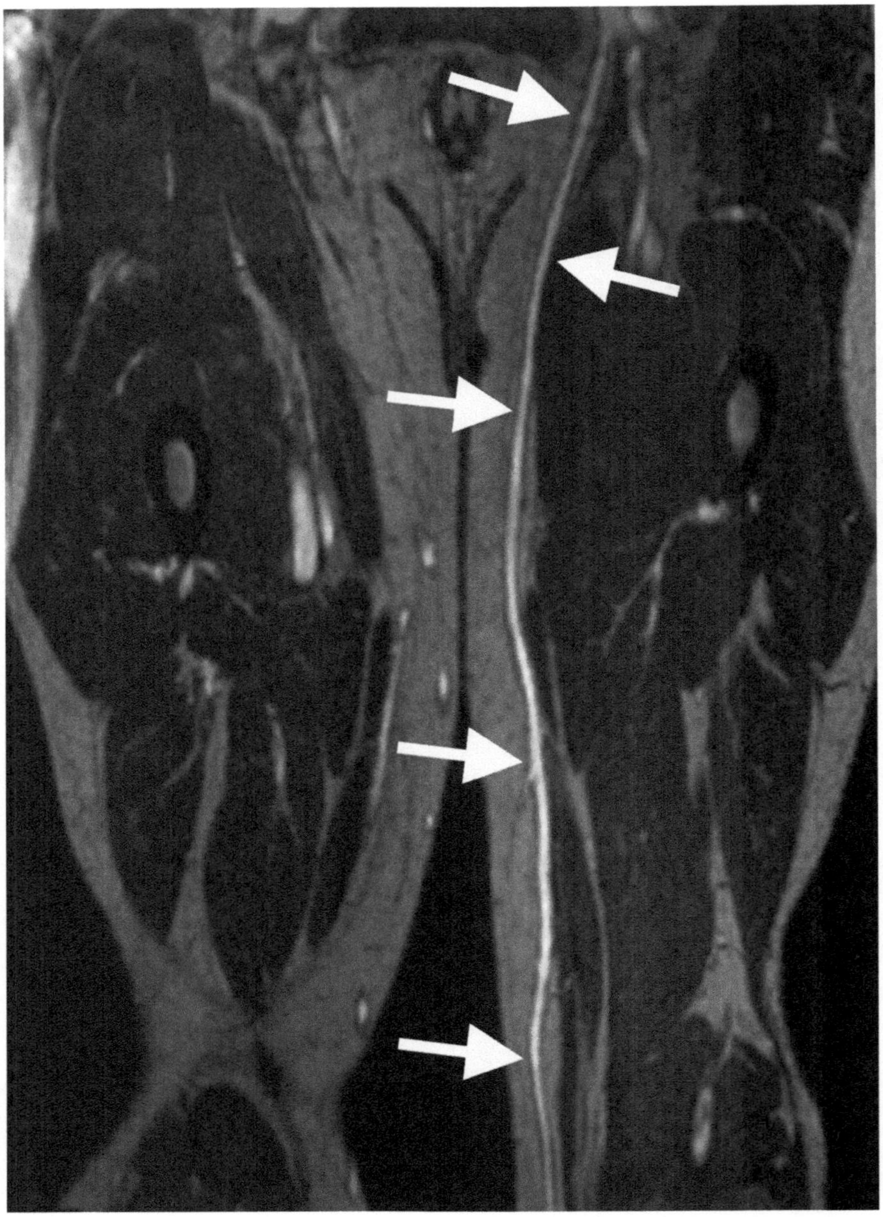

Figure 8. Multiplanar reformat of an MR-angiographic image of the great saphenous vein. The GSV displayed as a curved multiplanar reformat of high-spatial-resolution contrast-enhanced T1-weighted gradient-echo images during the steady-state of a 57 year old male patient suffering from PAOD stage III and thus being evaluated for bypass surgery.

27 of the 38 patients underwent subsequent bypass surgery. In all of these 27 patients, the MR-angiographic assessment and the independent sonographic evaluation showed the same results regarding the suitability of the vein which was considered as bypass conduit. A suitable saphenous vein was diagnosed in all of the 24/27 patients that received a venous bypass conduit. Intraoperative findings confirmed usability in these 24 patients (13 femoropopliteal, 6 popliteocrural and 5 femorocrural bypasses). Non-usability was found in 2/27 patients based on MRA/DUS: In one of these patients the diameter of the respective saphenous vein was too small, the second patient had nodular varicosities. A prosthetic graft was used for reconstruction in both patients. In 1/27 patients a prosthetic graft was utilized despite the usability of the great sapehnous vein based on MRA and DUS findings. This decision was taken by the surgeons due to the patients clinical condition and comorbidities (including coronary heart disease) in order to minimize the duration of the operation as well as to save the saphenous vein for a potential coronary bypass surgery. In 11 patients no bypass surgery was performed.

Discussion

Patients suffering from PAOD often present with concomitant venous disease [39].

In some patients that are evaluated for bypass surgery, veins or parts of them have already been removed due to varicosities or previous arterial surgery. Furthermore, the correct identification of a suitable vein helps to prevent unnecessary large dissections in already ischemic limbs [5], [40] and thereby reduces postoperative leg morbidity [13]. As such, the assessment of the usability of veins as a bypass graft is an indispensable part of the preoperative workup [41].

Our study demonstrates the diagnostic accuracy of MRA with a BPCA in comparison to DUS in the assessment of the luminal diameter of the GSV. Venous mapping was included in the MR-angiographic examination for arterial stenosis grading without the need of a change of examination parameters or any additional diagnostic step in the patient management. We compared sonographic and MR-angiographic measurements and tested the hypothesis that both modalities provide the same results concerning the usability of the GSV as a bypass conduit.

The visualization of the veins in the equilibrium phase of the MRA with Gadofosveset trisodium offered reliable results with regard to the luminal diameter of the GSV in our study population. Statistical analysis showed no significant differences between sonographic and MR-angiographic measurements. Usability (25/27) and non-usability (2/27) were diagnosed consistently by DUS as the standard of reference and MRA. Additionally, usability was verified by the intraoperative assessment of the vein in all patients that received a venous bypass conduit in subsequent bypass surgery.

MRA with the BPCA Gadofosveset trisodium has been proven to be safe, well-tolerated and highly efficient in patients with vascular disease [36], [42]. In 2000, a new disease which is now called nephrogenic systemic fibrosis (NSF) was first described [43]. In 2006, a link between NSF and the exposure to gadolinium-based contrast agents was observed [44], [45]. NSF is very rare and limited to patients with renal impairment [46], [47]. Following studies indicated that NSF almost exclusively occurs after administration of linear, non-ionic gadolinium-based contrast agents [44], [45]. Moreover a prolonged exposure to the contrast agent due to renal insufficiency is suggested as a factor in the pathogenesis of NSF [44], [45]. Although Gadofosveset trisodium is a gadolinium-based contrast agent with a linear structure and an extended plasma half life, so far no unconfounded cases of NSF after administration of a BPCA have been reported [44]. One reason for this might be the high efficiency of Gadofosveset trisodium which results in the use of a much lower Gadolinium concentration as compared to extracellular contrast agents [44]. Nevertheless, a responsible use of gadolinium-based contrast agents in patients with renal impairment is still obligatory.

The sequences needed for first pass and steady state MRA with a BPCA can be easily applied at any MR imaging system and allow for both arterial stenosis grading and the evaluation of venous diameters within the same scan with just a single-dose of contrast agent [35]. Traditionally, venous enhancement was considered a relative drawback of first-pass as well as of steady-state imaging because of impairment of arterial delineation [29], [30]. However, modern steady-state imaging with its increase in spatial resolution and the possibility to acquire isotropic voxels has proved to allow for a distinct analysis of arteries and veins without overlay [30], [31]. Our study lines with previous results that prove the potential of simultaneous visualization of arteries and veins, which was initially postulated in 1998 in view of examining the entire vasculature of the lower extremity in a single imaging procedure [29].

The accuracy of CE-MRA with a BPCA in arterial stenosis grading as compared with digital subtraction angiography (DSA) has already been demonstrated [31], [48]–[50]. Yet, few studies have investigated the inherent potential of the simultaneous visualization of arterial and venous structures in steady state imaging [33]–[35]. A recent study by Hadizadeh et al. showed that BPCA-MRA can reliably detect incidental venous thrombosis in patients undergoing peripheral MRA because of suspected PAOD [35]. Having demonstrated the reliability of BPCA-MRA in the venous diameter measurement and thus the assessment of the GSV as a bypass conduit, our findings support the usability of BPCA-MRA for simultaneously grading arterial stenosis and visualizing the peripheral veins of the lower extremities in a diagnostically conclusive way.

Our study has several limitations. In the first place, the comparison of the mean venous diameters for the three levels as well as the comparison of the single measurements point out, that MRA in comparison to DUS tends to somewhat over- or underestimate the vessel diameter. However, the fact that the diagnosis of usability versus non-usability by MRA and DUS was consistent in all cases indicates that these slight differences of BPCA-MRA and DUS can practically be neglected. Still, it has to be taken into consideration that a larger study population will increase statistical power. Secondly, the fact that the MRA was carried out as a routine examination for the evaluation of the arterial system, in some cases resulted in the MR technologist accidently excluding the saphenous vein from the scan volume, leading to a reduced number of available segments for comparisons of level 2 (54/76) and 3 (49/76) diameters in comparison to level 1 (58/76). In relation to DUS [19], an inherent limitation of the MR-angiographic examination is the inability to preoperatively mark the course of the veins on the skin as a guide for bypass surgery [10]. However, similar to conventional venography (phlebography), MRA offers a 'roadmap' of the entire vascular system of the lower extremity for treatment planning [21], especially if curved multiplanar reformats are reconstructed (figure 8). In combination with the option to examine the vascular system in different planes, diagnostic analysis and treatment planning are facilitated [21] even in cases of difficult sonographic evaluation due to obesity, previous surgical interventions, multiple collaterals or varicosities. Moreover, in contrast to phlebography, the depth of the saphenous vein as well as the distinction between deep and superficial veins is clearly evident. Yet, the currently limited access to post-processing workstations might hamper the surgeons first-hand preoperative look at the saphenous vein.

In this context, the benefits of DUS are well known: it is a noninvasive, relatively cheap, mobile and adjustable procedure free of ionizing radiation and contraindications and risks related to strong magnetic fields [21]. Keeping this in mind, BPCA-enhanced MRA for assessment of the GSV may appear a rather expensive and inconvenient approach in relation to DUS. However, the MR-angiographic assessment of the GSV vein is not proposed as a separate examination but as an adjunct to MRA which is anyway implemented for evaluation of the run-off arteries. Since the 'add-on' only relates to image analysis and not to the MRA procedure itself, most of the advantages of DUS mentioned above are outweighed. The duration of performing the bilateral image analysis of the GSV by the radiologist, which in our cohort was between 3 to 8 minutes, is actually the only additional time and cost factor caused by the MR-angiographic evaluation of the GSV. The bilateral sonographic examination took between 5 to 15 minutes without calculating the patient or equipment transport required. Moreover, the MRA technique is less examiner-dependent than DUS, can be documented in a standardized way and can be reanalyzed at any time. Furthermore, the ability to assess arteries and veins at the same time within one single diagnostic test, reduces the number of examinations, simplifies preoperative diagnostics as well as patient management and may thus shorten the length of the hospital stay [35].

Another limitation of this study was due to the surgical practice that a vein identified as unusable by DUS did not undergo an additional intraoperative evaluation. An intraoperative evaluation of such veins would generally not yield an assessment differing from the ultrasonographic evaluation, which renders them unsuitable for bypass surgery. Its intraoperative exploration would therefore cause unnecessary trauma to the patient.

A final limitation of our study is the fact that in the bypass surgeries performed, the use of the GSV was often not limited to its supragenual segment. In several cases the length of the bypass required resulted in the additional intraoperative dissection and use of the infragenual segment of the GSV. Intraoperatively, in three patients the diameter of the infragenual segment of the vein turned out to be too small to be used as a bypass conduit. In these cases the GSV of the contralateral lower leg, the small saphenous vein of the contralateral lower leg and a prosthetic graft were used respectively to complement the supragenual GSV in order to acquire a bypass conduit which is long enough. This observation does not hamper the validity or significance of our results but retrospectively highlights that an extension of our preoperative mapping to the infragenual GSV could have presented useful additional information for the surgeons.

In conclusion, the MR-angiographic assessment of the suitability of the saphenous vein as a bypass conduit corresponded with the sonographic evaluation in all of the patients who underwent peripheral MRA and subsequent bypass surgery. With BPCA-MRA, a reliable assessment of the venous diameter of the GSV is possible and shows no significant differences in comparison to DUS as the standard of reference. Consequently, in patients with PAOD who in the preoperative workup undergo peripheral MRA to evaluate the arterial status, the inherent MR-angiographic imaging of autogenous saphenous veins can offer additional information regarding the suitability of the veins as a bypass conduit without the need of an additive ultrasound examination.

Supporting Information

Table S1 Diameters of the great saphenous vein.

Author Contributions

Conceived and designed the experiments: ABJ AK WW. Performed the experiments: ABJ GK DH AK MSK WW. Analyzed the data: ABJ GK DH FT AK MSK FV WW HS. Wrote the paper: ABJ DH FT WW. Critical revision for important content: ABJ DH GK FT AK MSK FV HS WW.

References

1. Chaikhouni A (2010) The magnificient century of cardiothoracic surgery. Heart Views 11: 31–37.
2. Twine CP, McLain AD (2010) Graft type for femoro-popliteal bypass surgery. Cochrane Database Syst Rev CD001487. doi:10.1002/14651858.CD001487.pub2.
3. Klinkert P, Post PN, Breslau PJ, van Bockel JH (2004) Saphenous vein versus PTFE for above-knee femoropopliteal bypass. A review of the literature. Eur J Vasc Endovasc Surg 27: 357–362.
4. Schanzer A, Hevelone N, Owens CD, Belkin M, Bandyk DF, et al. (2007) Technical factors affecting autogenous vein graft failure: observations from a large multicenter trial. J Vasc Surg 46: 1180–1190.
5. Burnand KG, Senapati A, Thomas ML, Browse NL (1985) A comparison of preoperative long saphenous phlebography with operative dissection in assessing the suitability of long saphenous vein for use as a bypass graft. Ann R Coll Surg Engl 67: 183–186.
6. Mosley JG, Manhire AR, Raphael M, Marston JA (1983) An assessment of long saphenous venography to evaluate the saphenous vein for femoropopliteal bypass. Br J Surg 70: 673–674.
7. Shah DM, Chang BB, Leopold PW, Corson JD, Leather RP, et al. (1988) The anatomy of the greater saphenous venous system. J Vast Surg 3: 273–283. Tabrisky J, Christie SG, Nejdl RJ, Lindstrom RR (1976) The value of preoperative saphenous venography for graft evaluation in femoral arterial occlusive disease. J Can Assoc Radiol 27: 37–44.
8. Veith F, Moss C, Sprayregen S, Montefusco C (1979) Preoperative saphenous venography in arterial reconstructive surgery of the lower extremity. Surgery 85: 253–256.
9. Leopold PW, Shandall AA, Corson JD, Shah DM, Leather RP, et al. (1986) Initial experience comparing B-mode imaging and venography of the saphenous vein before in situ bypass. Am J Surg 152: 206–210.
10. McShane MD, Field J, Smallwood J, Chant AD (1988) Early experience with B mode ultrasound mapping of the long saphenous vein prior to femorodistal bypass. Ann R Coll Surg Engl 70: 147–149.
11. Buchbinder D, Semrow C, Friedell ML, Ryan T, Calligaro K, et al. (1987) B-mode ultrasonic imaging in the preoperative evaluation of saphenous vein. Am Surg 53: 368–372.
12. Luckraz H, Lowe J, Pugh N, Azzu AA (2008) Pre-operative long saphenous vein mapping predicts vein anatomy and quality leading to improved post-operative leg morbidity. Interact Cardiovasc Thorac Surg 7: 188–191.
13. Lemmer JH, Meng RL, Corson JD, Miller E (1988) Preoperative saphenous vein mapping for coronary artery bypass. J Card Surg 3: 237–240.
14. Head HD, Brown MF (1995) Preoperative vein mapping for coronary artery bypass operations. Ann Thor Surg 59: 144–148.
15. Seeger JM, Schmidt JH, Flynn TC (1987) Preoperative saphenous and cephalic vein mapping as an adjunct to reconstructive arterial surgery. Ann Surg 205: 733–739.
16. Leopold PW, Shandall A, Kupinski AM, Chang BB, Kaufman J, et al. (1989) Role of B-mode venous mapping in infrainguinal in situ veinarterial bypasses. Br J Surg 76: 305–307.
17. Towne JB, Schmitt DD, Seabrook GR, Bandyk DF (1991) The effect of vein diameter on patency of in situ grafts. J Cardiovasc Surg 32: 192–196.
18. Wengerter KR, Veith FJ, Gupta SK, Ascer E, Rivers SP (1990) Influence of vein size (diameter) on infrapopliteal reversed vein graft patency. J Vasc Surg 11: 525–531.
19. Puppinck P, Habi K, Ducasse E, Espagne P (1997) Evaluation of the venous network before arterial revascularization surgery. J Mal Vasc 22: 162–167.
20. Collins R, Cranny G, Burch J, Aguiar-Ibáñez R, Craig D, et al. (2007) A systematic review of duplex ultrasound, magnetic resonance angiography and computed tomography angiography for the diagnosis and assessment of symptomatic, lower limb peripheral arterial disease. Health Technol Assess 11: 1–184.
21. Lenhart M, Finkenzeller T, Paetzel C, Strotzer M, Mann S, et al. (2002) Contrast-enhanced MR angiography in the routine work-up of the lower extremity arteries. Rofo 174: 1289–1295.
22. Ruehm SG, Goyen M, Debatin JF (2002) MR angiography: first choice for diagnosis of the arterial vascular system. Rofo 174: 551–561.
23. Kroft LJ, de Roos A (1999) Blood pool contrast agents for cardiovascular MR imaging. J Magn Reson Imaging 10: 395–403.
24. Klessen C, Hein PA, Huppertz A, Voth M, Wagner M, et al. (2007) Firstpass whole-body magnetic resonance angiography (MRA) using the blood-pool contrast medium gadofosveset trisodium: comparison to gadopentetate dimeglumine. Invest Radiol 42: 659–664.
25. Maki JH, Wang M, Wilson GJ, Shutske MG, Leiner T (2009) Highly accelerated first- pass contrast-enhanced magnetic resonance angiography of the peripheral vasculature: comparison of gadofosveset trisodium with gadopentetate dimeglumine contrast agents. J Magn Reson Imaging 30: 1085–1092.
26. Frydrychowicz A, Russe MF, Bock J, Stalder AF, Bley TA, et al. (2010) Comparison of gadofosveset trisodium and gadobenate dimeglumine during time- resolved thoracic MR angiography at 3T. Acad Radiol 17: 1394–1400.
27. Lauffer RB, Parmelee DJ, Dunham SU, Ouellet HS, Dolan RP, et al. (1998) MS-325: albumin-targeted contrast agent for MR angiography. Radiology 207: 529–538.
28. Grist TM, Korosec FR, Peters DC, Witte S, Walovitch RC, et al. (1998) Steady-state and dynamic MR angiography with MS-325: initial experience in humans. Radiology 207: 539–544.
29. Goyen M (2008) Gadofosveset-enhanced magnetic resonance angiography. Vasc Health Risk Manag 4: 1–9.
30. Hadizadeh DR, Gieseke J, Lohmaier SH, Wilhelm K, Boschewitz J, et al. (2008) Peripheral MR angiography with blood pool contrast agent: prospective intraindividual comparative study of high-spatial-resolution steady-state MR angiography versus standard-resolution first-pass MR angiography and DSA. Radiology 249: 701–711.
31. Pfeil A, Betge S, Poehlmann G, Boettcher J, Drescher R, et al. (2012) Magnetic resonance VIBE venography using the blood pool contrast agent gadofosveset trisodium-An interrater reliability study. Eur J Radiol 81: 547–552.
32. Hoffmann U, Loewe C, Bernhard C, Weber M, Cejna M, et al. (2002) MRA of the lower extremities in patients with pulmonary embolism using a blood pool contrast agent: initial experience. J Magn Reson Imaging 15: 429–437.
33. Aschauer M, Deutschmann HA, Stollberger R, Hausegger KA, Obernosterer A, et al. (2003) Value of a blood pool contrast agent in MR venography of the lower extremities and pelvis: preliminary results in 12 patients. Magn Reson Med 50: 993–1002.

34. Hadizadeh DR, Kukuk GM, Fahlenkamp UL, Pressacco J, Schäfer C, et al. (2012) Simultaneous MR arteriography and venography with blood pool contrast agent detects deep venous thrombosis in suspected arterial disease. AJR Am J Roentgenol 198: 1188–1195.
35. Hartmann M, Wiethoff AJ, Hentrich HR, Rohrer M (2006) Initial imaging recommendations for Vasovist angiography. Eur Radiol 16 Suppl 2: B15–B23.
36. Goyen M (2007) Gadofosveset: the first intravascular contrast agent EU-approved for use with magnetic resonance angiography. Future Cardiol 3: 19–26.
37. Perreault P, Edelman MA, Baum RA, Yucel EK, Weisskoff RM, et al. (2003) MR angiography with gadofosveset trisodium for peripheral vascular disease: phase II trial. Radiology 229: 811–820.
38. Prandoni P (2007) Links between arterial and venous disease. J Intern Med 262: 341–350.
39. Cohn JD, Korver KF (2005) Optimizing saphenous vein site selection using Intraoperative venous duplex ultrasound scanning. Ann Thorac Surg 79: 2013–2017.
40. van Dijk LC, Wittens CH, Pieterman H, van Urk H (1996) The value of pre-operative ultrasound mapping of the greater saphenous vein prior to 'closed' in situ bypass operations. Eur J Radiol 23: 235–237.
41. Goyen M, Shamsi K, Schoenberg SO (2006) Vasovist-enhanced MR angiography. Eur Radiol 16 Suppl 2: B9–14.
42. Cowper SE, Robin HS, Steinberg SM, Su LD, Gupta S, et al. (2000) Scleromyxoedema-like cutaneous diseases in renal-dialysis patients. Lancet 356: 1000–1001.
43. Grobner T (2006) Gadolinium–a specific trigger for the development of nephrogenic fibrosing dermopathy and nephrogenic systemic fibrosis? Nephrol Dial Transplant 21: 1104–1108.
44. Marckmann P, Skov L, Rossen K, Dupont A, Damholt MB, et al. (2006) Nephrogenic systemic fibrosis: suspected causative role of gadodiamide used for contrast-enhanced magnetic resonance imaging. J Am Soc Nephrol 7: 2359–2362.
45. Breitschaft A, Stahlmann R (2009) Nephrogenic systemic fibrosis. Med Monatsschr Pharm 32: 377–382.
46. Braverman IM, Cowper S (2010) Nephrogenic systemic fibrosis. F1000 Med Rep 2: 84.
47. Anzidei M, Napoli A, Marincola BC, Nofroni I, Geiger D, et al. (2009) Gadofosveset-enhanced MR angiography of carotid arteries: does steady-state imaging improve accuracy of first-pass imaging? Comparison with selective digital subtraction angiography. Radiology 251: 457–466.
48. Bonel HM, Saar B, Hoppe H, Keo HH, Husmann M, et al. (2009) MR angiography of infrapopliteal arteries in patients with peripheral arterial occlusive disease by using Gadofosveset at 3.0 T: diagnostic accuracy compared with selective DSA. Radiology 253: 879–890.
49. Kos S, Reisinger C, Aschwanden M, Bongartz GM, Jacob AL, et al. (2009) Pedal angiography in peripheral arterial occlusive disease: first-pass i.v. contrast-enhanced MR angiography with blood pool contrast medium versus intraarterial digital subtraction angiography. AJR Am J Roentgenol 192: 775–784.

Indocyanine Green Video Angiography Predicts Outcome of Extravasation Injuries

Werner Haslik[1], Ursula Pluschnig[2], Günther G. Steger[2], Christoph C. Zielinski[2], K. F. Schrögendorfer[1], Jakob Nedomansky[1], Rupert Bartsch[2], Robert M. Mader[2]*

1 Division of Plastic and Reconstructive Surgery, Department of Surgery, Comprehensive Cancer Center of the Medical University of Vienna, Vienna, Austria, **2** Department of Medicine I, Clinical Division of Oncology, Comprehensive Cancer Center of the Medical University of Vienna, Vienna, Austria

Abstract

Background: Extravasation of cytotoxic drugs is a serious complication of systemic cancer treatment. Still, a reliable method for early assessment of tissue damage and outcome prediction is missing. Here, we demonstrate that the evaluation of blood flow by indocyanine green (ICG) angiography in the extravasation area predicts for the need of surgical intervention.

Methods: Twenty-nine patients were evaluated by ICG angiography after extravasation of vesicant or highly irritant cytotoxic drugs administered by peripheral i.v. infusion. Tissue perfusion as assessed by this standardized method was correlated with clinical outcome.

Results: The perfusion index at the site of extravasation differed significantly between patients with reversible tissue damage and thus healing under conservative management (N = 22) versus those who needed surgical intervention due to the development of necrosis (N = 7; $P = 0.0001$). Furthermore, in patients benefiting from conservative management, the perfusion index was significantly higher in the central extravasation area denoting hyperemia, when compared with the peripheral area ($P = 0.0001$).

Conclusions: In this patient cohort, ICG angiography as indicator of local perfusion within the extravasation area was of prognostic value for tissue damage. ICG angiography could thus be used for the early identification of patients at risk for irreversible tissue damage after extravasation of cytotoxic drugs.

Editor: Daniel Schneditz, Medical University of Graz, Austria

Funding: The authors have no support or funding to report.

Competing Interests: The authors have declared that no competing interests exist.

* Email: robert.mader@meduniwien.ac.at

Introduction

Extravasation as a complication of chemotherapy administration is defined as the unintended instillation or leakage of cytotoxic agents into the perivascular space or subcutaneous tissue. The incidence of extravasations ranges from 0.45% up to 6.4%, with higher figures observed in patients who had previously received multiple lines of chemotherapy [1,2]. The degree of local damage depends upon the toxic potential of the extravasated compound and the amount of drug delivered to the perivascular tissue [3].

Usually, three different classes of cytotoxic compounds are distinguished: i) non-vesicant substances which do not cause local irritations in case of extravasation; ii) irritant substances which cause pain, tissue irritation and swelling, but do not lead to tissue necrosis; iii) vesicant substances, which can cause ulcerations and necrosis necessitating surgical débridement and reconstruction with skin grafts, local flaps or even free flap coverage [4].

As the management of extravasations of cytotoxic drugs is mostly based upon retrospective evaluations of case reports and some data from animal models, the level of evidence of recommendations for clinical management of extravasation events is low. In addition, methods to objectively document the extent of tissue damage are based on photographic documentation alone. This technique is limited insofar, as sequelae including demarcation of skin, ulceration and necrosis may present weeks after the extravasation event. Typically, necrosis is detected 3–4 weeks after the extravasation event. Moreover, superficial alterations of the skin may not represent the true extent of subcutaneous tissue damage. Therefore, novel methods for the reliable identification of the extent of local tissue damage as well as early predictors of outcome are urgently warranted.

As extravasations are frequently associated with injury related venous thrombosis, one possibility to illustrate the extent of the affected extravasation area is to assess skin blood perfusion, which may be done by indocyanine green (ICG) angiography. This procedure is well-established in ophthalmology, burn and trauma management as well as surgical reconstruction for the assessment of tissue perfusion. The basic principle of all these applications is to enable an objective measurement of perfusion and to detect perfusion anomalies, which will eventually lead to necrosis. Therefore, ICG angiography has a predictive value, which is not available by clinical assessment only. In trauma management, ICG is able to predict occurrence of necrosis leading to a better management of the patients. In burn patients, ICG angiography was used for objectively estimating burn wound depth thereby assisting in the rational assessment of treatment options [5,6,7]. In oncology, the use of ICG angiography is so far limited to the detection of sentinel lymph nodes [8].

In contrast to non-vesicant and irritant cytotoxics, vesicants are prone to generate irreversible tissue damage at the extravasation site. Thus, extravasated vesicant cytotoxics define a subgroup of patients at high risk and in urgent need of an objective procedure to reliably assess extent and progress of local damage. In our department, decision-making for the treatment of extravasation injuries was based only on clinical assessment in the past. The aim of this study was to evaluate the impact of ICG angiography on determination of the extent of extravasation injuries and to assess its prognostic role with regards to clinical outcome.

Materials and Methods

Patients

Twenty-nine patients with extravasation of cytotoxics (vesicant or highly irritant agents) administered by peripheral i.v. infusion were included in this study. The study population included 22 female and seven male subjects (median age: 64 years, range: 33–81 years).

Inclusion criteria for the evaluation by ICG angiography were:

1. Patients with a substantial amount of extravasated compound (when a substantial part of the infusion volume was suspected to be administered in the subcutaneous space at that time), where the possibility of necrosis was highly suspected;
2. Patients with ongoing and persistent objective symptoms one or two weeks after the extravasation event or patients suffering from non-healing injuries.

The study was approved by the Institutional Review Board of the University Hospital Vienna. All patients gave written informed consent according to the institutional guidelines. Application of ICG for angiographic purposes was performed in accordance with the ethical regulations of the Medical University of Vienna.

ICG angiography

ICG angiography uses the tricarbocyanine dye ICG that binds quantitatively to plasma proteins. Due to this very rapid binding to plasma proteins after intravenous injection, there is no distribution into the interstitial space and ICG remains located exclusively in the intravascular space thereby allowing for the monitoring of superficial blood perfusion. With a plasma half-life of three to four min, ICG is metabolised by the liver and excreted into the bile. As described by Giunta and co-workers, the absorption and emission peaks in the near infrared spectral range (805 nm and 835 nm) lie within the optical window of the skin, enabling a penetration depth of at least three mm [9].

A single dose of 0.2 mg/kg ICG (ICG-Pulsion, Pulsion Medical Systems, Munich, Germany) was administered by intravenous bolus injection. The perfusion of the affected area was measured using dynamic laser-fluorescence-videography (IC-VIEW, Pulsion Medical Systems) [5,6]. This system contains a digital video camcorder combined with a near infrared light source. The results were recorded digitally allowing for real time viewing as well as quantitative evaluation performed by quantification software (IC-CALC, Pulsion Medical Systems). Different regions of interest (ROI) were defined: ROI 1 was centered in the middle of the extravasation lesion (red colour). ROI 2 was defined in the surrounding margin, but within the affected area of the lesion (blue colour). The fluorescence intensity of normal, well-perfused tissue (unaffected skin) was used for reference (green colour). Moreover, an ICG reference card (supplied by the manufacturer) was included in each measurement and used to normalize the recorded fluorescence data (yellow colour). Perfusion index and maximum pixel intensity of the defined ROI were calculated by IC-CALC software in each patient.

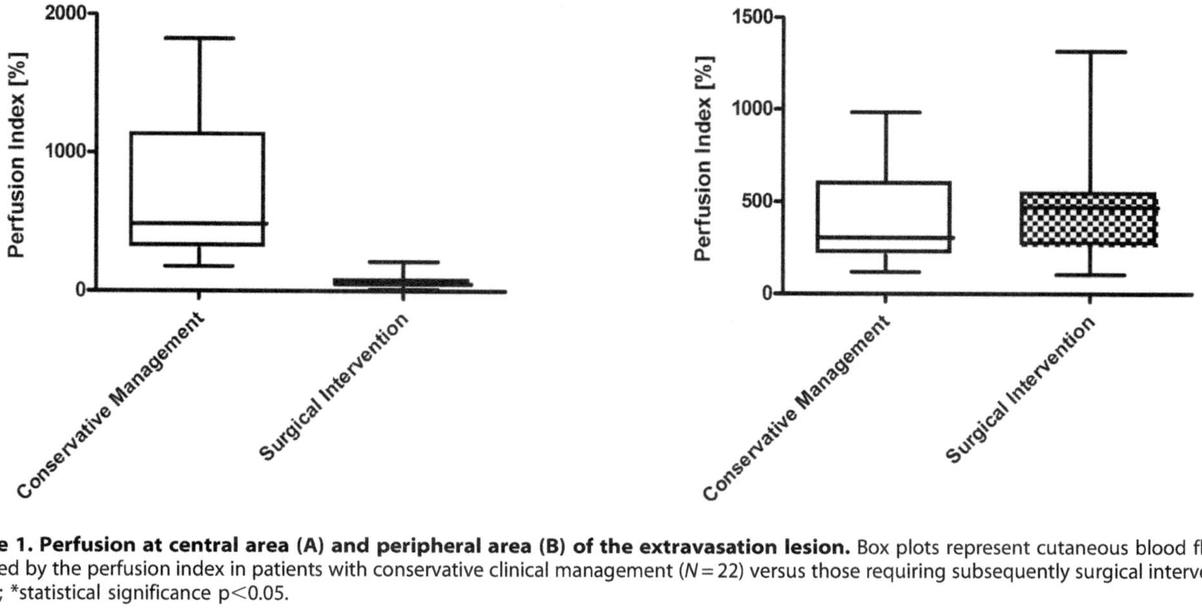

Figure 1. Perfusion at central area (A) and peripheral area (B) of the extravasation lesion. Box plots represent cutaneous blood flow as assessed by the perfusion index in patients with conservative clinical management ($N=22$) versus those requiring subsequently surgical intervention ($N=7$); *statistical significance $p<0.05$.

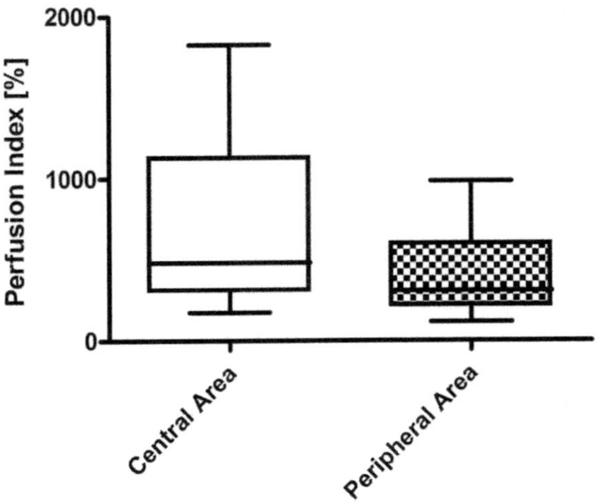

Figure 2. Perfusion in patients not requiring surgery: central area versus peripheral area of the extravasation lesion. Box plots represent cutaneous blood flow as assessed by the perfusion index in patients relying on conservative clinical management ($N = 22$).

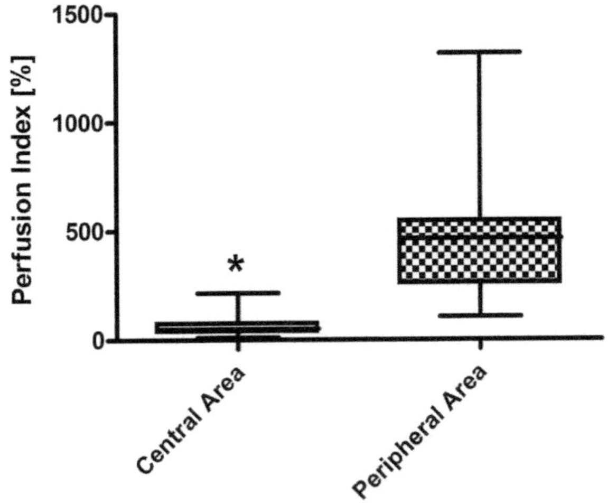

Figure 3. Perfusion in patients requiring surgery: central area versus peripheral area of the extravasation lesion. Box plots represent cutaneous blood flow as assessed by the perfusion index in patients requiring surgical intervention after extravasation of cytotoxics ($N = 7$); *statistical significance $p < 0.05$.

ICG fluorescence intensity throughout the measurement is drawn as a curve with affiliated slopes during signal increase. The software calculates the perfusion index in these regions as steepness of the curve of fluorescence intensity over time (pixel intensity per second) in comparison to the reference area (results in percent). The perfusion index is a parameter that gives more valid information on the quality of perfusion than the maximum ICG-fluorescence intensity alone. This parameter represents the information on the speed of filling with ICG, which correlates with the extent of blood supply [9]. The median period of time after the extravasation event during which patients were monitored for "conservative management" or "surgical intervention" outcomes was 44 days (range: 14–240 d).

Statistics

Outcome parameters obtained after ICG angiography, i.e. perfusion index and maximum pixel intensity, were compared by the Mann-Whitney test (patients with/without surgical intervention). According to the dependence of outcome variables, paired or non-paired statistical comparisons were calculated using GraphPad Prism version 4 software.

Results

In this exploratory study, 29 patients (female: 22; male: 7) with an extravasation of cytotoxic agents after i.v. administration were included. In 16 subjects, the extravasation was noted during infusion or on the same day, while in the reminders, the event was reported on the days thereafter. The ICG angiography took place within a median time-span of 12 days after the extravasation event. The extravasated compounds were mostly anthracyclines (epirubicin: 12, doxorubicin: 4, mitoxantrone: 1); other cases were caused by extravasations with vinorelbine ($N = 5$), platinum compounds ($N = 3$), trabectedin ($N = 2$), docetaxel ($N = 1$), and one not specified case (extravasation occurring during CHOP polychemotherapy). As all cytotoxics had the potential to cause severe tissue damage, there was no particular cytotoxic agent that was associated with more severe necrosis. The extravasation site was forearm ($N = 14$), dorsum of hand ($N = 9$), upper arm ($N = 3$), and antecubital fossa ($N = 3$).

Considering the perfusion index at extravasation areas, there was a highly significant difference between patients with conservative management ($N = 22$) and patient who needed surgical intervention ($N = 7$) due to irreversible tissue damage resulting in necrosis ($P = 0.0001$). This difference was restricted to the central area of the extravasation lesion at the injection site (Figure 1A) and was not observed in peripheral areas of the lesion (Figure 1B). Similarly, there was a highly significant difference between patients with conservative management and patients undergoing surgical intervention when considering another monitoring parameter, the maximum pixel intensity in the central area ($P = 0.0012$).

With regard to patients not requiring surgical interventions and thus healing under conservative management, the perfusion index was significantly higher in the central area of the lesion when compared with the peripheral area of the lesion indicative for a hyperaemic situation in the centre ($P = 0.0001$; Figure 2). In contrast, patients later requiring surgical intervention always showed a diminished perfusion index in the central area of the lesion when compared with the peripheral area ($P = 0.0156$) indicating a massive hypoperfusion as early indicator of irreversible tissue damage (Figure 3).

With a perfusion index set at a threshold level of 100%, a single patient undergoing later surgery presented with a higher perfusion index (sensitivity: 86%). Remarkably, there were no false positive patients as all patients with successful conservative management had perfusion indices higher than 100% in the central area of the lesion as well as in the peripheral area.

As we wanted to use the method as early predictive tool, we used only the first ICG evaluation for outcome reporting. In selected patients ($n = 8$), repeated measurements could be performed. In two of them, hypoperfusion in the central area of the lesion persisted throughout the observation period resulting eventually in necrosis and surgical intervention (range of the perfusion index: 36%–93%). In contrast, patients with conservative management, the perfusion index at the site of extravasation (central area) always considerably exceeded the threshold level of 100% (range of the perfusion index: 200%–1440%).

Discussion

This investigation was conducted in order to assess potential complications of chemotherapy extravasation by early prediction of sequelae, particularly irreversible tissue damage resulting in necrosis that will ultimately require surgical intervention and render conservative treatment futile. Tissue necrosis is a characteristic of vesicant cytotoxics, but has also sporadically been observed with compounds classified as irritant and even the less harmful group of non-vesicant agents. Therefore, the central issue to be addressed after extravasation is the early prediction of the necessity of surgical intervention as this knowledge determines intensity of follow-up visits, planning of surgery, and finally continuation of chemotherapy cycles with a minimum of delay. The exact extent of the extravasation area as well as the identification of irreversible tissue damage cannot be defined by macroscopic methods. Indeed, irreversible breakdown of subcutaneous tissue architecture may occur unnoticed well below the seemingly intact epidermal layer. In this region, spontaneous healing may no longer be expected.

Frequently, extravasation of vesicant agents is associated with thrombotic events thus further reducing local clearance of extravasated agents. In this context, thrombosis prevention with heparin has proven efficacious in an animal model by reducing extent and frequency of doxorubicin-related ulcerations, but was of limited effect in humans [10,11]. Enhanced tissue residence time of vesicants due to thrombosis in combination with higher subcutaneous concentrations of toxic compounds is therefore expected to pose a high risk for subsequent progression to tissue necrosis. We therefore hypothesised that early diagnosis of hypoperfusion of areas affected by extravasation would contribute to the prediction of an unfavourable clinical course. ICG angiography is a non-invasive technique to quantify skin perfusion down to a depth of approximately three millimetres. Upon several occasions, ICG angiography has proven to be a useful tool, which can be readily applied after burns and flap transplantation to discriminate perfused from non-perfused tissue areas. Other indications are assessment of liver function and cardiac output as well as ophthalmic examinations. This qualifies ICG angiography as a well-established and safe technique. As recording of blood flow is usually concluded within five minutes, the overall analysis time needed is approximately 30 minutes. As ICG angiography examines the upper layer of the skin, all dressings need to be removed and all measures, which may influence blood flow in the affected area are temporarily suspended including antidote administration [12]. In our experience, this is compatible with the current protocols of antidote administration (topical cooling, topical heat, application of DMSO or s.c. injection of hyaluronidase). The only contraindication against the use of ICG known so far is allergy against iodine.

In this study, we provide information about results of ICG angiography in two cohorts of patients after extravasation with vesicant cytotoxics. Of note, none of the patients with a perfusion index above 100% in the central area of the affected lesion developed subsequent tissue necrosis. This practically relevant information might be useful for further planning of the patient's follow-up visit and - if confirmed in a larger prospective series - may prove beneficial for all persons experiencing an extravasation. All other subjects not fulfilling this criterion may be considered at risk for developing severe sequelae such as necrosis and ultimately surgical intervention thus requiring a much closer attention and a more intense follow-up schedule.

As outlined, this observation may be explained by the fact that extravasations, particularly those of vesicants, are frequently associated with thrombosis in the affected tissue.

In contrast, a hyperaemic situation indicated an intact architecture of skin and blood vessels able to detoxify the extravasation area. This observation has been corroborated by histopathological examinations in our group (data not shown). This distinction cannot be made by macroscopic examination alone, which may even be misleading. Particularly in early stages of developing skin toxicity, a reasonable prediction of the imminent tissue damage based upon a purely macroscopic assessment is almost impossible even by experienced oncologic surgeons, but is feasible after ICG angiography. Despite these advantages, ICG angiography is limited in its predictive value to extravasations associated with local thrombotic events, which are frequently but not always observed. Due to the penetration depth of approximately three millimetres, deeper thrombosis and tissues obstruction in layers below the subcutaneous strata are likely to yield false negative results. Other issues to be elucidated in further investigations are the selection of patients, the predictive role in other compounds besides the investigated vesicants, the exact planning of ICG angiography and possible repetitions of ICG-based evaluations. A fine tuning of the cut-off values for discrimination may also be necessary, although the perfusion index above 100% may be considered a reasonable starting point for the follow-up management. As blood perfusion may also be examined by other techniques, non-invasive procedures such as the laser Doppler technique of skin blood measurement may pose an attractive alternative method [13,14]. This imaging technique is not dependent on the i.v. injection of a dye solution and may be performed in the absence of darkroom conditions.

Study limitations are that the two observers who were not independent from the treating team performed the ICG angiography and that ICG analyses were not performed in a blinded fashion. The relatively small number of 29 patients and the heterogeneity of the population can be considered another study limitation. However, given the fact that extravasation with a considerable amount of vesicant cytotoxics is a rare event and considering the highly significant difference between both treatment groups, 29 patients appear to be sufficient to postulate the value of ICG angiography in predicting the course of the extravasation event.

In conclusion, these data show for the first time that days after an extravasation event, a perfusion index $<100\%$ in the central area of the lesion is a strong indicator for patients later requiring surgical intervention. Likewise, a perfusion index $>100\%$ strongly predicts spontaneous healing under conservative management. The results of this prospective trial therefore indicate that ICG angiography objectively documents skin perfusion and helps defining the extent of injury after extravasation of cytotoxics. The early understanding of prognosis of subcutaneous skin injury may be very useful information to guide the decision for conservative or surgical intervention, the intensity of follow-up visits, and further planning of chemotherapy.

Author Contributions

Conceived and designed the experiments: WH UP GS CZ KS RM. Performed the experiments: WH UP KS RM. Analyzed the data: WH GS CZ KS JN RB RM. Contributed reagents/materials/analysis tools: WH RM. Contributed to the writing of the manuscript: WH UP GS CZ KS JN RB RM.

References

1. Barlock AL, Howser DM, Hubbard SM (1979) Nursing management of adriamycin extravasation. Am J Nurs 79: 94–96.
2. Laughlin RA, Landeen JM, Habal MB (1979) The management of inadvertent subcutaneous adriamycin infiltration. Am J Surg 137: 408–412.
3. Rudolph R, Stein RS, Pattillo RA (1976) Skin ulcers due to adriamycin. Cancer 38: 1087–1094.
4. Mader I, Furst-Weger P, Mader RM, Nogler-Semenitz E, Wassertheurer S (2010) Extravasation of cytotoxic agents. Wien New York: Springer.
5. Kamolz LP, Andel H, Auer T, Meissl G, Frey M (2006) Evaluation of skin perfusion by use of indocyanine green video angiography: Rational design and planning of trauma surgery. J Trauma 61: 635–641.
6. Kamolz LP, Andel H, Haslik W, Donner A, Winter W, et al. (2003) Indocyanine green video angiographies help to identify burns requiring operation. Burns 29: 785–791.
7. Yannuzzi LA (2011) Indocyanine green angiography: a perspective on use in the clinical setting. Am J Ophthalmol 151: 745–751.
8. Polom K, Murawa D, Rho YS, Nowaczyk P, Hunerbein M, et al. (2011) Current trends and emerging future of indocyanine green usage in surgery and oncology: a literature review. Cancer 117: 4812–4822.
9. Giunta RE, Holzbach T, Taskov C, Holm PS, Brill T, et al. (2005) Prediction of flap necrosis with laser induced indocyanine green fluorescence in a rat model. Br J Plast Surg 58: 695–701.
10. Askar I, Erbas MK, Gurlek A (2002) Effects of heparin fractions on the prevention of skin necrosis resulting from adriamycin extravasation: an experimental study. Ann Plast Surg 49: 297–301.
11. Petro JA, Graham WP, 3rd, Miller SH, Overholt T, Fallon T (1979) Experimental and clinical studies of ulcers induced with adriamycin. Surg Forum 30: 535–537.
12. Haslik W, Kamolz LP, Andel H, Winter W, Meissl G, et al. (2004) The influence of dressings and ointments on the qualitative and quantitative evaluation of burn wounds by ICG video-angiography: an experimental setup. Burns 30: 232–235.
13. Brown RF, Rice P, Bennett NJ (1998) The use of laser Doppler imaging as an aid in clinical management decision making in the treatment of vesicant burns. Burns 24: 692–698.

Epicardial Adipose Tissue Thickness Correlates with the Presence and Severity of Angiographic Coronary Artery Disease in Stable Patients with Chest Pain

Fabien A. Picard[1], Pascal Gueret[2], Jean-Pierre Laissy[3,4], Stéphane Champagne[2], Florence Leclercq[5], Didier Carrié[6], Jean-Michel Juliard[1], Patrick Henry[7], Ralph Niarra[8,9], Gilles Chatellier[8,9,10], Philippe Gabriel Steg[1,4,11]*

1 Cardiology Department, Assistance Publique-Hôpitaux de Paris, Hôpital Bichat, Université Paris-Diderot, Sorbonne-Paris Cité, Paris, France, **2** Cardiology Department, Assistance Publique-Hôpitaux de Paris, Hôpital Henri Mondor, Université Paris-Est-Créteil, Créteil, France, **3** Radiology Department, Assistance Publique-Hôpitaux de Paris, Hôpital Bichat, Université Paris-Diderot, Sorbonne-Paris Cité, Paris, France, **4** Département Hospitalo-Universitaire FIRE, INSERM U-1148, Assistance Publique-Hôpitaux de Paris, Hôpital Bichat, Université Paris-Diderot, Sorbonne-Paris Cité, Paris, France, **5** Cardiology Department, Centre Hospitalier Universitaire Arnaud de Villeneuve, Montpellier, France, **6** Cardiology Department, Centre Hospitalier Universitaire de Rangueil, Toulouse, France, **7** Cardiology Department, Assistance Publique-Hôpitaux de Paris, Hôpital Lariboisière, Université Paris-Diderot, Sorbonne-Paris Cité, Paris, France, **8** Epidemiology and Clinical Research Unit, Assistance Publique-Hôpitaux de Paris, Hôpital Européen Georges-Pompidou, Paris, France, **9** Unité INSERM Centre D'investigation Épidémiologique 4, Paris, France, **10** Université Paris Descartes, Sorbonne Paris Cité, Faculté de Médecine, Paris, France, **11** NHLI Imperial College, ICMS Royal Brompton Hospital, London, United Kingdom

Abstract

Objective: Epicardial adipose tissue (EAT) is suggested to correlate with metabolic risk factors and to promote plaque development in the coronary arteries. We sought to determine whether EAT thickness was associated or not with the presence and extent of angiographic coronary artery disease (CAD).

Methods: We measured epicardial fat thickness by computed tomography and assessed the presence and extent of CAD by coronary angiography in participants from the prospective EVASCAN study. The association of EAT thickness with cardiovascular risk factors, coronary artery calcification scoring and angiographic CAD was assessed using multivariate regression analysis.

Results: Of 970 patients (age 60.9 years, 71% male), 75% (n = 731) had CAD. Patients with angiographic CAD had thicker EAT on the left ventricle lateral wall when compared with patients without CAD (2.74±2.4 mm vs. 2.08±2.1 mm; p = 0.0001). The adjusted odds ratio (OR) for a patient with a LVLW EAT value ≥2.8 mm to have CAD was OR = 1.46 [1.03–2.08], p = 0.0326 after adjusting for risk factors. EAT also correlated with the number of diseased vessels (p = 0.0001 for trend). By receiver operating characteristic curve analysis, an EAT value ≥2.8 mm best predicted the presence of>50% diameter coronary artery stenosis, with a sensitivity and specificity of 46.1% and 66.5% respectively (AUC:0.58). Coronary artery calcium scoring had an AUC of 0.76.

Conclusion: Although left ventricle lateral wall EAT thickness correlated with the presence and extent of angiographic CAD, it has a low performance for the diagnosis of CAD.

Editor: Joseph Devaney, Children's National Medical Center, Washington, United States of America

Funding: The authors have no support or funding to report.

Competing Interests: The authors have declared that no competing interests exist.

* Email: gabriel.steg@bch.aphp.fr

Introduction

Epicardial adipose tissue (EAT) is a visceral adipose tissue surrounding the heart and the coronary arteries. Because of its endocrine and paracrine activity, secreting pro-inflammatory and anti-inflammatory cytokines and chemokines, it has been suggested to influence coronary atherosclerosis development [1–5]. The EVASCAN (EVAluation of CT SCANner) study [6] was recently performed to establish the diagnostic accuracy of computed tomography coronary angiography compared to conventional coronary angiography (CA) in a population of symptomatic patients with a clinical indication for anatomical coronary imaging.

Using EVASCAN data, which provided precise assessment of coronary artery disease by CA and the measure of EAT by cardiac computed tomography (CT) in a large cohort of patients, the current analysis was performed to clarify a possible link between EAT and CAD. Our hypothesis was that EAT, as measured by

CT scanner, was associated with the presence and extent of angiographic CAD.

Methods

Study population

We used EVASCAN data, which provided precise assessment of coronary artery disease by CA and the measure of EAT by cardiac CT to perform this study. Therefore, EVASCAN inclusion criteria were used. EVASCAN was a prospective study of correlation between CT angiography and conventional angiography in stable adults with chest pain referred for non-emergent invasive CA. Eligible patients were ≥18 years old with known or suspected CAD, able to undergo cardiac CT first, then CA within four days. The main exclusion criteria were: unstable clinical status, serum creatinine>150 µmol/L, atrial fibrillation, pregnancy and lactation. The protocol of this study complies with the Declaration of Helsinki, was approved by the institutional review board of Paris VI University and written informed consent was obtained from each patient. Classical CAD risk factors were recorded. The clinical characteristics of the patients are summarized in Table 1.

Cardiac CT and coronary angiography protocol

Patients underwent cardiac CT (684 (70.5%) patients had 64 row CT and 286 patients (29.5%) had 16 to 40 row CT) followed by conventional CA. Cardiac CT was performed using a standardized, optimized protocol for each system. All patients were in sinus rythm before cardiac CT. A beta-blocker was recommended if heart rate was>65 beats/minute.

Patients first underwent an unenhanced prospective ECG-gated acquisition for calcium scoring (Agatston score) and then a retrospective ECG-gated contrast-enhanced acquisition to explore the coronary tree and EAT. Scanning parameters varied according to the system used. Current intensity modulation was systematically applied to reduce radiation during systolic phases. The effective dose of the non-enhanced scan and the computed tomography coronary angiography was estimated from the product of the dose–length and a conversion coefficient ($k = 0.017 mSv/[mGy \times cm]$) for the chest as the investigated anatomic region [7].

A systematic reconstruction of the cardiac phases encompassing the RR interval (in 10% increments) was performed in all patients. Data were uploaded to dedicated workstations (Advantage Windows, GE; Brilliance, Philips; Leonardo, Siemens; Vitrea, Toshiba).

Conventional CA was performed using standard techniques via a femoral or radial approach [8]. All studies were performed using digital equipment. Multiple projections were obtained as deemed necessary by the angiographer.

Cardiac CT and CA interpretation

Cardiac CT and CA were analyzed visually in separate core laboratories in a blinded manner by experienced readers unaware of the patient's clinical information or the results of the other imaging technique.

For cardiac CT, EAT was defined as the adipose tissue between the surface of the heart and the visceral epicardium surrounding the 3 main coronary arteries. To determine EAT values, epicardial

Table 1. Population characteristics and comparison of the presence of significant angiographic coronary artery disease.

Characteristics	All patients (n = 970)	Presence of significant coronary artery disease: No N = 239	Yes N = 731	P
Men, n (%)	689 (71.03%)	122 (51.05%)	567 (77.56%)	**<0.0001**
Age (yrs), mean ± SD	60.85±11.36	57.19±12.29	62.05±10.77	**<0.0001**
BMI (kg/m2), mean ± SD	27.38±4.52	27.09±5.02	27.48±4.34	0.2614
Waist circumference (cm); mean ± SD	98.75±13.31	97.33±15.40	99.23±12.51	0.1601
Current smoker, n (%)	244 (25.15%)	59 (24.69%)	185 (25.31%)	0.8475
Diabetes, n (%)	244 (25.15%)	42 (17.57%)	181 (24.76%)	**0.0218**
Hypertension, n (%)	501 (51.65%)	95 (39.75%)	406 (55.54%)	**<0.0001**
Dyslipidemia, n (%)	427 (44.02%)	86 (35.98%)	341 (46.65%)	**0.0039**
Familial history of CAD; n (%)	660 (68.04%)	159 (66.53%)	501 (68.54%)	0.5631
Metabolic syndrome, n (%)	62 (6.39%)	11 (4.60%)	51 (6.98%)	0.1927
Total cholesterol (g/L), mean ± SD	2.09±1.04	2.09±0.92	2.09±1.07	0.9546
LDL cholesterol (g/L), mean ± SD	1.24±0.73	1.25±0.64	1.24±0.75	0.9163
HDL cholesterol (g/L), mean ± SD	0.54±0.29	0.59±0.32	0.53±0.28	**0.0255**
Calcium scoring, median [IQR]	15.50 [0.00; 331.00]	0.00 [0.00; 9.00]	82.00 [6.00; 626.00]	**<0.0001**
Calcium scoring; mean ± SD	379.72±840.59	72.43±275.58	539.28±980.08	**<0.0001**
LVLW EAT thickness (mm); mean ± SD	2.58±2.31	2.08±2.05	2.74±2.37	**0.0001**
RVLW EAT thickness (mm); mean ± SD	5.38±3.05	4.77±2.73	5.58±3.13	**0.0004**
LVLW EAT thickness ≥2.8 mm, n (%)	427 (44.02%)	83 (34.73%)	344 (47.06%)	**0.0009**
RVLW EAT thickness ≥5.3 mm, n (%)	405 (41.75%)	77 (32.22%)	328 (44.87%)	**0.0005**

BMI = body mass index; CAD = coronary artery disease; LDL = low-density lipoprotein; HDL = high-density lipoprotein; LVLW = left ventricle lateral wall; EAT = epicardial adipose tissue; RVLW = right ventricle lateral wall.

fat maximal thickness was measured at two different locations: on the left ventricle lateral free wall (LVLW) at the base of the ventricles in short-axis view and on the right ventricle lateral free wall (RVLW) at the base of the ventricles in short-axis view. Maximal thickness was measured from the visceral epicardium to the outside of the myocardium, and perpendicular to the surface of the heart. Maximal LVLW EAT thickness and maximal RVLW EAT thickness were used for analysis. EAT thickness was not measured at other sites (right atrioventricular groove, left atrioventricular groove, interventricular grooves...).

For CA, coronary arteries were scored using the American Heart Association coronary artery classification [9]. Each coronary segment was visually graded as: individually assessable or not; normal; non-significant stenosis (<50%); stenosis ≥50%; or total occlusion. In case of multiple lesions in a given segment or artery, the worst lesion was considered.

Baseline clinical and biological assessment

Baseline measurements were obtained for the following: total cholesterol, high-density lipoprotein cholesterol, low-density lipoprotein cholesterol, triglycerides; Body mass index (BMI) and waist circumference. Presence of high blood pressure, diabetes, coronary heredity and current or former smoker was recorded.

Biological samples were processed through local laboratories of each hospital.

Statistical analysis

Descriptive data are presented as frequencies and percentages. Continuous data are expressed as mean ± SD or median [IQR] according to the distribution of the parameter. Risk factors were compared between patients with and without CAD. Student's t test for independent groups was used to compare continuous variables, and chi-square test was used for categorical variables. The relation between cardiovascular risk factors and presence of CAD was assessed with univariate and multivariate logistic regression analysis. This relation was expressed by odds ratios (95% CIs). To determine the best cut-off of EAT thickness and calcium scoring, the Youden index (sensitivity + specificity −1) was calculated using the receiver operating characteristic (ROC) curve. The main aim of the Youden index is to find the best cut-off from the ROC curve, maximizing the difference between true positive rate (Sensitivity) and false positive rate (1-specificity). To determine the intra-observer variability of EAT measurements, one observer repeated the EAT data analysis for 25 randomly chosen CT-scanners on different days. Two observers measuring the already recorded image estimated inter-observer variability. The agreement for both intra- and inter-observer variability was evaluated by intra- and inter-class correlation coefficients (ICC). The ICC value is the ratio of the between-subject variance to the sum of the between-subject variance and the within-subject variance. The smaller the within-subject variance, the better the agreement and the higher the ICC. All statistical analyses were performed using SAS system version 9.2 (SAS Institute, Cary, NC, USA). A 2-tailed p-value <0.05 was considered statistically significant.

Results

Patients characteristics

Between June 2006 and June 2008, 40 centres prospectively enrolled 1254 patients; data from 970 were used in the present analysis. The patients excluded from the analysis had either incomplete, poor quality or missing Cardiac CT or CA, missing data for EAT thickness or withdrew consent. The baseline characteristics are shown in Table 1. The mean age was 61±11 years and 71% were male. The main cardiovascular risk factors were familial history of CAD in 68% of patients, treated hypertension in 52% of the patients, dyslipidaemia in 44% of the patients, current smoking in 25% of the patients and diabetes in 25% of the patients. Mean BMI was 27.4±4.5 kg/m2 and waist circumference was 99±13 cm.

EAT thickness measured by cardiac CT for the entire study sample was 2.58±2.31 mm for the LVLW and 5.38±3.05 mm for the RVLW.

The reproducibility of EAT measurements in our study was high both in terms of intra- and inter-observer variability (correlation coefficients: 0.89 and 0.74 respectively).

Epicardial fat thickness and presence of angiographic CAD

Seven hundred and thirty one patients (75%) were found to have significant CAD on coronary angiography. Their clinical and CT findings were compared to the remaining two hundred and thirty nine patients without significant CAD.

Baseline characteristics of the 2 groups (with or without CAD) are listed in Table 1.

Patients with angiographic evidence of CAD were more frequently males, older, with a higher prevalence of conventional risk factors (diabetes, hypertension, dyslipidaemia) although the prevalence of current smoking, the average BMI, waist circumference and metabolic syndrome were not different from patients without CAD. Total cholesterol and low-density lipoprotein cholesterol were similar among groups (probably because of a high prevalence of statin use). However, HDL levels were lower.

Patients with angiographic CAD had thicker EAT on both left and right ventricle lateral walls, when compared with patients without CAD (2.74±2.4 mm vs. 2.08±2.1 mm; $p=0.0001$ for LVLW and 5.58±3.1 mm vs. 4.77±2.7 mm; $p=0.0004$ for RVLW). Calcium scoring mean was also higher in patients with angiographic CAD (539.28±980.08 vs. 72.43±275.58; $p<0.0001$). (Table 1).

The odds ratio (OR) for a patient with a LVLW EAT value ≥ 2.8 mm to have CAD was 1.67 (95%CI 1.23 to 2.26). This relation remained significant after adjusting for CAD risk factors (OR = 1.46 [1.03–2.08], $p=0.0326$) (Table 2). Unlike LVLW EAT; the OR for a patient with a RVLW EAT value ≥5.3 mm to have CAD did not remain significant after adjusting for CAD risk factors (OR = 1.38 [0.97–1.98], $p=0.0757$).

The probability of a stenosis on angiography increased with increasing LVLW EAT thickness. In the first tertile of EAT thickness, the prevalence of at least one significant coronary artery stenosis was 68.9% (n = 221). In the second and the third tertiles, the prevalence rose to 75.9% (n = 249) and 81.3% (n = 261), respectively (P for trend = 0.0002) (Table 3 and Figure 1).

Simple linear regression analysis demonstrated that epicardial fat thickness was correlated with degree of coronary stenosis OR = 1.67, $p=0.0009$ but not with waist circumference: OR = 1.01, $p=0.16$ and BMI: OR = 1.02, $p=0.26$ in CAD subjects. The independent relation of epicardial fat thickness, waist circumference and BMI with coronary stenosis was then assessed by a multiple regression analysis in CAD subjects. Epicardial fat thickness was the most significant independent correlate of degree of coronary stenosis, dependent variable in CAD subjects. (Table 4).

Epicardial fat and extent of angiographic CAD

Increased LVLW EAT thickness correlated positively with the severity or extent of CAD (Figure 2): LVLW EAT thickness mean was 2.08±2.1 mm for the patients with no or minimal vessel

Table 2. Logistic regression analysis of the association between risk factors and presence of significant angiographic CAD.

	Univariate analysis			Multivariate analysis		
	OR	[95%CI]	P	OR	[95%CI]	P
Men	3.32	[2.44–4.51]	**<0.0001**	4.25	[2.98–6.05]	**<0.0001**
Age	1.04	[1.02–1.05]	**<0.0001**	1.04	[1.03–1.06]	**<0.0001**
BMI	1.02	[0.99–1.05]	0.2614	1.01	[0.98–1.05]	0.4632
Current smoker (yes vs. no)	1.03	[0.74–1.45]	0.8482	1.40	[0.92–2.14]	0.1139
Diabetes (yes vs. no)	1.54	[1.06–2.24]	**0.0226**	1.25	[0.79–1.98]	0.3469
Hypertension (yes vs. no)	1.90	[1.41–2.56]	**<0.0001**	1.89	[1.31–2.74]	**0.0007**
Dyslipidemia (yes vs. no)	1.56	[1.15–2.10]	**0.0041**	1.72	[1.22–2.42]	**0.0021**
Family history of CAD (yes vs. no)	1.10	[0.80–1.50]	0.5632	1.07	[0.75–1.53]	0.6985
Metabolic syndrome (yes vs. no)	1.55	[0.80–3.03]	0.1965	0.87	[0.39–1.92]	0.7241
LVLW EAT (≥2.8 vs. <2.8 mm)	1.67	[1.23–2.26]	**0.0009**	1.46	[1.03–2.08]	**0.0326**

OR = odds ratio; CI = confidence interval; other abbreviations as in Table 1.

disease, 2.43±2.4 mm for the patients with single vessel disease, 2.65±2.2 mm for patients with 2 vessel disease or left main disease and 2.95±2.5 mm for patients with 3 vessels disease or left main + right coronary artery disease (p for trend = 0.0001).

Moreover, patients with multivessel disease had more often a LV wall EAT thickness>2.8 mm. 83 (34.73%) patients with no or minimal vessel disease had LVLW EAT thickness>2.8 mm and 177 (51.45%) patients with three vessels disease had a LVLW EAT thickness>2.8 mm. This relation was better with calcium scoring (Figure 2).

Diagnostic performance of EAT and calcium scoring

On receiver operating characteristic (ROC) curve analysis, the best cut-off for LVLW EAT thickness to predict the presence of a significant coronary stenosis was 2.8 mm. LVLW EAT thickness ≥2.8 mm had a sensitivity of 46.1%, specificity of 66.5%, positive predictive value of 80%, and negative predictive value of 28.8%. The area under the curve was 0.58. The best cut-off for RVLW was 5.3 mm. RVLW EAT thickness ≥5.3 mm predicted the presence of significant coronary stenosis, with sensitivity of 45.1%, specificity of 67.9%, positive predictive value of 81.1%, and negative predictive value of 28.9%. The best cut-off for calcium scoring was 24 (Agatston score). Calcium scoring>24 predicted the presence of significant coronary stenosis, with sensitivity of 62.3%, specificity of 85.1%, positive predictive value of 89%, and negative predictive value of 54.2%. The area under the curve was 0.76 (Figure 3). Conventional cardiovascular risk factors ROC curve was determined and was added to LVLW EAT and calcium scoring measurement. Areas under the curve, sensibility, specificity, positive and negative predictive values are summarized in Table 5. LVLW EAT thickness and calcium scoring were statistically associated (p = 0.0125).

Discussion

The present study sought to determine the link between EAT and CAD using data from the EVASCAN study [6], a large multicenter prospective study originally performed to establish the diagnostic accuracy of CTCA compared to conventional coronary angiography in a population of symptomatic patients with a clinical indication for anatomical coronary imaging.

This study confirmed that EAT thickness of left ventricle wall was associated with CAD and an independent predictor of CAD. Interestingly, we found that, even though mean right ventricle wall EAT was thicker than left ventricle wall EAT, EAT of the left

Table 3. Association between angiographic coronary artery disease and left ventricle lateral wall EAT thickness tertiles.

	Tertile1	Tertile2	Tertile3	P
Men; n (%)	230 (71.65%)	223 (67.99%)	236 (73.52%)	0.2861
Age (yrs.); mean ± SD	57.34±11.77	61.36±10.92	63.91±10.38	**<0.0001**
BMI; mean ± SD	26.51±4.73	27.74±4.50	27.90±4.19	**0.0001**
Current smoker; n (%)	108 (33.64%)	67 (20.43%)	69 (21.50%)	**0.0001**
Diabetes; n (%)	66 (20.56%)	76 (23.17%)	81 (25.23%)	0.3700
Hypertension; n (%)	144 (44.86%)	179 (54.57%)	178 (55.45%)	**0.0170**
Dyslipidemia; n (%)	146 (45.48%)	149 (45.43%)	132 (41.12%)	0.4412
Metabolic syndrome; n (%)	14 (4.36%)	28 (8.54%)	20 (6.23%)	0.0931
Calcium scoring; median [IQR]	6.0 [0.0; 180.0]	24.0 [0.0; 422.0]	37.0 [0.0; 406.0]	**0.0024**
Presence of angiographic CAD; n (%)	221 (68.85%)	249 (75.91%)	261 (81.31%)	**0.0012**

Abbreviations as in Table 1 and 2.

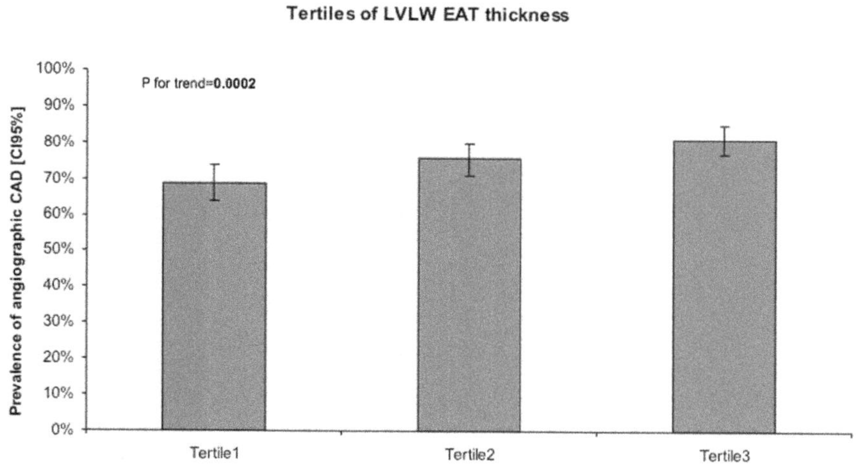

Figure 1. Association of angiographic coronary artery disease and left ventricle lateral wall (LVLW) epicardial adipose tissue (EAT) thickness tertile classification. CAD = coronary artery disease; LVLW = left ventricle lateral wall; EAT = epicardial adipose tissue. Prevalence of angiographic coronary artery disease and 95% confidence intervals [95% CIs] in LVLW EAT tertiles.

ventricle but not the right ventricle wall was associated to CAD. Whether this association is driven by a functional or mechanical cause is unclear and further physiopathological studies need to be done.

Second, EAT thickness was well correlated to the severity of angiographic CAD. The greater the LVLW EAT thickness, the greater the probability of multivessel disease. Thirdly, EAT thickness was not associated with BMI and waist circumference and was the best predictor of CAD. Finally, when studying EAT as a diagnostic screening tool, it had poor performance, lower than calcium scoring. Adding EAT measurement to calcium scoring did not improve significantly the ROC curve.

There are two main implications of the present results. First, from a pathophysiologic perspective, the association between EAT and angiographic CAD is consistent with the hypothesis that epicardial fat may play a role in the genesis of CAD. EAT is the visceral fat depot of the heart. It is a metabolically active organ with anatomical and functional contiguity to the myocardium as it is located along the coronary arteries on the surface of the ventricles and the apex of the heart [10]. Because of its close proximity, epicardial fat can locally affect the heart and coronary arteries through vasocrine or paracrine secretion of a number of bioactive molecules and pro-inflammatory cytokines [11–13]. In fact, excess accumulation of epicardial fat was reported to be a stronger coronary risk factor than the distribution of other body fat [14]. On the basis of these findings, several clinical studies have investigated EAT as a cause of CAD, finding that EAT thickness and volume strongly correlated with atherosclerosis and coronary artery calcium score, both of which are characteristic of plaques and CAD [1–5]. Echocardiographic studies have suggested that EAT was neither strongly associated with the incidence of major adverse cardiovascular events in patients with CAD, nor associated with coronary artery stenosis [15–17]. More recently, a meta-analysis by Xu et al. [18], of 15 case–control studies and one case sectional study (N = 2872 patients) found a positive association between EAT thickness and volume and the presence of CAD. Our study confirms this association.

In addition to being associated with the presence of CAD, EAT has also been associated with fatal and nonfatal coronary events in the general population, independently of conventional cardiovascular risk factors [19]. As such, the presence of EAT may complement information from cardiac computed tomography over and above the CAC scoring. These findings are consistent with the observation that EAT is strongly associated not only with the presence, but also with the severity of CAD. Whether this association is driven by functional or mechanical causes is still unclear and further physiopathological studies with molecular insights for this relation are needed. While additional information on the biological profile of our patients, including biomarkers of inflammation, would have been useful they were not available since our data were obtained in routine medical care. Nevertheless, recent studies have shown that increased EAT thickness was associated with low grade systemic *inflammation* [20] and that orosomucoid secretion by EAT could be a possible indicator of endothelial dysfunction in diabetes mellitus [21]. Moreover, Hirata et al. showed that inflammatory cell infiltration was

Table 4. Multivariable correlates of degree of coronary stenosis in CAD subjects.

	Univariate analysis			Multivariate analysis		
	OR	[95%CI]	P	OR	[95%CI]	P
BMI	1.02	[0.99–1.05]	0.2614	0.99	[0.92–1.06]	0.7239
Waist circumference	1.01	[0.99–1.03]	0.1604	1.01	[0.99–1.04]	0.3013
LVLW EAT (≥2.8 vs. 2.8 mm)	1.67	[1.23–2.26]	**0.0009**	1.67	[1.08–2.57]	**0.0197**

Abbreviations as in Table 1.

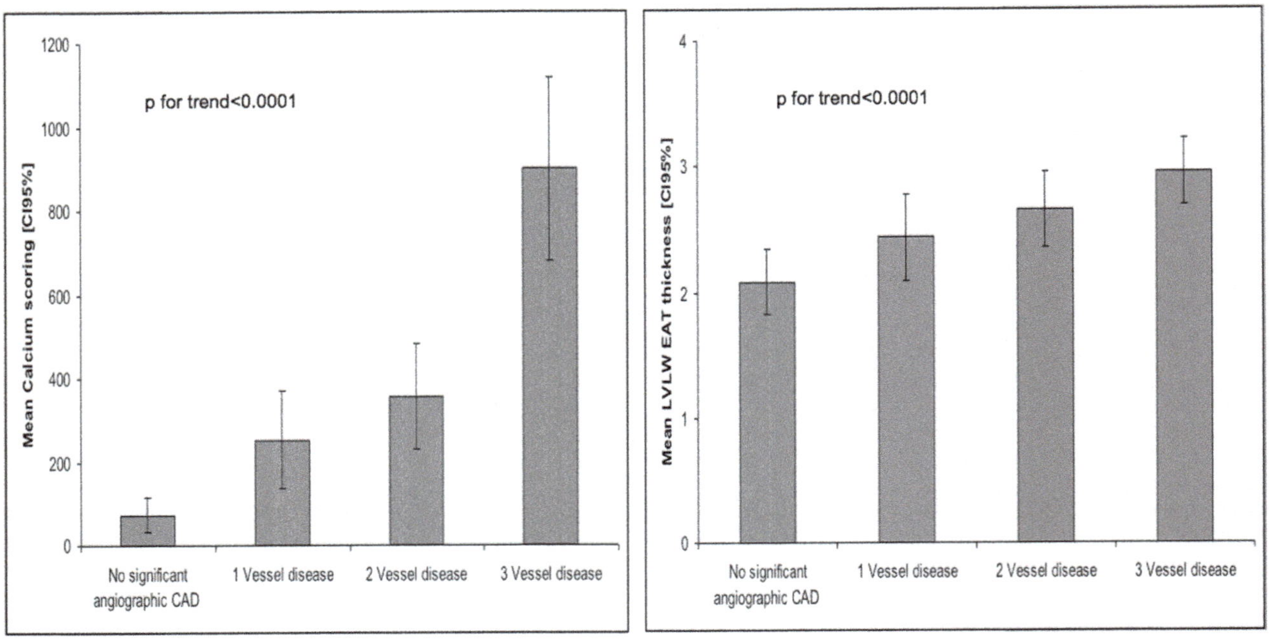

Figure 2. Association of left ventricle lateral wall (LVLW) epicardial adipose tissue (EAT) thickness and calcium scoring between patients with none or minimal coronary artery disease, 1, 2 or 3 vessel disease. Abbreviations as in Figure 1. Mean calcium scoring (Agatston score) and mean LVLW EAT thickness (mm) and 95% confidence intervals [95% CIs] in patients with no significant angiographic coronary artery disease, 1, 2 or 3 vessel disease.

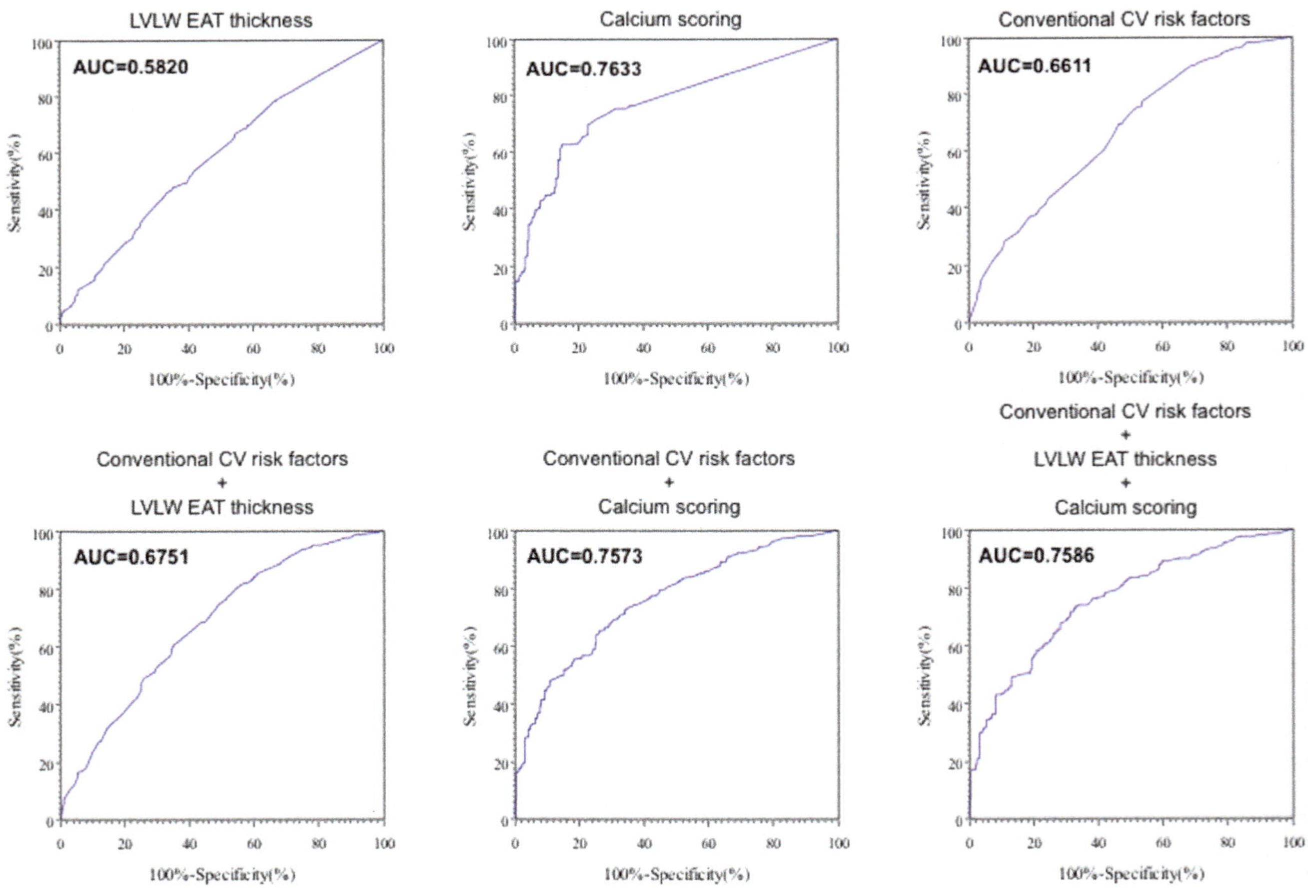

Figure 3. Receiver operating characteristic curves. Abbreviations as in Figure 1; CV= cardiovascular.

Table 5. Receiver operating characteristic curves: Areas under the curve, sensibility, specificity, positive and negative predictive values.

	AUC	Se	Sp	PPV	NPV
LVLW EAT thickness	0.5820	0.4610	0.6653	0.8081	0.2875
Calcium scoring	0.7633	0.6261	0.8514	0.8903	0.5418
Conventional CV risk factors	0.6611	0.7699	0.4635	0.8154	0.3956
Conventional CV risk factors + LVLW EAT thickness	0.6751	0.8061	0.4506	0.8187	0.4303
Conventional CV risk factors + calcium scoring	0.7573	0.6535	0.7352	0.8269	0.5230
Conventional CV risk factors + LVLW EAT thickness + calcium scoring	0.7586	0.7356	0.6706	0.8121	0.5672

AUC = area under the curve; Se = sensibility; Sp= specificity; PPV = positive predictive value; NPV = negative predictive value; CV = cardiovascular; other abbreviations as in Table 1.

enhanced in EAT, but not in subcutaneous fat, in patients with CAD [22]. Chronic inflammation in epicardial fat may participate in the pathogenesis of coronary atherosclerosis and therefore, it may be interesting to combine EAT abundance and biological markers to improve the identification of patient at risk of CAD events.

We reported an association between EAT and calcium scoring. Whether EAT could influence calcium scoring is unclear. Previous studies have shown that EAT correlates with the extent of CAC [23–25]. Alexopoulos et al. [3] found that larger EAT volumes were associated with the presence of plaques with a non-calcified component. However that study had a wide range of EAT volumes in patients with mixed plaques. Nevertheless, this observation suggests that the release of noxious agents from EAT may sustain an active atherosclerotic process as proven by the presence of non-calcified plaques. The presence of mere CAC, instead, could represent a more advanced and stable phase of the atherosclerotic process. In support of this hypothesis, Broedl et al. [26]. found that low levels of adiponectin, which is secreted locally by EAT, were associated with the presence of non-calcified or mixed coronary plaques, but not with the presence of calcified plaques. These concepts still remain speculative. It should also be noted that Greif et al. [27] found no relationship between EAT and any type of atherosclerotic plaque. However, these investigators did not adjust for differences in risk factor prevalence, likely confounding their ability to detect an effect of EAT volume.

The second important implication is that, although EAT is strongly correlated to the presence and extent of angiographic CAD, it is probably of little value as a diagnostic or screening tool since other methods such as calcium scoring or computed tomography coronary angiography have far superior sensibility and specificity. Moreover, adding EAT measurements to calcium scoring did not improve the diagnostic performance.

Limitations

The present study has some limitations. First, we measured EAT thickness rather than volume. However, even if multidetector CT measurements of volumetric EAT are considered more reproducible than multidetector CT measurements of EAT thickness [15,28], EAT thickness is easier to perform and less time-consuming compared to the labor-intensive work for measurements of volumetric EAT and therefore more suitable for research purposes. Consequently, we measured EAT thickness on the left and right ventricle free wall because of its accessibility and potential for use in clinical practice. We noted a strong positive association between EAT thickness and coronary atherosclerosis quantified by CA. Patients underwent mostly 64 row cardiac CT (684 (70.5%) patients) and the other 286 patients (29.5%) had 16 to 40 row CT. Nevertheless, even if 16 row cardiac CT are not used anymore (patients were included between June 2006 and June 2008), it does not affect EAT thickness measurement reliability. Second, this study was performed in symptomatic patients and not in an asymptomatic population undergoing screening, which could influence the results of EAT as a screening tool. However, this study was first performed on a pathophysiologic approach, not to prove the accuracy of EAT thickness measurement as a screening tool in an asymptomatic cohort. Thirdly, despite the independent association between epicardial thickness and CAD, our study did not provide direct molecular insights into this relation. Fourth, coronary angiography alone is not the most accurate method to estimate coronary stenosis degree and severity, especially in early lesions, due to outward remodeling of coronary vessels. However, coronary angiography represents the most widely used technique for assessing coronary anatomy. In the literature, significant stenosis is defined as>50% stenosis of the luminal diameter but this does not account for the presence of plaque instability, which may lead to acute coronary artery stenosis. Finally, we measured EAT in different parts of the heart, but the fact that it was not measured in right atrioventricular groove, left atrioventricular groove and interventricular groove could be a limitation.

Conclusions

From a pathophysiologic perspective, our study demonstrated a strong association between EAT and the presence and extent of angiographic CAD. It is consistent with the hypothesis that epicardial fat may play a role in the genesis of CAD, possibly due to paracrine or vasocrine mechanisms. Although EAT is correlated to CAD, it is probably of little value as a diagnostic or screening tool since other methods such as calcium scoring or computed tomography coronary angiography have far superior sensibility and specificity.

Author Contributions

Conceived and designed the experiments: FP PG PGS. Performed the experiments: JPL SC FL DC JMJ PH. Analyzed the data: RN GC. Contributed reagents/materials/analysis tools: FP PG PGS RN GC. Wrote the paper: FP PG PGS.

References

1. Wang TD, Lee WJ, Shih FY, Huang CH, Chen WJ, et al. (2010) Association of epicardial adipose tissue with coronary atherosclerosis is region-specific and independent of conventional risk factors and intra-abdominal adiposity. Atherosclerosis 213(1):279–87.
2. Bettencourt N, Toschke AM, Leite D, Rocha J, Carvalho M, et al. (2012) Epicardial adipose tissue is an independent predictor of coronary atherosclerotic burden. Int J Cardiol. 28;158(1):26–32.
3. Alexopoulos N, McLean DS, Janik M, Arepalli CD, Stillman AE, et al. (2010) Epicardial adipose tissue and coronary artery plaque characteristics. Atherosclerosis 210(1):150–4.
4. Oka T, Yamamoto H, Ohashi N, Kitagawa T, Kunita E, et al. (2012) Association between epicardial adipose tissue volume and characteristics of non-calcified plaques assessed by coronary computed tomographic angiography. Int J Cardiol. 161(1):45–9.
5. Eroglu S, Sade LE, Yildirir A, Bal U, Ozgul AS, et al. (2009) Epicardial adipose tissue thickness by echocardiography is a marker for the presence and severity of coronary artery disease. Nutr Metab Cardiovasc Dis. 19(3):211–7.
6. Gueret P, Deux JF, Bonello L, Sarran A, Tron C, et al. (2013) Diagnostic Performance of Computed Tomography Coronary Angiography (from the Prospective National Multicenter Multivendor EVASCAN Study). Am J Cardiol. 111(4):471–8.
7. Menzel HG, Shibilla H, Teunen D, editors (2000) European guidelines on quality criteria for computed tomography. Luxembourg: European Commission Publication. (No. EUR 16262 EN. 2000).
8. Smith SC, Feldman TE, Hirshfeld JW, Jacobs AK, Kern MJ, et al. (2006) ACC/AHA/SCAI 2005 guidelines update for percutaneous coronary intervention—summary article: a report of the American College of Cardiology/American Heart Association Task Force on Practice Guidelines (ACC/AHA/SCAI Writing Committee to Update the 2001 Guidelines for Percutaneous Coronary Intervention). J Am Coll Cardiol. 47(1):216–35.
9. Austen WG, Edwards JE, Frye RL, Gensini GG, Gott VL, et al. (1975) A reporting system on patients evaluated for coronary artery disease. Report of the Ad Hoc Committee for Grading of Coronary Artery Disease, Council on Cardiovascular Surgery, American Heart Association. Circulation 51(4 Suppl):5–40.
10. Sacks HS, Fain JN (2007) Human epicardial adipose tissue: A review. Am Heart J. 153(6):907–17.
11. Baker AR, Silva NF, Quinn DW, Harte AL, Pagano D, et al. (2006) Human epicardial adipose tissue expresses a pathogenic profile of adipocytokines in patients with cardiovascular disease. Cardiovasc Diabetol. 13;5: 1.
12. Rabkin SW (2007) Epicardial fat: properties, function and relationship to obesity. Obes Rev. 8(3):253–61.
13. Mazurek T, Zhang L, Zalewski A, Mannion JD, Diehl JT, et al. (2003) Human epicardial adipose tissue is a source of inflammatory mediators. Circulation 108(20):2460–6.
14. Taguchi R, Takasu J, Itani Y, Yamamoto R, Yokoyama K, et al. (2001) Pericardial fat accumulation in men as a risk factor for coronary artery disease. Atherosclerosis 157(1):203–9.
15. Chaowalit N, Somers VK, Pellikka PA, Rihal CS, Lopez-Jimenez F (2006) Subepicardial adipose tissue and the presence and severity of coronary artery disease. Atherosclerosis 186(2):354–9.
16. Albuquerque FN, Somers VK, Blume G, Miranda W, Korenfeld Y, et al. (2012) Usefulness of epicardial adipose tissue as a predictor of adverse cardiovascular events in patients with coronary artery disease. Am J Cardiol. 110(8):1100–5.
17. Parcon R, Kruk M, Kepka C, Pregowski J, Opolski MP, et al. (2011) Epicardial adipose tissue radiodensity is independently related to coronary atherosclerosis. A multidetector computed tomography study. Circ J. 75(2):391–7.
18. Xu Y, Cheng X, Hong K, Huang C, Wan L (2012) How to interpret epicardial adipose tissue as a cause of coronary artery disease: a meta-analysis. Coron Artery Dis. 23(4):227–33.
19. Mahabadi A, Berg M, Lehmann N, Kälsch H, Bauer M, et al. (2013) Association of Epicardial Fat With Cardiovascular Risk Factors and Incident Myocardial Infarction in the General Population: The Heinz Nixdorf Recall Study. J Am Coll Cardiol. 61(13):1388–95.
20. Tok D, Kadife I, Turak O, Ozcan F, Basar N, et al. (2012) Increased epicardial fat thickness is associated with low grade systemic inflammation in metabolic syndrome. Turk Kardiyol Dern Ars. 40(8):690–5.
21. Fandiño-Vaquero R, Fernández-Trasancos A, Alvarez E, Ahmad S, Batista-Oliveira AL, et al. (2014) Orosomucoid secretion levels by epicardial adipose tissue as possible indicator of endothelial dysfunction in diabetes mellitus or inflammation in coronary artery disease. Atherosclerosis 235(2):281–288.
22. Hirata Y, Kurobe H, Akaike M, Chikugo F, Hori T, et al. (2011) Enhanced inflammation in epicardial fat in patients with coronary artery disease. Int Heart J. 52(3):139–42.
23. Rosito GA, Massaro JM, Hoffmann U, Ruberg FL, Mahabadi AA, et al. (2008) Pericardial fat, visceral abdominal fat, cardiovascular disease risk factors, and vascular calcification in a community-based sample: the Framingham Heart Study. Circulation 117: 605–13.
24. de Vos AM, Prokop M, Roos CJ, Mejis MF, van der Schouw YT, et al. (2008) Peri-coronary epicardial adipose tissue is related to cardiovascular risk factors and coronary artery calcification in post-menopausal women. Eur Heart J. 29: 777–83.
25. Ding J, Kritchevsky SB, Harris TB, Burke GL, Detrano RC, et al. (2008) The association of pericardial fat with calcified coronary plaque. Obesity (Silver Spring) 16: 1914–9.
26. Broedl UC, Lebherz C, Lehrke M, Stark R, Greif M, et al. (2009) Low adiponectin levels are an independent predictor of mixed and non-calcified coronary atherosclerotic plaques. PLoS One 4:e4733.
27. Greif M, Becker A, von Ziegler F, Lebherz C, Lehrke M, et al. (2009) Pericardial adipose tissue determined by dual source CT is a risk factor for coronary atherosclerosis. Arterioscler Thromb Vasc Biol 29: 781–6.
28. Gorter PM, van Lindert AS, de Vos AM, Mejis MF, van der Graaf Y, et al. (2008) Quantification of epicardial and peri-coronary fat using cardiac computed tomography; reproducibility and relation with obesity and metabolic syndrome in patients suspected of coronary artery disease. Atherosclerosis 197(2):896–903.

Permissions

All chapters in this book were first published in PLOS ONE, by The Public Library of Science; hereby published with permission under the Creative Commons Attribution License or equivalent. Every chapter published in this book has been scrutinized by our experts. Their significance has been extensively debated. The topics covered herein carry significant findings which will fuel the growth of the discipline. They may even be implemented as practical applications or may be referred to as a beginning point for another development.

The contributors of this book come from diverse backgrounds, making this book a truly international effort. This book will bring forth new frontiers with its revolutionizing research information and detailed analysis of the nascent developments around the world.

We would like to thank all the contributing authors for lending their expertise to make the book truly unique. They have played a crucial role in the development of this book. Without their invaluable contributions this book wouldn't have been possible. They have made vital efforts to compile up to date information on the varied aspects of this subject to make this book a valuable addition to the collection of many professionals and students.

This book was conceptualized with the vision of imparting up-to-date information and advanced data in this field. To ensure the same, a matchless editorial board was set up. Every individual on the board went through rigorous rounds of assessment to prove their worth. After which they invested a large part of their time researching and compiling the most relevant data for our readers.

The editorial board has been involved in producing this book since its inception. They have spent rigorous hours researching and exploring the diverse topics which have resulted in the successful publishing of this book. They have passed on their knowledge of decades through this book. To expedite this challenging task, the publisher supported the team at every step. A small team of assistant editors was also appointed to further simplify the editing procedure and attain best results for the readers.

Apart from the editorial board, the designing team has also invested a significant amount of their time in understanding the subject and creating the most relevant covers. They scrutinized every image to scout for the most suitable representation of the subject and create an appropriate cover for the book.

The publishing team has been an ardent support to the editorial, designing and production team. Their endless efforts to recruit the best for this project, has resulted in the accomplishment of this book. They are a veteran in the field of academics and their pool of knowledge is as vast as their experience in printing. Their expertise and guidance has proved useful at every step. Their uncompromising quality standards have made this book an exceptional effort. Their encouragement from time to time has been an inspiration for everyone.

The publisher and the editorial board hope that this book will prove to be a valuable piece of knowledge for researchers, students, practitioners and scholars across the globe.

List of Contributors

Barbara Elisabeth Stähli, Lukas Andreas Altwegg, Christophe Wyss, Andreas Brauchlin, Thomas Michelle Frank, Felix Lüscher and Willibald Maier
Department of Cardiology, Cardiovascular Center, University Hospital Zurich, Zurich, Switzerland

Pierre-Alexandre Krayenbühl
Division of Internal Medicine, University Hospital Zurich, Zurich, Switzerland

Keiko Yonekawa
Department of Cardiology, Cardiovascular Center, University Hospital Zurich, Zurich, Switzerland
Division of Internal Medicine, University Hospital Zurich, Zurich, Switzerland

Danielle Hof and Arnold von Eckardstein
Institute of Clinical Chemistry, University Hospital Zurich, Zurich, Switzerland

Philipp Fischbacher anda Georg Schulthess
Department of Internal Medicine, Hospital Männedorf, Männedorf, Switzerland

Martin Hersberger
Institute of Clinical Chemistry and Biochemistry, Childrens Hospital Zurich, Zurich, Switzerland

Michel Neidhart and Steffen Gay
Center for Experimental Rheumatology, Department of Rheumatology, University Hospital Zurich, Zurich, Switzerland

Igor Novopashenny, Regine Wolters and Manfred Bernd Wischnewsky
FB Mathematics and Computer Science, University of Bremen, Bremen, Germany

Walter S. Speidl
Department of Internal Medicine II, Medical University of Vienna, Vienna, Austria

Svitlana Demyanets
Department of Internal Medicine II, Medical University of Vienna, Vienna, Austria
Department of Laboratory Medicine, Medical University of Vienna, Vienna, Austria

Katharina M. Katsaros, Konstantin A. Krychtiuk and Anna Wonnerth
Department of Internal Medicine II, Medical University of Vienna, Vienna, Austria
Ludwig Boltzmann Cluster for Cardiovascular Research, Vienna, Austria

Ioannis Tentzeris, Rudolf Jarai, Serdar Farhan, Thomas W. Weiss and Kurt Huber
3rd Medical Department for Cardiology and Emergency Medicine, Wilhelminenhospital, Vienna, Austria

Johann Wojta
Department of Internal Medicine II, Medical University of Vienna, Vienna, Austria
Core Facilities, Medical University of Vienna, Vienna, Austria
Ludwig Boltzmann Cluster for Cardiovascular Research, Vienna, Austria

Sei Komatsu, Tomoki Ohara, Yasuhiko Kobayashi and Kazuhisa Kodama
Cardiovascular Center, Amagasaki Central Hospital, Hyogo, Japan

Teruaki Kamata and Kazuaki Miyaji
Department of Diagnostic Imaging, Amagasaki Central Hospital, Hyogo, Japan

Atsuko Imai
Cardiovascular Center, Amagasaki Central Hospital, Hyogo, Japan
Department of Cardiology, Osaka University School of Medicine, Osaka, Japan

Po-Chao Hsu
Division of Cardiology, Department of Internal Medicine, Kaohsiung Medical University Hospital, Kaohsiung Medical University, Kaohsiung, Taiwan
Graduate Institute of Medicine, College of Medicine, Kaohsiung Medical University, Kaohsiung, Taiwan
Faculty of Medicine, College of Medicine, Kaohsiung Medical University, Kaohsiung, Taiwan

Ho-Ming Su
Division of Cardiology, Department of Internal Medicine, Kaohsiung Medical University Hospital, Kaohsiung Medical University, Kaohsiung, Taiwan
Faculty of Medicine, College of Medicine, Kaohsiung Medical University, Kaohsiung, Taiwan
Department of Internal Medicine, Kaohsiung Municipal Hsiao-Kang Hospital, Kaohsiung, Taiwan

Hsiang-Chun Lee
Division of Cardiology, Department of Internal Medicine, Kaohsiung Medical University Hospital, Kaohsiung Medical University, Kaohsiung, Taiwan
Graduate Institute of Medicine, College of Medicine, Kaohsiung Medical University, Kaohsiung, Taiwan

Suh-Hang Juo
Department of Medical Research, Kaohsiung Medical University Hospital, Kaohsiung Medical University, Kaohsiung, Taiwan
Medical Genetics, Kaohsiung Medical University, Kaohsiung, Taiwan
Center of Excellence for Environmental Medicine, Kaohsiung Medical University, Kaohsiung, Taiwan

Tsung-Hsien Lin, Wen- Chol Voon, Wen-Ter Lai and Sheng-Hsiung Sheu
Division of Cardiology, Department of Internal Medicine, Kaohsiung Medical University Hospital, Kaohsiung Medical University, Kaohsiung, Taiwan
Faculty of Medicine, College of Medicine, Kaohsiung Medical University, Kaohsiung, Taiwan

Jie Chen, Wei-Hai Xu, Li-Ying Cui and Shan Gao
Department of Neurology, Peking Union Medical College Hospital, Chinese Academy of Medical Sciences and Peking Union Medical College, Beijing, China

Jia Liu and Ren Xu
Shenzhen Institutes of Advanced Technology, Chinese Academy of Sciences, Shenzhen, China

Bo Hou
Department of Radiology, Peking Union Medical College Hospital, Chinese Academy of Medical Sciences and Peking Union Medical College, Beijing, China

Catriona Shaw
UK Renal Registry, Southmead Hospital, Bristol, United Kingdom
Department of Renal Sciences, Division of Transplantation Immunology and Mucosal Biology, Kings College London, London, United Kingdom

Dorothea Nitsch
London School of Hygiene and Tropical Medicine, London, United Kingdom

Retha Steenkamp
UK Renal Registry, Southmead Hospital, Bristol, United Kingdom

Cornelia Junghans
Department of Epidemiology and Public Health, University College London, London, United Kingdom

Sapna Shah
Department of Renal Medicine, Kings College Hospital, London, United Kingdom

Donal O'Donoghue
Department of Renal Medicine, Salford Royal NHS Foundation Trust, Salford, United Kingdom, Belfast, Northern Ireland, United Kingdom

Damian Fogarty
Department of Renal Medicine, Belfast Health and Social CareTrust

Clive Weston
Myocardial Ischaemia National Audit Project, College of Medicine, Swansea University, Swansea, Wales, United Kingdom

Claire C. Sharpe
Department of Renal Sciences, Division of Transplantation Immunology and Mucosal Biology, Kings College London, London, United Kingdom

Jian Wang
Department of Vascular Surgery, Union Hospital, Tongji Medical College, Huazhong University of Science and Technology, Wuhan, Hubei, China
National Research Council, Winnipeg, Manitoba, Canada
Department of Physiology, Faculty of Medicine, University of Manitoba, Winnipeg, Manitoba, Canada
Department of Cardiac Surgery, the First Affiliated Hospital, Harbin Medical University, Harbin, Heilongjiang, China

Bo Xiang and Ganghong Tian
National Research Council, Winnipeg, Manitoba, Canada
Department of Physiology, Faculty of Medicine, University of Manitoba, Winnipeg, Manitoba, Canada

Hung-Yu Lin
National Research Council, Winnipeg, Manitoba, Canada

Hongyu Liu
Department of Cardiac Surgery, the First Affiliated Hospital, Harbin Medical University, Harbin, Heilongjiang, China

Darren Freed and Rakesh C. Arora
National Research Council, Winnipeg, Manitoba, Canada
Department of Physiology, Faculty of Medicine, University of Manitoba, Winnipeg, Manitoba, Canada
Cardiac Science Program, Institute of Cardiovascular Sciences, St. Boniface General Hospital, Winnipeg, Manitoba, Canada

Shifeng Yang, Baoting Chao, Lebin Wu, Zhaoping Cheng, Yanhua Duan, Dawei Wu, Xiaopeng Ji, Pei Nie and Ximing Wang
Shandong Medical Imaging Research Institute, Shandong University, Jinan, Shandong, P.R. China

Xia Li
Departments of Ultrasound, Shandong Provincial Hospital, Jinan, Shandong, P. R. China

Yiqiang Zhan
Unit of Periodontology, University of Greifswald, Greifswald, Germany

Jiuhong Chen
CT Research Collaboration, Siemens Ltd., China, Beijing, P.R. China

Bo Liu
Healthcare Sector, Siemens Ltd., China, Shanghai, P.R. China

John W. Petersen and Carl J. Pepine
Division of Cardiovascular Medicine, University of Florida, Gainesville, Florida, United States of America

B. Delia Johnson and Sheryl F. Kelsey
Graduate School of Public Health, University of Pittsburgh, Pittsburgh, Pennsylvania, United States of America

Kevin E. Kip
College of Nursing, University of South Florida, Tampa, Florida, United States of America

R. David Anderson and Eileen M. Handberg
Division of Cardiovascular Medicine, University of Florida, Gainesville, Florida, United States of America

Barry Sharaf
Division of Cardiology, Brown University, Providence, Rhode Island, United States of America

Puja K. Mehta and C. Noel Bairey Merz
Division of Cardiology, Barbra Streisand Women's Heart Center, Heart Institute, Cedars-Sinai Medical Center, Los Angeles, California, United States of America

Sören Johst, Stephan Orzada, Anja Fischer, Lena C. Schäfer and Mark E. Ladd
Erwin L. Hahn Institute for Magnetic Resonance Imaging, University Duisburg-Essen, Essen, Germany
Department of Diagnostic and Interventional Radiology and Neuroradiology, University Hospital, University Duisburg-Essen, Essen, Germany

Kai Nassenstein, Lale Umutlu and Thomas C. Lauenstein
Department of Diagnostic and Interventional Radiology and Neuroradiology, University Hospital, University Duisburg-Essen, Essen, Germany

Stefan Maderwald
Erwin L. Hahn Institute for Magnetic Resonance Imaging, University Duisburg-Essen, Essen, Germany

Elin B. Brolin, Torkel B. Brismar, Jonaz Ripsweden and Kerstin Cederlund
Department of Radiology, Karolinska University Hospital Huddinge and Department of Clinical Science, Intervention and Technology, Division of Medical Imaging and Technology at Karolinska Institutet, Stockholm, Sweden

Tomas Jernberg and Loghman Henareh
Department of Medicine, Section of Cardiology, Karolinska University Hospital Huddinge and Karolinska Institutet, Stockholm, Sweden

Maria Daniel
Cardiology Unit, Department of Medicine, Karolinska University Hospital Solna and Karolinska Institutet, Stockholm, Sweden

Per Tornvall
Institution for Clinical Science and Education at Södersjukhuset, Karolinska Institutet, Stockholm, Sweden

Jeff Hsing, Benjamin R. Knowles and Mark E. Josephson
Department of Medicine, Cardiovascular Division, Beth Israel Deaconess Medical Center, Harvard Medical School, Boston, Massachusetts, United States of America

Dana C. Peters
Department of Medicine, Cardiovascular Division, Beth Israel Deaconess Medical Center, Harvard Medical School, Boston, Massachusetts, United States of America
Department of Radiology, Yale Medical School, New Haven, Connecticut, United States of America

Warren J. Manning
Department of Medicine, Cardiovascular Division, Beth Israel Deaconess Medical Center, Harvard Medical School, Boston, Massachusetts, United States of America
Department of Radiology, Beth Israel Deaconess Medical Center, Harvard Medical School, Boston, Massachusetts, United States of America

Wenlian Zhu
Division of Cancer Imaging Research, The Russell H. Morgan Department of Radiology and Radiological Science, The Johns Hopkins University School of Medicine, Baltimore, Maryland, United States of America

Yoshinori Kato and Dmitri Artemov
Division of Cancer Imaging Research, The Russell H. Morgan Department of Radiology and Radiological Science, The Johns Hopkins University School of Medicine, Baltimore, Maryland, United States of America
Department of Oncology, The Sidney Kimmel Comprehensive Cancer Center, The Johns Hopkins University School of Medicine, Baltimore, Maryland, United States of America

Chui Ming Gemmy Cheung and Tien Yin Wong
Vitreoretinal Service, Singapore National Eye Centre, Singapore, Singapore
Singapore Eye Research Institute, Singapore, Singapore
Department of Ophthalmology, Yong Loo Lin School of Medicine, National University of Singapore, Singapore, Singapore
Ophthalmology Academic Clinical Program, Duke-NUS Graduate Medical School, Singapore, Singapore

Xiang Li
Singapore Eye Research Institute, Singapore, Singapore
Department of Statistics and Applied Probability, National University of Singapore, Singapore, Singapore

Ranjana Mathur, Shu Yen Lee, Choi Mun Chan, Ian Yeo, Boon Kwang Loh, Edmund Yick-Mun Wong and Doric Wong
Vitreoretinal Service, Singapore National Eye Centre, Singapore, Singapore

Rachel Williams
Worldwide Epidemiology, R&D Projects, Clinical Platforms & Sciences, GlaxoSmithKline, Pennsylvania, United States of America

Jacob Palmer, Jinzhong Yang, Tinsu Pan and Laurence E. Court
Department of Radiation Physics, Unit 94, The University of Texas MD Anderson Cancer Center, Houston, Texas, United States of America

Min Li, Zhao-hui Peng, Juan Ding and Li Li
Department of Medical Imaging, Jinan Military General Hospital, Jinan, Shandong Province, China

Xiang-min Du
Department of Medical Engineering, Jinan Military General Hospital, Jinan, Shandong Province, China

Zhi-tao Jin
Department of Cardiology, General Hospital of the Second Artillery, Beijing, China

Na-Young Shin, Kyung-eun Kim, Mina Park, Dong Joon Kim, Sung Jun Ahn and Seung-Koo Lee
Department of Radiology, Severance Hospital, Yonsei University College of Medicine, Seoul, Korea

Young Dae Kim and Ji Hoe Heo
Department of Neurology, Severance Hospital, Yonsei University College of Medicine, Seoul, Korea

Johannes T. Kowallick, Jan M. Sohns, Martin Fasshauer, Wieland Staab and Joachim Lotz
Institute for Diagnostic and Interventional Radiology, Georg-August-University Göttingen, Göttingen, Germany
DZHK (German Centre for Cardiovascular Research), partner site Göttingen, Göttingen, Germany

Pablo Lamata
Department of Computer Science, University of Oxford, Oxford, United Kingdom
Division of Imaging Sciences and Biomedical Engineering, The Rayne Institute, St. Thomas' Hospital, King's College London, London, United Kingdom

Shazia T. Hussain
Papworth Hospital NHS Trust, Papworth Everard, Cambridgeshire, United Kingdom

Shelby Kutty
Children's Hospital and Medical Center, University of Nebraska College of Medicine, Omaha, Nebraska, United States of America

Michael Steinmetz
Department of Pediatric Cardiology and Intensive Care Medicine, Georg- August-University Göttingen, Göttingen, Germany
DZHK (German Centre for Cardiovascular Research), partner site Göttingen, Göttingen, Germany

Christina Unterberg-Buchwald and Gerd Hasenfuß
Department of Cardiology and Pneumology, Georg-August-University Göttingen, Göttingen, Germany
DZHK (German Centre for Cardiovascular Research), partner site Göttingen, Göttingen, Germany

Boris Bigalke
Division of Imaging Sciences and Biomedical Engineering, The Rayne Institute, St. Thomas' Hospital, King's College London, London, United Kingdom
Medizinische Klinik III, Kardiologie und Kreislauferkrankungen, Eberhard-Karls-Universität Tübingen, Tübingen, Germany

Andreas Schuster
Department of Cardiology and Pneumology, Georg-August-University Göttingen, Göttingen, Germany, Division of Imaging Sciences and Biomedical Engineering, The Rayne Institute, St. Thomas' Hospital, King's College London, London, United Kingdom
DZHK (German Centre for Cardiovascular Research), partner site Göttingen, Göttingen, Germany

Ying Song, Yang Wang, Chuanhui Li, Yanmin Wang, Shiqing Mu and Xinjian Yang
Department of Interventional Neuroradiology, Beijing Neurosurgical Institute and Beijing Tiantan Hospital, Capital Medical University, Beijing, China

William A. Mehan Jr., R. Gilberto González, Bradley R. Buchbinder, John W. Chen, William A. Copen,
Rajiv Gupta, Joshua A. Hirsch, George J. Hunter, Scott Hunter, Jason M. Johnson, Hillary R. Kelly, Mykol Larvie, Michael H. Lev, Stuart R. Pomerantz, Otto Rapalino, Sandra Rincon, Javier M. Romero, Pamela W. Schaefer and Vinil Shah
Neuroradiology Division, Massachusetts General Hospital, Harvard Medical School, Boston, Massachusetts, United States of America

Flora Hui1, Christine T. O. Nguyen, Phillip A. Bedggood, Zheng He, Algis J. Vingrys and Bang V. Bui
Department of Optometry and Vision Sciences, The University of Melbourne, Parkville, Victoria, Australia

Rebecca L. Fish and Rachel Gurrell
Neusentis, Pfizer Research and Development, Grant Park Science Park, Cambridge, United Kingdom

Lennart Nilsson, Marcus Gjerde, Eva Swahn and Lena Jonasson
Department of Medical and Health Sciences, Linköping University, Linköping, Sweden
Department of Cardiology, Linköping University, Linköping, Sweden

Wouter G. Wieringa and Gabija Pundziute
University of Groningen, University Medical Center Groningen, Department of Cardiology, Groningen, The Netherlands

Jan Engvall
Department of Medical and Health Sciences, Linköping University, Linköping, Sweden
Department of Clinical Physiology, Linköping University, Linköping, Sweden

Noemi Pavo, Georg Strebinger, , Gerald Maurer, Mariann Gyöngyösi
Department of Cardiology, Medical University of Vienna, Vienna, Austria

Andras Jakab
Department of Biomedical Imaging and Image-guided Therapy, Medical University of Vienna, Vienna, Austria

Maximilian Y. Emmert, Petra Wolint and Simon P. Hoerstrup
Swiss Centre for Regenerative Medicine, University of Zürich, Zürich, Switzerland
Division of Surgical Research, University Hospital of Zürich, Zürich, Switzerland
Clinic for Cardiovascular Surgery, University Hospital of Zürich, Zürich, Switzerland

Matthias Zimmermann
Department of Thoracic Surgery, Medical University of Vienna, Vienna, Austria

Hendrik Jan Ankersmit
Department of Thoracic Surgery, Medical University of Vienna, Vienna, Austria
Christian Doppler Laboratory for Cardiac and Thoracic Diagnosis and Regeneration, Vienna, Austria

Ann-Marie Bintu Munda Jah-Kabba, Guido Matthias Kukuk, Dariusch Reza Hadizadeh, Frank Träber, Hans Heinz Schild and Winfried Albert Willinek
University of Bonn, Dept. of Radiology, Germany

Arne Koscielny, Mustapha Sundifu Kabba and Frauke Verrel
University of Bonn, Dept. of Surgery, Germany

Werner Haslik, K. F. Schrögendorfer and Jakob Nedomansky
Division of Plastic and Reconstructive Surgery, Department of Surgery, Comprehensive Cancer Center of the Medical University of Vienna, Vienna, Austria

Ursula Pluschnig, Günther G. Steger, Christoph C. Zielinski, Rupert Bartsch and Robert M. Mader
Department of Medicine I, Clinical Division of Oncology, Comprehensive Cancer Center of the Medical University of Vienna, Vienna, Austria

Fabien A. Picard and Jean-Michel Juliard
Cardiology Department, Assistance Publique-Hôpitaux de Paris, Hôpital Bichat, Université Paris-Diderot, Sorbonne-Paris Cité , Paris, France

Pascal Gueret and Stéphane Champagne
Cardiology Department, Assistance Publique-Hôpitaux de Paris, Hôpital Henri Mondor, Université Paris-Est-Créteil, Créteil, France

Jean-Pierre Laissy
Radiology Department, Assistance Publique-Hôpitaux de Paris, Hôpital Bichat, Université Paris-Diderot, Sorbonne-Paris Cité , Paris, France
Département Hospitalo-Universitaire FIRE, INSERM U-1148, Assistance Publique-Hôpitaux de Paris, Hôpital Bichat, Université Paris-Diderot, Sorbonne-Paris Cité , Paris, France

Florence Leclercq
Cardiology Department, Centre Hospitalier Universitaire Arnaud de Villeneuve, Montpellier, France

Didier Carrié
Cardiology Department, Centre Hospitalier Universitaire de Rangueil, Toulouse, France

Patrick Henry
Cardiology Department, Assistance Publique-Hôpitaux de Paris, Hôpital Lariboisière, Université Paris-Diderot, Sorbonne-Paris Cité, Paris, France

Ralph Niarra
Epidemiology and Clinical Research Unit, Assistance Publique-Hôpitaux de Paris, Hôpital Européen Georges-Pompidou, Paris, France

Unité INSERM Centre D'investigation Épidémiologique 4, Paris, France

Gilles Chatellier
Epidemiology and Clinical Research Unit, Assistance Publique-Hôpitaux de Paris, Hôpital Européen Georges-Pompidou, Paris, France
Unité INSERM Centre D'investigation Épidémiologique 4, Paris, France
Université Paris Descartes, Sorbonne Paris Cité , Faculté de Médecine, Paris, France

Philippe Gabriel Steg
Cardiology Department, Assistance Publique-Hôpitaux de Paris, Hôpital Bichat, Université Paris-Diderot, Sorbonne-Paris Cité , Paris, France
Département Hospitalo-Universitaire FIRE, INSERM U-1148, Assistance Publique-Hôpitaux de Paris, Hôpital Bichat, Université Paris-Diderot, Sorbonne-Paris Cité , Paris, France
NHLI Imperial College, ICMS Royal Brompton Hospital, London, United Kingdom

Index